RECTAL CANCER – A MULTIDISCIPLINARY APPROACH TO MANAGEMENT

Edited by **Giulio Aniello Santoro**

Rectal Cancer – A Multidisciplinary Approach to Management
Edited by Giulio Aniello Santoro

Published by InTech
Janeza Trdine 9, 51000 Rijeka, Croatia

Publishing Process Manager Daria Nahtigal

Technical Editor Teodora Smiljanic

Cover Designer InTech Design Team

Additional hard copies can be obtained from orders@intechopen.com

Rectal Cancer – A Multidisciplinary Approach to Management,
Edited by Giulio Aniello Santoro
p. cm.
ISBN 978-953-307-758-1

For EU product safety concerns:
IN TECH d.o.o., Prolaz Marije Krucifikse Kozulić 3, 51000 Rijeka, Croatia,
info@intechopen.com or visit our website at intechopen.com.

Meet the editor

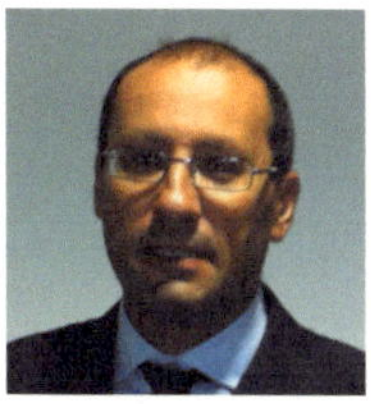

Dr. Giulio A. Santoro, MD, Ph.D., was educated at the University of Naples and at the University of Siena, Italy. He is Chief of the Pelvic Floor Unit and Consultant General Surgeon and Colorectal Surgeon, I°Department of Surgery at Treviso Regional Hospital, Italy. He also holds academic appointments as Professor of Gastrointestinal Surgery at University of Padua, Italy and Honorary Professor at Shandong University, China. Dr.Santoro is Director of the Italian School of Pelvic Floor Ultrasonography. He is board member of the Italian Society of Colorectal Surgery and member of the editorial board of World Journal of Gastrointestinal Surgery, Female Pelvic Medicine Reconstructive Surgery and Pelviperineology. He is also author of more then 200 chapters and articles published on peer-review journals as well as the author of three books. He was in the faculty of more than 300 international congresses, workshops and courses on imaging and management of Rectal Cancer, Benign Anorectal Diseases and Pelvic Floor Disorders.

Contents

Preface

Major developments in medicine over last few years have resulted in more reliable and accessible diagnostics and treatment of rectal cancer. Given the complex physiopathology of this tumor, the approach should not limit to a single specialty but involve a number of specialties (surgery, gastroenterology, radiology, biology, oncology, radiotherapy, nuclear medicine, physiotherapy) in an integrated manner. The subtitle of this book "Multidisciplinary Approach to Management" encompasses this concept. We have endeavored, with the help of an international group of contributors, to provide an up-to-date and authoritative account of the management of rectal tumor.

Our starting point (Section I) is the epidemiology of the rectal cancer, and this section addresses not only the evolution of rectal cancer epidemiology in the last years based on population-based cancer registry, but also the new AJCC staging classification. Development of screening models for colorectal cancer depends on disease risk stratification of individuals in the population. By performing opportunistic screening among high-risk populations, the average direct cost for each detected case of colorectal cancer is four times less than the cost of systematic screening.

Entire Section II is devoted to the various techniques (two-dimensional and three-dimensional endorectal ultrasonography, power-doppler ultrasound, conventional and dynamic magnetic resonance) that may be employed to image the rectal cancer. Endorectal ultrasound has been widely accepted as the reference method for local staging of rectal cancer, and is now proposed as mandatory for preoperative staging purposes in the guidelines of the main scientific societies. The technique has evolved, due to the systematic efforts of researchers, in defining the normal anatomy of rectal wall and perirectal anatomic structures, in differentiating early cancers from advanced neoplasm and in defining pathological from reactive perirectal nodes. The computer-assisted endosonographic Doppler and the immunohistochemical based methods represent rapid, reliable and reproducible ways for quantitative assessment of tumour vascularization. Rectal carcinoma with high angiogenic activity are more likely to have deeper tumor invasion, lymph node metastases and distant metastases. Due to its intrinsic multiparametricity and multiplanarity MRI is considered the most accurate modality in evaluating locally advanced rectal cancer and the presence of a positive circumferential resection margin. Dynamic Contrast Enhanced-Magnetic Resonance

Imaging is gaining a large consensus as a technique for diagnosis, staging and assessment of response to preoperative radiochemotherapy (RCT) due to its capability to detect the strict relationship that links tumor growth to angiogenesis.

The common use of total mesorectal excision (TME) and the shift from a postoperative to a preoperative RCT approach have substantially reduced the risk of local recurrences, increasing curative resection and the rate of anal sphincter preservation and improving local control and overall survival rates. The surgical principles in the treatment of rectal cancer are described in details in Section III, including combined modality treatment in early rectal cancer, single-incision laparoscopy, intraoperative sentinel lymph node mapping, neorectum for low rectal tumor, salvage surgery for local recurrence and causes and prevention of functional disturbances following low anterior resection.

Section IV is focused on neo-adjuvant and adjuvant treatments. The analysis of post-treatment tumor histological features helps to analyze if the mutational mechanisms, produced during tumor development, persist under therapy, and what changes the cells have undergone to be resistant to treatment. The response of rectal adenocarcinoma to neo-adjuvant RCT is limited to a defined group of patients. It is hoped in the future that the therapeutic course will be tailored to each patient based on analyses of initial pre-treatment biopsy assessment, thus minimizing unnecessary treatment for rectal cancer patients. Several microRNAs have been found to be involved in cancer response to therapy. High levels of miR-21 are associated with worse response to treatment, whereas patients bearing miR-21-low-level tumours have reduced risk of recurrent disease within a five-year follow-up period. In the setting of a complete tumor regression after neoadjuvant CRT, surgeons have searched for alternative management of patients in order to avoid the potential consequences of TME with or without abdominal perineal resection. Most patients with metastatic rectal cancer cannot be cured, although patients with liver and/or lung-limited disease are potentially curable with surgical resection of metastases. For other patients, palliative systemic chemotherapy is associated with an increase in survival and quality of life. Since the year 2000, new chemotherapy agents have been approved or are under evaluation in many clinical trials. Treatment must be individualized as always, taking into account goals therapy, and the toxicity profiles of each agent.

We wish to express our deep appreciation to InTech for supporting the idea of publishing a book in such an innovative form. Special thanks are due to Ms. Daria Nahtigal for her constant assistance throughout the development of the project, organizing every stage of the editorial work. Special acknowledgements must be given to the authors, who are among the foremost experts with outstanding qualifications in this complex field, and who have contributed to the many chapters of this volume. Without their experience and cooperation, this book would not have been possible.

We are confident that this book will be met with great interest from all clinicians involved in the care of patients suffering from rectal cancer.

August 2011

Giulio Aniello Santoro, M.D., Ph.D.,
Head, Pelvic Floor Unit
I Department of Surgery,
Regional Hospital, Treviso,
Italy

Honorary Professor,
Shandong University,
China

Part 1

Epidemiology

1

Rectal Cancer Epidemiology

Miguel Henriques Abreu[1], Eduarda Matos[2],
Fernando Castro Poças[3], Rosa Rocha[4] and Jorge Pinto[4]
[1]*Portuguese Institute of Oncology of Porto, Department of Medical Oncology*
[2]*ICBAS, University of Porto, Department of Health Community*
[3]*Porto's Hospital Centre, Santo Antonio's Hospital, Department of Gastroenterology*
[4]*Oncological Registry of Vila Nova de Gaia*
Portugal

1. Introduction

Colorectal cancer is the fourth most common cancer in men and the third most common one in women worldwide (Parkin, 2004; Parkin et al., 2005), accounting for approximately 436,000 incident cases and 212,000 deaths in 2008 (Quirke et al., 2011). This cancer has an important economic impact, estimating that in the initial, continuing and last year of life phases of care a total of more than $7 billion were spent (Yabroff et al., 2008). Randomized trials have shown that systematic screening of a target population of suitable age can reduce colorectal cancer by detecting asymptomatic lesions (Center et al., 2009).

Although there are differences in the etiologies and epidemiology of colon and rectal cancer (Giovannucci & Wu, 2006), the majority of the studies chose to examine colon and rectum cancers combined. However, a better understanding of these diseases nowadays, shows that these differences have an important impact in their approaches. First of all, the location of the tumours may determines different locations of metastisation. Unlike colon cancers, distal rectal tumours may first metastasize to the lungs because the inferior rectal veins drain into the inferior vena cava rather than into the portal venous system. The histological type can also vary. The vast majority of colorectal tumours are adenocarcinomas but 11-17% are mucinous carcinomas. This type, which has a penchant for the rectum and sigmoid colon, tends to be present at a more advanced stage (Consorti et al., 2000). The carcinoid tumours have a different clinical presentation too, depending on whether they appear in the rectum or in the colon (Marshall & Badnarchuk 1993; Spread et al., 1994). The rectum carcinoids develop at a young age, most of which are less than 2 cm and tend to be indolent. In contrast, colonic carcinoid tumours can be clinically aggressive and often metastise.

With a more accurate review, we can see that many habits could influence the development of rectal cancers and not colon cancers. Some studies support the view that family history, as well as the level of physical activity, is a stronger contributor to colon cancer relative to rectal cancer (Wei et al., 2004). The Women's Health Initiative (a large cohort study) (Paskett et al., 2007) also found a significant link between active cigarette smoking (not passive exposure to cigarette smoke) and rectal but not colon cancer.

These differences are important in terms of monitoring and have implications in treatment options, as well. Compared to colon cancers, the sensitivity of CT scan for detection of

malignant lymph nodes is higher for rectal cancers. Any perirectal adenopathy is presumed to be malignant since benign adenopathies are not typically seen in this area (Thoemi, 1997).
In a general form, rectal cancer shows predominance in male sex with a global worldwide incidence in this group of 13/100,000 by year. The incidence rates vary markedly worldwide with rates per 100,000 among males in the period of 1998-2002 reported to range from 2, 0 in India (New Delhi) to 31, 6 in Canada (Northwest Territories). In Europe the lowest rates in male were registered in Iceland (7, 6) followed by Italy- Salerno Providence (8, 1) and the highest in Czech Republic (27) followed by Slovak Republic (24, 4), (Curado et al., 2007).
A top ten ranking of age-standardized (world) incidence rates in Europe by sex and country can be seen in Table 1.

MEN			WOMEN		
Rank	**Country**	**Rate**	**Rank**	**Country**	**Rate**
1	Czech Republic	27,0	**1**	Czech Republic	12,1
2	Slovak Republic	24,4	**2**	Croatia	10,9
3	Croatia	20,9	**3**	Slovak Republic	10,5
4	Slovenia	20,5	**4**	Slovenia	10,1
5	Ireland	18,3	**4**	Norway	10,1
6	The Netherlands	17,6	**5**	The Netherlands	10,0
7	Germany	17,4	**6**	Denmark	9,8
8	Belgium	17,2	**7**	Russia	9,7
9	Denmark	16,6	**8**	Germany	9,1
10	Russia	16,6	**9**	Belgium	9,0
			10	Serbia	8,5

Data Source: Curado et al., 2007

Table 1. Top Ten Ranking (descending form) of age- standardized (world) incidence rates by sex and country.

Factors that may have contributed to the worldwide variation in incidence patterns include differences in the prevalence of risk factors and screening practices. Established and suspected modifiable risk factors for rectal cancer, including obesity, physical inactivity, smoking, heavy alcohol consumption, a diet high in red or processed meats and inadequate consumption of fruits and vegetables (Giovanucci, 2002; Schottemfeld & Fraumeni, 2006; Botteri et al., 2008), which are also associated with economic development or westernization (Popkin, 1994). For example, in Czech Republic, nearly 60% of men are cigarette smokers (Shafey et al., 2003) and more than 25% of adults are obese (Berghofer et al., 2008). In Japan, the increased intake of milk, meat, eggs and fat/oil over the past several decades has contributed to the increase in obesity in this country (Kuriki & Tajima, 2006; Matsushita et al., 2008).
In Portugal, particularly in the county of Vila Nova de Gaia (North of country) in the period of 2004- 2006 there were, on average 35 new cases per 100,000 inhabitants which, as showed, constitutes one of the highest rates in the world (Abreu et al., 2010).
In this chapter, the authors propose to examine the evolution of rectal cancer epidemiology based on the data of an active population- based cancer registry (The Cancer Registry of Vila Nova de Gaia). Given the near absence of studies focused only in rectal cancer, our data should also be further explored in other future population- based studies.

2. Patients and methods

2.1 Rectal Cancer Registry

The data were extracted from the Cancer Registry of Vila Nova de Gaia (ROG), founded in 1981 (Parkin et al., 2002). This registry, near the city of Porto, covers an area of 170 km^2, with a 2001 census population of 288 749 (139 808 men and 148941 women). The Cancer Registry of Vila Nova de Gaia uses active cases from different sources including hospitals, general practitioners, the health authority and the district death registration offices. The registry collects the cause of death in patient's death certificate and uses active follow-up to check the life status of apparently living patients avoiding the errors relating to incomplete ascertainment of death in registered patients with cancer and incomplete ascertainment of incident cases. The location of rectal tumours was classified according to the third edition of International Classification of Diseases for Oncology (Fritz et al., 1990). For the stage of the tumours, we used the 2002 version of the tumour node metastasis (TNM) system, with the stage III divided into three prognostic categories (A, B and C) (Greene et al., 2002). For each patient, rectal cancer treatment (surgery and/or chemotherapy and/or radiotherapy) was individualized according to protocols used at the time of diagnosis.

2.2 Statistical analysis

The study concerned the period 1995-2004 (399 cases) using the 1991 and 2001 census in the calculation of specific rates by age group, considering the following age groups (years) less than 44; 45-54; 55-64; 65-74 and 75 and above and the time periods 1995-1997; 1998-2000 and 2001-2004. Sex and age- standardized incidence rates were calculated using the European population and the ratio of the age- standardized rate between time periods, evaluated by a confidence interval of 95%. For both sexes, the tendency of evaluation were analysed by a Poisson regression model. χ^2 analysis was used to compare categorical variables.
Overall survival was calculated using the Kaplan- Meier method, and the curves were compared through a Log Rank test. The effect of topography and of histological type on survival was obtained, by controlling the stage disease, using a Cox proportional hazards regression model. Statistical significance was set to P value less than 0, 05. The statistical analyses were run in SPSS (version 15, 0; SPSS Inc, Chicago, Illinois, USA).

3. Results

There was a slight predominance of males (56.1%) compared with females which corresponds of a ratio of 1, 3. Patients' average age was 67 years old (standard deviation 12.5), with the youngest aged 22 years and the older aged 94 years. Rates increased with age over the three studied periods mainly in the older women (over age 65 years old) (Figs 1 & 2).
The crude rates calculated per 100 000 in the three periods analysed are: 17, 7; 18, 5; 16, 6 for men, and 9, 9; 12, 2; 15, 1 for women. The age-standardized rates are shown in Table 2. Upon analysing the comparison of standardized rate ratio, we conclude that in men the incidence had increased from the first period (1995-1997) to the second (1998-2000) in a nonsignificant way and decreased significantly during the next period (2001-2004). In women, the incidence rates of rectal cancer increased in the three periods, but in a nonsignificant way. The cumulative risk of developing rectal cancer before the age of 75 years in Vila Nova de Gaia was currently (2001-2005) estimated to be 1, 5 % in men and 1, 1% in women.

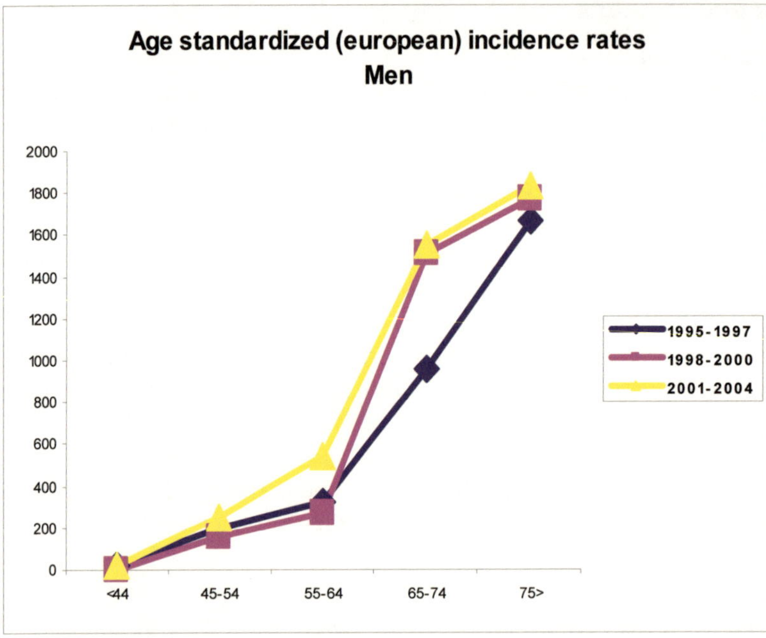

Fig. 1. Age- standardized incidence (European population) rates in men over the three periods

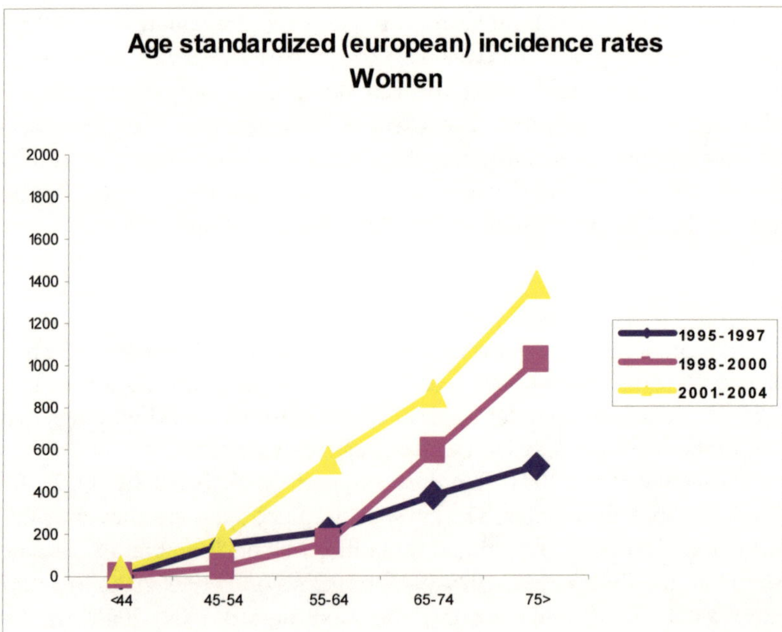

Fig. 2. Age- standardized incidence (European population) rates in women over the three periods

Men				
Period	**ASR**	**SE(ASR)**	**ASR2/ASR1**	**SRR: 95% CI**
1995-1997	23,08	2,444		
			1,21	0,970-1,506
1998-2000	27,90	2,789		
			0,67	0,510-0,894
2001-2004	18,26	1,923		
Women				
Period	**ASR**	**SE(ASR)**	**ASR2/ASR1**	**SRR:95% CI**
1995-1997	10,59	1,467		
			1,14	0,879-1,472
1998-2000	12,04	1,856		
			1,13	0,950-1,340
2001-2004	13,59	1,680		

ASR, age standardized rate; CI, confidence interval; SE, standardized error; SIR, standardized incidence ratio

Table 2. Standardized incidence rate ratio and 95% CI: comparison between the three time periods (1998-2000 versus 1995-1997 and 2001-2004 versus 1995-1997).

A Poisson regression model was carried out to check whether the presence of variables such as sex, age and period are linked to the risk (Table 3). The incidence of rectal tumours in men was higher, and a significant increase in all age groups (45-54; 55-64; 65-74; >75) was observed compared with the age group less than 44 years (reference group). Rectal tumours showed a nonsignificant increase in 1998-2000 and a nonsignificant decrease during the period 2001-2004. In 80% of cases, disease histology comprised adenocarcinomas, and 71, 9% of these were located in the rectum.

Variable	IRR (95% CI)
Gender	
Female	**Reference category**
Male	**1,77 (1,451-2,161)**
Age, years	
<44	**Reference category**
45-54	**10,44 (6,172-17,673)**
55-64	**21,88 (13,356-35,853)**
65-74	**61,790 (38,679-98,706)**
75+	**86,74 (53,845-139,747)**
Period	
1995-1997	**Reference category**
1998-2000	**1,16 (0,890-1,520)**
2001-2004	**0,98 (0,773-1,256)**

CI, confidence interval; IRR, incidence rate ratio

Table 3. Results of Poisson regression analysis

With regard to the stage, 25,1% of the tumours were diagnosed in stage I , 11,6% in stage II (A:8,3%; B:3,3%), 18,6% in stage III (A:3,0%; B:9,3%; C:6,3%), 13% in stage IV and 31,7% were unstaged. Upon analysing the stage by periods, we noticed that cases were not detected in earlier stages (Table 4).

	Period			
	1995-1997 n (%)	1998-2000 n (%)	2001-2004 n (%)	Total
Stage				
I	24 (24,0)	34 (34,0)	42 (42,0)	100 (100,0)
II	9 (19,6)	8 (17,4)	29 (63,0)	46 (100,0)
III	22 (29,7)	22 (29,7)	30 (40,5)	74 (100,0)
IV	10 (1,9)	18 (34,6)	24 (46,2)	52 (100,0)
Total	65 (23,9)	82 (30,1)	125 (46,0)	272 (100,0)

Table 4. Absolute and relative frequency distribution by stage disease (χ^2 =8, 949; d. f. = 6; *P*=0, 18)

3.1 Survival

Overall survival, which was 68% at the end of the first year and 50% at the end of 5 years, increased over the three periods being analysed (*P*=0,004; Fig.3).

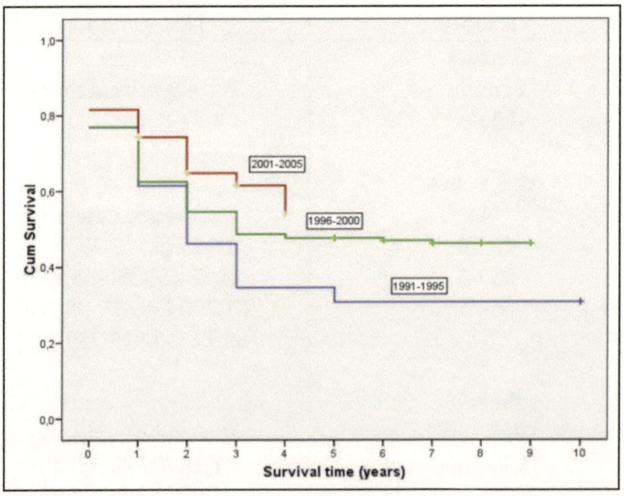

Fig. 3. Overall survival over the three analysed periods

Figure 4 shows that the difference in survival can be clearly seen for stage IV patients (*P*<0,001).

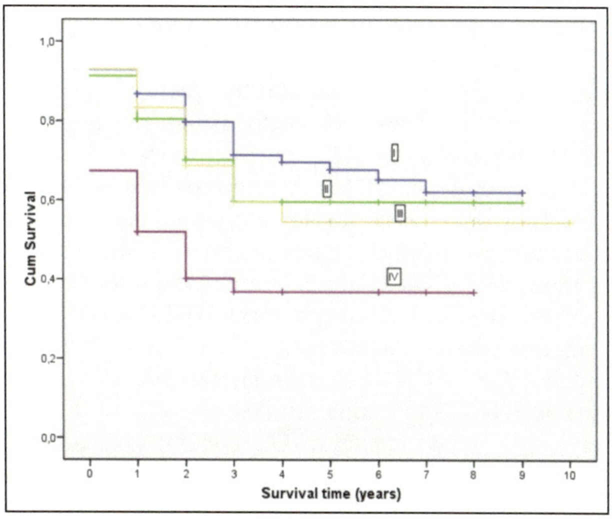

Fig. 4. Overall survival by disease stage

When analysing survival by subtypes in the 70 stage III patients, significant differences were not found (Log Rank test P=0.65). The location of the tumour (junction rectum- colon sigmoid versus rectum), after adjustment by stage, is not a significant factor in the prognosis for this cancer (Cox proportional hazards analysis: P=0.35). Overall survival is similar in adenocarcinomas versus others controlling the stage (Cox proportional hazards analysis: P=0.15).

4. Conclusion

The results of this study can be summarized as follows: first, there was a general increase in the incidence of rectal tumours during the analysed period in both sexes, with a predominance of male; second, tumours were considerably more frequent over the age of 45 years; third, the histological type and the locations analysed have not proven to be prognostic factors; finally, we did not observe an increase in early lesions (stage I/II) and approximately 20% of the individuals had distant metastatic disease at diagnosis. The primary prevention failed.

High- quality population- based cancer incidence data have been collected throughout the World since the early 1960s and published periodically in Cancer Incidence in Five Continents (Jemal et al., 2010). However, even in the last publication, the share of World population covered is only 11% (Curado et al., 2007). With the data available (Ponz de Leon et al., 2000, 2007) and according to our study, rectal cancer is more frequently observed in male patients, mainly in older ones (over 65 years). This reflects the expected increases in life expectancy and aging of the population (Thun et al., 2010). The differences between sexes tend to become smaller over time as it may suggest the slower adoption of certain risk behaviours associated with this cancer (Center et al., 2009). For instance, regular uptake of smoking worldwide traditionally lags several decades in women compared with men, with peak prevalence occurring at a much lower rate (Mackay & Amos, 2003). Additionally, the obesity related metabolic pathways that are implicated in rectal cancer are thought to be more heavily influenced by visceral abdominal fat that men tend to accumulate more of, compared with women in whom subcutaneous fat is more common (Frezza et al., 2006; Pischon et al., 2008).

In terms of mortality, many authors advocate that the quality of data vary by country, with a high accuracy of underlying cause of death noted in longstanding, economically developed countries and a lower accuracy reported in newly developed or economically transitioning countries (Center et al., 2009). Although the International Classification of the Diseases contains a carefully defined set of rules and guidelines that allow underlying cause to be selected in a uniform manner, interpretation of the concept probably varies considerably (Ferlay et al., 2007). The analysis of any apparent cancer mortality patterns is further complicated by the fact that mortality is influenced to a certain degree both by stage of the disease at diagnosis and by effectiveness of treatment. Hence the death rate for a cancer of equal incidence (i.e. of diagnosed cases) may be different from one country to another (Boyle & Smans, 2008). As in other studies, we noticed that rectal cancer survival varies, in an inversely way (Jessup et al., 1998; Gunderson et al., 2004) with the stage of the cancer (Harling et al., 2004; Rerink et al., 2004). Survival and disease relapse after surgery alone (Quirke et al., 1986; Adam et al., 1994) or combined with adjuvant treatment (Mohiuddin et al., 2000; Grann et al., 2001; Greene et al., 2001; Kapiteijn et al., 2001; Valentini et al., 2001; Tepper et al., 2002; Mohiuddin et al., 2006; Gunderson & Tepper, 2007) for rectal cancer patients are a function of both degree of bowel wall penetration of the primary lesion and nodal status. However nodal involvement alone is inadequate as the sole pathologic factor to predict survival and relapse rates (Quirke et al., 1986; Adam et al., 1994). Invasion through the bowel wall and number of involved lymph nodes are independent high- risk factors for both relapse and survival. For patients with a single high- risk factor of either direct tumor extension beyond the wall, nodes negative (T3N0), or positive nodes but primary tumor confined to the wall (T1-2N1-2), local relapse rates published in older surgical series have ranged from 20% to 40% (Gilbert, 1978; Rich et al., 1983). For patients with both positive nodes and extension beyond the wall (T3-4N1-2), the risk of pelvic relapse was nearly additive (40% to 65% in clinical series and 70% in a reoperative series) (Gilbert, 1978; Rich et al., 1983). The rate of systemic metastases is significantly higher for patients with both high- risk pathologic factors (extensive beyond rectal wall and positive nodes). In the sixth edition of American Joint Committee on Cancer (AJCC) staging (2002) , Stage II was subdivided into IIA (T3N0) and IIB (T4NO), and stage III was subdivided into IIIA (T1-2N1M0), IIIB (T3-4N1M0), and IIIC (any TN2M0)(14). A recently study, which validates the new AJCC staging (7th edition, 2009) for rectal cancer, based in a large cancer databases (Gunderson et al., 2009), demonstrates a more favorable prognosis of patients with T1-2N1-2 lesions (stage IIIC, AJCC sixth edition) in opposite of a less favorable prognosis of patients with T4N1 cancers (stage IIIB, sixth edition). This data supports the shift of T1-2N2 lesions from stage IIIC to an earlier stage of the disease (IIIA/IIIB) and T4N1 lesions from stage IIIB to IIIC and the subdivision of T4, N1 and N2 categories of disease. Patients with T4a lesions (penetrates to the surface of visceral peritoneum (revised definition, AJCC, seventh edition) have a better prognosis than patients with T4b lesions (directly invades or is adherent to other organs or structures) for each N category of disease (N0, N1 and N2). Patients with one positive node (N1a) have a better prognosis than patients with two to three positive nodes (N1b), and patients with four to five positive nodes (N2a) have a better prognosis than patients with seven or more positive nodes (N2b) by T category. In summary, the new AJCC seventh edition staging recommended the following changes: subdivide IIB into IIB (T4aN0) and IIC (T4bN0); shift more favorable

TN2 categories to either IIIA (T1N2a) or IIIB (T2N2a, T1-2N2b, T3N2a); and shift less favorable T4N1 lesions from IIIB to IIIC (T4bN1). For a better comprehension, the following two tables summarize the alterations of the last three AJCC staging based on TNM classifications (Table 5 &6).

Clinical classification		**5th edition (1997)**	**6th edition (2002)**	**7th edition (2009)**
T- primary tumour				
TX	Primary tumour cannot be assessed	+	+	+
T0	No evidence of primary tumour	+	+	+
Tis	Carcinoma in situ: intraepithelial or invasion of lamina propria	+	+	+
T1	Tumour invades submucosa	+	+	+
T2	Tumour invades muscularis propria	+	+	+
T3	Tumour invades through muscularis propria into subserosa or into non-perinealised pericolic or perirectal tissues	+	+	+
T4	Tumour directly invades into other organs or structures and/or perforates visceral peritoneum	+	+	+
T4a	Perforates visceral peritoneum	-	-	+
T4b	Directly invades other organs or structures	-	-	+
N- regional lymph nodes				
NX	Regional lymph nodes cannot be assessed	+	+	+
N0	No regional lymph node metastasis	+	+	+
N1	Metastasis in 1 to 3 regional lymph nodes	+	+	+
N1a	1 node	-	-	+
N1b	2-3 nodes	-	-	+
N1c	Satellites in subserosa, without regional nodes	-	-	+
N2	Metastasis in 4 or more regional lymph nodes	+	+	+
N2a	4-6 nodes	-	-	+
N2b	7 or more nodes	-	-	+
M- distant metastasis				
MX	Distant metastasis cannot be assessed	+	+	-
M0	No distant metastasis	+	+	+
M1	Distant metastasis	+	+	+
M1a	Metastasis confined to one organ (liver, lung, ovary, non- regional lymph node(s))	-	-	+
M1b	Metastasis in more than one organ on the peritoneum	-	-	+

Source: Quirke et al., 2011

Table 5. Comparative analysis of TNM classification of tumours of the rectum, 5th, 6th and 7th edition.

Stage	Stage grouping			5th edition (1997)	6th edition (2002)	7th edition (2009)
	T	N	M			
Stage 0	Tis	N0	M0	+	+	+
Stage I	T1, T2	N0	M0	+	+	+
Stage II	T3, T4	N0	M0	-	-	+
Stage IIA	T3	N0	M0	+	+	+
Stage IIB	T4	N0	M0	+	+	-
Stage IIB	T4a	N0	M0	-	-	+
Stage IIC	T4b	N0	M0	-	-	+
Stage III	Any T	N1, N2	M0	-	-	+
Stage IIIA	T1, T2	N1	M0	+	+	+
Stage IIIA	T1, T2	N1c	M0	-	-	+
Stage IIIA	T1	N2a	M0	-	-	+
Stage IIIB	T3, T4	N1	M0	+	+	-
Stage IIIB	T3, T4a	N1/N1c	M0	-	-	+
Stage IIIB	T2, T3	N2a	M0	-	-	+
Stage IIIB	T1, T2	N2b	M0	-	-	+
Stage IIIC	Any T	N2	M0	+	+	-
Stage IIIC	T4a	N2a	M0	-	-	+
Stage IIIC	T3, T4a	N2b	M0	-	-	+
Stage IIIC	T4b	N1, N2	M0	-	-	+
Stage IV	Any T	Any N	M1	+	+	-
Stage IVA	Any T	Any N	M1a	-	-	+
Stage IVB	Any T	Any N	M1b	-	-	+

T tumour, N node, M metastasis
Source: Quicke et al., 2011

Table 6. Comparative an analysis of TNM stage grouping of rectal cancer in the last three AJCC Staging editions

Unlike other studies (Ponz de Leon et al., 2004, 2007), during the three analyzed periods, we did not observe an increase in early lesions (stage I/II), as there were no statistically significant differences in the stages over time. This denotes that primary prevention failed even the screening for this cancer has been shown to be effective (Boyle, 1995; Faivre et al., 2004) and has been cited as one of the most important factors responsible for the recent decline in colorectal cancer rates in United States (Espey et al., 2007; Levin et al., 2008). On the time of the study, in Portugal, the screening programs were mostly opportunistic which is in agreement with the last International Agency for Research Cancer (IARC) publication that shows that colorectal cancer screening programs are responsible only for less than 15% of the incidence data source worldwide (Curado et al., 2007). Having this dramatic situation in mind, the Guidelines Committee of the World Gastroenterology Organization presented recently (Winawer et al., 2011), a new conceptual model of cascade colorectal cancer screening guidelines that is also evidence based but resource driven. The emphasis in this variation of the model is on colonoscopy resources at the top of the cascade for a screening goal of prevention by finding and removing the colorectal cancer precursor lesions, the adenoma, as well as early detection. The cascade concept says: “do what you can with what you have” rather than, “do it this way or no way”. The First Report of Cancer Screening in the European Union (Karsa et al., 2008), demonstrates that colorectal cancer programs are currently running or being established in 19 of the 27 Member States. Twelve of the Member States have adopted the population- based approach to program implementation recommended by the Council of the European Union (Cyprus, Finland, France, Hungary, Italy, Poland, Portugal, Romania, Slovenia, Spain, Sweden and the United Kingdom) (Klabunde et al., 2001) and seven have established non- population- based programs (Austria, Bulgaria, The Czech Republic, Germany, Greece, Latvia and the Slovak Republic). With these programs, a total of 70% of population aged 50-74, are covered (Fig. 5).

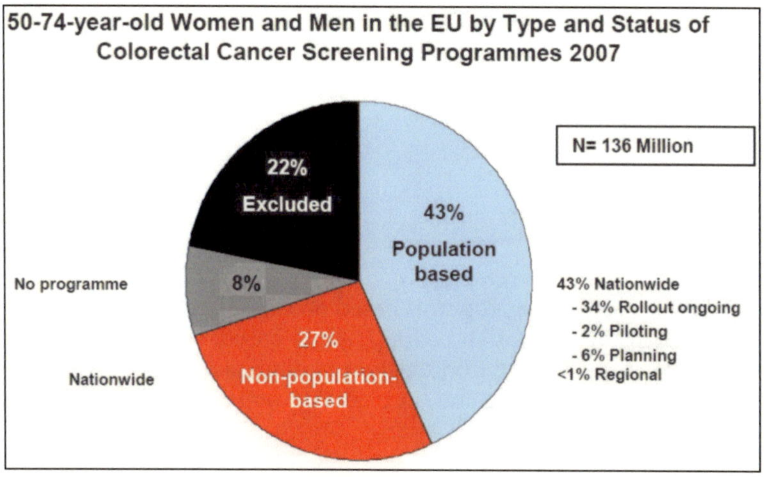

Source: Karsa et al. 2008

Fig. 5. Proportion of 50-74-year-old women and men targeted for colorectal cancer screening in the European Union in 2007, by program type and country implementation status, and women and men excluded due to age or lack of regional programs in countries with regional implementation status (proportions of 50-74-year-old persons in the EU population in %).

Variations between the Member States in the way colorectal screening is implemented is more pronounced than in other cancer screening like breast cancer. Out of the nineteen Member States running or establishing colorectal cancer screening programs in 2007, twelve (Bulgaria, Czech Republic, Finland, France, Hungary, Latvia, Portugal, Romania, Slovenia, Spain, Sweden, and the United Kingdom) have adopted only the non-invasive test specified in the Council Recommendation (fecal occult blood test- FOBT), six (Austria, Cyprus, Germany, Greece, Italy, Slovak Republic) use both the FOBT and an endoscopic test for primary screening and one (Poland) uses only an endoscopic test (colonoscopy) (Fig. 6&7). With the exception of Italy, in which flexible sigmoidoscopy is the endoscopic screening test used in seven loco- regional programs in 2007, the other Member States with endoscopic programs have adopted colonoscopy as the primary screening test. Out of 17 Member States for which information on the FOBT screening interval is available, 11 have adopted a 2-year interval for all participants with a negative test result. The recommended interval for colonoscopy is 5 years in Greece and 10 years in the four Member States which have adopted endoscopic screening programs. Due to the upper age limits of the respective target populations, the number of screening colonoscopies is limited to once or twice in a lifetime in Germany and Poland.

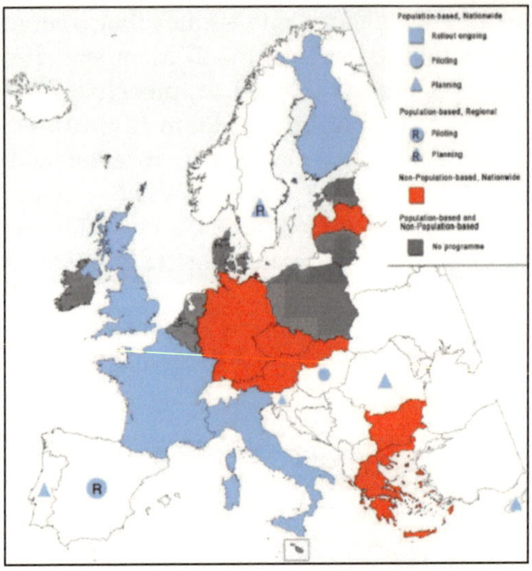

Source: Karsa et al., 2008

Fig. 6. Colorectal cancer screening programs based on FOBT (fecal occult blood test) in the European Union in 2007, by program type (population-based; non-population-based; no program) and country implementation status (population-based: nationwide or regional, rollout complete or ongoing, piloting and/or planning; non-population-based: nationwide or regional).

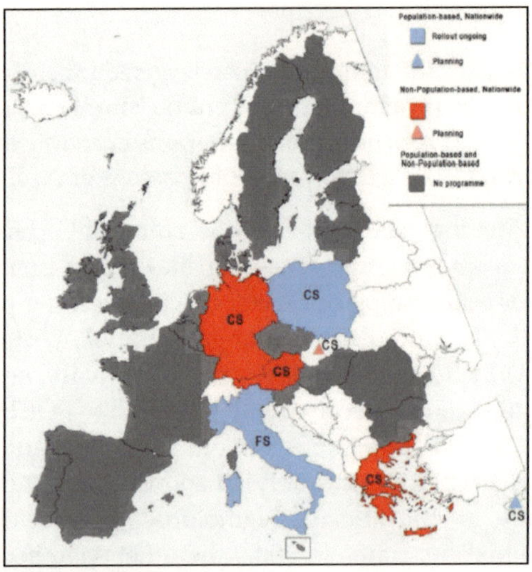

FS (flexible sigmoidoscopy), CS (colonscopy).
Source: Karsa et al., 2008

Fig. 7. Colorectal cancer screening programs based on novel screening tests still under evaluation (Endoscopy) in the European Union in 2007, by program type (population-based; non-population-based; no program) and country implementation status (population-based: nationwide or regional, rollout complete or ongoing, piloting and/or planning; non-population-based: nationwide or regional).

Despite the variations among countries, we hope that these measures will change in the medium term, the current patterns of incidence and mortality of rectal cancer.
Actually, this cancer remains a major public health problem worldwide.

5. Acknowledgment

The authors like to thank Prof. João Amado for reviewing of this chapter and Roche Farmacêutica Química, Lda (Portugal) for the financial support of this publication.

6. References

Abreu MH, Matos E, Poças FC, Rocha R, Pinto J & Lopes C. (2010). Staging and survival of rectal cancer in Vila Nova de Gaia, Portugal. *Eur J Gastroenterol Hepatol,* 22(2): 151-6.

Adam IJ, Mohamdee MO, Martin JG, *et al.* (1994). Role of circunferencial margin involvement in the local recurrence of rectal cancer. *Lancet,* 311:707-711.

Berghofer A, Pischon T, Reinhold T, Aprovian CM, Sharma AM & Willich SN. (2008). Obesity prevalence from a European perspective: a systematic review. *BMC Public Health,* 8:200.

Botteri E, Iodice S, Bagnardi V, Raimondi S, Lowenfels AB & Maisonneuve P. (2008). Smoking and colorectal cancer: a meta-analysis. *JAMA,* 300:2765-78.

Boyle P & Smans M. (Ed(s).). (2008). Cancer Mortality Patterns by Site, In: *Atlas of cancer mortality in European Union and The European Economic Area 1993-1997.* Lyon: IARC Scientific Publications, No. 159.

Boyle P. (1995). Progress in preventing death from colorectal cancer [Editorial]. Br J *Cancer,* 72:528-530.

Center MM, Jemal A, Smith RA & Ward E. (2009). Worldwide Variations in Colorectal Cancer. *CA Cancer J Clin,* 59 (6): 366-78.

Center MM, Jemal A, Ward E. (2009). International Trends in Colorectal Cancer Incidence Rates. *Cancer Epidemiol Biomarkers Prev,* 18(6):1688-1694.

Consorti F, Lorenzotti A, Midiri G, *et al.* (2000). Prognostic significance of mucinous carcinoma of colon and rectum: A prospective case- control study. *J Surg Oncol,* 73:70.

Curado MP, Edwards B, Shin H, *et al.* (2007). *Cancer Incidence in Five Continents,* Vol. IX. IARC Scientific Publications No 160. Lyon.

Espey DK, Wu XC, Swan J, *et al.* (2007). Annual report to the nation on the status of cancer, 1975-2004, featuring cancer in American Indians and Alaska Natives. *Cancer,* 110:2119-2152.

Faivre J, Dancourt V, Lejeune C *et al.* (2004). Reduction in colorectal cancer mortality by fecal occult blood screening in a French controlled study. *Gastroenterology,* 126(7): 1674-1680.

Ferlay J, Autier P, Boniol M, Heanue M, Colombet M & Boyle P. (2007). Estimates of the cancer incidence and mortality in Europe in 2006. *Ann Oncol,* 18(3): 581-92.

Frezza EE, Wachtel MS & Chiriva- Internati M. (2006). Influence of obesity on the risk of developing colon cancer. *Gut,* 55: 285-91.

Fritz A, Percy C, Jack A, Shanmugaratnam K, Sobin L, Parkin D & Whelan S. (1990). *International classification of diseases for oncology.* 3rd. Geneva: WHO.

Gilbert SB. (1978). The significance of symptomatic local tumor failure following abdominoperineal resection. *Int J Radiat Oncol Biol Phys,* 4:801-807.

Giovannucci E. (2002). Modifiable risk factors for colon cancer. *Gastroenterol Clin North Am,* 31:925-43.

Grann A, Feng C, Wong D, *et al.* (2001). Preoperative combined modality therapy for clinically resectable UT3 rectal cancer. *Int J Radiat Oncol Biol Phys*, 19:987-995.

Greene FL, Page DL, Fleming ID, Fritz A, Balch CM, Haller DG & Morrow M. (Ed(s).). (2002) *AJCC (American Joint Committee on Cancer) cancer staging manual.* 6th ed. New York: Springer- Verlag; p.114.

Greene FL, Stewart A & Norton HJ. (2001). New Tumor-node-metastasis staging strategy for node-positive (stage III) rectal cancer: An analysis. *J Clin Oncol,* 22:1778-1781.

Gunderson LL, Sargent D & Tepper J. (2004). Impact of T and N stage and treatment on survival and relapse in adjuvant rectal cancer. *J Clin Oncol*; 22: 1785-1796.

Gunderson LL & Tepper JE (Ed(s.)). (2007). Rectal cancer, In:*Clinical Radiation Oncology* (2nd ed). Philadelphia. PA. Churchill Livingstone/Elsevier, pp 1113.

Gunderson LL, Jessup JM, Sargent DJ, Greene FL & Stewart A. (2009). Revised Tumor and Node Categorization for Rectal Cancer Based on Surveillance, Epidemiology, and End Results and Rectal Pooled Analysis Outcomes. *J Clin Oncol,* 28:256-263.

Harling H, Bulow S, Kronborg O, Moller LN & Jorgensen T. (2004). Survival of rectal cancer patients in Denmark during 1994-1999. *Colorectal Dis,* 6: 153-157.

Jemal A, Center MM, Desantis C & Ward EM. (2010). Global Patterns of Cancer Incidence and Mortality Rates and Trends. *Cancer Epidemiology, Biomarkers and Prevention,* 19:1893-1907.

Jessup JM, Stewart AK & Menck HR. (1998). The National Cancer Data Base report on patterns of care for adenocarcinoma of the rectum, 1985-1995. *Cancer,* 83:2408.

Kapiteijn E, Marijnen CAM, Nagtegaal ID, *et al.* (2001). Preoperative radiotherapy combined with total mesorectal excision for resectable rectal cancer. *N Engl J Med,* 315:615-638.

Karsa L. (Ed(s).). (2008). Cancer Screening in the European Union, In: *First Report on the implementation of the Council Recommendation on cancer screening.* ISBN 978-92-79-08934-3.

Klabunde C, Bouchard F, Taplin S, Scharpantgen S & Ballard- Barbash R. (2001). Quality assurance for screening mammography: an international comparison. *J Epidemiol,* 55:57-204-212.

Kuriki K & Tajima K. (2006). The increasing incidence of colorectal cancer and the preventive strategy in Japan. *Asian Pac J Cancer Prev,* 7: 495-501.

Levin B, Lieberman DA, McFarland B, *et al.* (2008). Screening and surveillance for the early detection of colorectal cancer and adenomatous polyps, 2008: a joint guideline from the American Cancer Society, the Us MultiSociety Task Force on Colorectal Cancer, and the American College of Radiology. *CA Cancer J Clin,* 58:130-160.

Mackay J & Amos A. (2003). Women and tobacco. *Respirology,* 8: 123-30.

Marshall JB & Bodnarchuk. (1983). Carcinoid tumors of the gut: Our experience over three decades and review of literature. *J Clin Gastroenterol,* 16:123.

Matsushita Y, Takahashi Y, Mizoue T, Inoue M, Noda M & Tsugane S. (2008). Overweight and obesity trends among Japanese adults: a 10- year follow-up of the JPHC Study*: Int J Obes (Lond),* 32:1861-7.

Mohiuddin M, Hayne M, Regine WF, *et al.* (2000). Prognostic significance of postchemoradiation stage following preoperative chemotherapy and radiation for advanced/recurrent rectal cancers. Int J Radiat Oncol Biol Phys, 18:1075-1080.

Mohiuddin M, Winter K, Mitchell E, *et al.* (2006). Randomized phase II study of neoadjuvant combined-modality chemoradiation for distal rectal cancer: Radiation therapy Oncology Group trial 0012. *J Clin Oncol,* 24:650-655.

Parkin DM, Bray F, Ferlay J & Pisani P. (2005). Global cancer statistics, 2002. *CA Cancer J Clin,* 55: 74-108.

Parkin DM, Whelan SL, Ferlay J, Teppo L & Thomas DB. (2002). *Cancer Incidence in Five Continents.* Vol VIII. Lyon: IARC Scientific Publications, No. 155.

Parkin DM. (2004). International variation. *Oncogene,* 23: 6329-40.

Paskett ED, Reeves KW, Rohan TE, *et al.* (2007). Association between cigarette smoking and colorectal cancer in the Women's Health Initiative. *J Natk Cancer Inst,* 99: 1729.

Pischon T, Boeing H, Hoffman K, *et al.* (2008). General and abdominal adiposity and risk of death in Europe. *N Engl J Med,* 359: 2105-20.

Ponz de Leon M, Benatti P, Di Gregorio C, Fante R, Rossi G, Losi L, *et al.* (2000). Staging and survival of colorectal cancer: are we making progress? The 14- year experience of a specialized cancer registry. *Dig Liver Dis,* 32:312-317.

Ponz de Leon M, Marino M, Benatti P, Rossi G, Mengatti M, Pedroni M, et al. (2004). Trend of incidence, subsite distribution and staging of colorectal neoplasms in the 15-year experience of a specialized cancer register. *Ann Oncol,* 15:940-946.

Ponz de Leon M, Rossi G, Di Gregorio C, de Gaetani C, Rossi F, Ponti G, *et al.* (2007). Epidemiology of colorectal cancer: the 21- year experience of a specialized registry. *Intern Emerg Med,* 2:269-279.

Popkin BM. (1994). The nutrition transition in low-income countries: an emerging crisis. *Nutr Rev,* 52:285-98.

Quirke P, Durdey P, Dixon MF, *et al.* (1986). Local recurrence of rectal adenocarcinoma due to inadequate surgical resection: Histopathological study of lateral tumor spread and surgical excision. *Lancet,* 2: 996-999.

Quirke P, Risio M & Lambert R. (2011). Quality assurance in pathology in colorectal cancer screening and diagnosis- European recommendations. *Virchows Arch,* 458:1-19.

Reerink O, Mulder N, Botke G, Sluiter WJ, Szabó BG & Plukker JT. (2004). Treatment of locally recurrent rectal cancer, results and prognostic factors. *Eur J Surg Oncol,* 30:954-958.

Rich T, Gunderson LL, Gaidabini J, *et al.* (1983). Clinical and pathologic factors influencing local failure after curative resection of carcinoma of the rectum and rectosigmoid. *Cancer,* 52:1317-1329.

Schottenfeld D & Fraumeni J. (2006). Cancers of the colon and rectum, In: *Cancer Epidemiology and Prevention.* New York: Oxford University Press, 809-829.

Shafey O, Dolwick S & Guindon GE. (Ed(s.)). (2003). *Tobacco control country profiles.* 2nd ed. Atlanta (GA): American Cancer Society, WHO, International Union Against Cancer.

Spread C, Berkel H, Jewel L, *et al.* (1994). Colon carcinoid tumors: A population- based study. *Dis Colon Rectum,* 37:482.

Tepper JE, O'Connell MJ, Niedzwiecki D, *et al.* (2002). Adjuvant therapy in rectal cancer: Analysis of stage, sex and local control- Final report of Intergroup 0114. J *Clin Oncol,* 20:1744-1750.

Thoemi RF (1997). Colorectal cancer. Radiologic staging. *Radiol Clin North Am*; 35:457.

Thun MJ, DeLancey JO, Center MM, Jemal A & Ward EM. (2010). The global Burden of cancer: priorities for prevention. *Carcinogenesis*, 31; 100-10.

Valentini V, Coco C, Cellini N, *et al.* (2001). Ten years of preoperative chemoradiation for extraperitoneal T3 rectal cancer: Acyrate toxicity, tumor response and sphincter preservation in three consecutive studies. *Int J Radiat Oncol Biol Phys,* 51:371-383.

Wei EK, Giovannucci E, Wu K, *et al.* (2004). Comparasion of risk factors for colon and rectal cancer. *Int J Cancer*, 108:443.

Winawer SJ, Krabshuis J, Lambert R, O'Brien M & Fried M. (2011). Cascade colorectal cancer screening guidelines: a global conceptual model. *J Clin Gastroenterol,* 45(4): 297-300.

Yabroff KR, Mariotto AB, Feuer E & Brown ML. (2008). Projections of the costs associated with colorectal cancer care in United States, 2000-2020. *Health Economics,* 17(8): 947-959.

2

Opportunistic Screening for Colorectal Cancer

Xu An-gao
Huizhou Medicine Institute, Huizhou First Hospital, Guangdong
China

1. Introduction

Two major screening models are currently available in the world for colorectal cancer: systematic screening and opportunistic screening. Systematic screening covers all segments of the population in a certain area and requires the participation of specialized institutions and professionals as well as huge financial support. It is a population-based active screening. Opportunistic screening targets those who seek medical treatment and screens for disease of interest during patients' treatment or examination. Compared with systematic screening, opportunistic screening has the advantages of good compliance and no need for additional examination with slightly increased cost. The key to opportunistic screening for colorectal cancer is to identify the population at high risk for colorectal cancer and determine who need such screening. The criteria for identification of high-risk population for colorectal cancer include mainly family history, personal history, laboratory testing, and age: ① hereditary non-polyposis colorectal cancer (HNPCC) family members aged ≥ 10 years; ② individuals with first-degree relatives with familial polyposis aged ≥10 years; ③ individuals with first-degree relatives with colorectal cancer and aged ≥ (the age of the diagnosis of colorectal cancer in the affected relatives minus 10 years) (i.e. first-degree relatives who are 10 years younger than a colorectal cancer patient are at high risk for the cancer. For example, the first-degree relatives aged 50 years or older of a 60-year-old colorectal cancer patient are high-risk population for colorectal cancer.); ④ previous history of colorectal cancer or colorectal adenoma; ⑤ ulcerative colitis or Crohn's disease unhealed for more than 10 years; ⑥ history of biliary tract disease or cholecystectomy for more than 10 years; ⑦ history of lower abdominal radiotherapy for more than 10 years; ⑧ history of chronic schistosomiasis in the colon; ⑨ history of chronic appendicitis; ⑩ unexplained positive fecal occult blood test; ⑪ unexplained elevated serum CEA level; and ⑫ age of 50 years and older.

Development of screening models for colorectal cancer depends on disease risk stratification of individuals in the population. The risk of colorectal cancer development in individuals in a natural population with no symptoms of colorectal cancer is stratified into four levels: ① Level III high risk. Individuals in this subgroup have the highest risk and about 5% of colorectal cancer cases occur in this population, who should undergo screening every 3 months to 1 year. ② Level II high risk. About 15-20% of colorectal cancer cases occur in this population, who should undergo screening every 1 to 5 years. ③ Level I high risk. About 70% to 80% of colorectal cancer cases occur in this population, who should undergo screening at a frequency of 5 to 10 years. Stratifying the population at high risk for colorectal cancer into levels I, II, III high-risk subgroups will help choose screening methods and the timing of screening. ④ Low-risk subgroup. This population is at low risk for colorectal cancer and no screening is thus needed.

Major screening methods for colorectal cancer include digital rectal examination, fecal occult blood test, sigmoidoscopy, full colonoscopy and genetic testing. Full colonoscopy can serve as the preferred modality for opportunistic screening for colorectal cancer. If full colonoscopy is performed only after the discovery of distal colorectal tumor via sigmoidoscopy, there will be a missed diagnosis rate of 72.0%.

Our study shows that by performing opportunistic screening among high-risk populations, the average direct cost for each detected case of colorectal cancer is about 50,000 RMB yuan, four times less than the cost of systematic screening. For each detected case of colorectal tumor (cancer and adenoma combined), the direct cost of opportunistic screening on average is 2,000 RMB yuan. These data show favorable cost-effectiveness of opportunistic screening for colorectal cancer. In addition, of the colorectal cancers detected among high-risk populations, the proportion of colorectal cancers staged at Duke's A and B is 45% and 33% respectively. In contrast, of the colorectal cancers detected among symptomatic hospital-visiting patients, the proportion of colorectal cancers staged at Duke's A and B is 4% and 29%, respectively. Previous research has established that the 5-year survival rate following surgery of Dukes' A colorectal cancer can reach as high as 90%, which demonstrates the good social benefit of opportunistic screening.

Worldwide, the incidence rate of colorectal cancer ranks only after lung cancer and breast cancer. Overall, colorectal cancer accounts for 9% and 10% of malignant tumors in men and women respectively. Colorectal cancer thus poses a serous public health problem and increases greatly the burden of disease. In recent two decades, the incidence and mortality rates of colorectal cancer in the world increase significantly, with the incidence rate increasing from an annual average of about 2% to 6.4% and the average mortality rate increasing by 3.3% annually.

Currently, the incidence rate of colorectal cancer in China is 16.3/100,000 for men, 12.2/100,000 for women, and 14.2/100,000 for the whole population. The mortality rate of colorectal cancer in China is 8.0/100,000 for men, 5.9/100,000 for women, and 6.9/100,000 for the whole population. In recent years, with changes in lifestyle, dietary structure, and environment in China, the incidence and mortality rates of colorectal cancer are on the rise and its incidence rate ranks the fourth in malignant tumors. Its incidence rates in the 1990s increased by 31.9% in urban areas and 8.5% in rural areas as compared with the incidence rates in the 1990s. It is expected that colorectal cancer cases will be nearly doubled by 2030, with 400,086 new cases and 211,714 deaths.

Because colorectal cancer often presents no symptoms in the early stage, patients do not seek timely medical treatment. By the time clinical symptoms of colorectal cancer appear, their condition will usually have progressed to intermediate or advanced stages which are associated with increased disease burden and poor prognosis. Previous studies suggest that at least 80% of colorectal cancers derive from colorectal adenoma and that the transition from colorectal adenoma to colorectal cancer lasts over 5 years, with an average of 10 to 15 years, which makes early detection of lesions through screening possible. Considerable evidence based on research has confirmed that colorectal cancer screening in the population can identify precancerous disease and precancerous lesions of colorectal cancer as well as early colorectal cancer. Treatment can be prescribed, thereby reducing the incidence and mortality rates of colorectal cancer, and economic burden of colorectal cancer.

Population at risk of colorectal cancer has a likelihood of colorectal cancer development 2 to 4 times higher than the general population. High-risk population screening is an important part of secondary prevention of colorectal cancer. The focus of current medical model is shifting towards "early prevention". Strengthening the screening of colorectal cancer will contribute to "early prevention" and early diagnosis and early treatment, and will ultimately improve 5-year survival rate of colorectal cancer patients.

1.1 Overview

Two major screening models are currently available for colorectal cancer: systematic screening and opportunistic screening. Systematic screening covers all segments of the population in a certain area and requires the participation of specialized institutions and professionals as well as huge financial support. It is a population-based active screening. Opportunistic screening targets those who seek medical treatment and screens for disease of interest during patients' treatment or examination. Compared with systematic screening, opportunistic screening has the advantages of good compliance and no need for additional examination with slightly increased cost. Therefore, opportunistic screening among the population at high risk of colorectal cancer is feasible and also of great significance for early diagnosis of colorectal cancer. Opportunistic screening can be performed at outpatient departments or health examination centers, with no need of special financial support or additional personnel. Hence, it is individual-based passive screening. Our study shows that for each detected case of colorectal cancer, the average direct cost of systematic screening is about four times as much as that of opportunistic screening.

The main targets of opportunistic screening can be divided into three categories: ① individuals seeking health examination in the hospitals (community or health examination centers); ② individuals seeking medical treatment for disease other than colorectal cancer but having high risk factors for colorectal cancer (individuals present no clinical manifestations of colorectal tumors but have definite positive family history or personal history); ③ outpatients with no symptoms of colorectal cancer.

2. Definition of high-risk population for colorectal cancer

High-risk population refers to a group of individuals at high risk of a certain disease. Currently there is no unified definition of high-risk population for colorectal cancer in the international community. In general, identification of high-risk population for colorectal cancer is conducted by integrating family history, personal history, laboratory tests and age.

Family history

1. hereditary non-adenomatous colorectal cancer (HNPCC) family members aged ≥ 10 years;
2. first-degree relatives with familial polyposis aged ≥ 10 years;
3. individuals with first-degree relatives with colorectal cancer and aged ≥ (the age of the diagnosis of colorectal cancer in the affected relatives minus 10 years) (i.e. first-degree relatives 10 years younger than the colorectal cancer patient are high-risk population. For example, the first-degree relatives aged 50 years or older of a 60-year-old colorectal cancer patient are high-risk population for colorectal cancer.);

Personal History

4. previous history of colorectal cancer or colorectal adenoma;
5. ulcerative colitis or Crohn's disease unhealed for more than 10 years;
6. history of biliary tract disease or cholecystectomy for more than 10 years;
7. history of lower abdominal radiotherapy for more than 10 years;
8. history of chronic colonic schistosomiasis;
9. history of chronic appendicitis;

Laboratory tests

10. unexplained positive fecal occult blood test;
11. unexplained elevated serum CEA level;

Advanced age

12. age of 50 years and older.

Subjects presenting any one or more of the following symptoms are symptomatic of colorectal cancer and diagnostic testing is indicated. ①altered bowel habits (diarrhea, constipation, etc.); ② stool changes (thinning stool, blood stool, mucus stool, etc.); ③ tenesmus (feeling of unsatisfied defecation); ④abdominal mass; ⑤intestinal obstruction; ⑥ unexplained lower abdominal discomfort or abdominal pain; ⑦unexplained anemia; ⑧ unexplained weight loss or systemic cancer symptoms (such as fatigue, fever, etc.).

Subjects less than 50 years of age who do not meet the criteria of colorectal cancer high-risk populations and present no symptoms of colorectal cancer have low risk of colorectal cancer development and no screening is needed. If screening is required by an individual, fecal occult blood test in conjunction with colonoscopy can be employed.

3. Risk stratification of high-risk colorectal cancer populations

To achieve good cost-effectiveness and feasibility, screening can be performed in the population with high prevalence. Usually there are three ways of looking for population with high prevalence: ① questionnaire-based search for high-risk groups. High-risk populations are more likely to develop a certain disease than asymptomatic populations; ② conducting screening among a group of subjects with a particular clinical symptom or who are positive for a certain test; ③ conducting opportunistic screening at outpatient departments of hospitals or community medical centers. No matter which method is chosen, risk stratification of individuals is the first step of screening. On the basis of previous studies at home and abroad, we stratify the risk of asymptomatic individuals developing colorectal cancer into four levels. 1. Level III high risk. Individuals in this subgroup have the highest risk, who include ①HNPCC family members aged ≥ 10 years; ② individuals with first-degree relatives with familial polyposis aged ≥10 years; ③ ulcerative colitis or Crohns disease unhealed for more than 10 years. About 5% of colorectal cancer cases occur in the level III high-risk population. 2. Level II high risk. Subjects at level II high risk of colorectal cancer include: ① individuals with history of colorectal cancer; ② individuals with history of colorectal adenoma; ③ individuals with first-degree relatives with colorectal cancer and aged ≥ (the age of the affected relatives minus 10 years); ④ individuals with first-degree relatives with colorectal adenoma and aged ≥ (the age of the affected relatives minus 10 years);⑤ individuals with cholecystectomy performed more than 10 years ago; ⑥individuals with history of lower abdominal radiotherapy for more than 10 years; ⑦

individuals with chronic colonic schistosomiasis; ⑧ individuals with chronic appendicitis。About 15-20% of colorectal cancer cases occur in the level II high-risk population. 3. Level I high risk. Individuals at this risk level refer to a group of subjects who have an age of 50 years and older, present no colorectal cancer symptoms, and do not meet the criteria of levels II and III high-risk populations. About 70% to 80% of colorectal cancer cases occur in the level I high-risk population. Stratifying the population at high risk for colorectal cancer into levels I, II, III high-risk subgroups will help choose screening methods and the timing of screening. 4. Low-risk subgroup. Individuals at this risk level refer to a group of subjects under 50 years who have no symptoms of colorectal cancer and do not meet the criteria of levels II and III high-risk populations. This population is at low risk of colorectal cancer and no screening is thus needed.

4. Strategies of opportunistic screening for colorectal cancer

A complete colorectal cancer screening program should include determination of the population to be screened, the choice of screening methods, screening monitoring of different populations. There are various methods available for colorectal cancer screening and there is no generally accepted consensus worldwide as to which method is to be chosen and what program is most effective. American Cancer Society (ACS), United States Preventive Service Task Force (USPSTF), US Multisociety Task Force On Colorectal Cancer, American Society for Gastrointesinal Endoscopy (ASGE) and National Comprehensive Cancer Network (NCCN) have issued their own colorectal cancer screening guidelines [2-5]. The United Kingdom, Canada, and China also have developed their own screening guidelines. On the basis of these aforementioned guidelines, we developed an opportunistic screening program for colorectal cancer.

Risk stratification	Starting time of screening	Frequency of colonoscopy
I. Level I high risk		
1. More than 50 years old	50 years old	Every 10 years
II. Level II high risk		
2. Family history of colorectal cancer		
①First-degree relatives developing colorectal cancer at an age <60 years	40 years old or 10 years earlier than the age of onset of the youngest affected relative	Every 3-5 years if the first colonoscopy is normal
②First-degree relatives developing colorectal cancer at an age ≥60 years	40 years old	Every 3-5 years if the first colonoscopy is normal
3. Family history colorectal adenoma		
①First-degree relatives developing colorectal adenoma at an age <60 years	40 years old or 10 years earlier than the age of onset of the youngest affected relative	Every 5 years if the first colonoscopy is normal

Risk stratification	Starting time of screening	Frequency of colonoscopy
②First-degree relatives developing colorectal adenoma at an age ≥60 years	Individually determined	Every 10 years if the first colonoscopy is normal
4. Personal history of colorectal cancer ①Personal history of colon cancer	One year after surgical resection of the cancer	Re-examination at the 3rd year if the first one is normal and later every 5 years
②Personal history of rectal cancer	One year after surgical resection of the cancer	Re-examination at the 4th year if the first one is normal and later every 5 years Every 3-6 months in the first 2-3 years following low resection when no pelvic radiotherapy or mesorectal excision is performed
5. Personal history of colorectal adenoma ①Colonic adenomas ≤2, diameter <1cm and mild atypical hyperplasia	Not earlier than 5 years after surgery	Every 5 years
②Advanced tumors or adenomas >3	One year after surgery	Every 3 years
③Villous adenoma accompanied by possible incomplete excision	Within 2-6 months after surgery	Every 3 years
6. Cholecystectomy performed more than 10 years ago	At the time of knowledge	Every 5 years
7. History of lower abdominal radiotherapy performed more than 10 years ago	At the time of knowledge	Every 5 years
8. Chronic colonic schistosomiasis	At the time of knowledge	Every 5 years
9. Chronic appendicitis	At the time of knowledge	Every 5 years
III. Level III high risk		
HNPCC family history	20-25 years old or 10 years earlier than the age of onset of the youngest family member	Every 1-2 years and every 1 year after 40 years old
FAP family history ①Genetic test of FAP proband (+)		
Genetic test of FAP relatives (+)	10-12 years old	Every 1 year and, if no polyp is present, every 1 year until the age of 40 years. Then every 3-5 years.

Risk stratification	Starting time of screening	Frequency of colonoscopy
Genetic test of FAP relatives (-)	10-12 years old	Every 7-10 years until the age of 40 years. Then every 5 years.
②Genetic test of FAP proband (-)	10-12 years old	Every 1 year and, if no polyp is present, every 1 year until the age of 40 years.Thereafter, every 3-5 years.
Inflammatory bowel disease (ulcerative colitis or extensive Crohn's colitis)	10 years after onset	Every 1-2 years

Note: HNPCC: hereditary non-polyposis colorectal cancer; FAP: familial adenomatous polyposis

Table 1. Opportunistic screening programs for colorectal cancer

5. Screening methods and benefits

Screening methods for colorectal cancer mainly include digital rectal examination, fecal occult blood test, sigmoidoscopy, full colonoscopy and genetic testing. We recommend full colonoscopy as the preferred examination for opportunistic screening of the population at high risk of colorectal cancer. This recommendation is based on the following reasons. First, colonoscopy is needed to reach a definite diagnosis when other screening methods are positive. Second, colonoscopy is the only screening modality capable of both diagnosis and treatment. Third, if colonoscopy is performed only after distal colon cancer is found with sigmoidoscopy, there will be a missed diagnosis rate of 72.0%. If full colonoscopy cannot be used as the examination of choice for screening subjects, immunoassay fecal occult blood test can be performed daily for three consecutive days and, if positive, full colonoscopy can be then conducted.

A total of 3704 high-risk subjects were screened using full colonoscopy and 807 patients with colorectal tumors were identified, including 11 with colorectal cancer and 796 with colorectal adenomatous polyps, with a detection rate of colorectal tumor 22.8% and a detection rate of colorectal cancer 0.3%. Compared with the diagnosis of the 2675 subjects with colorectal cancer symptoms who sought medical help at the gastrointestinal departments, Dukes' A and B stage colorectal cancers accounted for 45% and 33% (78% combined) of the colorectal cancers detected in the high-risk population respectively whereas Dukes' A and B stage colorectal cancers accounted for 4% and 29% (33% combined) of the colorectal cancers detected in the symptomatic subjects seeking medical help at hospitals. This indicates that screening among high-risk population is an effective way for early detection of colorectal cancer. Previous research has established that the 5-year survival rate of Dukes' A colorectal cancer following surgery can reach as high as 90%, showing colorectal cancer screening will greatly enhance the survival rate of patients and yield good social benefits.

Our series of studies have shown that for every detected case of colorectal cancer, the average direct cost of systematic screening is 200,000 RMB yuan whereas the average direct cost of opportunistic screening is only about 50,000 RMB yuan, 4 times less than the cost of systematic screening. For each detected case of colorectal tumor (cancer and adenoma), opportunistic screening costs 2,000 RMB yuan on average. This shows the great economic benefit of opportunistic screening for colorectal cancer.

6. Issues and suggestions

Screening should cover more of the target population. The biggest drawback of opportunistic screening is that only those who seek medical help at hospitals or undergo health examination are screened while those potential patients who do not seek medical treatment are excluded from the screening. Therefore, some high-risk populations may be missed during the screening and the effectiveness of the screening is thus impaired. We can step up the publicity of screening programs, use information systems to manage residents' health records, keep track of personal information of those who do not undergo screening, and then invite them for screening. By doing so, more of the target population may be covered.

The awareness of the significance of screening on the part of patients and physicians needs to be improved. Adequate education and training are necessary for the success of opportunistic screening, which can raise the awareness of screening among patients and physicians, particularly the latter. Mandel et al. reported that with physicians' consultation and advice, 81% of FOBT-positive patients were willing to accept subsequent colonoscopy. Therefore, to improve screening efficiency, it is of considerable importance to educate general practitioners and gastroenterologists about the importance of screening. At present, most of the colorectal cancer screening work is done by community physicians and other first-line medical staff, who often lack knowledge and training in epidemiology. Studies have shown that community health providers in the U.S. often base their choice of colorectal cancer screening programs on patients' wishes, rather than following relevant national screening guidelines. Therefore, education among medical practitioners about the importance of screening and the establishment of specialized agencies responsible for guidance and monitoring of colorectal cancer screening may help clinicians to implement and enforce screening guidelines.

Government support is not enough. Many countries now have no comprehensive national statistics for colorectal cancer screening and thus can not develop a national screening strategy. The high cost of screening is also an important factor that reduces patients' compliance. Accordingly, we call upon the attention of our society and government for colorectal cancer screening, strive for the support of the national basic medical insurance, and advocate the coverage of colorectal cancer screening by medical insurance. These efforts will help us to carry out large-scale screening programs for colorectal cancer to achieve early diagnosis and early treatment.

7. Summary

Natural population screening and opportunistic screening are two screening models currently prevalent in many countries. Although both screening programs are intended to reduce cancer incidence and mortality rates, they are different in many aspects, especially in their anti-cancer strategy. Population-based screening programs have been mainly conducted as a preventive policy in local regions with government support. It needs responsibility for the program's implementation, such as population registration and quality assurance follow-up and evaluation. In this regard, natural population screening in many countries has not yet evolved into mature systematic screening. In contrast, opportunistic screening depends on individual members of a certain population requesting screening or their health advisors recommending screening. Although there is no conclusive evidence about its effectiveness, it has been implemented in clinical settings in different modes and holds great promise for clinical application.

8. References

[1] Burt RW, Barthel JS, Dunn KB, et al. NCCN clinical practice guidelines in oncology. Colorectal cancer screening. J Natl Compr Canc Netw[J], 2010, 8(1): 8-61.

[2] Half E, Bercovich D, Rozen P. Familiar adenomatous polyposis. Orphanet J Rare Dis[J], 2009, 4(1): 22.

[3] Wachsmannova-Matelova L,Stevurkova V,Adamcikova Z,et al. Different phenotype manifestation of familial adenomatous polyposis in families with APC mutation at codon 1309.Neoplasma[J], 2009, 56(6): 486-489.

[4] Terri Ades,Rick Alteri, Priti Bandi,et al. Colorectal Cancer Facts & Figures 2008-2010. Atlanta, GA: American Cancer Society, 2010:11

[5] Ahmedin Jemal, Rebecca Siegel, Jiaquan Xu,et al. Cancer Statistics, 2010. CA Cancer J Clin[J], 2010; 60(5):277-300.

[6 Melissa M. Center, Ahmedin Jemal, and Elizabeth Ward. RESEARCH ARTICLES: International Trends in Colorectal Cancer Incidence Rates.Cancer Epidemiol. Biomarkers Prev [J], Jun 2009; 18(6): 1688 - 1694.

[7] XU An-gao, JIANG Bo, ZHONG Xu-hui, et al. The trend of clinical characteristics of colorectal cancer during the past 20 years in Guangdong province. National Medical Journal of China [J], 2006, 86(4): 272-274

[8] XU An-gao, JIANG Bo, YU Zhi-jin, et al. Epidemiology investigation of colorectal cancer on community group in Guangdong province. National Medical Journal of China [J], 2007, 87(28): 1950-1953

[9] XU An-gao, YU Zhi-jin, ZHONG Xu-hui, et al. Screening of high-risk group with colorectal cancer. National Medical Journal of China [J], 2010,90(2): 116-118.

[10] XU An-gao, YU Zhi-jin, ZHONG Xu-hui, et al. Comparing three screening schemes of colorectal cancer in general population.Chinese Journal of Health Management [J], 2009, 3(3):155-158

[11] XU An-gao. The application of classification in high risk of colorectal cancer screening program. National Medical Journal of China[J], 2009,89(48):3385-3387.

[12] ASGE guideline: colorectal cancer screening and surveillance. Gastrointestinal Endoscopy[J], 2006,63 (4):546-557

[13] Robert A. Smith, Vilma Cokkinides, Durado Brooks, et al. Cancer screening in the United States, 2011: A Review of Current American Cancer Society Guidelines and Issues in Cancer Screening.CA Cancer J Clin[J], 2011; 61(8): 8 - 30.

[14] Fletcher RH. Colorectal cancer screening: for prevention or cure? J Epidemiol Community Health[J], 2009;63(7):505-506

[15] Hutchison B, Woodward CA, Norman GR, et al. Provision of preventive care to unannounced standardized patients. CMAJ[J]. 1998; 158(2):185-93.

[16] Mandel JS, Bond JH, Church TR, et al. Reducing mortality from colorectal cancer by screening for faecal occult blood. N Engl J Med[J], 1993; 328(19):1365-71

[17] Klabunde CN, Lanier D, Nadel MR, et al. Colorectal cancer screening by primary care physicians: recommendations and practices, 2006-2007. Am J Prev Med[J]. 2009,37(1):8-16.

[18] Chisato HA, Hiroshi SA,Tomio NA ,et al. The Standardized Development Method of the Japanese Guidelines for Cancer Screening. Jpn J Clin Oncol[J].2008,38(4):288 - 295.

3

Crohn's Disease and Colorectal Cancer

Andrea Denegri[1], Francesco Paparo[2] and Rosario Fornaro[3]
[1]University of Genoa, Department of Internal Medicine, Genova
[2]University of Genoa, Service of Diagnostic Imaging, Genova
[3]University of Genoa, Department of Surgery, Genova
Italy

1. Introduction

The etiology of Crohn's disease is still unknown. The most likely hypotesis is the alteration of the intestinal immune system with abnormal response to environmental factors and/or intrinsic factors in genetically predisposed individuals, with tissue destruction, chronic inflammation and fibrosis. There are many factors that could contribute to the onset of the disease, modulate clinical manifestations and influence the occurence of complications also post-operative: cigarette smoking is often associated with a more aggressive disease. The pathophysiological mechanism of this association is not yet clear. Crohn's disease is difficult to cure and even on the basis of this evidence, the therapeutic approach to patient can not be other than multidisciplinary. The most common complications of Crohn's disease are represented by stenosis, fistulas and abscesses that generally need a surgical therapy, despite drug treatment, newly with biological drugs have proved effective. Neoplastic degeneration is a terrible and feared complication in the long term. Although there is a substantial evidence that patients with ulcerative colitis are at increased risk of developing colorectal cancer, the prevalence of cancer in patients with Crohn's disease is also not so well defined even if it's now accepted that the risk of colorectal cancer is equivalent in both conditions. From a review of the literature it can be assumed that the number of cancer cases of large and small intestine associated with inflammatory bowel disease has increased both in patients with ulcerative colitis as well as in patients with Crohn's disease. The rectum, interested only in a small percentage of cases by Crohn's disease, does not seem to be subject to this consideration. Beside it the risk of developing extraintestinal tumors and lymphomas in patients with Crohn's disease appears to have increased in relation to the general population, but, at present, evidences to establish secure real causal link between these disorders are still lacking. The role of immunosuppressive therapies, often carried out on patients with Crohn's disease, also remains unclear. Cancer is often preceded by dysplasia in both patients with ulcerative colitis and in patients with Crohn's disease affection. Young patients who have severe Crohn's disease of long standing, with extensive colonic involvement may benefit from endoscopic surveillance for cancer, especially those affecting the large intestine. We're waiting for good screening methods more sensitive, less invasive and less costly in terms of economic cost and discomfort for the patient. An attitude of alertness may be stated as good: the onset of new symptoms in a patient with up till now stable disease should always be investigated.

2. Crohn's disease and cancer: History

For many years after the description of a chronic granulomatous intestinal disease dy Dalziel in 1913 (Dalziel, 1913) and, more fully, by Crohn, Ginzburg and Oppenheimer in 1931 (Crohn et al., 1932), it was considered that there was no relationship between Crohn's disease and cancer. The risk of developing cancer in patients with Crohn's disease, in fact, was subject of controversy since 1948, when Warren and Sommers reported the case of a colorectal carcinoma arising in a patient with Crohn's disease (Warren & Sommers, 1948). The testimony of some association between Crohn's disease and cancer remained for many years related to description of single case reports (Ginzburg et al., 1956; Buchanan et al., 1959; Zisk et al., 1960; Hoffert et al., 1963; Berman et al., 1964; Cantwell et al., 1968), until in 1973 Weedon et al. published an epidemiological study on the risk of cancer in patients with Crohn's disease compared with that of the general population (Weedon et al., 1973). While the evidence of an increased risk of colorectal cancer in patients with ulcerative colitis is yet another further confirmation in recent study (Eaden JA. et al., 2001; Freeman, 2008; Viennot et al., 2009; Lukas, 2010; Affendi et al., 2011), the risk of cancer in Crohn's disease on the other side is not so well defined, despite several investigations in this direction from 1973 to present. Based on the literature, however, it seems resonable to assume that there is an association between Crohn's disease and cancer of the large intestine (Greenstein, 2000; Zisman & Rubin, 2008; Xie & Itzkowitz, 2008; Kraus & Arber, 2009; Kiran et al., 2010; Katsanos et al., 2011). Eaden's meta-analysis has shown that the risk of colorectal cancer in ulcerative colitis increases more with long-standing disease (Lukas, 2010). The risk of developing colorectal cancer in patients with ulceratie colitis is 2% at 10 years, 8% at 20 years and 18% at 30 years of disase duration and this seems to happen also in Crohn's disease (Lukas, 2010; Kiran et al., 2010). The risk of developing cancer appears to be higher in patients with long-standing Crohn's diasease particulary if diagnosed before 25 years of age with extensive colonic involvement. Extent of disease, in fact, is another major risk factor (Lukas, 2010). Most cancer arise in patients with extensive disease, which is generally defined as extension of inflammation beyond the hepatic flexure but it was demonstred that proctitis and proctosigmoiditis posed no increased risk for patients with ulcerative colitis (Lukas, 2010). Recent data from numerous studies suggests that a degree between colonscopic and hystologically active inflammation are associated with an increased risk of cancer. The risk of lymphomas and extraintestinal neoplasms appears to be increased (Von Roon et al., 2007). Patients with Crohn's disease have a higher risk of gastrointestinal tract and an hematopoietic system cancers compared with that of the general population. Identify the most vulnerable groups of subjects may be useful for planning appropriate methods of surveillance and early detection. New clinical studies, basic, genetic and molecular research are needed in order to shed light on the complex pathogenetic mechanisms involved in cancer in patients with Crohn's disease.

2.1 Risk factors

The presence of an inflammatory bowel disease, especially if long standing, is in itself a risk factor for the development of malignancies (Eaden JA. et al., 2001; Jess et al., 2004; Jess T et al., 2005). Generally cancer develops through chronic inflammation leading to dysplasia, and then cancer but unlike sporadic colorectal cancer in the general population, the development of carcinogenesis in Crohn's disease does not always follow this sequential progression from low-grade dysplasia to high-grade dysplasia and finally cancer. In fact cancer can arise in patients with no prior dysplasia or without first progression from low-grade dysplasia to high-grade dysplasia even if they are therefore usually located in the region of the bowel affected by colitis and often, but not always, as the cancer grows in an exophytic sporadically, forming a "polyp", cancer that occurs on the mucosa affected by a chronic inflammatory process results in flat lesions that can affect the entire wall with circumferential stenosis (Ullman et al., 2009). Dysplasia is defined as the unequivocal neoplastic alteration of the epithelium without invasion into the lamina propria and macroscopically dysplastic lesions can range from flat lesions to plaque-like lesions even to raised localized or multifocal lesions. The onset of cancer is one of the most serious complications of inflammatory bowel disease and, moreover, the cause of 1/6 of deaths in patients with ulcerative colitis and 1/12 in patients with Crohn's disease (Jess et al., 2002). It is not easy to determine the potential role of the many factors involved in the development of cancer in patients with Crohn's disease. The risk estimates vary greatly in different studies, and this is due to differences in patient population, the statistical methods used and possibly to the different therapeutic approach to the disease. In this regard it should be noted the greater tendency in the Scandinavian countries to perform colectomy or proctocolectomy: this could justify a lower incidence of colorectal cancer in these regions than the United States or the United Kingdom (Von Roon et al., 2007). Nor should we forget the possible misinterpretation of the real incidence of cancer if you are referring only to studies in reference centers, which flow into the categories of patients at increased risk per se. The duration and the extent of anatomic disease (Von Roon et al., 2007), with a strong correlation between the intestinal segment affected by chronic inflammation and increased risk of cancer (Gyde et al., 1980; Greenstein et al., 1981; Ekbom et al., 1990; Gillen et al., 1994; Jess et al., 2004), younger age at diagnosis of Crohn's disease (Von Roon et al., 2007) , a positive family history for colorectal cancer (Askling et al., 2001), the Lynch syndrome (HNPCC) (Caruso et al., 1997), the presence of primary sclerosing cholangitis (Broomè et al., 2006), a positive drug history with immunomodulatory or immunosuppressive therapy (Bickston et al., 1999; Farrell et al., 2000; Bouhnik et al., 1996; Lewis et al., 2001; Bernstein et al., 2001), a history of oral contraceptive use (Lakatos et al., 2007), the habit of cigarette smoking at diagnosis of Crohn's disease and the persistence of this in subsequent years (Johnson et al., 2005; Von Roon et al., 2007, Jess et al., 2007;), and, ultimately, a less than optimal surgical approach to the disease (Greenstein et al., 1978; Greenstein, 2000), are all factors that can contribute also independently to the development of cancer in patients with Crohn's disease. Some studies testify the possibility that other factors may play a preventive action against the onset of cancer in patients with Crohn's disease. In this regard find space sporadic follow-up colonscopy or through office visites or hospital admissions (Jess et al., 2007), treatment with 5-aminosalicylates (Eaden J., 2003; Velayos et al., 2005; Jess et al., 2007), non steroidal anti-inflammatory drugs, folic acid and ursodeoxycholic acid (Itzkowitz, 2002), and finally cessation of cigarette smoking, labeled as the first step towards the possible therapeutic effects in the development of a cancer (Jess et al., 2007) and against the disease itself (Johnson et al., 2005). An appropriate surgical approach also plays an important role. A careful study of the role played by these factors could lead to the identification of groups of individuals at high risk of developing cancer, allowing you to plan methods of prevention or early detection practice.

The known association of dysplasia and colorectal cancer in Crohn's disease has been the basis for defining endoscopic screening and surveillance strategies. Surveillance strategy consists in the systematic search for dysplasia on endoscopic biopsies following a defined calendar. During endoscopic examination it is essential to examine the whole colon in search for all visible lesions preferably during the quiescent period of the disease to avoid histological confusion between dysplastic and regenerative lesions. In this case medical therapy is essential to reduce active inflammation and, once got it, plan short-term repeat colonscopy (Viennot et al., 2009). More numerous are the biopsies performed higher is the probability of detecting dysplasia. However this strategy is difficult, costs and involves a rate of morbidity which reduce its long-term observance. The ideal solution would be find other risk markers for neoplastic dengeneration, cheaper and better tolerated by patients. Chemoendoscopy is a new technique that involves the application of dye during colonscopy. Indigo carmine is a contrast dye that augments subtle mucosal alterations whereas methylene blue is an absorptive dye that is avidly taken up by mucosa but does not stain areas of inflammation or dysplasia, thereby creating a contrast gradient that enhances visualization. Chemoendoscopy seems to improve the sensitivity of detecting neoplasia and in addition to this offers potential to improve specifity as well, by facilitating enhanced endoscopic characterization of lesions. This allow the endoscopist to perform fewer biopsies more targeted. The combination of chemoendoscopy with magnification permits a detailed analysis of the mucosal helping to differentiate between benign and malignant lesions. Despite the promising information about this technique chemoendoscopy is not yet considered a standard of care approach to surveillance because of its cost and lack of training (Zisman & Rubin, 2008). 5-aminosalicylates are currently the most acknowledged treatment for colorectal cancer prevention in patients with Crohn's disease and the evidence of this protective role for 5-aminosalicylates against colitis-associated colorectal cancer is known since several years (Pinczowski et al., 1994; Viennot et al., 2009). Several recent studies confirmed this evidence (Van Staa et al., 2005; Velayos et al., 2005) even if not all authors are agree on this protective effect, because there is an important heterogeneity of individual study results and the best avaible data interpretation appears to be that of published meta-analysis (Viennot et al., 2009). Similar roles are played by non-steoroidal antinflammatory drugs and ursodeoxycholic acid (Itzkowitz, 2002). Is now generally accepted that Crohn's disease is associated with an increased risk of cancer. An increased risk of cancer in the intestinal tract is in fact detectable in patients with Crohn's disease, although not specifically have seen increases in incidence or relative risk of oropharynx, esophagus and stomach cancer than the general population; an upward trend has been documented for anus cancer. The risk of developing lymphoma is also increased. Controversial and difficult to interpret are the data on the association between Crohn's disease and other cancers.

2.1.1 Cancer of colon and rectum

The colorectal cancer in patients with Crohn's disease has particular characteristics that set it apart from sporadic cancer. Generally diffuse, with multiple characters, it may not be obvious macroscopic observation or involve the entire bowel wall with stricture formation, remaining silent with regard to the symptoms until an advanced stage: at this point is generally manifested by obstructive type symptoms , weight loss and presence of abdominal mass. Sometimes it can occur in association with fistulas or may occur in loops. The colorectal cancer in Crohn's disease frequently affects younger patients (48 vs. 70 years) and is localized preferably in the right colon (45% vs. 20% of cases), compared with the cancers arose de novo (Figure 1).

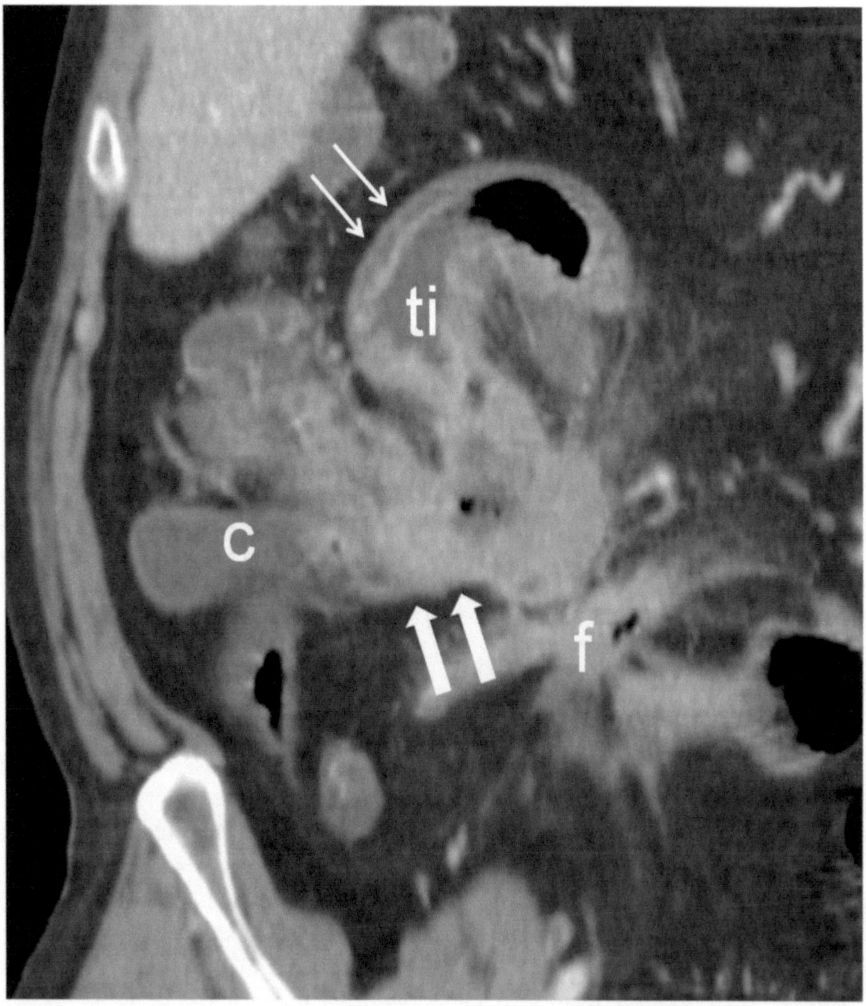

Coronal CT enterography reconstruction showing a severe stricturing form involving the ileocecal area in a 58 year-old male patient. Histological analysis of endoscopic biopsies demonstrated the presence of an invasive mucinous adenocarcinoma of the ileocecal valve. Legend: c = cecum; ti = terminal ileum; large arrows = ileocecal stricture; f = extra-enteric fistulous tract with internal air bubbles.

Fig. 1. Neoplasm of ileocecal valve

The risk of developing a colorectal cancer in patients with Crohn's disease is thus increased (Von Roon et al., 2007): this increased incidence is due to an increased incidence of only colon cancer, with regard to the rectum cancer; in fact, there are significant differences in risk than the general population (Von Roon et al., 2007; Figure 2).

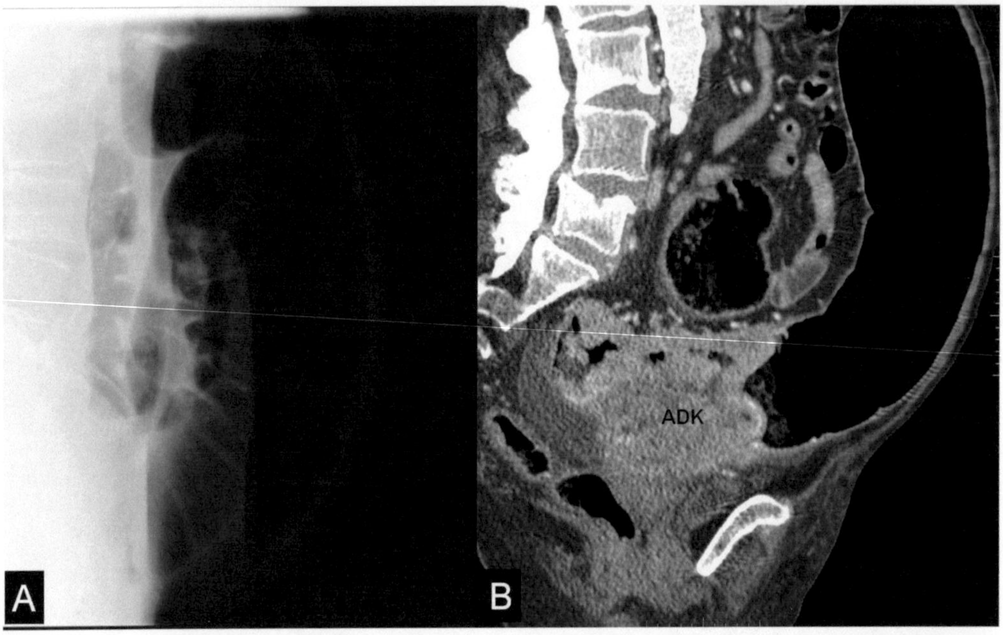

83 year-old female patient with a 40-year history of Crohn's disease and low intestinal obstruction signs. Supine trans-lateral radiography of the abdomen (A) demonstrates significant large bowel distension. The sagittal CT reconstruction (B) reveals the presence of a neoplastic stricture (ADK) which appears on CT images as a discrete circumferential thickening with inhomogeneous contrast enhancement of the sigmoid colon wall.

Fig. 2. Sigmoid colon tumor

This assumption could be attributed to the fact that Crohn's disease affects the rectum in a small percentage of cases. Intestinal segments affected by the disease are at increased risk (Gyde et al., 1980; Greenstein et al., 1981; Ekbom et al., 1990; Gillen et al., 1994; Jess et al., 2004;). While the risk of developing a colorectal cancer in patients with Crohn's disease confined to the small intestine appears to be similar to that of the general population (Von Roon et al., 2007), location of the large bowel disease is associated, however, a significant increase in the risk of cancer in this seat (Von Roon et al., 2007). The exact mechanism by which chronic inflammation results in carcinogenesis is unclear but it is believed that persistent inflammation result in increased cell proliferation as well as oxidative stress ending with the development of dysplasia (Itzkowitz & Yio, 2004). Probably the similar genetic mutations that result in sporadic colorectal cancer in the general population are also responsible for its development in Crohn's disease, but the sequence of events and frequency are altereted (Ullman et al., 2009). These events include microsatellite instability, inhibition of regulatory genes and loss of adenomatous polyposis coli, p53 and k-ras tumor specific suppressor function (Itzkowitz & Yio, 2004). For exemple in sporadic colorectal cancer loss of adenomatous polyposis coli gene function generally occur early and is frequent whereas p53 mutations occur late and are less frequent while in Crohn's disease associated colorectal cancer loss of adenomatous polyposis coli gene function generally occur late and is infrequent whereas p53 mutations occur early and are more frequent. Further studies are needed to explain this complex process (Ahmadi et al., 2009; Figure 3).

A diagnosis of Crohn's disease prior to age 25 is associated with an increased risk of cancer (Weedon et al., 1973; Greenstein et al., 1981), as well as a long-standing Crohn's disease (Fireman et al., 1989). Patients with severe Crohn's disease with extensive involvement of the large intestine and diagnosed before 25 years of age, not previously subjected to an intervention of prophylactic colectomy are at high risk for the development of a colorectal

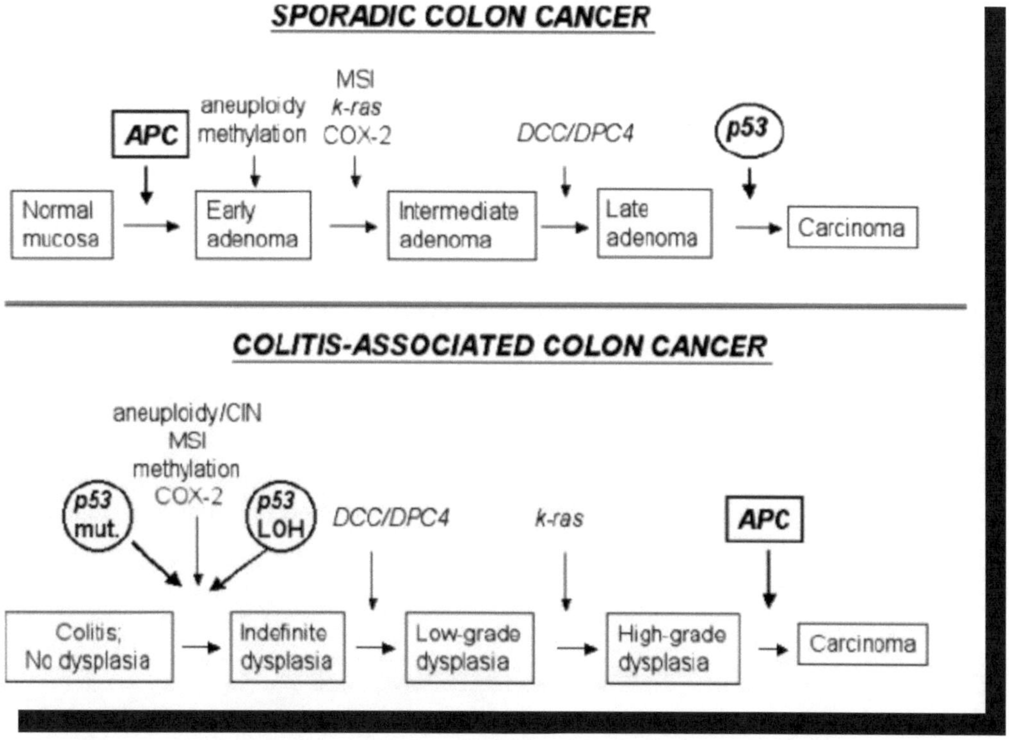

Fig. 3. Cancer in Crohn's disease: the role of k-ras, p53 and APC (Itzkowits & Yio, 2004).

cancer (Gillen et al., 1994; Sachar, 1994), these are precisely the patients who may benefit from an adequate surveillance program by endoscopy (Hamilton, 1985; Von Roon et al., 2007). The attitude of the surgeon facing a patient with Crohn's disease, which undergoes neoplastic transformation is borrowed from cancer surgery. Resection with wide margins on disease-free anastomosis accompanied by lymphadenectomy and possibly enlargement of the intervention in case of inflamed bowel in these cases are the primary target (Greenstein, 2000). In Crohn's colitis, unless you are facing a severe and extensive disease or the presence of perianal involvement, we prefer to perform, especially in young patients, segmental resection with immediate restoration of intestinal continuity with or without ileostomy possibly temporary. Other surgical procedures that are used in these patients: subtotal colectomy, the total proctocolectomy with end ileostomy or packaging of a J-pouch and palliative procedures (Fornaro et al., 2006; Fornaro et al., 2008; Fornaro et al., 2009). Contraindicated on the basis of the frequent recurrences reported in the literature, seems to be the ileoanal pouch (Greenstein, 2000). Screening colonscopy should be performed in patients with Crohn's disease after 8-10 years of disease and the interval between surveillance examinations is dependent on each individual's personal risk factors. In patients with a previous history of primary sclerosing cholangitis, active inflammation, dysplasia or stenosis, family history of bowel cancer annual surveillance is raccomanded (Kiran et al., 2010). Colectomy is strictly raccomanded for patients who were diagnosed with flat high-grade dysplasia or colorectal cancer and where diagnosis was confirmed by expert gastrointestinal pathologists. In patients with a biopsy indefinite for dysplasia, guidelines suggests colonscopy between 3 and 12 months. Multifocal low grade dysplasia is a stronger indication for colectomy. The optimal colonscopic surveillance interval for patients who were diagnosed with a flat low grade dysplasia is still unknown, but 3-6 months is often recommended (Lukas, 2010). Although guidelines currently exist, limitations of these guidelines indicate the need to continue research into the molecular pathogenesis of Crohn's disease associated colorectal cancer with the hope to identify targets for prevention. Advances in endoscopic imaging are alredy underway and may potentially aid in detection of dysplasia and improve surveillance. Management of dysplasia depends above all on the focality of dysplasia itself with the mainstay of involving proctocolectomy or continue endoscopic surveillance. Continued research on additional chemopreventive agents may reduce the incidence of Crohn's disease colorectal cancer but further studies are necessary to get this goal (Ahmadi et al., 2009).

2.1.2 Cancer of the small intestine

Most tumors of the small intestine in patients with Crohn's disease are composed of adenocarcinoma of the jejunum and terminal ileum, rarely diagnosed at an early stage likely to care (Fornaro et al., 1994, Figure 4).

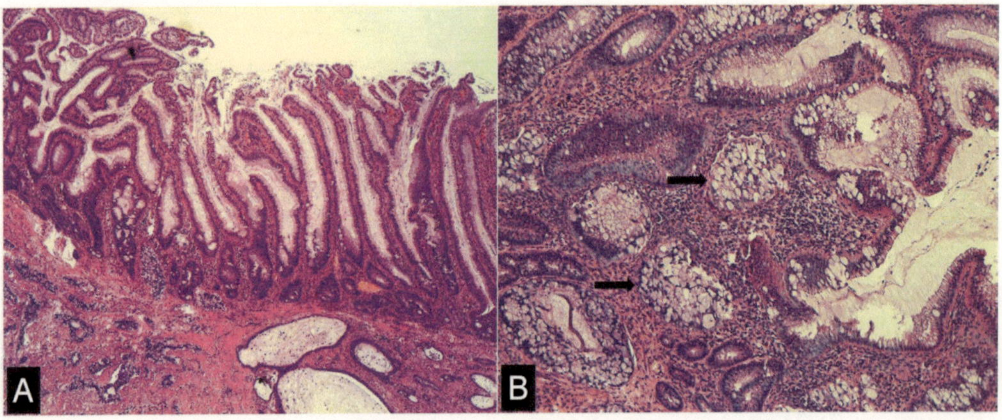

Histological microphotographs (A, B) of endoscopic biopsies taken from the proximal small bowel loop of an ileocolic anastomosis in a patient with Crohn's disease recurrence. Image A demonstrates superficial adenomatous transformation of small bowel mucosa, which was adjacent to an area of invasive mucinous adenocarcinoma. Image B shows neoplastic nests of small bowel mucinous adenocarcinoma (black arrows).

Fig. 4. Dysplasia-carcinoma sequence in the small bowel.

The most common clinical presentation of small bowel cancer is intestinal obstruction (Greenstein et al., 1978). Other important symptoms are diarrhea, weight loss and fistulae. They, too, such as colorectal cancer, differ from the adenocarcinomas occurred de novo in several respects. The mean age of patients is generally lower (45 vs. 60 years), the cancer occurs more often distally with multiple characters (76% vs. 20% of cases) or in loops (Greenstein et al., 1978), attributable to the postoperative life even reduced to 8 months (Greenstein, 2000). Sarcomas are rarely seen in the small intestine in patients with Crohn's disease: these rather represent a third of cancers arose de novo. Risk factors for developing carcinoma in small bowel segments of involved mucosa in patients with Crohn's disease are poorly defined but numerous case reports document them in strictured mucosa and fistulae. Surgery must be considered if it's difficult to examine fistulae and strictures or if symptoms worsen (Xie & Itzkowitz, 2008). A long-standing history of Crohn's disease is most frequently associated with the appearance of small intestine tumors. Small intestine cancers occurs, as told above, in two thirds of cases with symptoms of obstructive (Greenstein et al., 1978; Greenstein, 2000); diarrhea, weight loss, fistulas, abdominal masses, may also be present. A delay in diagnosis may be partly justified by a non-specific accompanying symptoms and the presence of such symptoms in patients with quiescent Crohn's disease for a long time, however, must lead early on the implementation of appropriate diagnostic tests. The prognosis of small intestine cancer in patients with Crohn's disease is poor (Crohn et al., 1932). The relative risk of developing small intestine cancer in Crohn's disease patients is higher than in the general population (Von Roon et al., 2007), increasing in relation to the anatomical segment affected by chronic inflammation (Greenstein et al., 1981; Jess et al., 2004). Patients with Crohn's disease exclusively localized to the ileum only have a higher risk of developing a small intestine cancer (Von Roon et al., 2007). Although the risk of developing small intestine cancer is higher in patients with Crohn's disease compared with that found in the general population, it remains, in absolute terms, rather than restricted. In fact the absolute number of cases of small bowel adenocarcinoma is low because of the rarity of this cancer in the general population but in patients with Crohn's disease the risk is greater than in the general population. This risk vary in the different studies reported in literature. Based on the stated, hypothesis of a correlation between a chronic inflammation and cancer seems reasonable (Itzkowitz & Yio 2004). The different modes of clinical presentation, with symptoms often generic and nonspecific, and the difficulties of endoscopic evaluation of the small intestine, now partly overcome by modern techniques videocapsulo-tele-endoscopy, the difficult exploration of strokes or bypassed affected by stenosis or possibility of an occult malignancy are important limitations to the surveillance of these patients. Outpatient visits, with particular emphasis on examination of the abdomen and the perineal skin, accompanied by a careful anamnestic investigation aims to investigate the occurrence or the modification of old and new symptoms, especially if it occurred after a long period of quiescence of the disease, could be a viable alternative to more cumbersome methods of surveillance. Segmental resection is preferable to surgery in patients with Crohn's disease complicated by small intestine carcinoma (Greenstein, 2000).

2.1.3 Other intestinal tumors

The risk of developing squamous cell carcinoma of the anus is increased (Von Roon et al., 2007). Worsening perianal symptoms in these patients should warrant vigilance for this tumor which often requires examination under anesthesia for adequate tissue diagnosis. An increased risk for hepatobiliary cancers in patients with primary sclerosing cholangitis (Xie

& Itzkowitz, 2008). There is nothing, however, statistically significant increases with regard to the oropharynx , esophagus and stomach cancer. These data find ample confirmation in the literature (Mellemkjaer et al., 2000; Von Roon et al. 2007). There is also an association between Crohn's disease and carcinoid tumors, found primarily in the appendix (Fornaro et al 1998; Szabo et al. 1999; Fornaro et al., 2007). The onset of cancer in loops is described in the literature (Greenstein et al., 1978): This complication has led to the abandonment of the internal bypass interventions, largely carried out until the 60s, now played only in exceptional cases, urgently. Patients with perianal Crohn's disease out to meet the development of squamous cell carcinoma of the anus are usually treated with an abdominal-perineal resection (Greenstein, 2000; Sjodahl et al., 2003), or alternatively can be treated with local excision surgery preceded by radiotherapy and chemotherapy, especially if they are in early stage squamous cell carcinoma (Greenstein, 2000).

2.1.4 Lymphomas and leukemias

The risk of lymphoma in patients with Crohn's disease is increased compared with that of the general population (Mellemkjaer et al., 2000; Arsenau et al., 2001; Von Roon et al., 2007), particularly in patients who undergo immunosuppressive therapy with corticosteroids or other immunomodulatory agents (Bernstein et al., 2001; Lakatos L. & Lakatos PL., 2007). The risk of hematopoietic cancer in patients with Crohn's disease has been a growing concern. In Crohn's disease, in fact, there is an increased risk of lymphoma specially in the first years of follow-up. Immunosuppressive therapy, which are often carried out on patients with Crohn's disease, influence the occurrence of hematopoietic disorders (Bouhnik et al., 1996; Bickston et al., 1999; Farrell et al., 2000). Following the introduction of tumors necrosis factor inhibitors in the treatment of Crohn's disease, subsequent reports indicated an excess of malignant lymphoma among treated patients with a raised fear of iatrogenic lymphoma. Studies examining the risk of lymphoma associated with azathioprine and 6-mercaptopurine reported variable results. Heterogeneity in the type, the dose and duration of immunomodulatory therapy may be responsible for this discrepancy (Xie & Itzkowitxz, 2008). The association between Crohn's disease and lymphoma is confirmed by numerous case reports (Perosio et al., 1992; Brown et al., 1992; Vazquez et al., 1993; Vanbockrijck et al., 1993; Larvol et al., 1994; Veldman et al., 1996; Kelly et al., 1997; Woodley et al., 1997; Charlotte et al., 1998; Kashyap et al., 1998; Parasher et al., 1999; Musso et al., 2000; Li et al., 2001; Martinez Tirado et al., 2001; Calvo-Villas et al., 2003; Hall et al., 2003; Sivarajasingham et al., 2003; Losco et al., 2004; Garcia-Sanchez et al., 2006;). In 60% of cases, lymphomas occur in the small and large intestine (Figure 5, 6). An association between Crohn's disease and leukemia has been described in literature (Caspi et al., 1995), but the data do not reach statistical significance. It seems difficult to implement methods of monitoring the patients at high risk of developing cancer: hospital visits, set carefully on history of symptoms and physical examination, could be a viable alternative to costly and unnecessary diagnostic tests. For intestinal lymphomas is primarily surgical excision (Greenstein, 2000). Surgery may be followed by radiation therapy when indicated, or chemotherapy, which is the definitive therapeutic approach for this type of cancer.

2.1.5 Extraintestinal malignancies

The risk of extraintestinal malignancy in patients with Crohn's disease is slightly increased compared with that of the general population (Von Roon et al., 2007; Figure 7). Hardly,

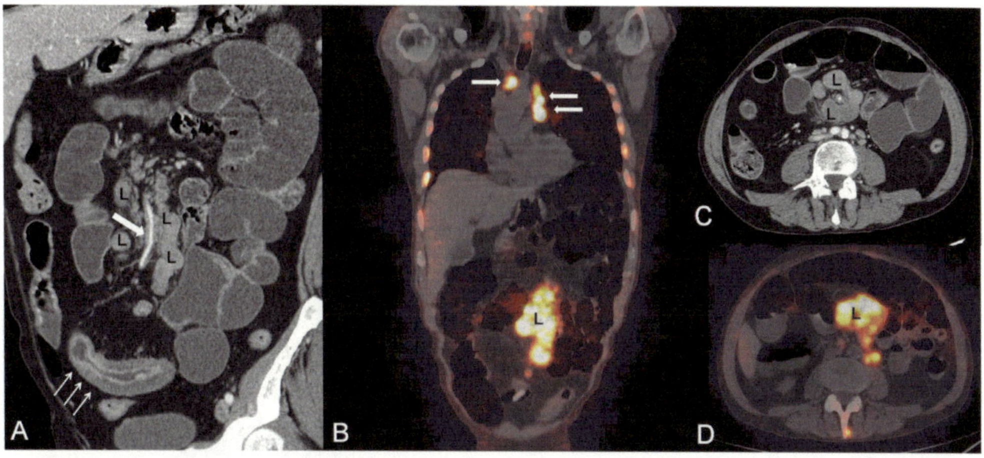

Imaging findings in a 60 year old man with lymphoma and long standing Crohn's disease. Coronal CT enterography reconstructed image (A) showing multiple, large mesenteric adenopathies (L) along the course of the superior mesenteric artery (large white arrow) and a small bowel inflamed segment with the typical bilaminar stratification of Crohn's disease (white arrows). Coronal PET-CT (fused) reconstructed image (B) which demonstrates 18F-FDG-glucose uptake of mesenteric adenopathies (L) and the presence of concomitant mediastinal adenopathies characterized by an high SUV (standard uptake value) (large white arrows). Axial CT enterography image (C) and corresponding PET-CT fused image (D) showing the mesenteric lymphadenopathies (L) surrounding the superior mesenteric artery.

Fig. 5. Lymphoma

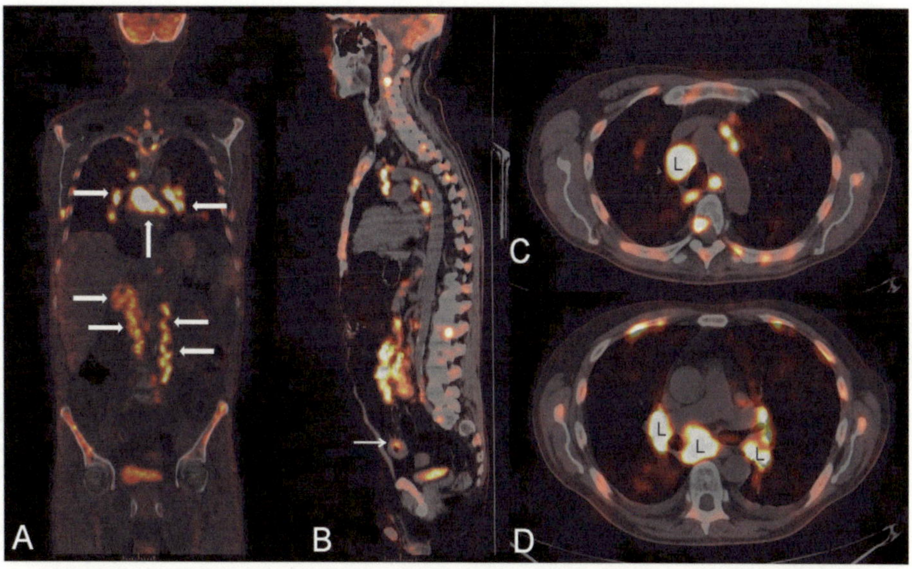

Coronal PET-CT reconstructed image (A) which demonstrates the presence of several lymphadenopathies in mediastinal and abdominal para-aortic nodal stations (large arrows). In the sagittal PET-CT reconstructed (fused) image (B) a moderate 18F-FDG-glucose uptake is appreciable on a small bowel loop with signs of inflammation (white arrow). Two axial PET-CT fused images focused on the mediastinal lymphadenopathies (L).

Fig. 6. Same patient of Figure 5

however, studies reported in this sense in literature don't reached statistical significance and the association-Crohn's disease tumor may be entirely random (Mellemkjaer et al., 2000). Cases are reported in the literature of malignancies arising on fistula, stricture or stoma (Grenstein 2000), and also for this reason, actions of palliation are to be preferred to resection (Askling et al., 2001). Monitoring of cancer in these patients is very complex and a screening is not feasible. Attention is directed to the symptoms: a history and physical examination can direct accuratly to the most appropriate diagnostic methods.

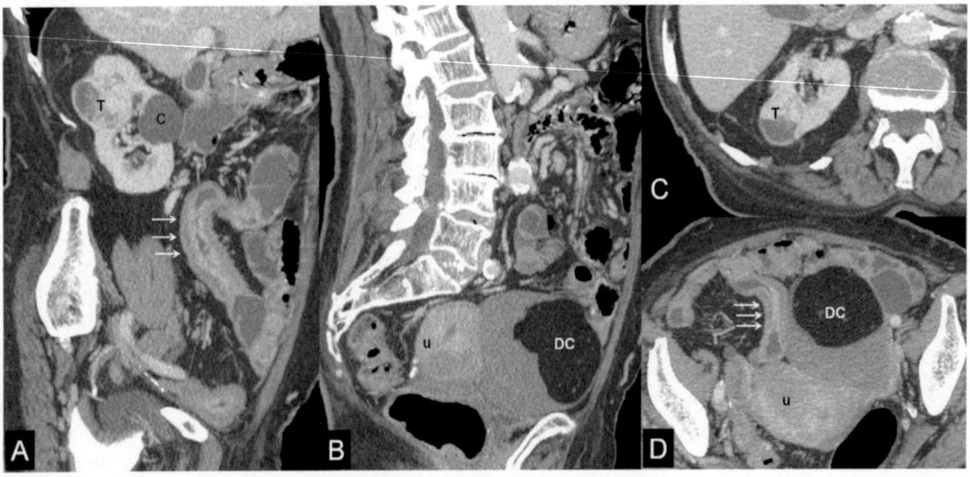

Two sagittal reconstructed CT enterography images (A, B) and two axial CT enterography images (C, D) in a 75 year old woman with a long standing Crohn's disease. Image A reveals the presence of a solid nodular lesion on the upper pole of the right kidney with unhomogeneous contrast enhancement (T), and a small bowel loop affected by Crohn's disease (white arrows), which is characterized by typical bilaminar stratification of its wall.
In the same patient a large left ovarian dermoid cyst (DC), with a prominent fat component, is well appreciable in image B. Image C shows the solid nodular lesion of the right kidney which demonstrated to be a clear cell carcinoma at histological analysis. An inflamed small bowel loop (white arrows) can be seen adjacent to the right lateral aspect of the ovarian lesion in image D. Legend: T = renal tumor; C = renal cyst; white arrows = small bowel loop affected by Crohn disease; u = uterus; DC = dermoid cyst.

Fig. 7. Kidney tumor in long-standing Crohn's disease

3. Conclusion

Patients with Crohn's disease are at increased risk of colon, small bowel and hematopoietic cancers with and increased risk of lymphoma or extraintestinal malignancies (although lower). The risk of developing a colorectal cancer is mainly increased in patients with diffuse and severe colic, especially if arose at a young age, with a Crohn's disease diagnosis made before 25 years of age. These patients appear to be at particularly high risk of developing a colorectal cancer and are therefore ideal candidates for surveillance with repeated colonoscopies. In particular young patients could benefit from regular endoscopic screening. However, since only one study in literature has stratified patients for extent of disease (Gillen et al., 1994), you can not make recommendations or determine a cut-off extension of disease above which it is legitimate to begin screening for colorectal cancer even if there are now guidelines that recommend a screening after 8-10 years of Crohn's

Crohn BB., Ginzburg L. & Oppenheimer GD. (1932). Regional ileitis: a pathological and clinical entity. JAMA, 99, Oct 1932, 1323-29.
Dalziel TK. (1913). Chronic interstitial enteritis. BMJ 2, 1913, 1068-70.
Eaden JA., Adams KR. & Mayberry JF. (2001). The risk of colorectal cancer in patients with ulcerative colitis: a meta-analysis. Gut, 48, Apr 2001, 526-35.
Eaden J. (2003). Review article: the data supporting a role for aminosalicylates in the chemoprevention of colorectal cancer in patients with inflammatory bowel disease. Aliment Pharmacol Ther, 18, Sep 2003, 15-21.
Ekbom A., Helmick C., Zack M. & Adami O. (1990). Increased risk of large bowel cancer in Crohn's disease with colonic involvement. Lancet, 336, Aug 1990, 357-9.
Farrell RJ., Ang Y., Keeling P., 0'Brien DS., Kellher D., Keeling PW. & Weir DG. (2000). Increased risk of non-Hodgkin's lymphoma in inflammatory bowel disease patients on immunosuppressive therapy but overall risk is slow. Gut, 47, Oct 2000, 514-9.
Fireman Z., Grossman A., Lilos P., Hacohen D., Bar Mei S., Roxen P. & Gilat T. (1989). Intestinal cancer in patients with Crohn's disease. A population study in central Israel. Scand J Gastroenterol, 24, Apr 1989, 346-50.
Fornaro R., Bertoglio C., Cambiaso C., Carissimi T., Borzone E. & Ferrarsi R. (1994). Adenocarcinoma of the small intestine. A case report and the clinico-therapeutics considerations. G Chir, 15, Oct 1994, 437-9.
Fornaro R., Secco GB., Terrizzi A., Boaretto R., Fardelli R., Cataletti M., Baldi E., Pastorino A & Ferraris R. (1998). Adenocarcinoid of the appendix: a case report and anatomo-pathological and clinico-therapeutic considerations. G. Chir., 19, Apr 1998, 165-9.
Fornaro R., Secco GB., Picori E., Stabilini C., FrascioM., Ricci B., Mandolino F., De Salvo L. & Gianetta E. (2006). Surgical treatment of Crohn's disease complications. Our experience. G Chir, 27, Jan-Feb 2006, 21-6.
Fornaro R., Frascio M., Sticchi C., De Salvo L., Stabilini C., Mandolino F., Ricci B. & Gianetta E. (2007). Appendicectomy or right hemicolectomy in the treatment of appendicela carcinoid tumors?. Tumori, 93, Nov-Dec 2007, 587-90.
Fornaro R., Frascio M., Stabilini C., Sticchi C., Barberis A., Denegri A., Ricci B., Mandolino F., Lazzara F. & Gianetta E. (2008). Crohn's disease surgery: problems of post-operative recurrence. Chir Ital, 60, Nov-Dec 2008, 761-81.
Fornaro R., Frascio M., Denegri A., Stabilini C., Imperatore M., Mandolino F., Lazzara F & Gianetta E. (2009). Crohn's disease and cancer. Ann Ital Chir, 80, Mar-Apr 2009, 119-25.
Freeman. (2008). Colorectal cancer in Crohn's disease. World J Gastroenterol, 14, Mar 2008, 1810-1.
Garcia-Sanchez M., Poyato-Gonzalez A., Giraldez-Jimenez M., et al. (2006). MALT lymphoma in a patient with Crohn's disease:a causal or incidental association?. Gastroenterol Hepatol, 29, Feb 2006, 74-6.
Gillen CD., Andrews AH., Prior P. & Allan RN. (1994). Crohn's disease and colorectal cancer. Gut, 35, May 1994, 651-5.
Gillen CD., Walmsley RS., Prior P., Andrews HA. & Allan RN. (1994). Ulcerative colitis and Crohn's disease: a comparision of the colorectal cancer risk in estensive colitis. Gut, 35, Nov 1994, 1590-2.
Ginzburg L., Schneider K., Dreizin D. & Levison C. (1956). Carcinoma of the jejunum occurring in a case of regional enteritis. Surgery, 39, Feb 1956, 347-51.

Greenstein AJ., Sachar D., Pucillo A., Kreel I., Geller S., Janowitz HD. & Aufses A. (1978). Cancer in Crohn's disease after diversionary surgery: a report of seven carcinomas occuring in excluded bowel. Am J Surg, 135, Jan 1978, 86-90.

Greenstein AJ., Sachar DB., Smith H., Janowitz HD. & Aufses AH. Jr. (1981). A comparison of cancer risk in Crohn's disease and ulcerative colitis. Cancer, 48, Dec 1981, 2742-5.

Greenstein AJ., Gennuso R., Sachar DB, Heimann T., Smith H., Janowitz HD & Aufses AH. Jr. (1985). Extraintestinal cancers in inflammatory bowel disease. Cancer, 56, Dec 1985, 2914-21.

Greenstein AJ. (2000). Cancer in inflammatory bowel disease. Mt Sinai J Med, 67, May 2000, 227-40.

Gyde SN., Prior P., Macartney JC., Thompson H., Waterhouse JA. & Allan RN. (1978). Malignancy in Crohn's disease. Gut, 21, Dec 1980, 1024-9.

Hall CH. Jr. & Shamma M. (2003). Primary intestinal lymphoma complicating Crohn's disease. J Clin Gastroenterol, 36, Apr 2003, 332-6.

Hamilton SR. (1985). Colorectal carcinoma in patients with Crohn's disease. Gastroenterology , 89, Aug 1985, 398-407.

Hoffert P., Weingarten L., Friedman L. & Morecki R. (1963). Adenocarcinoma of the terminal ileum in a segment of bowel with coexisting active enteritis. N J Med, 63, May 1963, 1567-71.

Itzkowitz S.H. (2002). Cancer prevention in patients with inflammatory bowel disease. Gastroenterology Clin N Am, 31, Dec 2002, 1133-1144.

Itzkowitz SH & Yio X. (2004). Inflammation and cancer IV. Colorectal cancer in inflammatory bowel disease: the role of inflammation. Am J Physiol Gastrointest Liver Physiol, 287, Jul 2004, 7-17.

Jess T., Winther KV., Mukholm P., Langholz E. & Binder V. (2002). Mortality and causes of death in Crohn's disease:follow-up of a population-based cohort in Copenhagen County, Denmark. Gastroenterology, 122, Jun 2002, 1808-14.

Jess T., Winther KV., Munkholm P., Langholz E. & Binder V. (2004). Intestinal and extra-intestinal cancer in Crohn's disease: follow-up of a population-based cohort in Copenhagen County, Denmark. Aliment Pharmacol Ther, 19, Feb 2004, 287-93.

Jess T., Gamborg M., Matzen P., Munkholm P. & Sorensen TI. (2005). Increased risk of intestinal cancer in Crohn's disease: a meta-analysis of population-based cohort studies. Am J Gastroenterol, 100, Dec 2005, 2724-9.

Jess T., Loftus EV. Jr., Velayos FS., Whinter KV., Tremaine WJ., Zinsmeister AR., Scott Harmsen W., Langholz E., Binder V., Mukholm P. & Sandborn WJ. (2007). Risk factors for colorectal cancer neoplasia in inflammatory bowel disease: a nested case-control study from Copenhagen County, Denmark and Olmested County, Minnesota. American Journal of Gastroenterology, 102, Apr 2007, 1-8.

Johnson CJ., Cosens J. & Mansfield JC. (2005). Review article: smoking cessation as primary therapy to modify the course of Crohn's disease. Aliment Pharmacol Ther, 21, Apr 2005, 921-31.

Kashyap A. & Forman SJ. (1998). Autologous bone marrow transplanation for non Hodgkin's lymphoma resulting in a long-term remission of coincidental Crohn's disease. Br. J. Haematol, 103, Dec 1998, 651-2.

Katsanos KH., Stamou P., Tatsioni A., Tsianos VE., Zoumbas S., Kavvadia S., Giga A., Vagias I., Christodoulou DK. & Tsianos EV; Northwest Greece IBD Study Group. (2011). Prevalence of inflammatory bowel disease related dysplasia and cancer in 1500 colonscopies from a referral center in northwestern Greece. J Crohns Colitis, 5, Feb 2011, 19-23.

Kelly MD., Stuart M., Tschuchnigg M., Turner J. & Tydd T. (1997). Primary intestinal Hodgkin's disease complicating ileal Crohn's disease. ANZ J Surg, 67, Jul 1997, 485-9.

Kraus S. & Arber N. Inflammation and colorectal cancer. (2009). Curr Opin Pharmacol, 9, Aug 2009, 405-10.

Kiran RP., Khoury W., Church JM., Lavery IC., Fazio VW & Remzi FH. (2010). Colorectal cancer complicating inflammatory bowel disease: similarities and differences between Crohn's disease and ulcerative colitis based on three decades of experience. Ann Surg, 252, Aug 2010, 330-5.

Lakatos L. & Lakatos PL. (2007). Changes in the epidemiology of ibd. Orv Etil, 148, Feb 2007, 223-8.

Larvol L., Soule JC. & Le Tourneau A. (1994). Reversibile lymphoma in the setting of azathioprine therapy for Crohn's disease. N Engl J Med, 331, Sep 1994, 883-4.

Lewis JD., Bilker WB., Brensinger C., Deren JJ., Vaughn DJ. & Strom BL. (2001). Inflammatory bowel disease is not associated with an increased risk of lymphoma. Gastroenterol, 121, Nov 2001, 1080-7.

Li S. & Borowitz MJ. (2001). Primary Epstein-Barr virus-associated Hodgkin disease of the ileum complicating Crohn's disease. Arch Pathol Lab Med, 125, Mar 2001, 424-7.

Losco A., Gianelli U., Cassani B., Baldini L., Cont D. & Basilico G. (2004). Epstein-Barr virus-associated Lymphoma in Crohn's disease. Inflamm Bowel Dis, 10, Jul 2004; 425-9.

Lukas M. (2010). Inflammatory bowel disease as a risk factor for colorectal cancer. Dig Dis, 28, Nov 2010, 619-24.

Martinez Tirado P., Redondo Cerezo E., Gonzalez Aranda Y. & Cabello Tapia M. (2001). Ki-Lymphoma of the skin in a patient with Crohn's disease undergoing treatment with azathioprine. Gastroenterol Hepatol, 25, May 2001, 271-2.

Mellemkjaer L., Johansen C., Gridley G., Linet MS., Kruger Kjaer S. & Olsen JH. (2000). Crohn's disease and cancer risk, Denmark. Cancer Causes and Control, 11, Feb 2000, 145-150.

Moody GA., Jayanthi V., Probert CS., Mac Kay H. & Mayberry JF. (1996). Long-term therapy with sulphasalazine protects against colorectal cancer in ulcerative colitis: a retrospective study of colorectal cancer risk and compliance with treatment in Leicestershire. Eur J Gastroenterol Hepatol, 8, Dec 1996, 1179-83.

Musso M., Porretto F., Crescimanno A., Bondi F., Polizzi V. & Scalone R. (2000). Crohn's disease complicated by relapsed extranodal Hodgkin's lymphoma: prolonged complete remission after unmanipulated PBPC autotransplant. Bone Marrow Transplant, 26, Oct 2000, 921-3.

Parasher G., Jaswal S., Golbey S., Grinberg M. & Iswara K. (1999). Extraintestinal non-Hodgkin's lymphoma presenting as obstructive jaundice in a patient with Crohn's disease. Am J Gastroenterol, 94, Jan 1999, 226-8.

Perosio PM., Brooks JJ., Saul SH. & Haller DG. (1992). Primary intestinal lymphoma in Crohn's disease: minute tumor with a fatal outcome. Am J Gastroenterol, 87, Jul 1992, 894-8.

Pinczowski D, Ekbom A & Baron J. (1994). Risk factors for colorectal cancer in patients with ulcerative colitis: a case-control study. Gastroenterology, 107, Jul 1994; 117-20.

Sachar DB. (1994). Cancer in Crohn's diseeae: dispelling the myths. Gut, 35, Nov 1994, 1507-8.

Sivarajasingham N., Adams SA., Smith ME. & Hosie KB. (2003). Perianal Hodgkin's lymphoma complicating Crohn's disease. Int J Colorectal Dis, 18, Mar 2003, 174-6.

Sjodahl RI., Myrelid P. & Soderholm JD. (2003). Anal and rectal cancer in Crohn's disease. Colorectal Dis, 5, Sep 2003, 490-5.

Szabo CG., Barta Z., Kerekes L. & Szackal S. (1999). Association of carcinoid tumor of the appendix and Crohn's disease. A case report and review of literature Orv Hetil, 140, Jul 1999, 1635-9.

Ullman T., Odze R. & Farraye FA. (2009). Diagnosis and management of dysplasia in patients with ulcerative colitis and Crohn's disease of the colon. Inflamm Bowel Disease, 15, Apr 2009, 630-655.

Van Staa TP., Card T., Logan RF. & Leufkens HG. (2005). 5-Aminosalicylate use and colorectal cancer risk in inflammatory bowel disease: a large epidemiological study. Gut, 54, Nov 2005, 1573-8.

Vanbockrijck M., Cabooter M., Casselman J., Vanvuchelen J., Van Hoof A. & Michielssen P. (1993). Primary Hodgkin's disease of the ileum complicating Crohn's disease. Cancer, 72, Sep 1993, 1784-9.

Vazquez C. & Desaive C. (1993). Malignant lymphoma comlicating Crohn's disease of the ileum. A propos of a case. J Chir (Paris), 130, Aug-Sep 1993, 364-6.

Velayos FS., Terdiman JP. & Walsh JM. (2005). Effect of 5-aminosalicylate use on colorectal cancer and displasya risk: a systematic review and meta-analysis of observational studies. Am J Gastroenterology, 100, Jun 2005, 1345-53.

Veldman W., Van Beek M., Keuning JJ. & Driessen WM. (1996). Regional enteritis complicating malignant lymphoma. Neth J Med, 49, Aug 1996, 82-5.

Viennot S., Deleporte A., Moussata D., Nancey S., Flouriè B & Reimund JM. (2009). Colon cancer in inflammatory bowel disease: recent trends, questions and answers.Gastroenterol Clin Biol, 33, Jun 2009, 190-201.

Warren S & Sommers SC. (1948). Cicatrizing enteritis (regional enteritis) as a pathological entity: analysis of one hundred and twenty cases. Am J Pathol, 24, May 1948, 475-501.

Weedon DD., Shorter RG., Ilstrup DM., Huizenga KA. & Taylor WF. (1973). Crohn's disease and cancer. N Engl J Med, 289, Nov 1973, 1099-103.

Woodley HE., Spencer JA. & MacLennan KA. (1997). Small bowel lymphoma complicating long-standing Crohn's disease. AJR Am. J. Roentgenol, 169, Nov 1997, 1462-3.

Xie J. & Itzkowitz SH. (2008). Cancer in inflammatory bowel disease. World J Gastroenterol, 14, Jan 2008, 378-89.

Zisk J., Shore J., Rosoff L. & Friedman N. (1960). Regional ileitis complicated by adenocarcinoma of the ileum: a report of two cases. Surgery, 47, Jun 1960, 970-4.

Zisman TL & Rubin DT. (2008). Colorectal cancer in inflammatory bowel disease. World J Gastroenterol, 14, May 2008, 2662-9.

Part 2

Imaging

4

Preoperative Staging of Rectal Cancer: Role of Endorectal Ultrasound

Miro A.G.F.[1], Grobler S.[2] and Santoro G.A.[3]
[1]*Department of General Surgery, Ascalesi Hospital, Naples*
[2]*Department of Surgery, Universital Hospital, Bloemfontein,*
[3]*Department of Surgery, Regional Hospital, Treviso*
[1,3]*Italy*
[2]*South Africa*

1. Introduction

Preoperative staging of rectal cancer by endorectal ultrasonography (ERUS) was first described by Feifel and Hildebrandt in 1985 (1). Since then, ultrasonographic imaging of rectal wall has been widely accepted as the reference method for local staging of rectal cancer, and is now proposed as mandatory for preoperative staging purposes in the guidelines of the main scientific societies (2-7).

The technique has witnessed a constant evolution due to the systematic efforts of researchers in defining the normal anatomy of rectal wall and perirectal anatomic structures, in differentiating early cancers from advanced neoplasms and in defining pathological from reactive perirectal nodes. ERUS is faced with the challenge of improved imaging of the perirectal structures. The relationship of the tumor to the mesorectal fascia has emerged as one of the most powerful risk factors of outcome in terms of local relapse as the tumor distance from the mesorectal fascia is predictor of circumferential resection margin (CRM) (8).

2. Equipment

ERUS is an operator-dependent examination whose accuracy closely relates to the operator experience. It is an easy-to-learn procedure for accurate staging (9). ERUS has many advantages over CT and MRI. Firstly, ERUS probe is placed in close proximity to the area to be studied so that resolution and imaging quality are greatly enhanced. Secondly, it is an office procedure of short time consuming and is well tolerated by patients. Thirdly, it is relatively low cost.

In order to obtain meaningful images, the operator must have an overall understanding and therefore correct use of the controls of the ultrasound device and of the probe. Many types of ultrasound probes have been used to evaluate the rectal wall and the anal canal. Most of these were developed to examine the prostate gland and are not ideal for evaluating the wall of the rectum and the adjacent structures. Images of the rectal wall and of the adjacent structures are best achieved with radial probes with a 360° field of view with a frequency range of 6-16 MHz and a focal length (depth of penetration) of 2-5cm. We currently use a BK medical scanner (BK Medical A/S, Mileparken 34, DK-2730 Herlev, Denmark), with mechanical anorectal transducers types 2050 and 2052. Inside the head of the these probes, two crystals are assembled back to back. The assembly can rotate inside the transducer to give a 360° field of view and can be moved inward and outward for a distance of 60mm for a 3D automatic acquisition. The full length of acquisition is achieved by touching two buttons at the base of the transducer, without any discomfort for the patient and without any movement of the transducer. The probe is long enough (270mm) to cover the entire length of the rectum and to reach into the sigmoid colon.

In routine clinical scanning, the operator works in a two-dimensional (2D) plane. Newer probes, with automatic three-dimensional (3D) acquisition and special dedicated software (BK 3Di), give a spatial, high-resolution, 3D reconstruction combining a series of closely spaced 2D images. The advantages of 3D imaging is that the 3D volume can be freely rotated, rendered, tilted and sliced to allow the operator to infinitely vary the different section parameters and visualize the lesion at different angles and in different planes (coronal, frontal, axial) to get the most information from the data. After 3D acquisition, it is immediately possible to select coronal as well as sagittal views. The data can be saved, exported, reviewed and manipulated to derive comprehensive images of the study area. Multiplanar reformatting is probably the most useful mean of displaying the structures. With 3D reconstruction it is then possible to measure the tumor size and to evaluate the relations of the tumor with respect to bowel layers and perirectal anatomic structures. In addition the 3D dataset can be manipulated to render images with enhanced surface features (surface render mode) as well as depth features (opacity, luminance, thickness and filter settings), so as to best delineate the tumor and it surroundings.

3. Technique

ERUS is usually performed with the patient positioned in the left lateral decubitus (Sims position). Before inserting the probe into the rectum, a digital rectal examination must be performed to identify size, morphology and location of the tumor, if it is low enough. If there is a stenotic annular lesion, the finger can determine whether it will allow easy passage of the probe (11, 12). The transducer is covered by a latex balloon (water standoff condom) that is held in place over a transducer collar by two round rubber rings. Before starting the procedure, the balloon is filled with degassed water to remove air bubbles. Inflating the balloon with degassed water during the procedure (at varying volumes, due to different diameters of rectal ampulla) allows acoustic coupling between the transducer and the rectal wall. When using the 2050 probe, it is mandatory to introduce the transducer through a dedicated proctoscope, inserted into the rectum to pass the proximal border of the rectal mass. This also ensures distension of the balloon around the tip of ultrasound probe as it extends from the distal tip of the proctoscope. Reusable metal sigmoidoscopes or disposable proctoscope (A.4522, Sapimed, Alessandria, Italy) (13) are available. The use of dedicated proctoscope facilitates the positioning of the probe or easy passage of the probe into strictures as well as observation of its exact localization with respect to the distance from the anal verge.

The entire shaft of the balloon-covered probe is coated with a layer of warm ultrasound gel. The probe tip is gently inserted through the proctoscope to reach the base and the balloon inflated with water. The patient should be instructed before the examination that no pain should be experienced. Under no circumstances should force be used to advance the probe.

The examiner should never try to push the tip through a narrow stenotic lesion. However, in most instances, passage can be achieved although the volume of the fluid in the balloon should be substantially reduced in order to withdraw the probe through the stenotic portion of a lesion. In some instances it may be necessary to use a smaller probe, 7mm in diameter (vs. 17mm of the 2050 B-K probe). The amount of water used to fill the balloon is usually 50-60 ml, but sometimes it may be increased to provide complete acoustic coupling with the rectal wall. The examiner should never distend the balloon with more than 150ml of degassed water, as it may rupture. If this occurs, the probe must be removed from the rectum and cleaned, a new balloon installed, and the whole procedure restarted. If air, blood or stool gets between the balloon and the rectal wall, it will prevent correct visualization of the rectal wall. To avoid this, we administer an enema two hours before the examination. The rectum can also be gently irrigated prior to passage of the probe. It may, however, be necessary to remove the probe to further irrigate the rectum under direct vision to achieve the complete cleansing of the rectum. The proctoscope and ultrasound probe may then be reintroduced to repeat the ultrasound examination with optimal images.

With the patient is in the Sims position, by convention, we report the image in a clockwise manner; the anterior aspect of the rectum will be superior (12 o'clock) on the screen, right lateral will be left (9 o'clock) on the screen, left lateral will be right (3 o'clock) on the screen, and posterior will be inferior (6 o'clock) on the screen (as in the image on the axial CT scan). Once the 20cm scored mark on the shaft of the probe is at the proximal end of the proctoscope, the proctoscope is then pulled back on the probe as far as possible, thus exposing the transducer for at least 4 cm beyond the end of the proctoscope. The balloon is then instilled with 30-60cc of water, the volume of fluid usually needed to gain optimal imaging. Higher frequencies provide better resolution of the sphincter muscles and of the rectal wall layers, whereas pararectal tissue and lymph nodes are more accurately assessed using lower frequencies. To achieve the most accurate staging, biopsy should be performed after ERUS or at least three weeks before, otherwise, the accuracy of the exam could be significantly altered by edema or clots that could interfere with the correct evaluation of the case, understaging or overstaging the neoplasm (14). For a correct examination it is of particular importance to keep be probe at the center of the rectal ampulla, with the balloon filled. The entire tumor should be scanned because depth of infiltration could vary at different points of the tumor itself. The perirectal fat is examined for suspicious lymph nodes. The search for lymph nodes should be made in the proximal part of the tumor (15). 3D spatial reconstruction will aid in the differentiation between nodes and vascular structures. Images are usually obtained using an ultrasound frequency of 10 to 16MHz, depending on which part of the rectum is being examined. Higher frequencies provide better resolution of the sphincter muscles and the rectal wall layer, whereas pararectal tissues and lymph nodes are more accurately assessed using lower frequencies (16). Complications of this technique have not been reported. Manipulation of the tumor by a transducer often exacerbates tumor bleeding for a short period. The possibility of perforation through the tumor by a rigid probe is always an hazard, but so far, it has not been reported.

4. Ultrasound anatomy

Sonographic characteristics of the rectal wall have been well described (1, 17). It consists of five layers, three hyperechoic layers separated by two hypoechoic layers (Figure 1). Debate continues over how these two sets of layers correspond. The first hyperechoic line correspond to the interface between the balloon and the mucosa. The second hypoechoic line corresponds to the mucosa, muscularis mucosa, and submucosa. The third hyperechoic line represents an interface between the submucosa and muscularis propria. The fourth hypoechoic line represents the muscularis propria. The fifth hyperechoic line represents an interface between the muscularis propria and perirectal fat/serosa (17). Good visualization depends on maintaining the probe in the centre of lumen of the rectum and having adequate distension of the water-filled balloon with good acoustic contact with rectal wall. Attention must be focused on the third hyperechoic layer. Once it has been ascertained that the middle hyperechoic line is broken, then an invasive lesion is recognised and attention is then turned to the thickness of the muscularis propria and the integrity of the outer hyperechoic line to see if the perirectal fat is invaded. Rectal tumors appears as hypoechoic lesions that infiltrate, interrupt and distort different wall layers and are staged according to the level of invasion through the rectal wall. The fibrofatty tissue surrounding the rectum contains blood vessels, nerves and lymphatics and has an inhomogeneous echo pattern. Very small, 2-3mm, round to oval hypoechoic lymph nodes may be seen and must be distinguished from blood vessels, which are also circular hypoechoic areas, but when followed longitudinally, they are seen to extend further than the corresponding diameter and can often be seen to branch and elongate in a longitudinal fashion, confirming that this is a blood vessel and not a node.

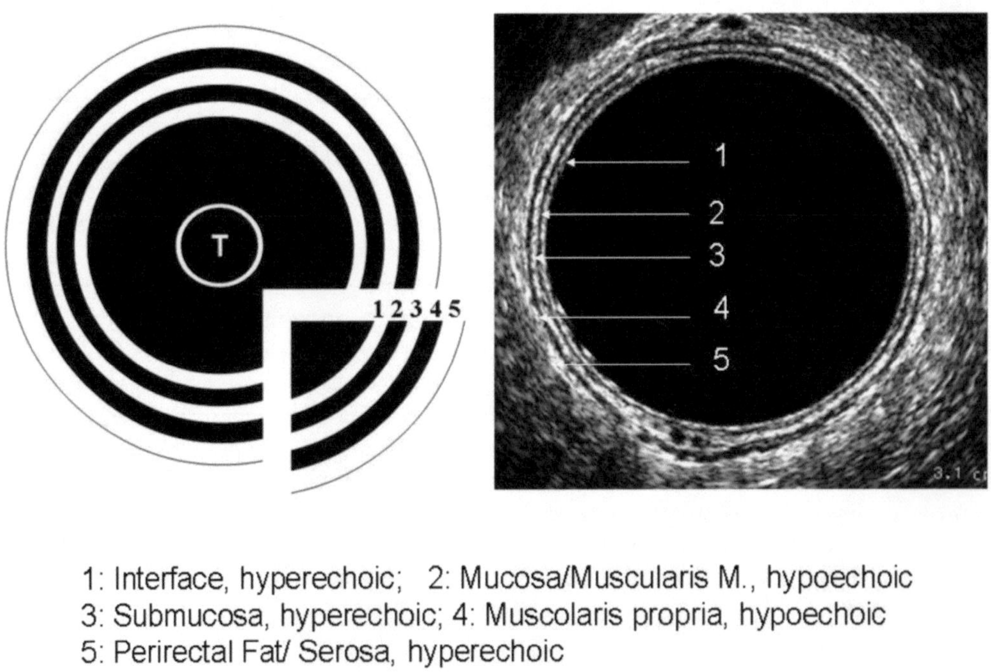

Fig. 1. The sonographic five-layer structure of the rectal wall consists of three hyperechoic layers separated by two hypoechoic layers

Metastatic lymph nodes appear as hypoechoic round masses in mesorectal fat. They tend to be larger, not homogeneus and more round, with well-defined borders. Rifkin has suggested that if nodes measure more than 3mm they are suspicious for metastatic disease (18). The pattern, however is not specific, and lymph nodes enlarged by inflammation may have an identical pattern (1). Normal lymph nodes are probably not visualized. Prominent draining veins are also hypoechoic, but in some instances can mimic a node, although their branching configuration makes the vascular structures easily detectable with 3D reconstruction. If there is any doubt, it can be used probe that can provide Doppler interrogation. In addition, with appropriate wire guides, needle aspirates for cytological assessment (FNAC) can be obtained. ERUS also may visualize perirectal anatomical structures. The upper anal canal has as landmark the puborectalis muscle. Additional structures that may be seen include the seminal vessels, prostate, bladder, and urethra in males and the vagina, uterus and bladder in females. Loops of small bowel may occasionally be noted.

Tranperineal and endovaginal ultrasound may be complementary modalities of imaging, but are more useful in assessing structural and functional aspects of the pelvic floor.

5. Rectal cancer staging

On ERUS, rectal tumors are staged according to the level of invasion through the rectal wall, corresponding to the stages of the TNM classification. To differentiate between ultrasonographic staging and pathologic staging, ultrasound stages are labeled with the prefix "u". Hildebrandt (1) was the first to propose an ultrasonographic staging of rectal cancer according to the TNM classification (Table 1). In this staging were proposed only two N stages: N0 if no nodes involved are present and N1 if metastatic nodes are identified.

uT0	Benign lesion or in situ neoplasm
uT1	Cancer infiltrating submucosa
uT2	Cancer infiltrating muscularis propria
uT3	Cancer infiltrating the rectal wall through serosa or perirectal fat
uT4	Cancer infiltrating perirectal organs or structures
uN0	No regional metastatic nodes
uN1	Metastatic nodes

Table 1. Ultrasonographic staging of rectal cancer by Hildebrandt and Feifel

In general ultrasonographic practice, it can be very difficult to make a clear distinction between a deep tumor of one T-stage and an early tumor of the next T-stage. For this reason, a revised ultrasonographic rectal staging was proposed by the Sloan Kettering Cancer Center (19). Sub-stages for indeterminate depth of tumor invasion (T) were described and the presence of perirectal nodes was defined as: definite, probable, or equivocal (Table 2).

uT0	Benign lesion or in situ neoplasm
uTw	Benign lesion or cancer initially infiltrating submucosa
uT1	Cancer infiltrating submucosa
uTx	Advanced T1 or early T2 tumor
uT2	Cancer infiltrating muscularis propria
uTy	Advanced T2 or early T3 tumor
uT3	Cancer infiltrating the rectal wall through serosa or perirectal fat
uTz	Advanced T3 or early T4 tumor
uT4	Cancer infiltrating perirectal organs or structures
uN0	No regional metastatic nodes
uN1	<3 malignant perirectal lymph nodes
uN2	>3 malignant perirectal lymph nodes
uNx	Perirectal nodes not evaluable

Table 2. Ultrasonographic staging of rectal cancer by Sloan Kettering Cancer Center

5.1 Stage uT0: Villous adenoma

Sonographic evaluation of a villous rectal lesion is useful in determining the presence of infiltrating tumor. The presence of an intact hyperechoic submucosal interface indicates lack of tumor invasion into the submucosa (Figure 2). Heintz et al. (20) believe that ERUS cannot distinguish between villous adenoma and invasive cancers because neither the muscularis mucosae nor the submucosa are sonographically visible and the first hypoechoic layer corresponds anatomically to the mucosa and the submucosa. They suggest that uT0 and uT1 tumors, which manifest as a broadening of the first hypoechoic layer, should be classified together. Instead, Adams and Wong (21) disagree with this interpretation and consider the first hypoechoic layer as the mucosa and muscularis mucosae and the middle hyperechoic layer as the submucosa. Consequently, these authors consider lesions that expand the inner hypoechoic layer but are surrounded by a uniform middle hyperechoic layer to be villous adenoma; lesions that expand the inner hypoechoic layer and have distinct echo defects of the middle hyperechoic layer are considered uT1 tumors. Technical difficulties associated with scanning villous adenoma may be due to very large lesions that tend to attenuate rectal layers and lesions with a very large exophytic component (Figure 3). In large carpeting lesions, careful evaluation of the entire tumor is necessary to ensure that a small area of invasion has not been overlooked. In some polyps, the complex structure produces fixed artefacts over a portion of the rectal wall, obscuring the image. Snare biopsy of lesions before referral to ERUS produces a burn artifact, that may lead to tumor overstaging.

5.2 Stage uT1: Submucosal invasion

If a tumor arises in a polyp it is important to determine whether the stalk is invaded. Differences in classification are reported between Western and Japanese pathologists. In 1985 Haggit et al. (22) divided the depth of invasion into four levels:

Level 0, carcinoma in situ or intramucosal carcinoma;

Level 1, carcinoma invading through the muscularis mucosa into the submucosa but limited to the head of the polyp;

Level 2, carcinoma invading the level of the neck of the adenoma;

Level 3, carcinoma invading any part of the stalk;
Level 4, carcinoma invading into the submucosa of the bowel wall below the stalk of the polyp. By definition, all sessile polyps with invasive adenocarcinoma are Level 4.
They studied 129 patients with pTis to pT1 colorectal tumors and noted that Level 4 invasion was a statistically significant factor ($p<0.001$) predicting positive nodes. Similar results were reported by Nivatvongs et al. (23) on 151 patients with pT1 colorectal tumors undergoing bowel resection in which invasion into the submucosa of the bowel wall at the base of the stalk (Level 4) was the single most significant risk factor for positive nodes. For sessile polyps the risk was 10% and for pedunculated polyps 27%. Suzuky et al. (24) determined the risk of lymph node metastases in 65 patients having Haggitt's Level 4 invasion into the submucosa. Lymph node metastasis was noted in 11 (16.9%) of the 65 patients, however the width of submucosal invasion was significantly greater in node-positive than in node-negative patients ($p=0,001$). When 5mm wide submucosal invasion was used as an indicator for intestinal resection, 37 patients were found to have indications for bowel resection and 11 (29.7%) had lymph node metastases. The positive predictive value increased from 17 to 30% when the width of submucosal invasion was added to Haggitt's Level 4 as an indicator for bowel resection. Seitz et al. (25) suggested that Haggitt's classification applies well for pedunculated polyps, however it should not be used for malignant sessile polyps.

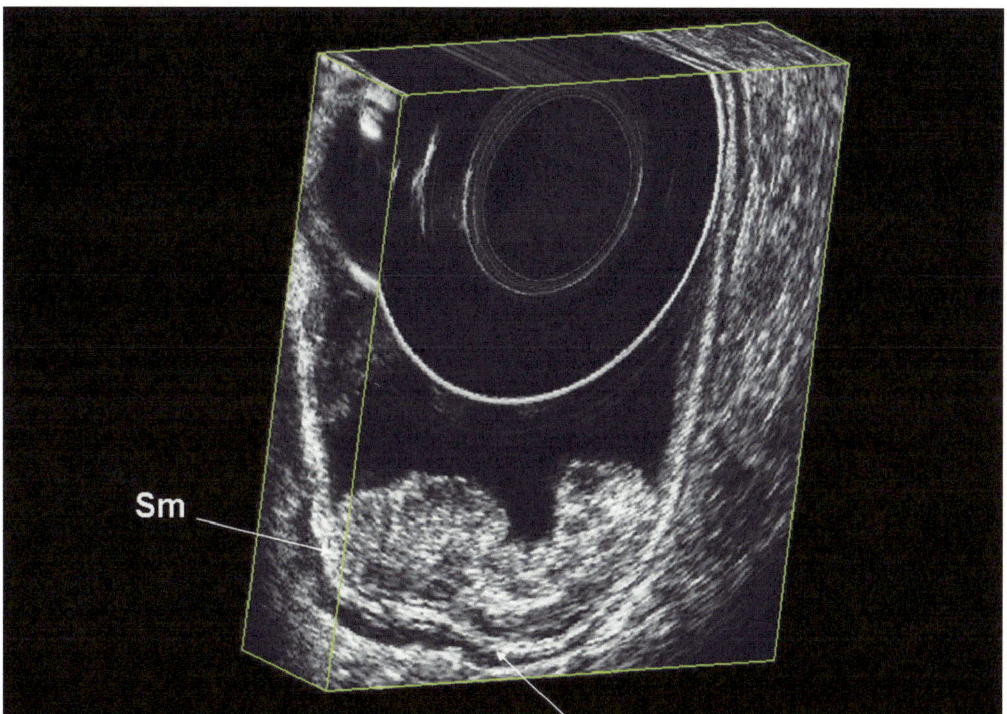

Fig. 2. Villous rectal lesion are characterized at ultrasonography by a broadening of the first hypoechoic layer and an intact hyperechoic submucosal interface

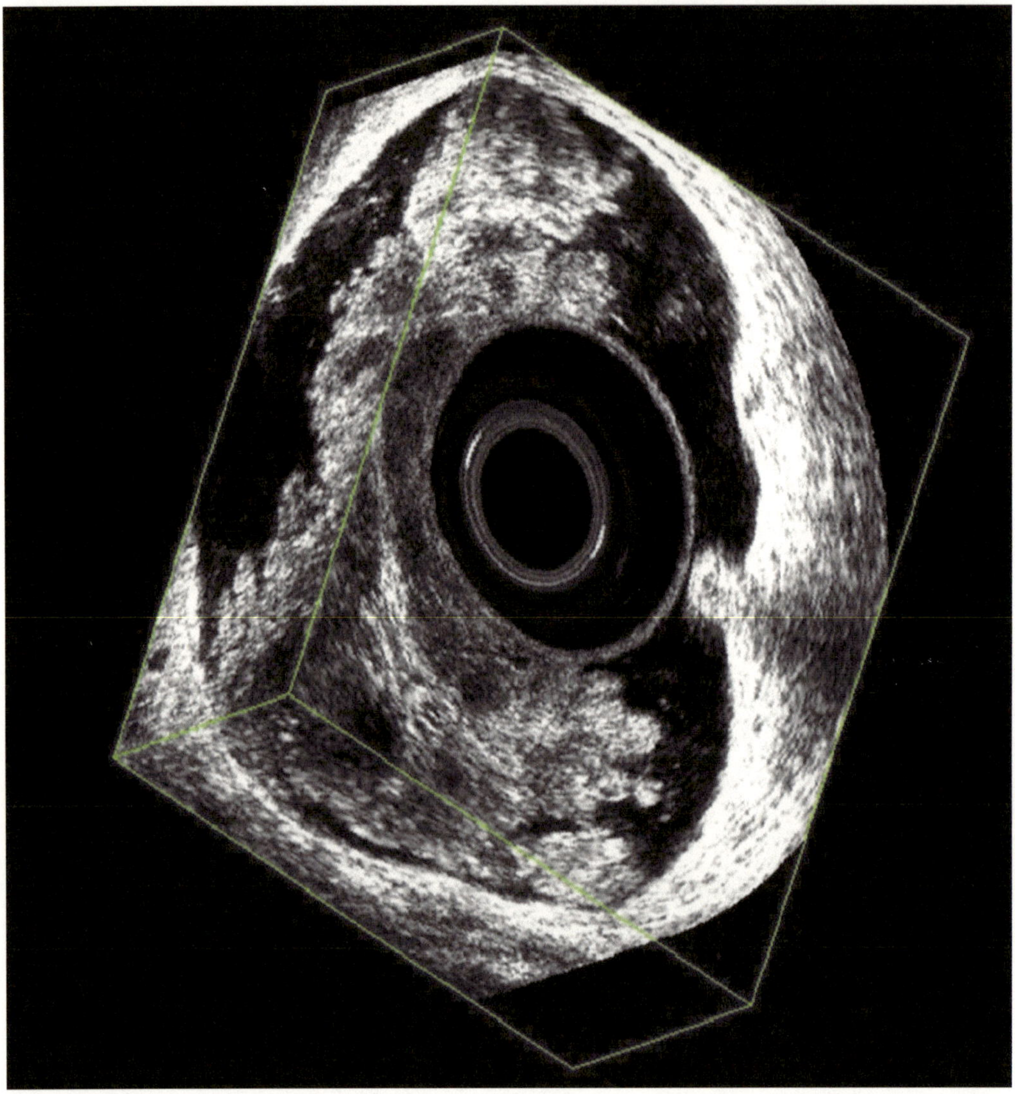

Fig. 3. Very large exophytic villous adenoma may cause technical difficulties during scanning

Kudo et al. (26) were the first to differentiate three different types of early invasive cancers:
1. SM-1 tumor, invading the superior third of the submucosa;
2. SM-2 tumor, invading the superficial two thirds of the submucosa;
3. SM-3 tumor, invading the deep third of the submucosa.

Type SM-1 tumors were further subdivided in three subtypes:
1. SM-1a: invasion is <1/4 of the submucosa;
2. SM-1b: invasion is <1/2 of the submucosa;
3. SM-1c: invasion is >1/2 of the submucosa.

Kikuchi et al. (27) found that the risk of lymph node metastasis was 0% for SM-1 lesions, 10% for SM-2 lesions and 25% for SM-3 lesions (p<0.001). In their study the SM-3 was the only independent risk factor for lymph node metastasis. Akasu et al. (28) recently proposed a classification of the depth of submucosal cancer into two groups:

1. SM-slight (SM-s), tumor invasion limited to the upper third of the submucosa;
2. SM-massive (SM-m), tumor invasion extended to the middle or lower third of the submucosa.

In their series, the prevalence of lymph node metastasis in pTis, pT1-slight and pT1-massive were 0%, 0% and 22%, respectively. Thus massive submucosal invasion can be considered a risk factor for lymph node metastasis. They suggested that patients with massive submucosal invasion are best treated by radical surgery. A recent study from Mayo Clinic confirmed these data (29). Among patients with T1 carcinoma in the middle or lower third of the rectum the multivariate risk factors for long-term, cancer-free survival was invasion into the lower third of the submucosa. For lesions with SM-3 invasion, the radical surgical resection group had lower rates of distant metastasis and better survival compared with patients who underwent local excision (29, 30). Therefore a decision whether to perform radical surgery or local excision or polypectomy should be based principally on assessment of submucosal invasion depth.

Our ERUS criteria to determine the depth of tumor invasion are as follows:

1. benign lesion (uT0): hypoechoic mass within the second hypoechoic mucosal layer. The submucosal hyperechoic layer remains intact around the entire breadth of the tumor; Carcinoma in situ (pTis) is included in this group because it cannot be differentiated from benign adenoma by ultrasound imaging alone;
2. submucosal cancer (uT1): tumor invading the submucosal layer. These lesions are stratified into two subtypes: uT1-slight (slightly irregularity of the submucosa) (Figure 4) and uT1-massive (massive irregularity) (Figure 5). Small focal disruption of the submucosal layer but with the fourth hypoechoic muscular layer intact are also classified as uT1-massive tumor;
3. lesions with distinct break of the submucosal layer and invasion of the muscular layer (uT2).

Over- and under-staging of rectal tumors continues to be a problem with ERUS due to a variety of well-documented causes as reported by Adams and Wong (21) and Kim et al. (31). A source of error can be due to the compression of the rectal wall by the water-filled balloon. To prevent any distortion of the lesion or separation of the balloon from the rectal wall with the interposition of non-conductive air between the probe and the rectum, a sufficient quantity of water can be instilled to fill the entire rectum. In this case the transducer is covered with a condom that does not cause compression of the rectal wall as with the balloon. A source of errors in the evaluation of early rectal cancer by ERUS can also frequently be caused by examiner misinterpretation or a tendency to overestimate a malignant lesion because of concern for under-treatment despite clear ERUS imaging.

5.3 Stage uT2: Invasion of the muscular layer

Sonographic diagnosis of tumor invasion of the muscularis propria is based on thickening of this layer (Figure 6). The muscularis propria is represented by a thin hypoechoic layer adjacent to the hyperechoic submucosal interface. As the tumor is also hypoechoic, early muscular invasion is difficult to detect. The surrounding hyperechoic layer corresponding to the perirectal fat interface remains intact. Lymph node metastases occur in approximately 15-20% of patients with T2 tumors. ERUS is important to distinguish uT2 and uT1 lesions, because local therapy is not routinely recommended for uT2 rectal lesions (30).

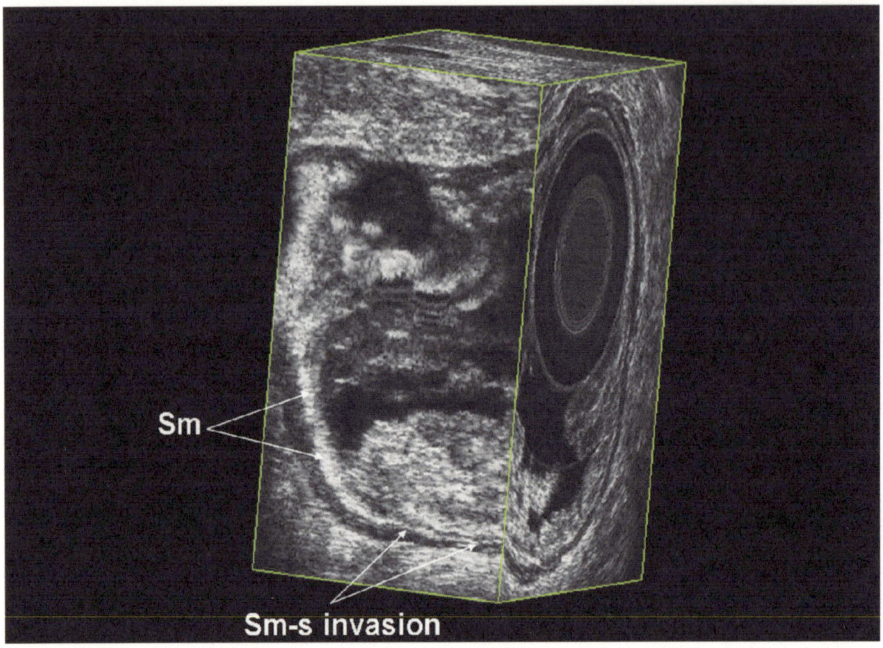

Fig. 4. uT1-slight cancer are characterized at ultrasonography by a broadening of the first hypoechoic layer and a slightly irregularity of the hyperechoic submucosal interface

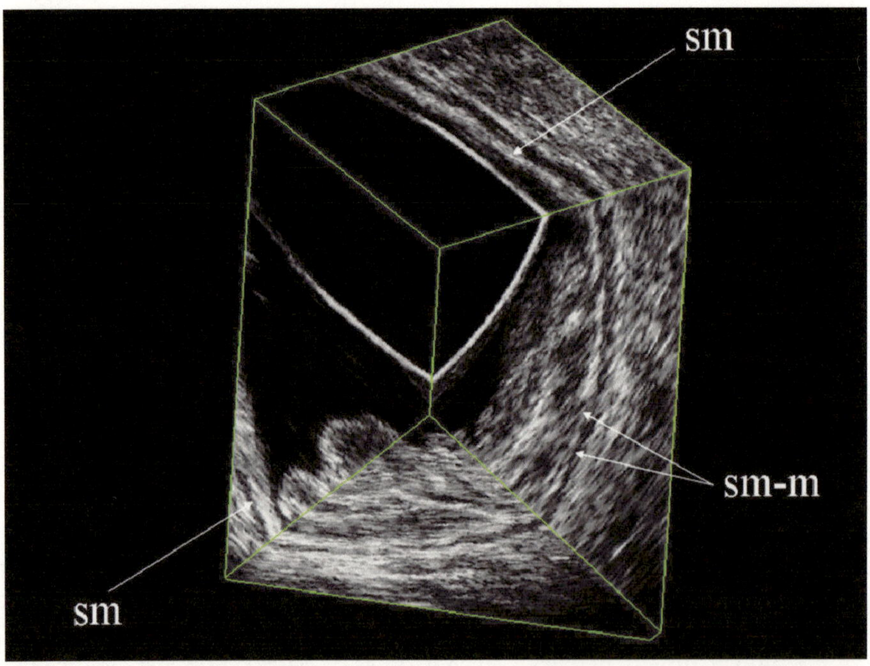

Fig. 5. uT1-massive cancer are characterized at ultrasonography by a broadening of the first hypoechoic layer and a massive irregularity or a small focal disruption of the hyperechoic submucosal interface. The fourth hypoechoic muscular layer appears intact

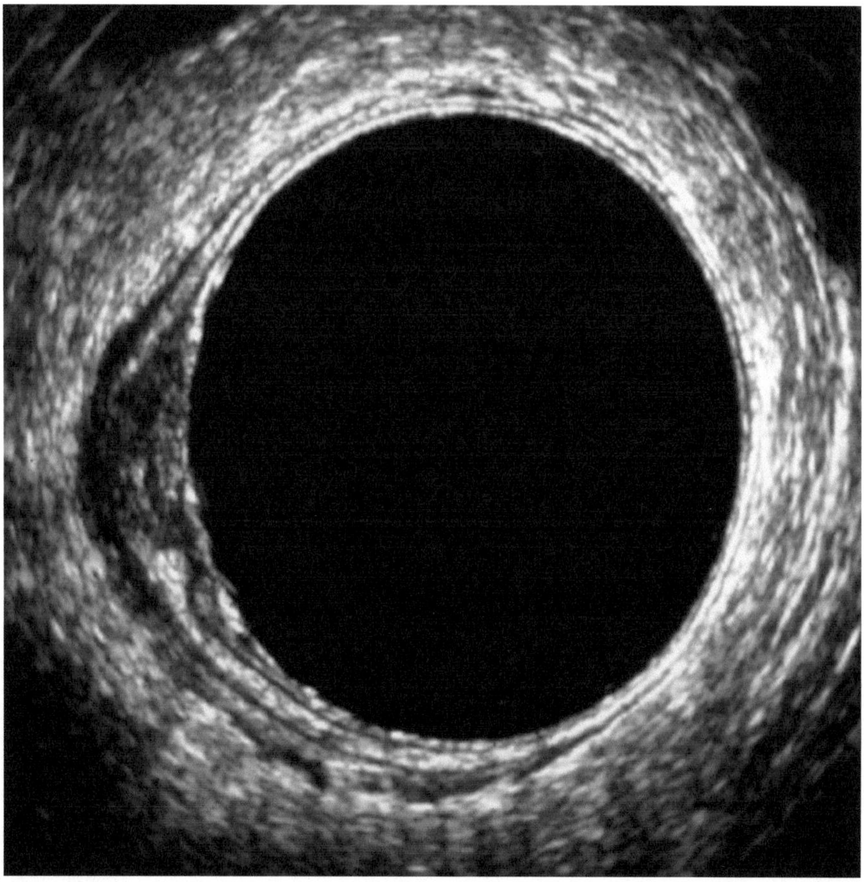

Fig. 6. Sonographic diagnosis of tumor invasion of the muscularis propria (uT2) is based on thickening of this layer

Overstaging is a particular problem with T2 tumors. Among the interpretative errors, severe inflammatory infiltrate underlying a tumor, which is sonographically indistinguishable from malignant tissue, can prohibit accurate evaluation of tumor invasion and appears to cause inevitable errors (32, 33). Understaging, on the other hand, may be caused by a failure to detect microscopic cancer infiltration owing to the limits of resolution of the equipment (32, 33, 34).

5.4 Stage uT3: Perirectal fat invasion

Perirectal fat invasion is diagnosed sonographically by the presence of irregularity of the outer hyperechoic layer that corresponds to the perirectal fat interface. These findings should be associated with disruption of the hyperechoic layer corresponding to the submucosa and thickening of the hyperechoic layer representing the muscularis propria (Figure 7). Contiguous organs are not involved. About 10% of such tumors are, however, accompanied by a narrowing of the lumen or angulation that may render it difficult or impossible to advance the probe proximal to the tumor. To perform a complete staging by ERUS, a residual lumen of 2cm is necessary. Under these circumstances the study may be incomplete and the presence of enlarged lymph nodes may not be ascertained accurately because nodes are often located proximal to the tumor. The prevalence of regional lymph node metastases in uT3 tumors is approximately 30-50%.

The recognition of perirectal fat invasion is an important determination to select appropriate patients for pre-operative combined chemotherapy and radiation therapy followed by surgery. One of the most important drawbacks in endosonographic staging is the distinction between T2 tumors invading most of the muscularis propria and T3 tumor which slightly invades the perirectal fat. Indeed most errors are understaging of small pT3 tumors or overstaging of pT2 tumors (35, 36).

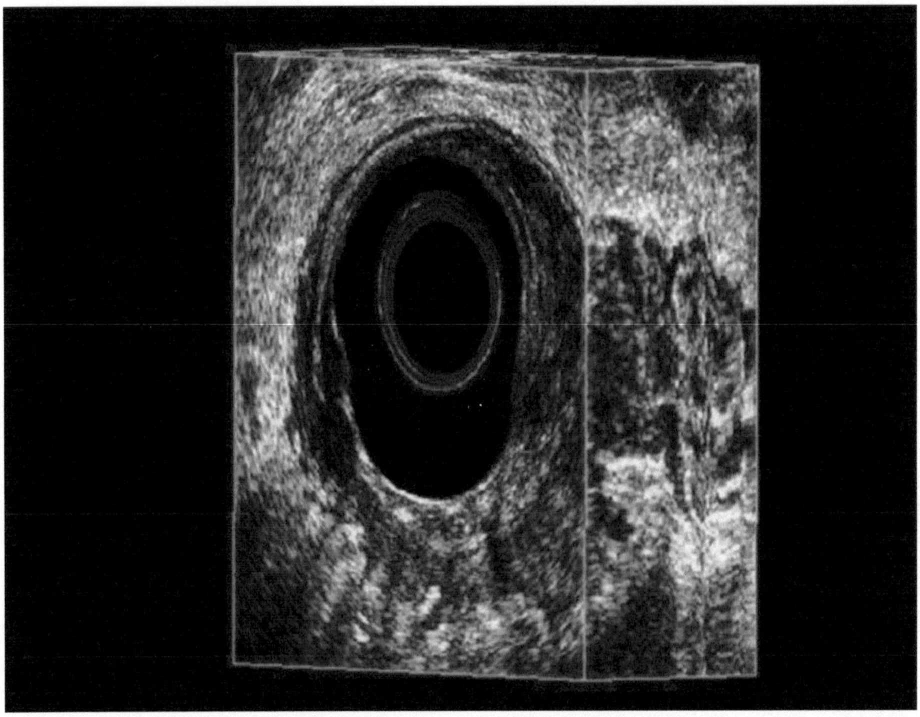

Fig. 7. Perirectal fat invasion (uT3) is diagnosed sonographically by the presence of irregularity of the outer hyperechoic layer that corresponds to the perirectal fat interface

5.5 Stage uT4: Extensive local invasion

uT4 lesions are locally invasive into contiguous organs such as bladder, uterus, cervix, vagina, prostate and seminal vesicles (Figure 8). These advanced lesions are clinically fixed or tethered. Sonographically there is a loss of the normal hyperechoic interface between the tumor and the adjacent organ. The inability of ERUS to distinguish between malignant infiltration or peritumoral inflammation results in a somewhat lower staging accuracy with regard to T4 cancers. Frank stenosis also precludes precise endosonographic evaluation and angulation of the probe to the tumor axis also can cause misinterpretation.

5.6 Stage uN1-2: Lymph node metastases

Metastatic involvement of the mesorectal lymph nodes is a major independent prognostic factor. It has been observed that the presence of more than three nodes is associated with a poor prognosis. Moreover, identification of a metastatic perirectal lymph node is important as these patients may benefit from pre-operative adjuvant radiotherapy and some of the early T1 or T2 lesions with mesorectal node involvement are not suitable for local excision.

Sonographic evaluation of lymph node metastases is somewhat less accurate than depth of invasion (16, 18, 19, 34, 35). Undetectable or benign appearing lymph nodes are classified as uN0. Malignant appearing lymph nodes are classified as uN1 (<3 lymph nodes) or uN2 (>3 lymph nodes). Normal, non-enlarged perirectal nodes are not usually seen on ERUS. The criteria used to identify metastatic lymph nodes in most of the studies are echogenicity, border demarcation and node diameter. Inflamed, enlarged lymph nodes appear hypoechoic, with ill defined borders. Most of the sound energy is reflected because the lymphatic tissue has not changed. In contrast, metastatic lymph nodes that have been completely replaced by the tumor do not provide the normal tissue architecture and appear hypoechoic with an echogenicity similar to the primary tumor. Malignant lymph nodes tend to be round in shape rather than oval, have discrete borders and are most commonly found adjacent to the primary tumor or in the mesorectum proximal to the tumor (15) (Figure 9).

The sonographic features of lymph nodes generally can be distinguished into four groups:

1. if lymph nodes are not visible by ultrasound, the probability of lymph node metastasis is low;
2. hyperechoic lymph nodes are often benign and result from non-specific inflammatory changes;
3. hypoechoic lymph nodes larger than 5mm are highly suggestive for lymph node metastasis;
4. lymph nodes larger than 5mm with mixed echogenic patterns cannot be classified accurately but should be considered metastatic.

On size characteristic alone, sonographically detected nodes in the mesorectum greater than 5mm in diameter have a 50-70% chance of being involved, whereas those smaller than 4mm have less than 20% chance. However, up to 20% of patients have involved nodes of less than 3mm, limiting the accuracy of the technique. Hulsmans et al (37) studied several features by correlating pathologic and sonographic findings in the lymph nodes of specimens obtained from a series of 21 consecutive patients with resected rectal cancer. These features included ratio of long axis to short axis diameter, referred as to roundness index; lobulations (multiple notches); echogenicity; not homogeneous; border delineation; presence of an echo-poor rim (the outer rim being more hypoechoic than the rest of the node); presence of a peripheral halo; and presence of a hilar reflection. The authors showed that three ultrasonographic features of a node significantly correlated to it being benign or malignant at histopathologic examination are: short axis diameter, degree of inhomogeneity and the presence or absence of hilar reflection.

Overstaging and understaging may occur during assessment of lymph node involvement. Edematous lymph nodes transmit more sound energy and have an echogenicity similar to metastases. The cross-sectional appearance of blood vessels in the perirectal fat may be commonly confused with positive lymph nodes. The sonographic continuity of hypoechoic vessels over a distance greater than the cross-sectional diameter is the criterion used to distinguish vessels from hypoechoic lymph nodes. With careful scanning, blood vessels appear to branch or extend longitudinally. In addition, it may be difficult to differentiate islands of tumor outside the bowel wall from involved nodes. With careful scanning, one can demonstrate continuity with the main tumor that may not have been recognised initially. Even with an improved understanding of the characteristic of malignant lymph node and utilizing criteria of shape, echogenicity and border features, micrometastases and granulomatous inflammation will remain difficult, if not impossible, to differentiate by ERUS. If a whole node is replaced by tumor or the node is enlarged secondary to it, detection is more likely. However, if only a small deposit or a micrometastasis is present in a node, the characteristics of the node are unlikely to be sufficiently altered to allow detection. This explains in part the lower accuracy rate for lymph node detection with current, conventional ultrasonography. Grossly malignant lymph nodes located at a distance from the primary tumor also remain undetected if they exceed the depth of penetration of the transducer. This is particularly true for nodes in the proximal mesorectum out of the length of the probe. To obtain high sensitivity and high specificity, the combination of a small cutoff value and ERUS-guided fine needle aspiration biopsy may be helpful.

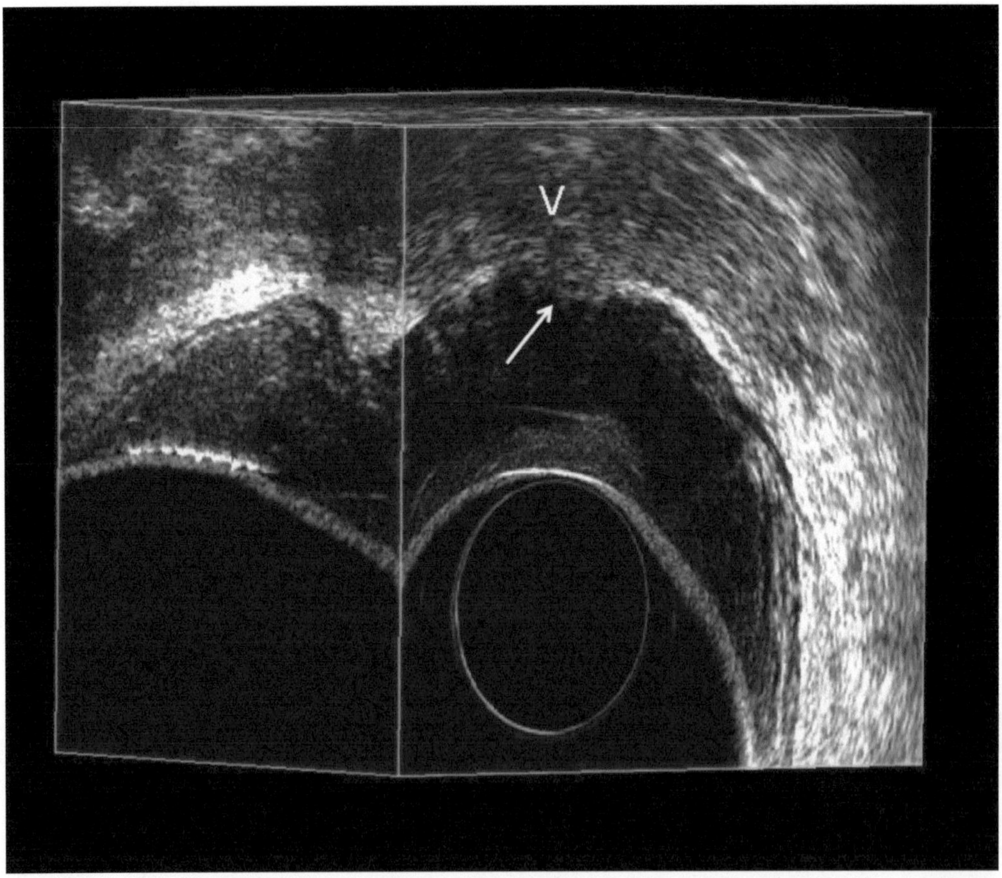

Fig. 8. uT4 lesion with invasion of the vaginal wall

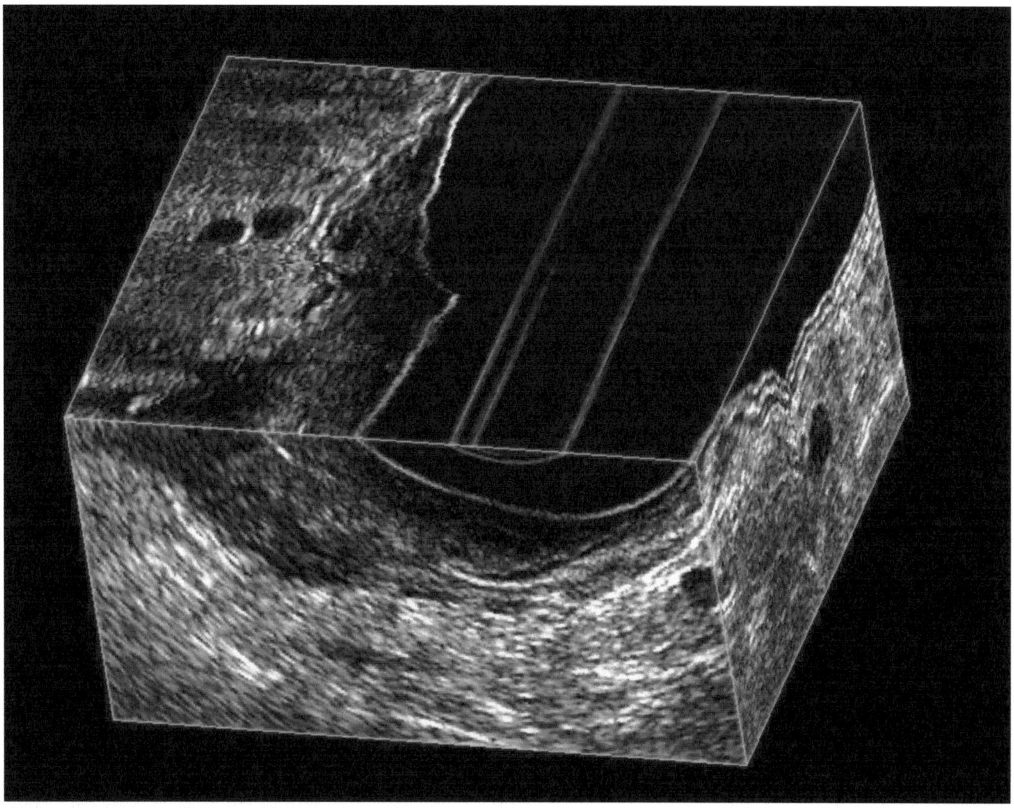

Fig. 9. Malignant lymph nodes appear as round hypoechoic structure, with discrete borders, adjacent to the primary tumor

6. Discussion

The improved understanding of rectal cancer biologic behavior mandates for a correct staging of the disease to allow tailored treatment in relation to the stage of the tumor. There is general agreement that villous adenomas with focal areas of carcinoma in situ and early T1 rectal cancers are best treated with local surgery, whereas advanced T1 and T2 rectal cancers because of the well known risk of associated nodal metastases, are best cured with radical surgery. Early T3 cancers may be safely treated with radical surgery alone or a short course of preoperative radiotherapy, while advanced T3, T3N1-2, T4N0-1-2 lesions mandate neoadjuvant chemotherapy-radiotherapy regimens to attempt to downstage the tumours (38, 39). Furthermore, staging is linked to ultimate prognostic outcome of the patient.

Systemic staging of rectal cancer is best achieved by contrast-enhanced thoraco-abdomino-pelvic multidetector CT scan. This is justified by the general availability of the device, the costs and the short duration time of the examination required to achieve good quality images and for the ability to reconstruct images into planes other than the axial plan alone (e.g. sagittal, frontal, oblique planes). For local staging of rectal cancer, CT accuracy is limited by the intrinsic difficulty to define the layers of rectal wall and thus the depth of penetration of the lesion. In the study of Rifkin et al. (18), 81 patients underwent CT and ERUS for staging purposes of rectal cancer; the accuracy of CT in assessing depth of rectal wall invasion was 53%, compared with 72% for ERUS. Beynon et al. (40) compared ERUS to CT for the evaluation of mesorectal nodal status; they found that the accuracy of CT was only 57%, compared with 87% for ERUS. More recently Herzog et al. (41) examined 87 patients who underwent both CT and ERUS; they found accuracy of CT to be 74.7%, whereas ERUS had an accuracy of 90.,8%. In the study of Goldman et al. (42) the accuracy in defining perirectal fat invasion was 52% for CT scanning vs. 81% for ERUS; the accuracy was respectively 64% vs. 68% for lymph node metastases. The best results in rectal staging with CT scan are reported by Civelli et al. (43) with an accuracy of 86.8% for T3 stage, a sensitivity of 100% and a specificity of 78.7%. In lymph node staging, the referred accuracy was 73.6%, sensitivity was 52.6% and specificity was 85.3%. In summary, the accuracy of CT is highly variable and should not be used as a sole method of staging rectal cancer (42).

ERUS is currently the most widely used and effective staging modality in the local assessment of rectal cancer. Its accuracy in numerous trials ranges from 80 to 95% for T-staging and 70 to 75% for N-staging, levels that are slightly higher than the respective 75 to 85% and 60 to 70% reported with MRI (44). In experienced hands, ERUS can accurately measure size, circumference and distance of the tumor from various anatomic landmarks (e.g. sphincters, prostate, vagina, seminal vesicles, mesorectal fascia, etc.) and gives indications to radiotherapists to plan irradiation fields (depth and length of infiltration). Furthermore it is capable of examining the anal sphincters for defects as well as tumor infiltration, allowing the surgeon to decide whether a sphincter-saving resection is safe or feasible (45). The accuracy of ERUS has been assessed in many studies and the main evidence emerged has been that T-staging accuracy varies relative to tumor stage. ERUS tends to be less accurate in staging T2 rectal cancers that are often overstaged (44, 46, 47). Orrom et al. (48) evaluated 59 patient who underwent ERUS and radical resection for rectal cancer. The patients were divided into three categories chronologically based on user experience. Group 1 had no standardization of the operator who performed the exam. The accuracy of this group was only 58%, with 37% of lesions that were overstaged and 4% of tumors that were understaged. Group 2 was based on a better standardization in the performance of the exam. In this group a proctoscope was used to improve localization of the rectal cancer. The accuracy increased to 77%, with 20% of cancers overstaged and 3% understaged. Group 3 adopted the widely accepted division of rectal wall into five layers. Accuracy rate increased to 95% with only 5% overstaging and no understaging. Garcia-Aguilar et al. (47) undertook a large retrospective study to assess the accuracy of ERUS on 545 patients, who underwent rectal surgery without neoadjuvant treatment. The overall accuracy of ERUS in assessing depth of penetration of the tumor into the rectal wall was 69%, with 18% of tumors overstaged and 13% understaged. Furthermore, ERUS correctly staged most villous adenomas (accuracy 87%) but less than half of T1 tumors (accuracy 47%). A selection bias of this study is represented by the exclusion from the final analysis of all patients (270 patients) who received neoadjuvant radiation/chemotherapy. A systematic literature review from Worrell et al. (49) showed that ERUS correctly established a cancer diagnosis in 81% of 62 biopsy-negative rectal adenomas which had focal carcinoma on histopathology. Beynon (50) examined 111 patients, of whom 100 undewent surgical resection; the accuracy was 93% for tumor staging, and the sensitivity for T3 and T4 stage was 98.7%. Overstaging occurred in 5% cases and understaging occurred 2% of cases. Two recent meta-analysis, based the first on 11 studies reported that the sensitivity of ERUS in correctly staging T1, T2, T3, T4 rectal cancers was 84%, 76%, 88%, 87% respectively (51). The second recent meta-analysis comprised 31 studies and reported ERUS sensitivity rate related to the stage of 76%, 75%, 88% and 87% respectively (52).

The sensitivity and specificity of ERUS in staging rectal cancer after polypectomy was evaluated in two papers. Garcia-Aguilar et al. (53) assessed 63 patients with malignant rectal polyps removed by snare excision at colonoscopy. ERUS accuracy in evaluating the presence of residual cancer in the rectal wall was 54%, with 39% of positive predictive value and 65% of negative predictive value. Furthermore ERUS accurately identified metastatic lymph nodes in two of three patients who had radical surgery. ERUS was more useful than polyp morphologic and histologic criteria to determine the presence of residual cancer in the rectal wall. Kruskal et al. (54) reported 18 patients who had ERUS staging before surgical resection for adenocarcinoma discovered in polypectomy specimens (5 transanal surgery, 13 endoscopic surgery). ERUS correctly predicted T stage in eight patients (44%); seven tumors (39%) were overstaged and three tumors (17%) were understaged. In this study, ERUS showed a sensitivity of 94%, specificity of 50%, accuracy of 89%, positive predictive value of 94% and negative predictive value of 50%. They concluded that ERUS facilitates surgical planning and should be considered the technique of choice in staging this patient population, always keeping in mind the limits of ERUS staging when performed after biopsy or polypectomy (edema, blood clots, and inflammatory reaction) could interfere with a good imaging, leading to over- or understaging the tumor.

A recent study (55) evaluated 142 patients to characterize slight or massive irregularity of the hyperechoic submucosal layer to differentiate uT1-slight or uT1 massive tumors. ERUS correctly detected the depth of invasion in 87.2% of patients with a concordance between ultrasonographic and histopathologic staging of kappa 0.81 (95% confidence interval). The recognition of early from massive T1 rectal cancers consequently selected the appropriate management in 95.2% of cases. Akasu et al. (28) reported the result of a study on 154 patients with early stage rectal cancer preoperatively evaluated with ERUS. Sensitivity, specificity and overall accuracy rates for detection of slight or massive submucosal invasion were 99%, 74%, 96% and 98%, 88%, 97% respectively. Pikarsky (56) from Cleveland Clinic showed that ERUS confirmed the histopathologic diagnosis of rectal villous tumor without evidence of malignancy in 26 out of 27 patients. Konishi et al. (57) reported that the overall accuracy of ERUS-based evaluation of tumor invasion depth was 60% in villous lesions and 91% in non-villous lesions. In differentiating mucosa neoplasias (M)/ submucosal cancers with slight invasion (SM-s) from non M/SM-s the accuracy of ERUS in villous and non-villous lesions was 66% and 96%, respectively. Akahoshi et al. (58) improved the accuracy of ERUS by using a high-frequency ultrasound probe (12MHz). The depth of invasion was correctly assessed in 87% (46/53) of pT1 tumors. Stark et al. (59) reported their experience with high multifrequency probes. The sensitivity of ERUS with regard to invasion was 89% (16/18), specificity 88% (37/42), and accuracy 88% (53/60). They concluded that rectal endosonography can distinguish between benign rectal lesions and early invasive rectal cancers. Similar results were reported by Hunerbein et al. (60) with a high frequency miniprobe in the staging of colonic tumors. The infiltration depth was correctly classified in 78 of 88 patients (accuracy, 87%). We conducted a prospective study to compare accuracy of 3D-ERUS with high frequency probe to conventional 2D-ERUS in the preoperative staging of early invasive rectal cancer (61): eighty-nine consecutive patients with rectal villous lesions were examined using both 3D-ERUS and conventional 2D-ERUS. All lesions were resected either endoscopically or surgically. Malignant transformation was found in 35 rectal villous adenomas at histological examination. 2D-ERUS correctly determined the depth of invasion of villous polyps in 6 of 7 M neoplasias (85.7%), 8 of 12 SM-s lesions (66.6%) and 12 of 16 SM-m lesions (75%), whereas the accuracy of 3D-ERUS was 85.7% for M neoplasias, 83.3% for SM-s and 87.5% for SM-m lesions. Overall accuracy of the 2D-ERUS based evaluation of villous lesions was lower than that of 3D-ERUS based evaluation (27/35, 77.1%, vs. 30/35, 85.7%), however there was no significant difference (p=0.5). In the evaluation of SM-s lesions the accuracy of 3D-ERUS was significantly superior to 2D-ERUS based evaluation (p<0.029). Tumor location and gross morphology (sessile or pedunculated did not correlate with the accuracy of the T-staging. Eight of 54 pT0 tumors (14.8%) were overstaged by 2D-ERUS, while 5 of 54 (9.2%) were overstaged by 3D-ERUS. The prevalence of lymph node metastases in M, SM-s and SM-m lesions were 0%, 0% and 12.5%, respectively. These findings showed 3D-ERUS to have a significant advantage over 2D-ERUS for the accurate evaluation of superficial submucosal cancer invasion. Stereoscopic visualization provided easier and more complete understanding of depth of submucosal invasion.

Overstaging is a particular problem with T2 tumors. Peritumoral inflammation and desmoplastic changes are commonly causes of error, as both are difficult to differentiate from actual tumor borders. Overstaging may also be the result of preoperative biopsies, that can create hematomas, edema, clots due to bleeding and disrupt sonographic anatomy. Fear of understaging is another cause that has been described as responsible of overstaging in T2 rectal cancers (63). In general, the time interval between performance of diagnostic tests and the reference test (pathology on surgical specimen) should be short. A longer period between the performance of the diagnostic test and the reference test will lead to a greater change in the disease status and decrease in the discriminatory power of the diagnostic test. Potential bias of several studies is that the time elapsed between test and surgery was not described or was longer than the ideal of one week. In a prospective study Sailer et al. (62) examined the value of ERUS in the preoperative staging of 160 rectal tumors. For T2 tumors, the sensitivity was only 41% and the specificity 92% as the majority of pT2 rectal cancers were overstaged (uT3). The authors concluded that ERUS is not helpful in the assessment of T2 carcinomas. Katsura et al (64) reported that the predictive value of positive rate in the assessment of rectal wall invasion by ERUS was 96.2% in uT1 and 87.5% in uT2.

3D-ERUS offers a significant advantage over conventional 2D-ERUS for the accurate evaluation of rectal cancer. In a preliminary study, Kim et al. (65) showed that the accuracy of 3D-ERUS was 90.9% for pT2 whereas that of 2D-ERUS was 84.8%. It is of note that the classification system is highly reproducible through the use of cut-off points that are usually straightforward histologically, such as the distinction between T2 and T3 tumor depending on the invasion of the mesorectum or not. This does not always easily transfer to staging through imaging. All imaging methods are good enough to show the bulk of the tumor, but have difficulty in predicting the microscopic invasion of an interface. It is therefore unrealistic to expect 100% accuracy from imaging technology in predicting a histologic classification (66). Glaser et al. (67) reported that the sensitivity of ERUS for detection of perirectal fat infiltration (uT3) was 97%, specificity was 90% and positive predictive value was 90%. The inability of ERUS to distinguish between fat infiltration or peritumoral inflammation results in somewhat lower staging accuracy with regard to T4 cancers. In conclusion, the overall agreement between uT-stage and pTstage in the larger studies is 63% to 69%, with 12% to 15% understaging and 18% to 24% overstaging (44, 47, 68, 69). In these series there was understaging of uT1 between 6% to 24%, and of uT2 tumor from 16% to 30%. Overstaging in uT3 occurred in 20% to 28% of cases.

There is a marked reduction in survival rate in patients with rectal cancer and nodal metastases. Ultrasonographic criteria for distinguishing malignant from inflammatory lymph nodes are a source of controversy. The criteria of echogenicity and border characteristics are subjective, although at least one study has shown that as many as 72% of nodes with hypoechoic patterns are metastatic (70). Nodal size as a criterion to consider a node to be metastatic is a matter of debate. Whilst metastatic lymph nodes tend to be larger than normal nodes, the 3 to 5mm diameter used as a cutoff is quite arbitrary. Kim et al. (51) reported that roughly 18% of nodes measuring less than 5mm in diameter harboured metastases. Akasu et al. (28) found that the incidence of metastasis in nodes with diameter around 2mm, 3 to 5mm and >6mm was 9.5%, 47% and 87%, respectively. These data suggest that ERUS can miss up to 20% of these smaller nodes. The accuracy of ERUS in assessing lymph node involvement varies from 58% to 86% (35). In a recent meta-analysis by Puli et al. (71), in which only studies confirmed by surgical histology were selected, the sensitivity of ERUS in diagnosing nodal involvement by rectal cancers was 73.2% and specificity was of 75.8%. In this meta-analysis was evaluated also the influence of fine needle aspiration (FNA) during the procedure that resulted in very low or not complications. However, there were not enough studies to draw definitive conclusions on the accuracy of FNA. The potential bias of this meta-analysis was that all the studies were either retrospective or consecutive, but no prospective studies were included. The authors concluded that sensitivity and specificity of ERUS for nodal involvement was moderate. It performs better when there is no anatomic nodal invasion than in the presence of anatomic nodal invasion. Further refinement in ERUS technologies and re-evaluation of diagnostic criteria based on prospective studies are needed to improve our diagnostic accuracy. The theoretic additional value of ERUS-guided FNA on suspicious nodes, was addressed by Siddiqui et al. (71). They found no benefits in using FNA, because all perirectal node large enough to be visualized by ERUS were confirmed to harbour metastases. In their initial experience of ultrasonographic rectal staging, Holdsworth et al. (72) used a 5.5MHz transducer. They identified lymph node metastases with a sensitivity of 57% and specificity of 64%, concluding that the technique is not reliable to identify metastases. With the growing experience of the operator, the modernization of the probes (introduction of multifrequencies probes) and with the introduction of 3D-dedicated software, Kim et al. (65) reported that lymph node metastases were accurately predicted by 3D-ERUS in 84.8% of patients, whereas 2D-ERUS predicted the disorder in 66.7%. Although their findings did not show 3D-ERUS to have a statistically significant advantage over 2D-ERUS, stereoscopic visualization provided easier and more complete understanding of lymph nodes.

Accuracy of ERUS is highly dependent on operator experience. The capability to perform an accurate examination is crucial for the acquisition of high quality images and for the interpretation of the study. The presence of an uniform acoustic contact is essential for the production of good ultrasonographic images. The position of the probe in relation to the tumor is critical. Whether tumor site (in terms of height) and position (with respect to rectal circumference) has an influence on the reliability of ERUS staging is not settled as yet. Sentovich et al. (74) and Senesse at al. (75) reported significantly better result for tumors of the distal third. The reason for the less accurate staging in the lower rectum is a technical one, because it is the difficult to reach all sites of the rectum with a rigid probe. This consideration prompted us to develop a new dedicated proctoscope to allow easy passage of the probe above the rectal lesion. We performed a prospective study to determine whether tumor site and tumor position would influence the accuracy of 3D-ERUS staging. (13). ERUS was performed on 173 consecutive patients with primary rectal cancer. In 65 patients the tumor was located 0.1-6cm from the anal verge (lower rectal tumor), 77 patients had tumors 7-12cm from the anal verge (middle rectal tumor) and 31 tumors were 13-18cm form the anal verge (upper rectal tumors). With regard to position, 46 tumors were situated anteriorly, 30 in the left lateral wall, 43 posteriorly and 42 in the right lateral wall. In 12 patients the tumor occupied two-thirds of the rectal circumference. All lesions were resected either endoscopically or surgically. ERUS correctly predicted the depth of invasion in 62/65 (95.3%) lower rectal tumors, 74/77 (96.1%) middle rectal tumors and 28/31 (90.3%) upper rectal tumors. With regard to position, accuracy was 93.4% for tumors located anteriorly, 90.4% for tumors in the right lateral rectal wall, 90.6% for tumors located posteriorly and 86.6% for tumors in the left lateral rectal wall. The accuracy of 3D-ERUS for lymph node metastases, assessed in 142 patients, was 44/46 (95.6%) for lower rectal tumors, 61/65 (93.8%) for middle rectal tumors and 28/31 (90.3%) for upper rectal tumors. Our analysis showed that there was no difference between the different positions, which means that all tumors are equally amenable to ERUS staging if they are within reach of the probe. Tumors situated on the haustral folds are often overstaged because of artifacts induced by tangential imaging. Air bubbles trapped from unfilled space in the rectal vault due to insufficient inflation, produce strong acoustic shadowing and prevent visualization of deeper tissues (75). The impact of tumor level on ERUS accuracy is controversial. Sailer et al. (76) have suggested impaired visualization of tumors located in both the proximal and distal rectum. In their study, 162 tumors were divided into three groups based on tumor location. Reduced accuracy in the staging of low rectal tumors has been attributed to the anatomy of the rectum, who makes it difficult to maintain uniform acoustic contact and properly orientation of the probe. Another explanation is poor definition of the five sonographic layers just above the dentate line, particularly along the posterior wall (47, 75).

A number of comparative studies have been performed to assess the efficacy of ERUS and MRI. Some studies have shown clear supremacy of ERUS, whereas other have shown little difference. MRI as with CT, is accurate in assessing spread of the tumor beyond the rectal wall, invasion of contiguous structures, spread to regional lymph nodes or distant metastases. The lateral pelvic nodes, such as the obturator nodes, are located too far from the rectum to be imaged effectively with ERUS. Therefore, possible advantages of MRI may lie with assessment of the lateral pelvic lymph nodes, pelvic wall invasion and involvement of levator ani muscle. Previously, MRI was not able to delineate the layers of the rectal wall. With high resolution techniques, thin slice MRI can be used to measure the depth of extramural spread accurately, with good correlation with corresponding pathology measurement in surgical specimens (78). Furthermore the relationship of tumor to the mesorectal fascia can be evaluated so that CRM positive status can be predicted when tumor is imaged within 1mm from the mesorectal fascia. Brown et al. (79) evaluated the effectiveness of digital examination, ERUS and MRI in staging rectal cancer in 98 patients undergoing total mesorectal excision with pathology as the gold standard. ERUS correctly identified 14 out of 31 (45%) tumors with favorable prognosis (in two cases extramural depth was overestimated; in the remaining 15 patients, failure to reach the tumor using the EUS probe resulted in inability to assess tumor depth). In this category of patients, MRI correctly identified all patients. In the preoperative identification of tumors with unfavorable prognosis, ERUS correctly identified 32 out of 39 (82%) patients and MRI correctly identified 33 out of 39 (85%) tumors. In the preoperative identification of locally advanced tumors (28 cases), only one was successfully identified using ERUS; in 12 patients, tumor could not be assessed because not reached by the probe or because of pain experienced by the patient. In 15 patients, tumor deposits involving the mesorectal fascia had not been identified. MRI successfully identified 22 out of 28 patients with locally advanced tumors. In four patients, nodes close to the mesorectal fascia had not been detected. In each of these cases, nodes were partially replaced by small tumor foci that were not resolved on MR images. In two patients tumor was thought to have breached the wall anteriorly by <1mm, but histopathologic examination showed stage pT4 peritoneal infiltration by the tumor. In a meta-analysis by Bipat et al (80), ERUS was found to be the most accurate staging modality when compared to CT and MRI imaging for evaluation of local invasion of rectal cancer. For lymph node involvement, the results were comparable, with low sensitivity values. ERUS was used to evaluate only perirectal or mesorectal lymph nodes, whereas CT and MRI were also used to evaluate iliac and mesenteric or retroperitoneal lymph nodes. In a large recent European multicenter study (81), MRI showed an agreement in T-staging of 57% with 19% overstaging and 24% understaging. It was also very accurate in predicting the extramural depth of tumor invading the mesorectum. MRI was able to identify large T3 and T4 tumors and invasion of the mesorectal fascia. Because of the accurate depiction of large tumoral mass, it is often said that with MRI "what you see is what you get" (66). Most failures of MRI occur in the differentiation between T1 and T2 lesions and between T2 and borderline T3 lesions. A T1 tumor cannot be reliably distinguished from T2 because the submucosal layer is generally not visualized on phased array MRI. Like ERUS, MRI has some difficulty in differentiating lesions on the border of T2 and T3 from a desmoplastic reaction. MRI with endorectal coils has been studied in a number of small size studies for the evaluation and staging of rectal tumors (82). With the addition of endorectal surface coils to conventional MR imaging, spatial resolution has increased and anatomic definition improved. T2-weighted turbo spin-echo sequences allow to distinguish the five layers of the rectal wall. Rectal carcinoma in T2-weighted turbo spin-echo sequences has medium-to-low signal intensity, higher than the muscular layer. MRI and ERUS demonstrate similar efficacy in the preoperative staging of rectal tumors. Overall accuracy rates of 70-90% have been reported for staging of rectal tumors using MRI with endorectal coils. However, coils are too expensive and not used worldwide. A further limitation of MRI with endoanal coils is the inability to advance the coil through a stricture caused by advanced rectal cancer. In the evaluation of lymph nodes, MRI does not offer significant improvement in accuracy rates compared with ERUS.

In conclusion, ERUS is currently the best modality for the preoperative staging of rectal cancer. It is not alternative, but rather complementary to high-resolution MRI. Future improvements may include the possibility to visualize the mesorectal fascia or to better evaluate lymph nodes less than 5mm in diameter. ERUS is much less expensive than MRI and it can be readily used in the office, immediately providing important information for treatment planning. MRI has the advantage, over ERUS, that the images can be more easily interpreted and evaluated by other radiologists, clinicians and oncologists. The images can also be used by radiotherapists for planning the radiotherapy fields and by surgeons to guide the resection in advanced cases.

7. References

[1] Hildebrandt U, Feifel G. Preoperative staging of rectal cancer by intrarectal ultrasound. Dis Colon Rectum 1985; 28: 42-46

[2] Benson AB 3rd, Choti MA, Cohen AM, et al. NCCN practice guidelines for colorectal cancer. Oncology 2000; 14: 203-212

[3] Glimelius B, Oliveira J. Rectal cancer: ESMO clinical recommendations for diagnosis, treatment and follow-up. Ann Oncol 2008; 19 (Suppl 2): ii31- ii32

[4] Van Cutsem E, Dicato M, Haustermans K, et al. The diagnosis and management of rectal cancer: expert discussion and recommendations derived from the 9th World Congress on Gastrointestinal Cancer, Barcelona 2007. Ann Oncol 2008; 19 (Suppl 6): vi1-vi8

[5] Engstrom PF, Arnoletti JP, Benson AB 3rd et al. NCCN clinical practice in oncology: rectal cancer. J Natl Compr Canc Netw 2009; 7: 838-881

[6] DCCG Danish national guidelines for rectal cancer treatment 2009. http://www.kirurgiskselskab. dk/dks/krc.htm#top

[7] Association Francaise de Chirurgie. French national guidelines for rectal cancer treatment. Gastroenterol Clin Biol 2007; 31:1s9-1s22

[8] Norwegian Gastrointestinal Cancer Group. Kontrollopplegg ved kolorectalcancer (Norwegian Guidelines) 2007. Available at http//www.ngicg.no/gronnbok/gronnbok.htm

[9] Glimelius B, Beets-Tan R, Blomqvist L, et al. Mesorectal fascia instead of circumferential resection margin in preoperative staging of rectal cancer. J Clin Oncol 201; 29: 1-2

[10] Li JC, Liu SY, Lo AW, et al. The learning curve for endorectal ultrasonography in rectal cancer staging. Surg Endosc 2010; 24: 3054-3059

[11] Lohnert MSS, Doniec JM, Henne-Bruns D. Effectiveness of endoluminal sonography in the identification of occult local rectal cancer recurrences. Dis Colon Rectum 2000; 43: 483-491

[12] Saclarides TJ. Endorectal ultrasound. Surg Clin North Am 1998; 78: 237-249

[13] Santoro GA, D'Elia A, Battistella G, Di Falco G. The use of a dedicated rectosigmoidoscope for ultrasound staging of tumours of the upper and middle third of the rectum. Colorectal Dis 2007; 9: 61-66

[14] Goertz RS, Fein M, Sailer M. Impact of biopsy on the accuracy of endorectal ultrasound staging of rectal tumors. Dis Colon Rectum 2008; 51: 1125-1129

[15] Koh DH, Brown G, Temple L et al. Distribution of mesorectal lymph nodes in rectal cancer: in vivo MR imaging compared with histopathological examination: initial observation. Eur Radiol 2005; 15: 1650-1657

[16] Shaffazin DM, Wong WD. Endorectal ultrasound in the preoperative evaluation of rectal cancer. Clin Colorectal Cancer 2004; 4: 124-132

[17] Kim HJ, Wong WD. Role of endorectal ultrasound in the conservative management of rectal cancers. Semin Surg Oncol 2000; 19: 358-366

[18] Rifkin MD, Ehrlich SM, and Marks G. Staging of rectal carcinoma: prospective comparison of endorectal US and CT. Radiology 1989; 170: 319-322

[19] Rivadeneira DE, Wong WD. Preoperative staging of rectal cancer. Clin Colon Rectal Surg 2002; 1: 17-26

[20] Heintz A, Buess G, Frank K, et al. Endoluminal ultrasonic examination of sessile polyps and early carcinomas of the rectum. Surg Endosc 1989; 3: 92-95

[21] Adams WJ, Wong WD. Endorectal ultrasonic detection of malignancy within rectal villous lesions. Dis Colon Rectum 1995; 38: 1093-1096
[22] Haggit RC, Glotzbach RE, Soffer RE, Wrouble LD. Prognostic factors in colorectal carcinomas arising in adenomas: implications for lesions removed by endoscopic polypectomy. Gastroenterology 1985; 89: 328-336
[23] Nivatvongs S, Rojanasakul A, Reiman HM et al. The risk of lymph node metastasis in colorectal polyps with invasive adenocarcinoma. Dis Colon Rectum 1991; 34: 323-328
[24] Suzuki T, Sadahiro S, Marukoyama S, et al. Risk of lymph node and distant metastases in patients with early invasive colorectal cancer classified as Haggit's level 4 invasion: image analysis of submucosal layer invasion. Dis Colon Rectum 2003; 46: 203-208
[25] Seitz U, Bohnacker S, Seewald S, et al. Is endoscopic polypectomy an adequate therapy for malignant colorectal adenomas? Presentation of 114 patients and review of the literature. Dis Colon Rectum 2004; 47: 1789-1797
[26] Kudo S. Endoscopic mucosal resection of flat and depressed types of early colorectal cancer. Endoscopy 1993; 25: 455-461
[27] Kikuchi R, Takano M, Takagi K et al. Management of early invasive colorectal cancer: risk of recurrence and clinical guidelines. Dis Colon Rectum 1995; 38: 710-717
[28] Akasu T, Kondo H, Moriya Y et al. Endorectal ultrasonography and treatment of early stage rectal cancer. World J Surg 2000; 24: 1061-1068
[29] Nascimbeni R, Nivatvongs S, Larson DR, Burgart LJ. Long-term survival after local excision for T1 carcinoma of the rectum. Dis Colon Rectum 2004; 47: 1773-1779
[30] Mellgren A, Sirivongs P, Rothenberger DA, et al. Is local excision adequate therapy for early rectal cancer? Dis Colon Rectum 2000; 43: 1064-1071
[31] Kim J, Yu CS, Jung HY et al. Source of error in the evaluation of early rectal cancer by endoluminal ultrasonography. Dis Colon Rectum 2001; 44: 1302-1309
[32] Maier AG, Barton PB, Neuhold NR et al. Peritumoral tissue reaction at transrectal US as a possible cause of overstaging in rectal cancer: histopathologic correlation. Radiology 1997; 203: 785-789
[33] Hulsmans FJH, Tio TL, Fockens P et al. Assessment of tumor infiltration depth in rectal cancer with transrectal sonography: caution is necessary. Radiology 1994; 190: 715-720
[34] Solomon MJ, McLeod RS, Cohen EK et al. Reliability and validity studies of endoluminal ultrasonography for anorectal disorders. Dis Colon Rectum 1994; 37: 546-551
[35] Santoro GA, Di Falco G. Endorectal ultrasound in the preparative staging of rectal cancer. In: Santoro GA, Di Falco G (eds). Atlas of endoanal and endorectal ultrasonography. Springer-Verlag Italia, Milan 2004: 11-21
[36] Muthusamy VA, Chang KJ. Optimal methods for staging rectal cancer. Clin Cancer Res 2007; 13: 6877-6884
[37] Hulsmans FJ, Bosma PA, Mulder PJ et al. Perirectal lymph nodes in rectal cancer: in vitro correlation of sonographic parameters in histologic findings. Radiology 1992; 184: 553

[38] Janjan NA, Crane C, Feig BW, et al. Improved overall survival among responders to preoperative chemoradiation for locally advanced rectal cancer. Am J Clin Oncol 2001; 24: 107-112
[39] Sitzler PJ, Seow-Choen F, Ho YH, et al. Lymph node involvement and tumor depth in rectal cancers: an analysis of 805 patients. Dis Colon Rectum 1997; 40: 1472-1476
[40] Beynon J, Mortensen NJ, Foy DM, et al. Preoperative assessment of mesorectal lymph node involvement in rectal cancer. Br J Surg 1989; 76: 276-279
[41] Herzog U, von Flue M, Tondelli P, et al. How accurate is endorectal ultrasound in the preoperative staging of rectal cancer? Dis Colon Rectum 1993; 36: 127-134
[42] Goldman S, Arvidsson H, Norming U, et al. Transrectal ultrasound and computer tomography in preoperative staging of lower rectal adenocarcinoma. Gastrointest Radiol 1991; 16: 259-263
[43] Civelli EM, Gallino G, Mariani L, et al. Double-contrast barium enema and computerized tomography in the preoperative evaluation of rectal carcinoma: are they still useful diagnostic procedures? Tumori 2000; 86: 389-392
[44] Ptok H, Marush F, Meyer F, et al. Feasibility and accuracy of TRUS in the pre-treatment staging for rectal carcinoma in general practice. Eur J Surg Oncol 2006; 32: 420-425
[45] Rieger N, Tjandra J, Solomon M. Endoanal and endorectal ultrasound: applications in colorectal surgery. ANZ J Surg 2004; 74: 671-675
[46] Kim NK, Kim MJ, Yun SH, et al. Comparative study of transrectal ultrasonography, pelvic computerized tomography, and magnetic resonance imaging in preoperative staging of rectal cancer. Dis Colon Rectum 1999; 42: 770-775
[47] Garcia-Aguilar J, Pollack J, Lee SH, et al. Accuracy of endorectal ultrasonography in preoperative staging of rectal tumors. Dis Colon Rectum 2002; 45:10-15
[48] Orrom WJ, Wong WD, Rothenberger DA, et al. Endorectal ultrasound in the preoperative staging of rectal tumors. A learning experience. Dis Colon Rectum 1990; 33: 654-659
[49] Worrell S, Horvath K, Blakemore T, Flum D. Endorectal ultrasound detection of focal carcinoma within rectal adenomas. Am J Surg 2004; 187: 625-629
[50] Baynon J. An evaluation of the role of rectal endosonography in rectal cancer. Ann R Coll Surg Engl 1989; 71: 131-139
[51] Kim JC, Kim HC, Yu SC, et al. Efficacy of 3-dimensional endorectal ultrasonography compared with conventional ultrasonography and computed tomography in preoperative rectal cancer staging. Am J Surg 2006; 192: 89-97
[52] Assenat T, Thézenas S, Samalin E, et al. The value of endoscopic rectal ultrasound in predictingthe lateral clearance and outcome in patients with lower third rectal adenocarcinoma. Endoscopy 2007; 39: 309-313
[53] Garcia-Aguilar J, Hernàndez de Anad E, Rothenberger DA et al. Endorectal ultrasound in the management of patients with malignant rectal polyps. Dis Colon Rectum 2005; 48: 910-917
[54] Kruskal JB, Sentovich SM, Kane RA. Staging of rectal polyps after polypectomy: usefulness of endorectal US. Radiology 1999; 211: 31-35
[55] Santoro GA, Gizzi G, Pellegrini L et al. The value of high-resolution three-dimensional endorectal ultrasonography in the management of submucosal invasive rectal cancer. Dis Colon Rectum 2009; 52: 1837-1843

[56] Pikarsky A, Wexner S, Lebensart P, et al. The use of rectal ultrasound for the correct diagnosis and treatment of rectal villous tumors. Am J Surg 2000; 179: 261-265
[57] Konishi K, Akita Y, Kaneko K, et al. Evaluation of endoscopic ultrasonography in colorectal villous lesions. Int J Colorectal Dis 2003; 18: 19-24
[58] Akahoshi K, Yoshinaga S, Soejima a, et al. Transit endoscopic ultrasound of colorectal cancer using 12MHz catheter probe. Br J Radiol 2001; 74: 1017-1022
[59] Starck M, Bohe M, Simanaitis M, Valentin L. Rectal endosonography can distinguish benign rectal lesions and invasive early rectal cancers. Colorectal Dis 2003; 5: 246-250
[60] Hunerbein M, Handke T, Ulmer C, Shlag PM. Impact of miniprobe ultrasonography on planning of minimally invasive surgery for gastric and colonic tumors. Surg Endosc 2004; 18: 601-605
[61] Santoro GA, Bara Egan D, Di Falco G. Three dimensional endorectal ultrasonography in the evaluation of early invasive rectal cancer. Colorectal Dis 2004; 6 (Suppl 2): 20
[62] Sailer M, Leppert R, Kramer M, et al. The value of endorectal ultrasound in the assessment of adenomas, T1- and T2-carcinomas. Int J Colorectal Dis 1997; 12: 214-219
[63] Massari M, De Simone M, Cioffi U, et al. Value and limits of endorectal ultrasonography for preoperative staging of rectal carcinoma. Surg Laparosc Endosc. 1998; 8: 438-444
[64] Katsura Y, Yamada K, Ishizawa T et al, Endorectal ultrasonography for the assessment of wall invasion and lymph node metastasis in rectal cancer. Dis Colon Rectum 1992; 35: 362-368
[65] Kim JC, Cho YK, Kim SY, et al. Comparative study of three-dimensional and conventional rectal ultrasonography for the assessment of wall invasion and lymph node metastasis in rectal cancer. Surg Endosc 2002; 16: 1280-1285
[66] Beets GL, Beets-Tan RGH. Pretherapy imaging of rectal cancers: ERUS or MRI? Surg Oncol Clin N Am 2010; 19: 733-741
[67] Glaser F, Shlag P, Herfarth CH. Endorectal ultrasonography for the assessment of invasion of rectal tumors and lymph node involvement. Br J Surg 1990; 77: 883-887
[68] Marusch F, Koch A, Schmidt U, et al. Routine use of transrectal ultrasound in rectal carcinoma: results of a prospective multicenter study. Endoscopy 2002; 34: 385-390
[69] Kauer WK, Prantl L, Ditter HJ et al. The value of endosonographic rectal carcinoma staging in routine diagnostics: a 10-year analysis. Surg Endosc 2004;18: 1075-1078
[70] Badger SA, Devlin PB, NeillyPJ, Gilliand R. Preoperative staging of rectal carcinoma by endorectal ultrasound: is there a learning curve? Int J Colorectal Dis 2007; 22: 1261-1268
[71] Puli SR, Reddy JBK, Bechtold ML, et al. Accuracy of endoscopic ultrasound to diagnose nodal invasion by rectal cancers. a meta-analysis and systematic review. Ann Surg Oncol 2009; 16: 1255-1265
[72] Siddiqui AA, Fayiga Y, Huerta S. The role of endoscopic ultrasound in the evaluation of rectal cancer. Int Semin Surg Oncol 2006; 3: 36-42
[73] Holdsworth PJ, Johnston D, Chalmers AG et al. Endoluminal ultrasound and computer tomography in the staging of rectal cancer. Br J Surg 1988; 75: 1019-1022
[74] Sentovich S, Blatchford G, Falk P et al. Transrectal ultrasound of rectal tumore. Am J Surg 1993; 166: 638-641

[75] Senesse P, Khemissa F, Lemanski C, et al. Contribution of endorectal ultrasonography in preoperative evaluation for very low rectal cancer. Gastroenterol Clin Biol 2001; 25: 24-28

[76] Edelman BR, Weiser MR. Endorectal ultrasound: its role in the diagnosis and treatment of rectalcancer. Clin Colon Rectal Surg 2008; 21: 167-177

[77] Sailer M, Leppert R, Bussen D, et al. Influence of tumor position on accuracy of endorectal ultrasound imaging. Dis Colon Rectum 1997; 40: 1180-1186

[78] Brown G, Radcliffe AG, Newcombe RG et al. Preoperative assessment of prognostic factors in rectal cancer using high resolution magnetic resonance imaging. Br J Surg 2003; 90: 355-364

[79] Brown G, Davies S, Williams GT et al. Effectiveness of preoperative staging in rectal cancer: digital rectal examination, endoluminal ultrasound or magnetic resonance imaging? Br J Cancer 2004; 91: 23-29

[80] Bipat S, Glas AS, Slors FJM, et al. Rectal cancer: local staging and assessment of lymph node involvement with endoluminal US, CT and MR imaging. a meta-analysis. Radiology 2004; 232: 773-783

[81] MERCURY Study Group. Extramural depth of tumor invasion at thin-section MR in patients with rectal cancer: results of the MERCURY study. Radiology 2007; 243: 132-139

[82] Meyenberger C, Huch Boni RA, Bertschinger P et al. Endoscopic ultrasound and endorectal magnetic resonance imaging: a prospective, comparative study for preoperative staging and follow-up of rectal cancer. Endoscopy 1995; 27: 469-479

5

Dynamic Contrast Enhanced Magnetic Resonance Imaging in Rectal Cancer

Roberta Fusco[1], Mario Sansone[1], Mario Petrillo[2], Antonio Avallone[3], Paolo Delrio[3] and Antonella Petrillo[3]
[1]*Department of Biomedical, Electronics and Telecommunications Engineering University 'Federico II' of Naples*
[2]*Department of Radiology, Second University of Naples*
[3]*IRCCS National Cancer Institute, Fondazione Pascale, Naples*
Italy

1. Introduction

In the last few years the clinical management of rectal cancer has become very complex. A wide spectrum of therapeutic options is available. Magnetic Resonance Imaging (MRI) could play a pivotal rule in the prognostic and therapeutic assessment of rectal cancer (Chen et al., 2005).

As known, MRI can provide information about the stage of the disease according to TNM classification focussing on the depth of mesorectal invasion and on lymph node involvement inside and outside the mesorectum (Beets-Tan & Beets, 2004; Gunderson et al., 2004). Due to its intrinsic multiparametricity and multiplanarity MRI is considered the 'gold standard' particularly in differentiating between intramural and extramural disease, and in the management of Locally Advanced Rectal Cancer (LARC) (Beets-Tan & Beets, 2004; Petrillo et al., 2006).

The common use of total mesorectal excision (TME) and the shift from a postoperative to a preoperative chemo-radiotherapy (pre-CRT) approach have substantially reduced the risk of local recurrences, increasing curative resection and the rate of anal sphincter preservation and improving local control and overall survival rates (Avallone et al., 2006; 2011; Delrio et al., 2005; 2003).

Although morphological tumour assessment performed by MRI has been repeatedly shown to be the most accurate modality in evaluating the presence of a positive circumferential resection margin (CRM), MRI is considered not to be conclusive in pre-CRT tumor response evaluation since histopathological downstage is not always associated with tumour effective reduction (Petrillo et al., 2007). The main difficulty regarding post-chemoradiation MRI includes discrimination of active tumour and post-treatment fibrosis, particularly when differentiating stage T2 and stage T3 carcinomas, according to different recurrence and overall survival rates between Low Risk (T1/T2N0) and Intermediate Risk (T3/N0) as reported by Gunderson et al. (2002; 2004).

Previous considerations support a Dynamic Contrast Enhanced-Magnetic Resonance Imaging (DCE-MRI) approach that could gain a renewed role to MRI adding functional data to the morphological examination. DCE-MRI has been reported by many authors as a tool potentially able to permit an evaluation of pre-CRT effectiveness basing on the strict relationship between tumor growth and angiogenesis (Ceelen et al., 2006; de Lussanet et al., 2005; Kremser et al., 2007).

DCE-MRI is gaining a large consensus as a technique for diagnosis, staging and assessment of therapy response for different types of tumours, due to its capability to detect highly active angiogenesis. It is well known that angiogenesis is a key factor in the growth and dissemination of cancer; characterisation of the angiogenic status of the tumour on an individual patient basis could allow for a more targeted approach to treatment of rectal cancer (Goh et al., 2007; Kapse & Goh, 2009).

More specifically, in the case of rectal cancer, previous trials have provided the proof of principle that inhibition of angiogenesis has the potential to enhance the effectiveness of the treatment for this disease. In vivo imaging techniques capable to assess tumour perfusion have the potential to improve the management of treatment for patients with rectal cancer (Chen et al., 2005; de Vries et al., 2000; 2001; 2003; Kremser et al., 2007).

The aim of this chapter is to review the main issues concerning the assessment of the angiogenic status of rectal cancer by means of DCE-MRI. More specifically, the aim of this chapter is to present:

- a review of the widespread methodologies used for DCE-MRI data acquisition and analysis;
- the main findings of scientific literature concerning DCE-MRI evaluation of rectal cancer.

2. DCE-MRI basis

Cancer can develop in any tissue of the body that contains cells capable of division. The earliest detectable malignant lesions, referred to as *cancer in situ*, are often a few millimeters or less in diameter and at an early stage are commonly avascular. In avascular tumours cellular nutrition depends on diffusion of nutrients and waste materials and places a severe limitation on the size that such a tumour can achieve. The maximum diameter of an avascular solid tumour is approximately $150 - 200\mu m$, and is governed effectively by the maximum diffusion distance of oxygen. Conversion of a dormant tumour in situ to a more rapidly growing invasive neoplasm, may take several years and is associated with vascularization of the tumour. The development of neo-vascularization within a tumour results from a process known as angiogenesis.

There are positive and negative regulators of angiogenesis. Release of a promoter substance stimulates the endothelial cells of the existing vasculature close to the neoplasia to initiate the formation of solid endothelial sprouts that grow toward the solid tumour (Knopp et al., 1999). Vascular endothelial growth factor (VEGF) also known as vascular permeability factor (VPF), induces angiogenesis and strongly increases microvascular permeability to plasma proteins. As vascular growth factors are released, proteases are also induced to degrade perivascular tissue, allowing the endothelial cells to proliferate and form primitive, immature, and, therefore, leaky vessels (Dor et al., 2001; Guetz et al., 2006). Figure 1 summarizes the main phases of tumor vasculature development.

Therefore, the morphology of the neo-vascular network in tumours can differ significantly from that seen in normal tissue. Tumour vasculature is often highly heterogeneous, and the capillaries are extremely coarse, irregularly constricted or dilated and distorted.

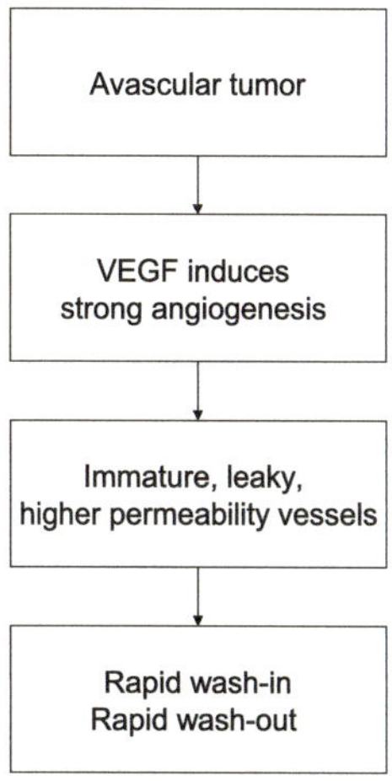

Fig. 1. A summary of the main phases of tumor vasculature development (angiogenesis) and the effects that are measurable by means of DCE-MRI.

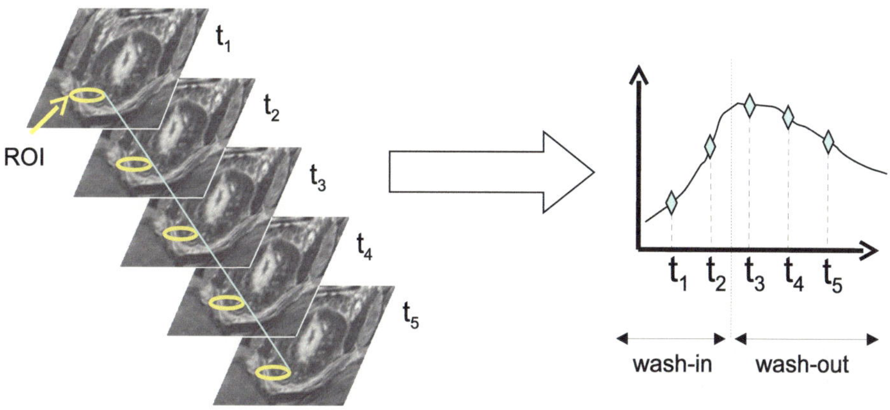

Fig. 2. DCE-MRI in rectal cancer: a series of T_1-weighted images before and after CA injection; the time-intensity curve of the selected region of interest (ROI) is also shown.

Angiogenic inhibitors can reduce both the number of vessels (particularly nonfunctional vessels) and their permeability. Some therapies, such as anti-vascular endothelial growth factor antibody (antiVEGF Ab), are specifically directed against a growth factor (VEGF) and are thought to regulate vascular maturation and permeability (Lichtenbeld et al., 1999).
While avascular tumours are not detectable by MRI (Choyke et al., 2003), DCE-MRI can help to characterise vascularized cancers (Leach et al., 2005). After intravenous injection, the contrast agent (CA) pass through the tumor vasculature and immediately leaks through the vessels walls accumulating in the extravascular extracellular space (EES) because of the concentration gradient (wash-in phase, see fig. 2). Hereafter, CA concentration within plasma will return lower than EES and backflow will occur (wash-out phase). Using specific T_1-weighted pulse sequences the accumulation of CA causes an increase of signal intensity (enhancement) on images (fig. 2). Malignant tumors generally show faster and higher levels of enhancement than is seen in normal tissue. DCE-MRI is currently widely used in the study of tumour angiogenesis and in the development and trial of anti angiogenic drugs.

3. DCE-MRI data acquisition

Several issues of data acquisition should be taken into account when developing protocols for DCE-MRI, both to facilitate the integration of results from multiple institutions and to ensure that the data reflect the underlying physiology as accurately as possible (Ashton, 2010; Evelhoch, 1999; Leach et al., 2005).
In particular, the type of data acquisition affects the data analysis procedure: while semi-quantitative model-free analysis (see section 4) can be performed without accurate measurement of CA concentration, a full model-based approach requires accurate CA quantification.
Key factors affecting DCE-MRI of rectal cancer include: type of contrast agents and the relationship between CA concentration and signal enhancement; constraints concerning spatial and temporal resolution; the impact of patient motion.

3.1 Relationship between contrast agent concentration and signal enhancement

It is generally assumed that the relaxation rate ($R_1 = 1/T_1$) of soft tissues is linearly related to the mean tissue CA concentration (C_T) via the Bloembergen and Solomon equation:

$$R_1 = \frac{1}{T_1} = \frac{1}{T_{1,0}} + r_1 C_T = R_{1,0} + r_1 C_T \tag{1}$$

where $T_{1,0}$ and $R_{1,0}$ are, respectively, the relaxation time and the relaxation rate of the tissue in absence of CA and the proportionality constant r_1 is called 'relaxivity'.
Main properties concerning the relaxivity include: it depends upon the macromolecular environment; it is dependent on the type of macromolecule to which the Gd ion is attached; it decreases with external magnetic field; it increases with temperature; and it is also dependent on the pH of the solution (Stanisz & Henkelman, 2000).
However, most studies assume that r_1 is constant at a given temperature and magnetic field and that it is independent on the tissue environment. The typical value used for r_1, estimated in pure saline water, is 4.5 L/mmol/s per kg of water (Stanisz & Henkelman, 2000).
In typical DCE-MRI experiments, T_1-weighted spoiled gradient-echo sequences are used. In this case the signal intensity S has the following expression (Sourbron, 2010):

$$S = \rho \cdot g \cdot \frac{\sin\alpha \cdot (1 - \exp(-T_R/T_1))}{1 - \cos\alpha \cdot \exp(-T_R/T_1)} \cdot \exp(-T_E/T_2^*) \tag{2}$$

where ρ is the proton density, g is a constant determined by system receiver and image reconstruction settings, α is the flip angle, T_R is the repetition time, T_E is the echo time, T_2^* is the transverse relaxation time taking into account field inhomogeneity .
If it is assumed that Gd ions have no effect on ρ and that the T_E is so short to neglect the influence of T_2 (or, more importantly, changes in T_2^* during the series), then the Gd ions can influence the signal intensity only by means of their effect on T_1 (decrease of T_1). Under these assumptions, and as α approaches 90° and $T_R \ll T_1$ the relationship between signal intensity and $1/T_1$ becomes approximately linear:

$$S \approx \rho \cdot g \cdot \frac{T_R}{T_1} \tag{3}$$

this relationship remains approximately valid across a range of values for T_R/T_1 and α.
Therefore, an estimate of CA concentration can be obtained using eq. (1) and eq. (3):

$$[Gd] = \frac{1}{r_1}\left(\frac{1}{T_1} - \frac{1}{T_{1,0}}\right) \approx \frac{S - S_0}{r_1 \cdot \rho \cdot g \cdot T_R} \tag{4}$$

where S_0, S, $T_{1,0}$ and T_1 are the signal intensities and spin-lattice relaxation times before and after administration of contrast agent respectively. The difference $S - S_0$ is called *signal enhancement*.

The difficulty in comparing different studies comes from the nature of g: in fact, the loading of the coil, the receiver settings at the MR console and image reconstruction parameters can be different among several studies.

Therefore, it could be more advantageous to normalise with respect to the pre-contrast signal intensity:

$$[Gd] \approx \frac{S - S_0}{S_0}\frac{1}{r_1 \cdot T_{1,0}}. \tag{5}$$

The quantity $(S - S_0)/S_0$ is called *relative signal enhancement*. Consequently, the concentration of CA is related to both r_1 and $T_{1,0}$ of tissue.

As observed before, the relaxivity r_1 can be considered fixed for soft tissues. As far as the longitudinal relaxation time prior to contrast injection ($T_{1,0}$) it can be easily measured before CA administration using opportune pulse sequences (Collins & Padhani, 2004).

One common method for $T_{1,0}$ estimation is to use several gradient-echo (GRE) images with variable flip angles. In fact, rearranging eq. (2) that equation yields (Parker et al., 1997):

$$Y(\alpha) = X(\alpha) \cdot \exp(-T_R/T_{1,0}) - \rho g(1 - \exp(-T_R/T_{1,0}))\exp(-T_E/T_2^*) \tag{6}$$

where $Y(\alpha) = S_\alpha/\sin\alpha$ and $X(\alpha) = S_\alpha/\tan\alpha$. Hence a plot of $Y(\alpha)$ against $X(\alpha)$ for several (typically three or more) flip angles will result in a straight line and $T_{1,0}$ can be calculated from the slope (via standard linear regression).

3.2 Spatial and temporal resolution

The requirements for temporal and spatial resolution for a particular oncologic application often are in direct conflict. Both the importance for high temporal resolution to accurately characterize contrast kinetics and the need for high spatial resolution to identify distinguishing features of lesion morphology have been investigated in several studies (Cheng, 2008; Dale et al., 2003; Evelhoch, 1999; Henderson et al., 1998).

In general, it can be stated that for an accurate estimation of tracer kinetics parameters, a short interval between samples must be used, especially for the analysis of the wash-in phase. For example, Henderson et al. (1998) found that this interval should be approximately less than 16 s in the case of breast DCE-MRI. In the wash-out phase, this requirement could be relaxed (de Vries et al., 2003; Kremser et al., 2007).

A high temporal resolution can be difficult to obtain because the acquisition of a single volume could require several seconds as a large part of the whole abdomen is scanned. One approach to overcome this problem is to choose a single slice containing the tumor, so that the sampling interval can be maintained below a few seconds (Blomqvist et al., 1998; Ceelen et al., 2006; de Lussanet et al., 2005). However, this approach is not able to manage with the heterogeneity of the tumour (Jackson et al., 2007). An hybrid approach could involve a rapid imaging with low spatial resolution in the wash-in phase while a slow, high-resolution imaging could be adopted in the wash-out phase (de Vries et al., 2000; 2003).

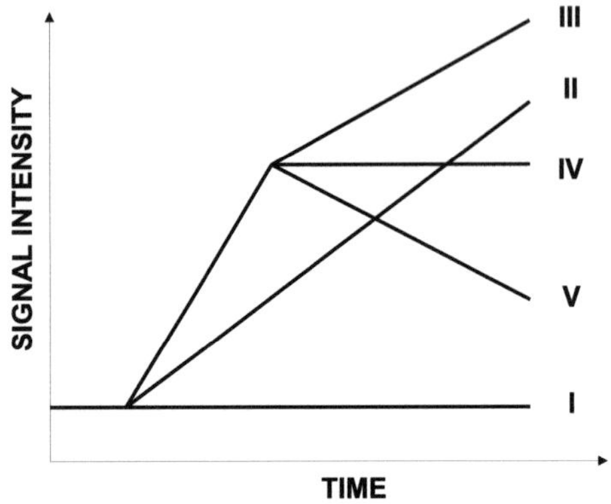

Fig. 3. Classification system for semi-quantitative of the TICs. The level of angiogenesis is supposed to increase with the number of the curve-type: (I) no enhancement; (II) slow sustained enhancement; (III) rapid initial and sustained late enhancement (persistent); (IV) rapid initial and stable late enhancement (plateau); (V) rapid initial and decreasing late enhancement (wash-out). Curves from (I) to (III) are typically associated to normal or benign tissues; type (IV) can be classified as suspicious and (V) as malignant.

3.3 Patient motion

Since the TIC is sampled over several minutes, patient motion can become a serious obstacle to an accurate evaluation of kinetic parameters. Motion correction should be applied before any tracer kinetics analysis is performed (Fei et al., 2002). However, 2D or 3D registration is difficult because the signal intensity of a pixel can change over time both because of spatial displacement and CA absorption. Therefore, DCE-MRI specific methods are currently being developed for simultaneous iterative registration and tracer kinetics analysis (Buonaccorsi et al., 2007; Melbourne et al., 2007; Xiaohua et al., 2005).

4. DCE-MRI data analysis

Different methods for DCE-MRI data analysis have been proposed, ranging from simple semi-quantitative inspection of the time-intensity curves (TICs) to more sophisticated tracer kinetics modelling (Brix et al., 2010; Sourbron, 2010). The different methods were designed to capture the biologically relevant components from the dynamic MR signal and to relate them to the underlying pathophysiological processes taking place in the tissue.

In principle, the derivation of physiological data from DCE-MRI relies on the application of appropriate tracer kinetics models to describe the distribution of contrast media following its systemic administration. However, the application of these techniques is still complex and they cold not be widely available outside specialist centres. In response to this, many semi-quantitative approaches for the classification of enhancement curve shapes have been described and are now in relatively common use in clinical settings.

Both semi-quantitative and full-quantitative data analysis can be performed on a region of interest (ROI) basis or on a pixel-by-pixel basis. We will briefly describe the two approaches.

4.1 Semi-quantitative analysis

Semi-quantitative analysis can help the radiologist in classifying the TIC shape as normal, benign, malignant (see fig. 3). Classification of TICs according to this scheme can achieve very

good diagnostic performance in differentiating malignant from benign lesions as described in the case of breast lesions (Daniel et al., 1998; Kuhl, 2007; Nishiura et al., 2011).
As regards the rectal cancer, many papers explored the possibility to apply a semi-quantitative approach to lesion classification. Different TIC features have been used by the different authors, the aim being to extract as much physiological information as possible.
The approaches can be roughly subdivided in two classes. In a first type of approach, the classification of the TIC is performed by means of several features having, on an intuitive basis, a link with physiological characteristics (see fig. 4). As an example, Tuncbilek et al. (2004) used the maximal relative enhancement within the first minute (MSD_{1min}), the maximal relative enhancement of the entire study (MSD), the steepest slope (WIS_{max}). Similarly, Blomqvist et al. (1998) and Dicle et al. (1999) used MSD and WIS_{max}.
Another approach is to extract TIC features that are associated to tracer kinetics theory (see section 4.2). Within this framework de Lussanet et al. (2005); de Vries et al. (2000; 2001; 2003); Kremser et al. (2007) used, as a first step in quantitative assessment of tumor perfusion, the steepest slope of the TIC during contrast medium uptake (WIS_{max}), and, on the base of the work by Miles (1991) they evaluated the Perfusion Index (PI) as:

$$\begin{aligned} PI &= \frac{1}{\sigma_{tumor}} \left[\frac{dC_{tumor}/dt|_{max}}{C_{art}|_{max}} \right] \\ &= \frac{1}{\sigma_{tumor}} \left[\frac{WIS_{max}}{C_p(t)|_{max}} \right] \end{aligned} \tag{7}$$

where σ_{tumor} is tissue density. Although PI is an approximated parameter, it combines two important quantities: tissue perfusion and extraction fraction (Brix et al., 2010; Sourbron, 2010).
When calculated on a pixel-by-pixel basis the above parameters can be displayed graphically as pseudo-coloured maps superimposed on the corresponding morphological MR images (see section 4.3, fig. 7).
Figure 4 shows the most important parameters that have been used in several studies. The definitions of the several quantities are not always in accordance. Therefore we have tried to use a unifying terminology for semi-quantitative parameters (see tab. 1):

TTK time between the beginning of dynamic acquisition and the maximum enhancement;

TWI time between the onset of enhancement and the maximum enhancement;

TWO time between the maximum enhancement and the end of the acquisition;

MSD the maximum signal level with respect to the baseline;

WIS slope of the wash-in phase (increase in signal intensity between enhancement onset and maximum enhancement divided by time to peak);

WOS slope of the wash-out phase (decrease in signal intensity between maximum enhancement and the signal intensity at the end of acquisition divided by time TWO);

WII intercept of the wash-in straight-line with the y-axis;

WOI intercept of the wash-our straight-line with the y-axis;

AUCWI area under gadolinium curve in the was-in phase;

AUCWO are under gadolinium curve in the wash-out phase;

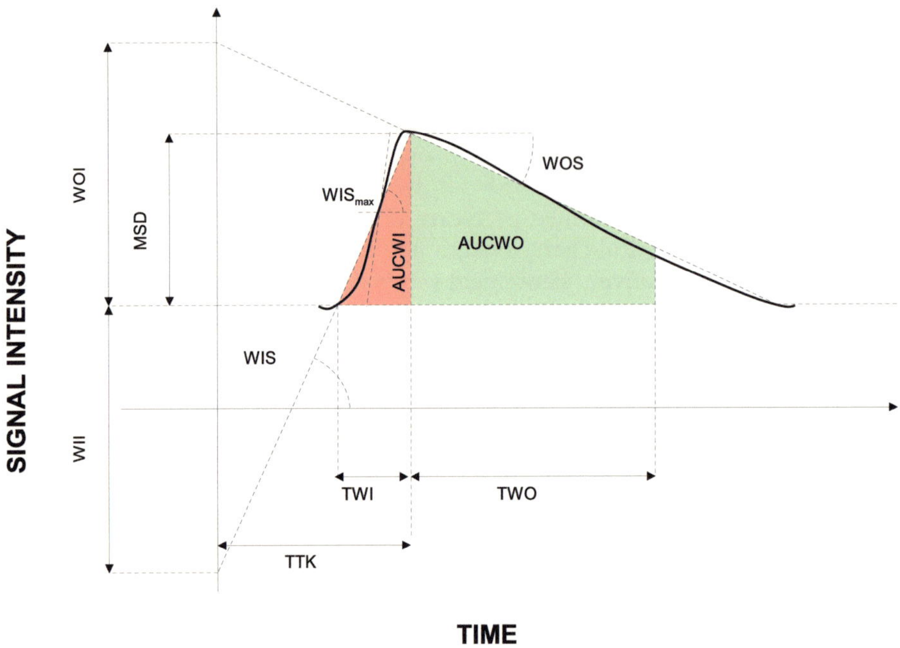

Fig. 4. Semi-quantitative analysis: illustration of the parameters calculated from the TIC. See table 1 for definition of terms.

Parameter	Definition
TTK	Time To Knee
TWI	Time of Wash-In
TWO	Time of Wash-Out
WII	Wash-In Intercept
WOI	Wash-Out Intercept
WIS	Wash-In slope
WOS	Wash-Out slope
MSD	Maximum Signal Difference
AUCWI	Area Under Wash-In
AUCWO	Area Under Wash-Out

Table 1. Semi-quantitative analysis: definition of terms in fig. 4

4.2 Tracer kinetics modelling

The flow of CA within the tissue of interest can be described using compartmental modelling. Different tracer kinetics modelling approaches have been proposed (Brix et al., 2010; Sourbron, 2010). The most widespread one is the two-compartments model (Tofts, 1997). The advantage of tracer kinetics modelling over semi-quantitative analysis is that it provides an estimate of physiological parameters directly related to vessels permeability and to blood flow (and therefore to the angiogenic status of the tissues).

In order to model CA kinetics in terms of physiologically meaningful parameters we first need to define the elements within the tissue and the functional processes that affect the distribution of the tracer. It is customary to represent the tissue as comprising three or four compartments (fig. 5). Major compartments are: the vascular plasma space, the extra-cellular extra-vascular

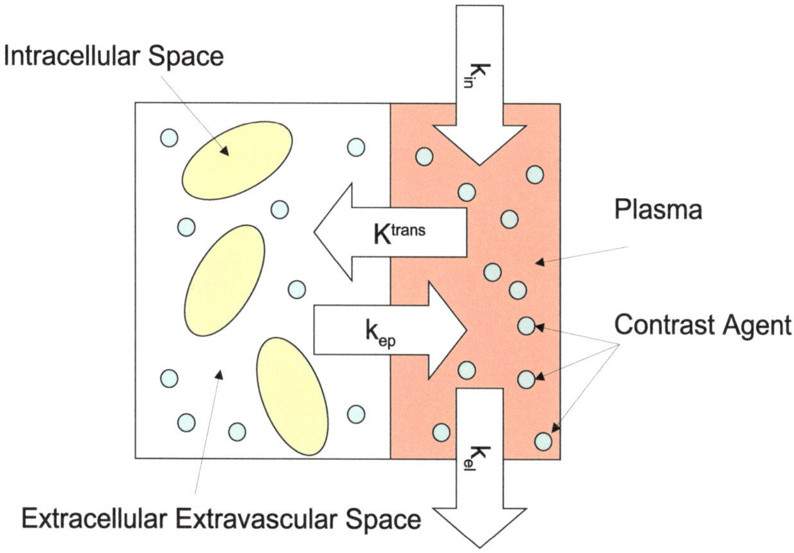

Fig. 5. Major compartments and functional variables involved in the distribution of the contrast agent in the tissue.

space (EES), and the intracellular space. A fourth tissue component forms a catch-all for all the other microscopic tissue components, such as membranes, fibrous tissues, etc.

All clinically utilised MRI contrast agents, and most experimental agents, do not pass into the intracellular space of the tissue, due to their size, inertness, and non-lipophilicity, making the intra-cellular space un-probable using DCE-MRI; for this reason, the intra-cellular and 'other' volumes are usually lumped together as a loosely defined 'intra-cellular' space.

We will indicate the quantities associated to the EES, plasma and intra-cellular compartments with the subscripts e, p and i respectively. The quantities associated to the whole tissue will be marked by a subscript T. The volume occupied by the different compartments may be expressed either as an absolute value (V_e,V_i,V_p,V_T) or as fractions (v_e,v_i,v_p) of V_T. They must satisfy the constraint:

$$v_e + v_p + v_i = 1. \tag{8}$$

All the models make some basic assumptions related to concepts in tracer kinetics. The most important are: the *linearity* of the tissue (the flux of CA between compartments is proportional to the difference of CA concentrations in the two compartments); the *stationarity* of the tissue (the parameters describing the compartments are constant during data acquisition); and the tissue is formed of *well-mixed compartments* (a compartment is said to be well-mixed when the CA immediately distributes over the whole compartmental volume). Under these assumptions the rate of wash-in and wash-out of the CA in the EES can be described by a modified general rate equation (Kety, 1951):

$$v_e \frac{dC_e}{dt} = K^{trans}(C_p(t) - C_e(t)), \tag{9}$$

where C_e and C_p are the CA concentrations [mmol/L] in V_e and V_p respectively; K^{trans} [min^{-1}] is the volume transfer constant between V_p and V_e (see fig. 5) (Tofts, 1997).

There exist a fundamental relationship between K^{trans} and v_e (Tofts et al., 1999):

$$k_{ep} = K^{trans}/v_e, \tag{10}$$

where k_{ep} is the *rate constant* (see fig. 5). The rate constant can be derived from the *shape* of the TIC.

The other two parameters in fig. 5 represent the input function from the injection of gadolinium based contrast (k_{in}) and the clearance rate (k_{el}) (Choyke et al., 2003).

Both blood plasma flow and blood perfusion (capillary permeability) contribute to the value of K^{trans}. If the flow of CA to the tissue is large, K^{trans} is dominated by the capillary wall permeability (permeability surface area, PS); if the delivery of CA to the tissue is insufficient, blood perfusion will be the dominant factor, and K^{trans} will be proportional to the blood flow F (volume of blood per unit time):

$$K^{trans} = F \cdot E \tag{11}$$

where E is the extraction fraction of the tracer $E = 1 - \exp(-\frac{PS}{F})$ (PS is the permeability surface area product).

The relationships described above form the basis of the models used to describe contrast agent kinetics by a number of researchers, and the conventions for the names and symbols used are now generally accepted (Tofts et al., 1999).

In normal tissues, the vascular volume is a small fraction $v_p \approx 0$ of the total tissue volume V_T (approximately 5% , although it can be considerably higher in some tissues), and it is sometimes assumed (largely as a matter of convenience) that the tracer concentration in the tissue as a whole, C_T, is not influenced to a large degree by the concentration in the vessels (i.e. $C_T = v_p C_p + v_e C_e \simeq v_e C_e$).

While this assumption is acceptable in abnormalities with small increase in blood volume, that are located in tissues with a relatively low normal blood volume, it is not valid in many contexts, especially because blood volume can largely increase in tumours.

Perhaps the most straightforward approach is to extend eq. 9 to include the concentration of contrast agent in the blood plasma, giving $C_T = v_p C_p + v_e C_e$. Using this relationship and eq. 9 we have the extended Tofts' model (see fig. 6):

$$C_T(t) = v_p C_p(t) + K^{trans} \int_0^t C_p(\tau) \exp\left(-\frac{K^{trans}}{v_e}(t-\tau)\right) d\tau, \tag{12}$$

More comprehensive models, such as the one proposed by St Lawrence & Lee (1998) can allow direct quantification of flow (F), extraction fraction (E), v_e and mean capillary transit time (MTT). Here, rather than defining a composite parameter K^{trans}, it is possible to separately estimate F and PS (permeability surface area product). As this model has many parameters, successful application requires a high temporal resolution and an accurate measurement of C_T, which limits its application in clinical trials. The tissue concentration is given by the following equation (St Lawrence & Lee, 1998):

$$C_T(t) = F \int_0^{MTT} C_p(t-u)du + E \cdot F \int_{MTT}^t C_p(u) e^{-\frac{E \cdot F}{v_e}(t-u-MTT)} du \tag{13}$$

In general, the aim of the compartmental analysis is to estimate the parameters K^{trans},v_p and v_e from DCE-MRI data (Leach et al., 2005). This problem can be seen either as a *system identification* problem or as a *non linear regression* problem (Sourbron, 2010). The limited scope of this chapter does not allow for a deep description of these techniques. We will instead discuss in further detail an important issue that is prominent whichever approach is used: the influence of $C_p(t)$, the arterial input function (AIF).

4.2.1 Influence of the arterial input function

>From eq. (12) it is clear that the C_T can be seen as the output of a linear system whose impulse response is determined by the tracer kinetics parameters K^{trans} ad v_e and whose input is the AIF. Therefore, errors in estimation of AIF can seriously affect the parameters estimates.
AIF can be obtained by direct measurement of blood flux (Yang et al., 2004). For example, Larsson et al. (1996) utilised an AIF measured from blood samples drawn from the brachial artery at intervals of 15 s during the DCE-MRI data acquisition. This method is not suitable for clinical practice and other approaches have been proposed.
One of the simplest methods was proposed by Brix et al. (1991): they assumed that AIF followed a mono-exponential model and included it as a third parameter directly into the TIC model (se fig. 6 (b)). Another approach for modelling of arterial flux was based on population parameters: the early application proposed by Tofts (1997) assumed a bi-exponential form of the AIF as previously found in normal population (Weinmann et al., 1984). Also multi-exponential modelling by means of nonlinear fitting of arterial flux measured directly on the images on a patient by patient basis has been investigated (Larsson et al., 1996).
Exponential modelling has shown to be only applicable when the sampling rate is relatively slow and there is a negligible plasma fraction. When the plasma fraction is non-negligible, this approach tends to over-estimate the volume transfer constant K_{trans}. To overcome this problem, Parker et al. (2006) measured a high temporal resolution population AIF on a large number of individuals and estimated the parameters of a sophisticated model. Later, Orton et al. (2008) proposed a computationally efficient version of this model decomposing the input function into a bolus model and a body transfer function:

$$C_p(t) = A_B t e^{-\mu_B t} + A_G(e^{-\mu_G t} - e^{-\mu_B t}). \tag{14}$$

A similar model for AIF has been previously proposed by Simpson et al. (1999):

$$C_p(t) = A \cdot t \cdot e^{-t \cdot B} + C[1 - e^{-t \cdot D}] \cdot e^{-t \cdot E} \tag{15}$$

where A, B, C, D, E were estimated on an individual basis.
Also, other approaches based on reference tissues have been proposed (Walker-Samuel et al., 2007; Yankeelov et al., 2005). The development of many analysis methods has proceeded in tandem with specific data acquisition programmes, and the modelling assumptions frequently reflected limitations imposed by the data. Care must therefore be taken in applying these methods in settings other than those originally intended and in comparing apparently compatible results from different studies using different models and/or data acquisitions.

4.3 ROI vs pixel-by-pixel

Region Of Interest (ROI)-based analysis involves the selection (manual or [semi]-automatic) of a ROI and subsequently averaging of the TICs over the ROI (fig. 2). The data-analysis is then applied on the averaged TIC. ROI-based analysis has the advantages of speed and ease of use; moreover, if the ROI is opportunely chosen the SNR can be increased. However, it has the disadvantage of intra-observer variability; moreover, ROI-based analysis could be unable to catch heterogeneity within the tumour (Jackson et al., 2007). Further, inappropriate selection

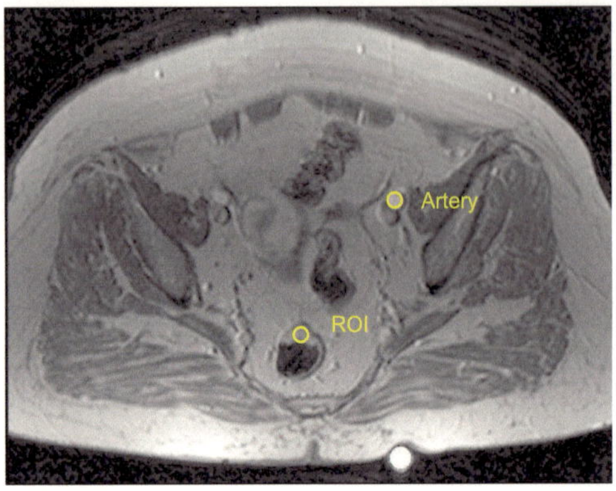

(a)

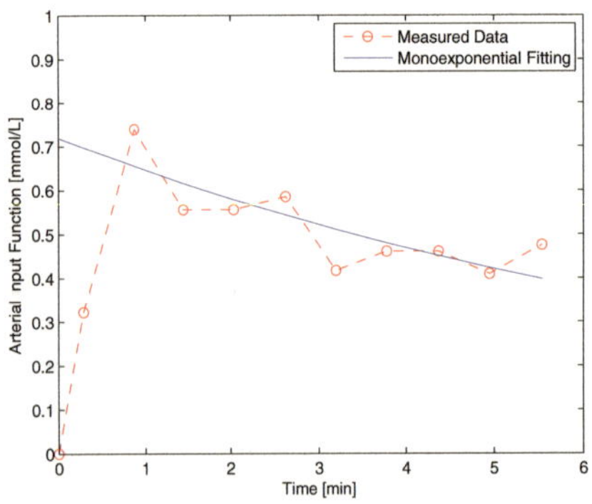

(b)

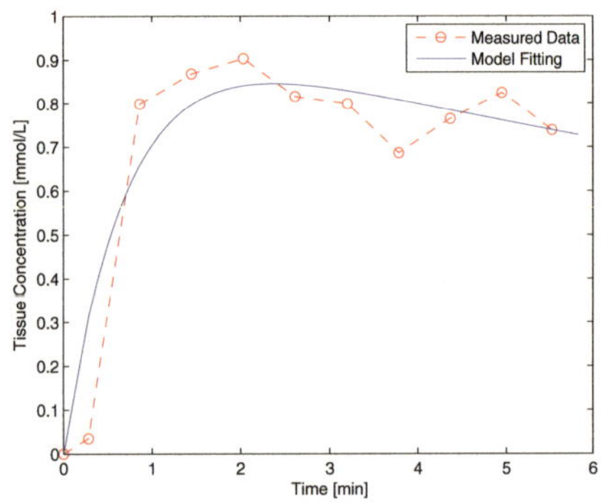

(c)

Fig. 6. a) The ROIs selected by an expert radiologist on the artery and on the tissue of interest; b) the time intensity curve of AIF; c) Curve fitting using the Tofts model.

of the ROI, so that it includes both enhancing and necrotic or non-enhancing components of the tumour, could give misleading interpretation.

These shortcomings can be addressed applying the data-analysis on a pixel-by-pixel basis obtaining a map for each chosen parameter (Fig. 7). Pixel by pixel analysis deals specifically with tumour heterogeneity and potentially provides a far wider range of information concerning tumour behaviour than is available from ROI analysis. Summary values within a ROI can subsequently be obtained averaging the parametric map. Unfortunately, the use of parametric images imposes significant further demands on the acquisition and analysis techniques. In particular, the use of pixel by pixel analysis assumes that there is negligible motion at the spatial resolution of the individual voxel.

An hybrid approach consists in using parametric maps for ROI selection and subsequent application of data analysis to the ROI. This approach can potentially benefit from both ROI-based and pixel-by-pixel processing (Sourbron, 2010).

Also, semi-automatic approaches for model-based segmentation of DCE-MRI images are currently being developed (Buonaccorsi et al., 2007; Kelm et al., 2009; Sansone et al., 2011; Schmid et al., 2006; Xiaohua et al., 2005)

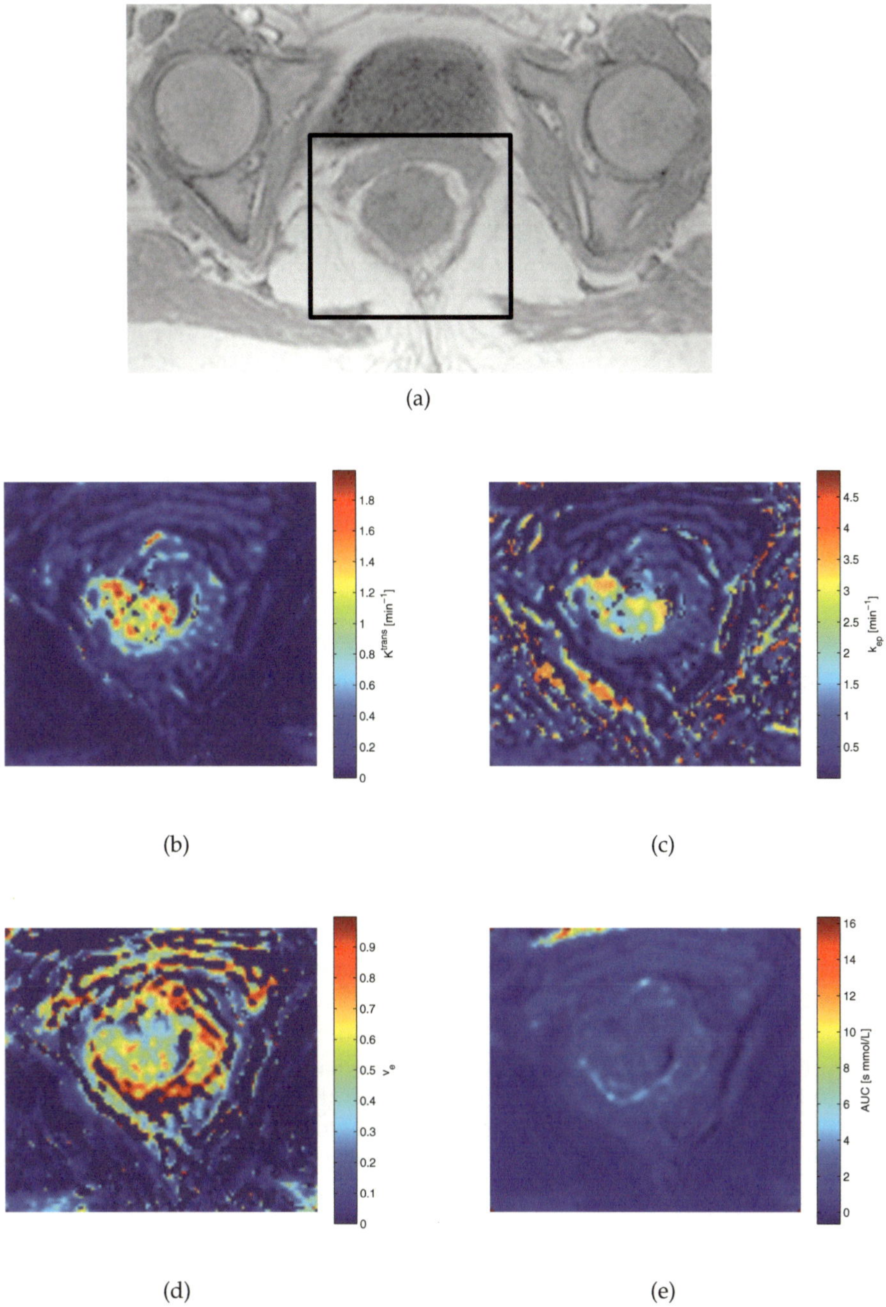

Fig. 7. Example of parametric maps. The pulse sequence had TE/TR/FlipAngle=4.76ms/9.8ms/25°, pixel resolution 0.6 x 0.6 mm x mm, sampling interval of 34 s. a) T_1-weighted image: the rectangle surrounds the ROI chosen by a radiologist; b) K^{trans} map; c) k_{ep} map; d) v_e map. e) Area under the Gd curve (AUC);

5. DCE-MRI in rectal cancer

In this section we will discuss a number of studies reporting findings concerning the application of DCE-MRI to rectal cancer. Mainly, DCE-MRI has been applied for both cancer staging and therapy response evaluation. Studies can be grouped according to the approach used: either semi-quantitative or full-quantitative (see section (4)).

As discussed in section (4), in principle, a full model-based approach should provide information directly related to vessels permeability and blood flow, thus evidencing vasculature modification caused by chemo-radiotherapy. However, drawbacks of this approach include: a great accuracy is required for gadolinium quantification; model choice is not always clear; parameters estimation is affected by the specific algorithm chosen. The semi-quantitative approach, instead, although providing summary information, roughly related to the patophysiology of the cancer, could be more robust in clinical settings.

Blomqvist et al. (1998) proposed a piecewise linear fitting of the TIC. The TIC was divided into three parts: the first part was characterised by the time needed for the contrast medium to reach the ROI; the second part was characterised by the rapid increase in signal intensity (wash-in); the third part presented little or no increase in CA. In their study, none of the parameters in the piecewise linear approximation were found to significantly help discriminating malignant from benign. WOI was the only parameter that was significantly different between the malignant and benign groups.

Preoperative TNM staging of rectal cancer using endorectal coil and dynamic contrast enhancement, was performed by Drew et al. (1999) using visual inspection based on the pattern of the enhancement: they found a substantial tumour over-staging when compared to pathological specimens.

Dicle et al. (1999) evaluated the accuracy of DCE-MRI in the differentiation of malignant and benign pelvic lesions during follow-up of patients with treated colorectal tumours, using a semi-quantitative approach. They calculated the maximum change in relative enhancement E_{max} (which is related to MSD), the acceleration rate of the TIC (which can be identified approximately as WIS) and the ratio of the signal intensity of the lesions to the signal intensity of the iliac artery at 60 s ($(S_L/S_A)_{60}$). The acceleration rate of the TIC and $(S_L/S_A)_{60}$ were found to be valuable in the differential diagnosis; E_{max} showed no capability to differentiate benign from malignant lesions. Sensitivity was 83% for each calculated parameter. $(S_L/S_A)_{60}$ had the highest specificity and accuracy among the parameters.

de Vries et al. (2000) have monitored 11 patients with cT3 rectal carcinoma who underwent preoperative chemoirradiation. They looked for a relationship between the PI (eq. 7) with therapy outcome. They used a short sampling interval of 14s in the wash-in phase (first 10 minutes of acquisition) followed by a longer interval (2 min) in the subsequent period (up to 50 min). They found that PI increased after the 1st and 2nd week of treatment. Monitoring of PI values before therapy seemed to have a prognostic value: they found a significant correlation between PI before therapy and N downstaging.

After, de Vries et al. (2001) evaluated 17 patients using a similar methodology. Moreover in this study they evaluated also the tumor heterogeneity. They found similar results.

Later, the same research group de Vries et al. (2003) observed further 34 patients with primary rectal carcinoma and preoperative chemoirradiation. They found that the PI of non-responders before therapy was higher than responders. They showed the possible role of an increased angiogenic activity in aggressive tumour cell clusters that resulted in reduced nutrient supply and higher fraction of intratumoral necrosis.

Study	Parameters	Final Diag.	Nr. Pat.	Nr. Images	Time interval [s]
Blomqvist et al. (1998)	TTP, WIS, WOI, WOS	TNM	30	60	4
Drew et al. (1999)		TNM	29		
Dicle et al. (1999)	MSD, $(S_L/S_A)_{60}$	biopsy	19		from 5s to 10 min
de Vries et al. (2000)	PI	TNM	11	31 + (15)	14 + (2 min)
de Vries et al. (2001)	PI	TNM	17		
de Vries et al. (2003)	PI	TNM	34	31 + (15)	14 + (2 min)
Kremser et al. (2007)	PI	TNM	58	15	13
Tuncbilek et al. (2004)	MSD_{1min},MSD,$\%/s$,TWI	MVD	21	8	30
Zhang et al. (2008)	ER_{peak},TTP,T_{first},uptake rate	MVD,VEGF	38	15-20	13-18
Müller-Schimpfle et al. (1993)	K^{trans},v_e	needle biopsy	18	24	25
George et al. (2001)	K^{trans}	VEGF	31	42	10
Torricelli et al. (2003)	relative enhanchement	biopsy/surgery	36	11-13	30
de Lussanet et al. (2005)	K^{trans}, k_{ep},v_e,PI	MVD,CD31,CD34	17	250	
Atkin et al. (2006)	K^{trans},v_e,MSD	MVD,CD31,VEGF	14	40	12
Ceelen et al. (2006)	K^{trans},v_e	MVD,VEGF,pO_2	11 (rats)	500	1.1
Mross et al. (2009)	K^{trans}, AUC	VEGF	22	106	3
Yao et al. (2011)	K^{trans},v_e , k_{ep}	MVD,TNM	26	25	8
Gu et al. (2011)	K^{trans},v_e , k_{ep}	TNM	26	10	6.3

Table 2. Summary of the main characteristics of the examined DCE-MRI rectal cancer studies. Per each study the table reports: the parameters examined; the method used for final diagnosis; the number of patients; the number of images and the time interval between them.

In line with these results, the same researchers published another paper (Kremser et al., 2007) in which they examined, using similar methodology, 58 patients before chemo-radiotherapy . Once again they found that PI is a good predictor of therapy outcome, being, before therapy, the PI of non-responders lower than responders.
Torricelli et al. (2003) elaborated dynamic images with a semi-quantitative postprocessing by plotting TICs and calculating the percentage of signal increase at the end of the first postcontrast dynamic sequence. The pelvic lesions were classified as recurrent or not recurrent by applying the following diagnostic criteria: (a) morphology and signal intensity of the lesion in unenhanced sequences and (b) percentage of enhancement in dynamic enhanced sequences. Unenhanced MRI had 80% sensitivity and 86% specificity. Analysis of the percentage of enhancement showed 87% sensitivity and 100% specificity.
Tuncbilek et al. (2004) studied 21 consecutive patients without radiotherapy (RT). They observed that TTP, WII_{max} and $E_{max/1}$ were strong correlated with microvessel density (MVD). As regards prognostic value, they found that histologic grade and $E_{max/1}$ correctly predicted metastases in 66.7% and 90.5 % of cases respectively.
Using a 3T scanner and basing on a semi-quantitative approach Zhang et al. (2008) found that rectal carcinoma had higher ER_{peak}, higher uptake rate ER_{peak}/T_{peak}, earlier T_{peak}, earlier $T_{firstenhanceent}$, than normal rectal wall.
All the previous studies showed that a semi-quantitative approach is feasible and can have good performances. In particular the perfusion index (PI) has shown to be a simple and robust prognostic factor.
On the other side, general guidelines for tracer kinetics approach have been indicated by Leach et al. (2005). Primary (K^{trans}, AUC) and secondary (v_e, k_{ep}) endpoints have been recommended.
Tracer kinetics modelling has been applied to the rectal cancer by Müller-Schimpfle et al. (1993) who reported 91-100 % sensitivity in differentiating benign from malignant lesions in pelvic lesions. Furthermore, they demonstrated that malignant lesions showed faster and greater enhancement compared with benign lesions and claimed that a more accurate differentiation with the usage of dynamic gadolinium-enhanced MRI could be obtained than with standard contrast-enhanced MRI.
As regards the therapy response, George et al. (2001) showed a correlation between K_{trans} and VEGF tumour expression showing that tumours having higher permeability seemed to better respond to pre-CRT than tumours having lower permeability.
de Lussanet et al. (2005) evaluated radio-therapy related microvascular changes in locally advanced rectal cancer (LARC) by DCE-MRI quantitative approach and histology. This study showed that K^{trans} values presents significant radio-therapy related reductions in microvessel blood flow in locally advanced rectal cancer. They studied tumor heterogeneity using histograms of K^{trans}, v_e and evaluating medina tumor values and median tumor/muscle ratio. Radiation therapy damages all blood vessels, but specific effects depend on vessel size, location, and dose-time-volume factors. Although acute effects of RT are marked by increased microvascular permeability, related to endothelial cell damage and local inflammation, longer term effects are marked by decreased permeability, resulting from basement membrane thickening and extracapillary fibrosis. The DCE-MRI volume fraction EES (v_e) showed some increased variation after Rt. Cell destruction caused by radiation may have increased the relative EES to which the CA can leak. In other part of the tumor infiltration of inflammatory cells can decrease EES.

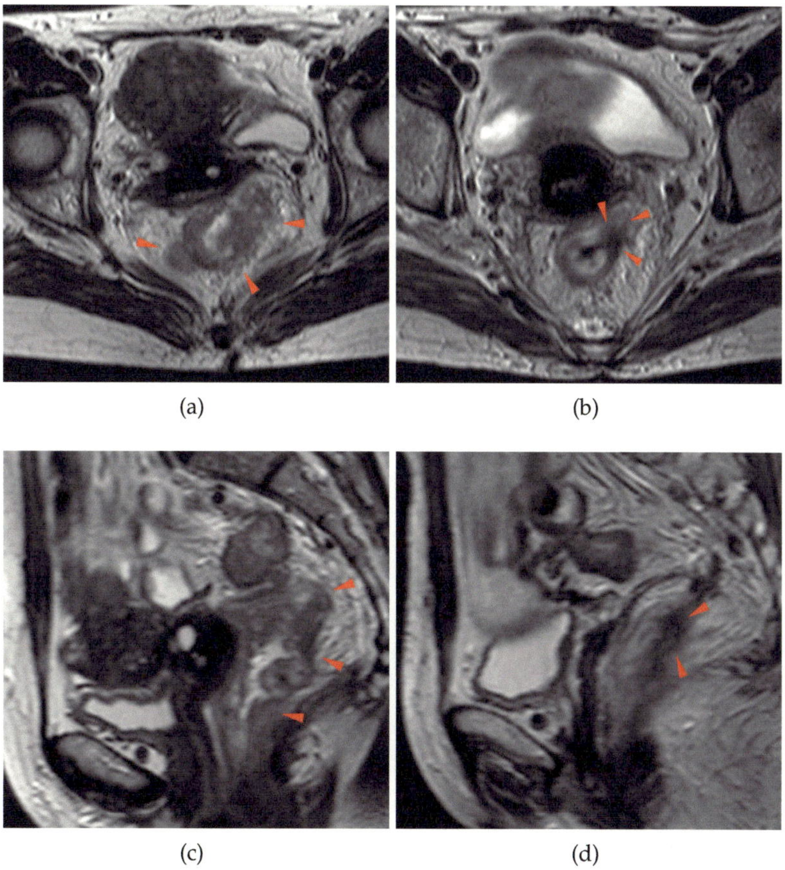

Fig. 8. (a) A heterogeneous irregular thickening along the entire rectal wall is well shown on T2w axial pre-pCRT scan (arrowheads). (b) After pCRT, a hypo-intense spiculated area with thin digitations into peri-rectal fat is visible on T2w axial scan (arrowheads). (c) In the same patient, multiple irregular rectal wall thickening are shown on T2w sagittal pre-pCRT scan (arrowheads). (d) A single hypo-intense area, showed also in (b) is pointed by arrowheads, suspecting for a residual post-pCRT tumor focus (arrowheads).

Controversially, Atkin et al. (2006) analysed 14, by preoperative DCE-MRI, patients that had not undergone any previous chemo-radioherapy. They reported a negative correlation between transfer constant K^{trans} with CD31. They noticed that this correlation is paradoxical because K^{trans} should be posiively coupled to blood flow,microvessel permeability and surface area. They suggested that this paradox could be related to the high level of maturation of vessels within rectal cancers, with mature vessels demonstrating relatively low permeability. Moreover, they reported no correlation of DCE-MRI with other measures such as MVD (which provide anatomical data only). Therefore they concluded that DCE-MRI does not simply reflect static histological vascular properties in patients with rectal cancer.
Monitoring 11 rats before and after fractionated short-term radiotherapy (Ceelen et al., 2006) observed a significant reduction of K^{trans} and v_e, while in non irradiated muscle tissue no changes were observed. After RT, pO_2 levels were inversely related to both K^{trans} and v_e. No

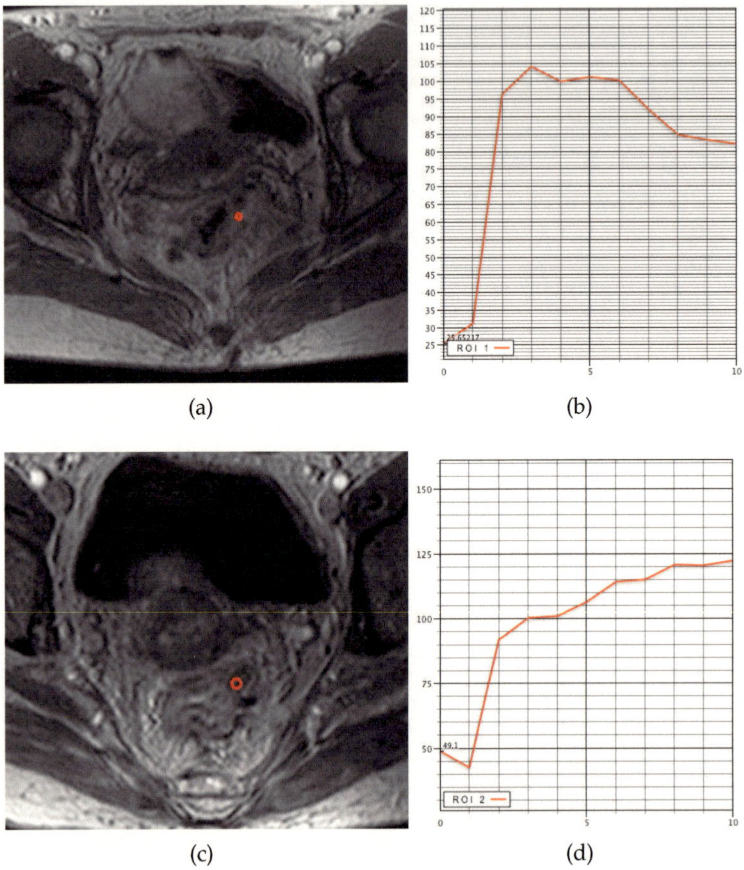

Fig. 9. T1w post-contrast scan obtained on the same patient in fig. 8, before (a)-(b) and after (c)-(d) pre-CRT. The analysis of TIC calculated on a ROI, drawn outside the rectal wall where on T2w scans (fig. 8) tumor clearly spreads into peri-rectal fat pad, confirm this suspect showing a rapid CA intake and a fast discharge (b). After pre-CRT, on the same areas showed on T2w scans (fig. 8) no pathological CA uptake is present confirming that hypo-intense tissue visible on T2w scans are tumor nests but only residual inflammation due to pre-CRT. This patient was considered as a Responder. Histopathology showed a TRG 1.

correlation was found between DCE-MRI parameters and histologic parameters (MVD, VEGF expression). MVD did not differ significantly between RT-trated and control animals.
Mross et al. (2009) proposed an hybrid approach including AUC and K^{trans} for evaluating the response to treatment of 22 patients.
Yao et al. (2011) reported moderate and strong relationship between K^{trans} and clinicopathological elements, K^{trans} might be the prognostic indicator of rectal cancer.
Gu et al. (2011) found a positive correlations between k_{ep} and SUV values in primary rectal adenocarcinomas suggesting an association between angiogenesis and metabolic activity and further reflecting that angiogenic activity in washout phase is better associated with tumor metabolism than the uptake phase.
Although these encouraging results, the evaluation after neo-adjuvant therapy remains actually difficult in borderline cases where an overestimation is the most common drawback.

This phenomenon has been addressed to the presence of inflammatory tissue still mostly vascularized so as tumour residual areas (see fig. 8 and 9).
In conclusion, DCE-MRI can be considered a valuable tool for clinical investigation of rectal cancer, in particular for re-staging and therapy evaluation. Further improvements should involve the underestimation phenomenon, a clinically relevant problem, frequently observed on morphologic MRI that is not yet been solved because of the presence of small areas of tumors within poorly vascularized fibrotic tissue under the spatial resolution of DCE-MRI technique.

6. References

Ashton, E. (2010). Quantitative MR in multi-center clinical trials, *J Magn Reson Imaging* 31(2): 279–288.

Atkin, G., Taylor, N. J., Daley, F. M., Stirling, J. J., Richman, P., Glynne-Jones, R., d'Arcy, J. A., Collins, D. J. & Padhani, A. R. (2006). Dynamic contrast-enhanced magnetic resonance imaging is a poor measure of rectal cancer angiogenesis, *Brit J Surg* 93(8): 992–1000.

Avallone, A., Delrio, P., Guida, C., Tatangelo, F., Petrillo, A., Marone, P., Cascini, L. G., Morrica, B., Lastoria, S., Parisi, V., Budillon, A. & Comella, P. (2006). Biweekly oxaliplatin, raltitrexed, 5-fluorouracil and folinic acid combination chemotherapy during preoperative radiation therapy for locally advanced rectal cancer: a phase I-II study, *Brit J Cancer* 94(12): 1809–1815.

Avallone, A., Delrio, P., Pecori, B., Tatangelo, F., Petrillo, A., Scott, N., Marone, P., Aloi, L., Sandomenico, C., Lastoria, S., Iaffaioli, V. R., Scala, D., Iodice, G., Budillon, A. & Comella, P. (2011). Oxaliplatin plus dual inhibition of thymidilate synthase during preoperative pelvic radiotherapy for locally advanced rectal carcinoma: long-term outcome, *Int J Radiat Oncol* 79(3): 670–676.

Beets-Tan, R. G. H. & Beets, G. L. (2004). Rectal cancer: review with emphasis on MR imaging, *Radiology* 232(2): 335–346.

Blomqvist, L., Fransson, P. & Hindmarsh, T. (1998). The pelvis after surgery and radio-chemotherapy for rectal cancer studied with Gd-DTPA-enhanced fast dynamic MR imaging, *Eur Radiol* 8(5): 781–787.

Brix, G., Griebel, J., Kiessling, F. & Wenz, F. (2010). Tracer kinetic modelling of tumour angiogenesis based on dynamic contrast-enhanced CT and MRI measurements, *Eur J Nucl Med Mol Imaging* 37 Suppl 1: S30–51.

Brix, G., Semmler, W., Port, R., Schad, L. R., Layer, G. & Lorenz, W. J. (1991). Pharmacokinetic parameters in CNS Gd-DTPA enhanced MR imaging, *J Comput Assist Tomogr* 15(4): 621–628.

Buonaccorsi, G. A., O'Connor, J. P., Caunce, A., Roberts, C., Cheung, S., Watson, Y., Davies, K., Hope, L., Jackson, A., Jayson, G. C. & Parker, G. J. (2007). Tracer kinetic model–driven registration for dynamic contrast-enhanced MRI time-series data, *Magnet Reson Med* 58(5): 1010–1019.

Ceelen, W., Smeets, P., Backes, W., Damme, N. V., Boterberg, T., Demetter, P., Bouckenooghe, I., Visschere, M. D., Peeters, M. & Pattyn, P. (2006). Noninvasive monitoring of radiotherapy-induced microvascular changes using dynamic contrast enhanced magnetic resonance imaging (DCE-MRI) in a colorectal tumor model, *Int J Radiat Oncol* 64(4): 1188–1196.

Chen, C., Lee, R., Lin, J., Wang, L. & Yang, S. (2005). How accurate is magnetic resonance imaging in restaging rectal cancer in patients receiving preoperative combined chemoradiotherapy?, *Dis Colon Rectum* 48(4): 722–728.

Cheng, H. M. (2008). Investigation and optimization of parameter accuracy in dynamic contrast-enhanced MRI, *J Magn Reson Imaging* 28(3): 736–743.

Choyke, P. L., Dwyer, A. J. & Knopp, M. V. (2003). Functional tumor imaging with dynamic contrast-enhanced magnetic resonance imaging, *J Magn Reson Imaging* 17(5): 509–520.

Collins, D. J. & Padhani, A. R. (2004). Dynamic magnetic resonance imaging of tumor perfusion, *IEEE Eng Med Biol Mag* 23(5): 65– 83.

Dale, B. M., Jesberger, J. A., Lewin, J. S., Hillenbrand, C. M. & Duerk, J. L. (2003). Determining and optimizing the precision of quantitative measurements of perfusion from dynamic contrast enhanced MRI, *J Magn Reson Imaging* 18(5): 575–584.

Daniel, B. L., Yen, Y. F., Glover, G. H., Ikeda, D. M., Birdwell, R. L., Sawyer-Glover, A. M., Black, J. W., Plevritis, S. K., Jeffrey, S. S. & Herfkens, R. J. (1998). Breast disease: dynamic spiral MR imaging, *Radiology* 209(2): 499–509.

de Lussanet, Q. G., Backes, W. H., Griffioen, A. W., Padhani, A. R., Baeten, C. I., van Baardwijk, A., Lambin, P., Beets, G. L., van Engelshoven, J. M. A. & Beets-Tan, R. G. H. (2005). Dynamic contrast-enhanced magnetic resonance imaging of radiation therapy-induced microcirculation changes in rectal cancer, *Int J Radiat Oncol* 63(5): 1309–1315.

de Vries, A. F., Griebel, J., Kremser, C., Judmaier, W., Gneiting, T., Debbage, P., Kremser, T., Pfeiffer, K. P., Buchberger, W. & Lukas, P. (2000). Monitoring of tumor microcirculation during fractionated radiation therapy in patients with rectal carcinoma: preliminary results and implications for therapy, *Radiology* 217(2): 385–391.

de Vries, A. F., Griebel, J., Kremser, C., Judmaier, W., Gneiting, T., Kreczy, A., Ofner, D., Pfeiffer, K. P., Brix, G. & Lukas, P. (2001). Tumor microcirculation evaluated by dynamic magnetic resonance imaging predicts therapy outcome for primary rectal carcinoma, *Cancer Res* 61(6): 2513–2516.

de Vries, A. F., Kremser, C., Hein, P. A., Griebel, J., Krezcy, A., Ofner, D., Pfeiffer, K. P., Lukas, P. & Judmaier, W. (2003). Tumor microcirculation and diffusion predict therapy outcome for primary rectal carcinoma, *Int J Radiat Oncol* 56(4): 958–965.

Delrio, P., Avallone, A., Guida, C., Lastoria, S., Tatangelo, F., Cascini, G. M., Marone, P., Petrillo, A., Budillon, A., Marzo, M. D., Palaia, R., Albino, V., Rosa, V. D. & Parisi, V. (2005). Multidisciplinary approach to locally advanced rectal cancer: results of a single institution trial, *Suppl Tumori* 4(3): S8.

Delrio, P., Lastoria, S., Avallone, A., Ravo, V., Guida, C., Cremona, F., Izzo, F., Palaia, R., Ruffolo, F., Puppio, B., Guidetti, G. M., Cascini, G. L., Casaretti, R., Tatangelo, F., Marone, P., Rossi, G. B., Budillon, A., Petrillo, A., Rosa, V. D., Comella, G., Morrica, B., Tempesta, A., Botti, G. & Parisi, V. (2003). Early evaluation using PET-FDG of the efficiency of neoadjuvant radiochemotherapy treatment in locally advanced neoplasia of the lower rectum, *Tumori* 89(4 Suppl): 50–53.

Dicle, O., Obuz, F. & Cakmakci, H. (1999). Differentiation of recurrent rectal cancer and scarring with dynamic MR imaging, *Brit J Radiol* 72(864): 1155–1159.

Dor, Y., Porat, R. & Keshet, E. (2001). Vascular endothelial growth factor and vascular adjustments to perturbations in oxygen homeostasis, *Am J Physiol Cell Physiol* 280(6): C1367–1374.

Drew, P. J., Farouk, R., Turnbull, L. W., Ward, S. C., Hartley, J. E. & Monson, J. R. (1999). Preoperative magnetic resonance staging of rectal cancer with an endorectal coil and dynamic gadolinium enhancement, *Brit J Surg* 86(2): 250–254.

Evelhoch, J. L. (1999). Key factors in the acquisition of contrast kinetic data for oncology, *J Magn Reson Imaging* 10(3): 254–259.

Fei, B., Wheaton, A., Lee, Z., Duerk, J. L. & Wilson, D. L. (2002). Automatic MR volume registration and its evaluation for the pelvis and prostate, *Phys Med Biol* 47(5): 823–838.

George, M. L., Dzik-Jurasz, A. S., Padhani, A. R., Brown, G., Tait, D. M., Eccles, S. A. & Swift, R. I. (2001). Non-invasive methods of assessing angiogenesis and their value in predicting response to treatment in colorectal cancer, *Brit J Surg* 88(12): 1628–1636.

Goh, V., Padhani, A. R. & Rasheed, S. (2007). Functional imaging of colorectal cancer angiogenesis, *Lancet Oncol* 8(3): 245–255.

Gu, J., Khong, P., Wang, S., Chan, Q., Wu, E. X., Law, W., Liu, R. K. & Zhang, J. (2011). Dynamic contrast-enhanced MRI of primary rectal cancer: quantitative correlation with positron emission tomography/computed tomography, *J Magn Reson Imaging* 33(2): 340–347.

Guetz, G. D., Uzzan, B., Nicolas, P., Cucherat, M., Morere, J., Benamouzig, R., Breau, J. & Perret, G. (2006). Microvessel density and VEGF expression are prognostic factors in colorectal cancer. meta-analysis of the literature, *Brit J Cancer* 94(12): 1823–1832.

Gunderson, L. L., Sargent, D. J., Tepper, J. E., O'Connell, M. J., Allmer, C., Smalley, S. R., Martenson, J. A., Haller, D. G., Mayer, R. J., Rich, T. A., Ajani, J. A., Macdonald, J. S. & Goldberg, R. M. (2002). Impact of T and N substage on survival and disease relapse in adjuvant rectal cancer: a pooled analysis, *Int J Radiat Oncol* 54(2): 386–396.

Gunderson, L. L., Sargent, D. J., Tepper, J. E., Wolmark, N., O'Connell, M. J., Begovic, M., Allmer, C., Colangelo, L., Smalley, S. R., Haller, D. G., Martenson, J. A., Mayer, R. J., Rich, T. A., Ajani, J. A., MacDonald, J. S., Willett, C. G. & Goldberg, R. M. (2004). Impact of T and N stage and treatment on survival and relapse in adjuvant rectal cancer: a pooled analysis, *J Clin Oncol* 22(10): 1785–1796.

Henderson, E., Rutt, B. K. & Lee, T. (1998). Temporal sampling requirements for the tracer kinetics modeling of breast disease, *Magn Reson Imaging* 16(9): 1057–1073.

Jackson, A., O'Connor, J. P. B., Parker, G. J. M. & Jayson, G. C. (2007). Imaging tumor vascular heterogeneity and angiogenesis using dynamic contrast-enhanced magnetic resonance imaging, *Clin Cancer Res* 13(12): 3449–3459.

Kapse, N. & Goh, V. (2009). Functional imaging of colorectal cancer: positron emission tomography, magnetic resonance imaging, and computed tomography, *Clin Colorectal Cancer* 8(2): 77–87.

Kelm, B., Menze, B., Nix, O., Zechmann, C. & Hamprecht, F. (2009). Estimating kinetic parameter maps from dynamic Contrast-Enhanced MRI using spatial prior knowledge, *IEEE Trans Med Imaging* 28(10): 1534–1547.

Kety, S. S. (1951). The theory and applications of the exchange of inert gas at the lungs and tissues, *Pharmacol Rev* 3(1): 1–41.

Knopp, M. V., Weiss, E., Sinn, H. P., Mattern, J., Junkermann, H., Radeleff, J., Magener, A., Brix, G., Delorme, S., Zuna, I. & van Kaick, G. (1999). Pathophysiologic basis of contrast enhancement in breast tumors, *J Magn Reson Imaging* 10(3): 260–266.

Kremser, C., Trieb, T., Rudisch, A., Judmaier, W. & de Vries, A. (2007). Dynamic t(1) mapping predicts outcome of chemoradiation therapy in primary rectal carcinoma: sequence implementation and data analysis, *J Magn Reson Imaging* 26(3): 662–671.

Kuhl, C. (2007). The current status of breast MR imaging part i. choice of technique, image interpretation, diagnostic accuracy, and transfer to clinical practice, *Radiology* 244(2): 356 –378.

Larsson, H. B. W., Fritz-Hansen, T., Rostrup, E., Sondergaard, L., Ring, P. & Henriksen, O. (1996). Myocardial perfusion modeling using MRI, *Magnet Reson Med* 35(5): 716–726.

Leach, M. O., Brindle, K. M., Evelhoch, J. L., Griffiths, J. R., Horsman, M. R., Jackson, A., Jayson, G. C., Judson, I. R., Knopp, M. V., Maxwell, R. J., McIntyre, D., Padhani, A. R., Price, P., Rathbone, R., Rustin, G. J., Tofts, P. S., Tozer, G. M., Vennart, W., Waterton, J. C., Williams, S. R. & Workman, P. (2005). The assessment of antiangiogenic and antivascular therapies in early-stage clinical trials using magnetic resonance imaging: issues and recommendations, *Brit J Cancer* 92(9): 1599–1610.

Lichtenbeld, H. C., Ferarra, N., Jain, R. K. & Munn, L. L. (1999). Effect of local anti-VEGF antibody treatment on tumor microvessel permeability, *Microvasc Res* 57(3): 357–362.

Melbourne, A., Atkinson, D., White, M. J., Collins, D., Leach, M. & Hawkes, D. (2007). Registration of dynamic contrast-enhanced MRI using a progressive principal component registration (PPCR), *Phys Med Biol* 52(17): 5147–5156.

Miles, K. A. (1991). Measurement of tissue perfusion by dynamic computed tomography, *Brit J Radiol* 64(761): 409–412.

Müller-Schimpfle, M., Brix, G., Layer, G., Schlag, P., Engenhart, R., Frohmuller, S., Hess, T., Zuna, I., Semmler, W. & van Kaick, G. (1993). Recurrent rectal cancer: diagnosis with dynamic MR imaging, *Radiology* 189(3): 881–889.

Mross, K., Fasol, U., Frost, A., Benkelmann, R., Kuhlmann, J., Büchert, M., Unger, C., Blum, H., Hennig, J., Milenkova, T. P., Tessier, J., Krebs, A. D., Ryan, A. J. & Fischer, R. (2009). DCE-MRI assessment of the effect of vandetanib on tumor vasculature in patients with advanced colorectal cancer and liver metastases: a randomized phase i study, *J Angiogenes Res* 1: 5.

Nishiura, M., Yasuhiro, T. & Murase, K. (2011). Evaluation of time-intensity curves in ductal carcinoma in situ (DCIS) and mastopathy obtained using dynamic contrast-enhanced magnetic resonance imaging, *Magn Reson Imaging* 29(1): 99–105.

Orton, M. R., d'Arcy, J. A., Walker-Samuel, S., Hawkes, D. J., Atkinson, D., Collins, D. J. & Leach, M. O. (2008). Computationally efficient vascular input function models for quantitative kinetic modelling using DCE-MRI, *Phys Med Biol* 53(5): 1225–1239.

Parker, G. J. M., Roberts, C., Macdonald, A., Buonaccorsi, G. A., Cheung, S., Buckley, D. L., Jackson, A., Watson, Y., Davies, K. & Jayson, G. C. (2006). Experimentally-derived functional form for a population-averaged high-temporal-resolution arterial input function for dynamic contrast-enhanced MRI, *Magnet Reson Med* 56(5): 993–1000.

Parker, G. J., Suckling, J., Tanner, S. F., Padhani, A. R., Revell, P. B., Husband, J. E. & Leach, M. O. (1997). Probing tumor microvascularity by measurement, analysis and display of contrast agent uptake kinetics, *J Magn Reson Imaging* 7(3): 564–574.

Petrillo, A., Catalano, O., Delrio, P., Avallone, A., Guida, C., Filice, S. & Siani, A. (2007). Post-treatment fistulas in patients with rectal cancer: MRI with rectal superparamagnetic contrast agent, *Abdom Imaging* 32(3): 328–331.

Petrillo, A., Filice, S., Avallone, A., Delrio, P., Guida, C., Tatangelo, F., Marone, P., Nunziata, A. & Siani, A. (2006). Staging of locally advanced rectal cancer (LARC): proposal of a one-stop magnetic resonance (mr) imaging-based protocol, *Eur Radiol Supplements* 16: 321–494.

Sansone, M., Fusco, R., Petrillo, A., Petrillo, M. & Bracale, M. (2011). An expectation-maximisation approach for simultaneous pixel classification and tracer kinetic modelling in dynamic contrast enhanced-magnetic resonance imaging, *Med Biol Eng Comput* 49(4): 485–495.

Schmid, V. J., Whitcher, B., Padhani, A. R., Taylor, N. J. & Yang, G. (2006). Bayesian methods for pharmacokinetic models in dynamic Contrast-Enhanced magnetic resonance imaging, *IEEE Transactions on Medical Imaging* 25(12): 1627–1636.

Simpson, N. E., He, Z. & Evelhoch, J. L. (1999). Deuterium NMR tissue perfusion measurements using the tracer uptake approach: I. optimization of methods, *Magnet Reson Med* 42(1): 42–52.

Sourbron, S. (2010). Technical aspects of MR perfusion, *Eur J Radiol* 76(3): 304–313.

St Lawrence, K. S. & Lee, T. Y. (1998). An adiabatic approximation to the tissue homogeneity model for water exchange in the brain: I. theoretical derivation, *J Cereb Blood Flow Metab* 18(12): 1365–1377.

Stanisz, G. J. & Henkelman, R. M. (2000). Gd-DTPA relaxivity depends on macromolecular content, *Magnet Reson Med* 44(5): 665–667.

Tofts, P. S. (1997). Modeling tracer kinetics in dynamic Gd-DTPA MR imaging, *J Magn Reson Imaging* 7(1): 91–101.

Tofts, P. S., Brix, G., Buckley, D. L., Evelhoch, J. L., Henderson, E., Knopp, M. V., Larsson, H. B., Lee, T. Y., Mayr, N. A., Parker, G. J., Port, R. E., Taylor, J. & Weisskoff, R. M. (1999). Estimating kinetic parameters from dynamic contrast-enhanced t(1)-weighted MRI of a diffusable tracer: standardized quantities and symbols, *J Magn Reson Imaging* 10(3): 223–232.

Torricelli, P., Pecchi, A., Luppi, G. & Romagnoli, R. (2003). Gadolinium-enhanced MRI with dynamic evaluation in diagnosing the local recurrence of rectal cancer, *Abdom Imaging* 28(1): 19–27.

Tuncbilek, N., Karakas, H. M. & Altaner, S. (2004). Dynamic mri in indirect estimation of microvessel density, histologic grade, and prognosis in colorectal adenocarcinomas, *Abdom Imaging* 29: 166–172.

Walker-Samuel, S., Leach, M. O. & Collins, D. J. (2007). Reference tissue quantification of DCE-MRI data without a contrast agent calibration, *Phys Med Biol* 52(3): 589–601.

Weinmann, H. J., Laniado, M. & Mützel, W. (1984). Pharmacokinetics of GdDTPA/dimeglumine after intravenous injection into healthy volunteers, *Physiol Chem Phys Med NMR* 16(2): 167–172.

Xiaohua, C., Brady, M., Lo, J. L. & Moore, N. (2005). Simultaneous segmentation and registration of contrast-enhanced breast MRI, *Information Processing in Medical Imaging: Proceedings of the ... Conference* 19: 126–137.

Yang, C., Karczmar, G. S., Medved, M. & Stadler, W. M. (2004). Estimating the arterial input function using two reference tissues in dynamic contrast-enhanced MRI studies: Fundamental concepts and simulations, *Magnet Reson Med* 52(5): 1110–1117.

Yankeelov, T. E., Luci, J. J., Lepage, M., Li, R., Debusk, L., Lin, P. C., Price, R. R. & Gore, J. C. (2005). Quantitative pharmacokinetic analysis of DCE-MRI data without an arterial input function: a reference region model, *Magnet Reson Imaging* 23(4): 519–529.

Yao, W. W., Zhang, H., Ding, B., Fu, T., Jia, H., Pang, L., Song, L., Xu, W., Song, Q., Chen, K. & Pan, Z. (2011). Rectal cancer: 3D dynamic contrast-enhanced MRI; correlation with microvascular density and clinicopathological features, *Radiol Med* 116(3): 366–374.

Zhang, X. M., Yu, D., Zhang, H. L., Dai, Y., Bi, D., Liu, Z., Prince, M. R. & Li, C. (2008). 3D dynamic contrast-enhanced MRI of rectal carcinoma at 3T: correlation with microvascular density and vascular endothelial growth factor markers of tumor angiogenesis, *J Magn Reson Imaging* 27(6): 1309–1316.

6

Tumour Angiogenesis in Rectal Cancer- Computer-Assisted Endosonographic and Immunohistochemical Methods for Assessment

Tankova Ludmila[1], Daniel Kovatchki[2], Georgi Stoilov[3], Antonina Gegova[4] and Ivan Terziev[5]
[1]*Clinical Centre of Gastroenterology, Clinic of Gastroenterology, University Hospital „Queen Joanna", Sofia*
[2]*Golden Cross Private Clinic, Vienna*
[3]*Institute of Mechanics, Bulgarian Academy of Sciences, Sofia*
[4]*Department of Pathology, Medical Faculty, University „Kliment Ohridski", Sofia*
[5]*Department of Pathology, University Hospital „Queen Joanna", Sofia*
[1,3,4,5]*Bulgaria*
[2]*Austria*

1. Introduction

Angiogenesis is an essential process in tumour growth, invasion, metastasis and recurrence. The conventional way of quantifying angiogenesis requires a biopsy or tissue specimens applying specific immunohistochemical or molecular biological tests. The evaluation of the microvessel density is a gold standard in the assessment of the tumour neovascularisation. The determination of the vascular endothelial growth factor (VEGF) expression of the tumour sections is an alternative method of estimating the angiogenic activity of the tumour. Doppler ultrasound is an attractive modality for imaging angiogenesis in vivo which can be repeated without exposing the patient to any risk (Chen et al., 2002; Ogura et al., 2001; Yang et al., 2002). Because of its high sensitivity in measuring slow flows and the improved detailed information about the curved and irregular vessel ways, power Doppler is a suitable technique for depicting the vessels inside the tumour. Nevertheless, the evaluation of the tumour angiogenesis has not still become routine, which might be explained by the lack of an accurate method for angiogenesis assessment (Pietra et al., 2000).

2. Aim

Aim of the current study was to evaluate the rectal cancer angiogenesis with Doppler endosonography and immunohistochemistry and to compare the results with computer-assisted methods

3. Material and methods

3.1 Patients

One hundred ninety five patients (123 males, 72 females; mean age 61.5 ± 11 years) with histologically proved rectal cancer were included in the study. The age of the patients ranged from 27 to 83 years. The patients were operated and staged according to the criteria of *World Health Organization* (WHO) for colon and rectum as follows: in stage I - 36 patients (18.5%), stage II - 53 (27.2%), stage III - 84 (43%), and stage IV - 22 patients (11.3%) (Hamilton et al., 2000). Immunohistochemical studies were performed in 110 rectal tumour samples. The distribution of the stages was as follows: Stage I – 20 patients (18.2%); Stage II - 29 patients (26.4%); Stage III – 47 patients (42.7%), Stage IV – 14 patients (12.7%).
The patients were followed up for a mean period of 30.4 ± 17.6 months (from 6 to 82 months) after the operation.

3.2 Assessment of angiogenesis by Doppler endosonography

All patients were examined on Toshiba, Nemio SSA 550A, Japan apparatus with a biplane convex transversal and end-fire scanning probe PVM-740RT (5.0/7.5/10 MHz/144°) capable of pulse colour and power Doppler. Every patient was prepared by small enema two hours before endosonography. The examination was performed with the patient in left lateral position. The probe was inserted 12-15cm and then was pulled out to the tumour level. pulse colour (cut-off wall filter: 50-100Hz; pulse repetition frequency: 4kHz) and power Doppler were used to estimate tumour vascularisation. Power Doppler settings were set to detect low velocity flow without artefacts (frequency 5MHz, power Doppler gain 20 (range: 1-30); dynamic range: 20-40dB, pulse repetition frequency: 1kHz).

3.2.1 Pulse colour and power Doppler

The semi quantitative assessment of angiogenesis was done by pulse colour Doppler, measuring the peak systolic velocity (PSV, cm/s) and the resistance index (RI) of the arterial flow in the tumour. The highest value for PSV was recorded, as well as the lowest value for RI. By using power Doppler endosonography tumour vascularisation was determined subjectively according to the following classification: poor vascularisation - absent or isolated colour signals; abundant vascularisation - abundance of chaotic vessels in the periphery and/or the central part of the tumour.

3.2.2 Computer-assisted power Doppler examination

The power Doppler was used for the digital tumour vascularisation assessment. The colour window was set to include the lesion and a small part of the surrounding normal tissues. Afterwards, three tumour slices with maximal colour signal numbers were chosen. The tumour image was traced with the pointer, followed by a computer-assisted calculation of the percentage ratio of the number of the coloured pixels within a delineated tumour section to the number of total pixels in that specific tumour section (Fig. 1.). The term Power Doppler Vascularisation Index (PDVI) was introduced, showing the mean of the three consecutive results.

3.3 Assessment of angiogenesis by immunohistochemistry

The histological assessment of the microvessel density (MVD) and the level of the VEGF expression in the tumour specimens were determined in 110 patients (71 males; 39 females;

mean age 62 years). The sections were taken from the point of greatest tumour penetration into the rectal wall.

The LSAB2 method (Labelled Streptavidin-Biotin2) was applied using streptavidin-biotin-peroxidase technique.

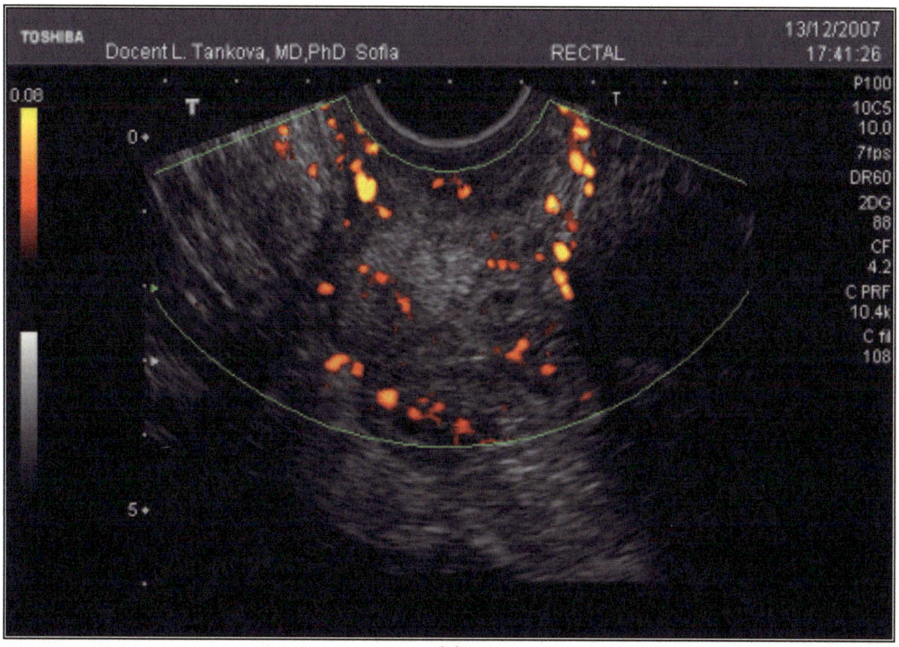

(a)

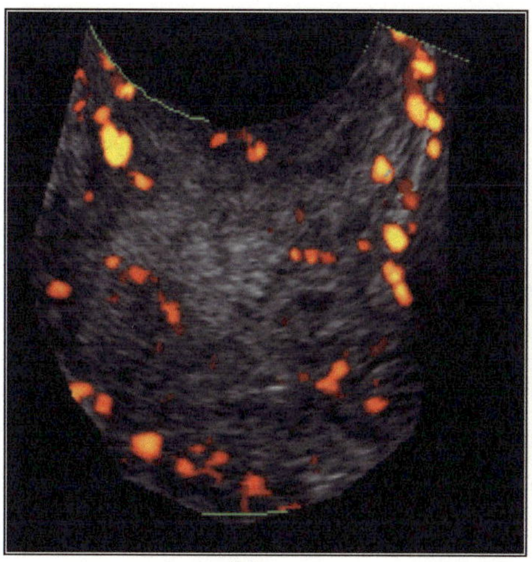

(b)

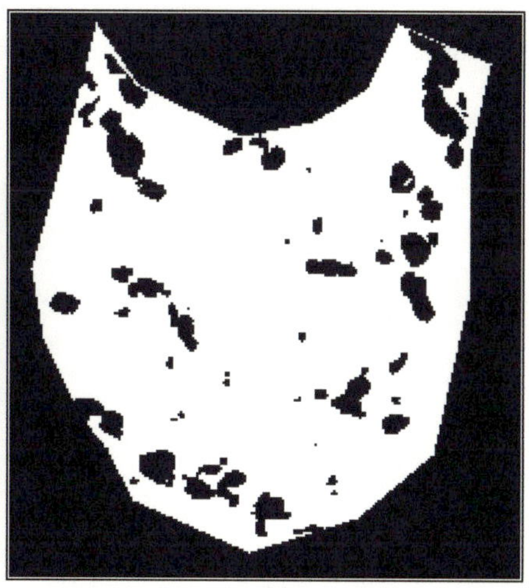

(c)

Fig. 1. (a) - Power Doppler image of tumour hypervascularisation. (b) and (c) - Determination of Power Doppler Vascularisation Index (PDVI) as the ratio of the colour pixels within a marked tumour section to the number of total pixels in that specific tumour section.

Four µm-thick sections of formalin-fixed, paraffin-embedded resection specimens were prepared. The sections were mounted on clean slides, previously coated with poly-L-lysin adhesive, then deparaffinized using xylol and rehydrated in graded alcohols. Antigen retrieval was done using target retrieval solution (citrate buffer, pH 6, DakoCytomation code S1700 for CD31 and code S2368 for VEGF) in a water bath at 95-98^{0}C for 20min. Thereafter, the endogenous peroxidase was deactivated by soaking the slides in 3% hydrogen peroxidase for 5min to block endogenous peroxidase. Antibodies were purchased from DakoCytomation, Inc, Carpinteria, California: Mouse Monoclonal anti-CD31 antibody (code N1596, clone JC/70A, ready for use dilution 1:20), Monoclonal Mouse Anti-Human VEGF (code M7273, clone VG1, dilution 1:25). The binding reaction was detected by DAB (diaminobenzidine) Substrate Chromogen System. Finally, the sections were counterstained with haematoxylin and mounted using aqueous mounting medium. All immunostaining processes were carried based on the manufacturers' recommendations.

3.3.1 Determination of microvessel density

MVD was determined via the method proposed by Weidner et al. (Weidner et al., 1991).
The regions with the most intensive vascularisation (hot spots) were defined by scanning the entire tumour section at low magnification (x40 or x100) with a selection of three fields (Fig. 2.). These were the fields with highest density of the brown coloured CD31+ cells. The individual microvessels were counted at high magnification of x200 (20x objective, 10x eyepiece) or x250 (25x objective, 10x eyepiece). The pictures were realized with the optical microscope Nikon 800E or Leica DM1000, coupled to a colour video camera.
Each image corresponded to a microscope field with an area of 0,29mm^2. The counting of the microvessels was done manually by calculating the average number for the three selected fields and dividing this number by 0.29, thus obtaining the number of microvessels per mm^2. Any brown-stained endothelial cell or endothelial cell cluster that was clearly separated from adjacent microvessels, tumour cells and connective elements was counted as one microvessel, independent of the presence of a vascular lumen or erythrocytes.

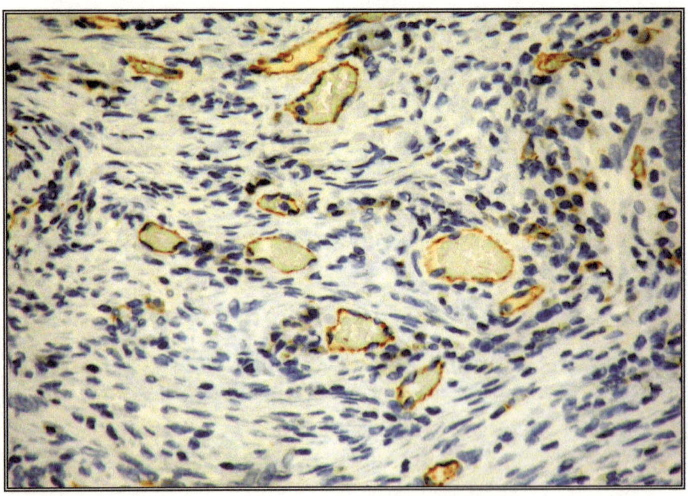

Fig. 2. CD31 immunostaining. Representative cases of „hot spot" of tumor specimens with high MVD (original magnification x 100)

3.3.2 Computer-assisted method for endothelial area assessment

Computer-assisted method for endothelial area determination was applied by imaging analysis software. The quality of the colouring varies since archive paraffin blocks were used for the immunohistochemical tests and the samples were prepared at different conditions. Because of that, several steps were needed to equalise the colour image quality before the automatic calculation of the coefficient of vascularisation (CV):

- Equalization of the image colour temperatures. Figure 3. shows two images, shot at different conditions with different spectral curves.

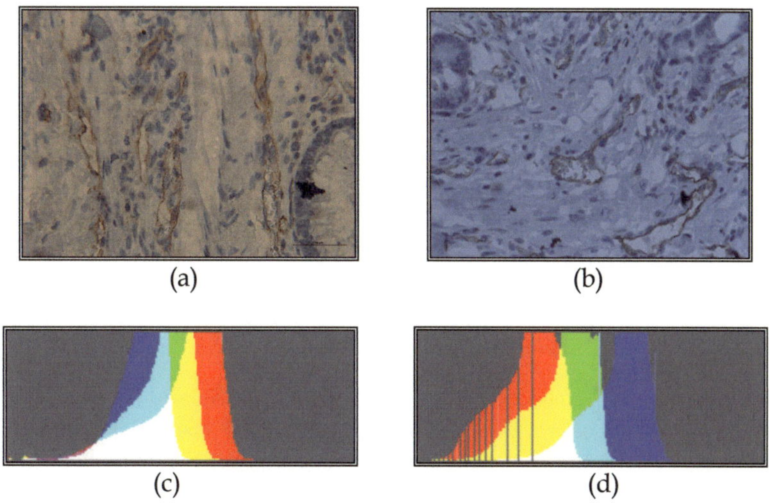

Fig. 3. (a) (b) - Images shot at different conditions. (c) (d) - Corresponding spectral curves

- After their colour temperatures have been equalized (Fig. 4.), the images had the same colours, but different contrast and brightness, depending on the optical characteristics of the microscope and the camera.

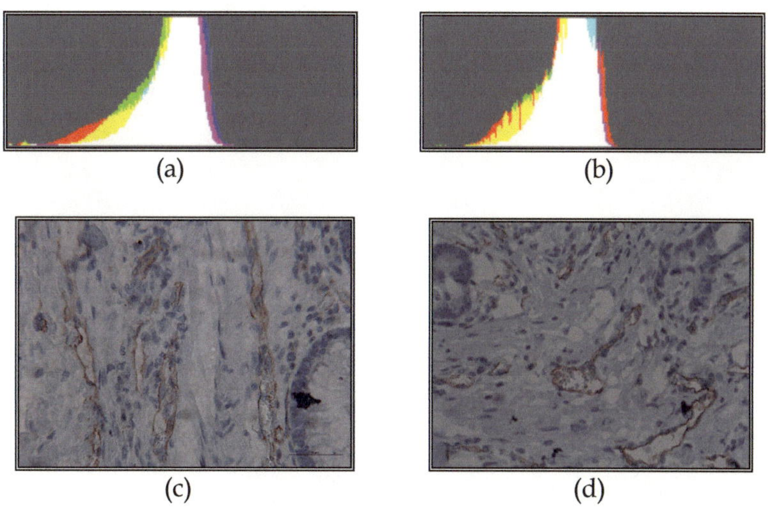

Fig. 4. (a)(b) - Equalized spectral curves. (c)(d) – Corresponding images

- The contrast was increased, so that the intensity histogram filled the whole usable dynamic range, yielding images with close colour properties and contrast (Fig. 5.).

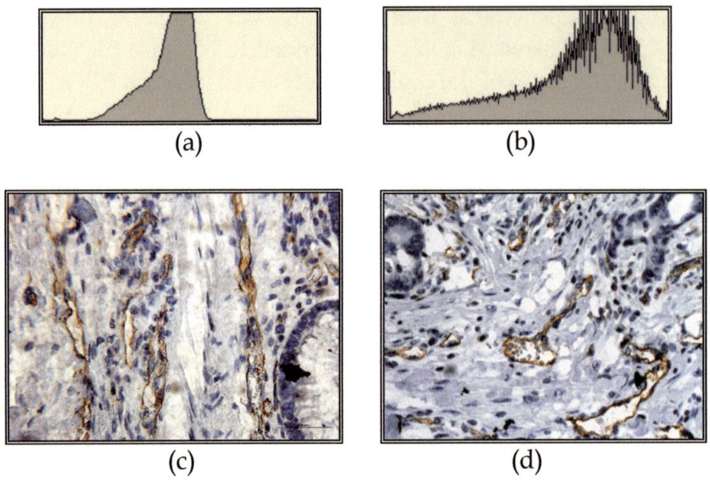

Fig. 5. (a) - Histogram of the contrast (b) - Histogram of the contrast with an extended dynamic range. (c) (d) - Equalized images

The brown marked endothelial cells were determined by imaging analysis software with high accuracy (Fig. 6.). In order to exclude non-endothelial structures a computer-assisted method was used, in which a qualified researcher-pathologist observed the marked areas before the final estimation. The endothelial area was measured automatically and the coefficient of vascularisation was calculated. The coefficient of vascularisation (CV) depicts the percentage of the endothelial area (CD31+ areas) in relation to the total image surface. The mean value of the coefficient from measurements in three areas was chosen.

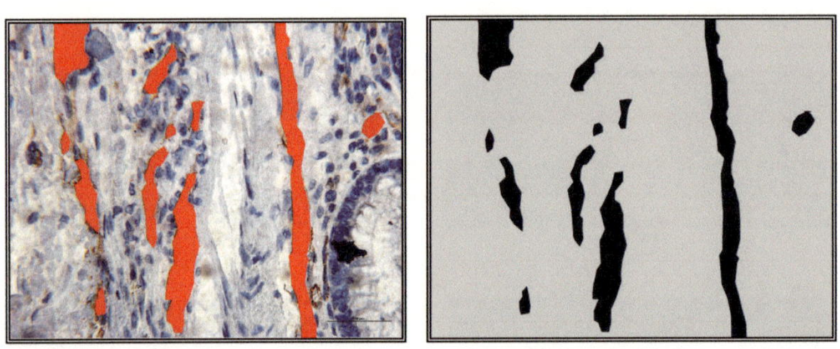

Fig. 6. Computer-assisted selection of the vessels and calculation of the coefficient of vascularisation.

- The data were entered automatically in a database for statistical processing.

3.3.3 Immunohistochemistry for VEGF

The VEGF immunoreactivity was estimated at magnification of x200 or x250. Only the clear brownish staining of the cytoplasm and/or the membrane of the tumour cells was counted as positive. The intensity value was given on a scale from 0 to 3 (0 – no staining, 1 – weak staining in <25% of tumour cells, 2 - moderate cytoplasm staining in >25% of cells; 3 - strong cytoplasm staining). In order to facilitate the correlative analyses, values 0 and 1 were defined as negative staining, whereas values 2 and 3 were considered positive staining. Even if a small part of the tumour had a high staining intensity, the whole tumour was regarded as with high intensity.

3.4 Statistical methods

The data was entered and processed with the statistical package SPSS for Windows version 17. The degree of significance, for which the zero hypotheses was rejected, was chosen as $p < 0.05$. The following statistical methods were used: Descriptive analysis; Variation analysis; Student's t-test; Single factor dispersion analysis (ANOVA) - parametric method to test hypotheses for differences between several independent subsets; Mann-Whitney non-parametric test - to test hypotheses for differences between two independent subsets; Kaplan-Meier's method for survival curves estimation; Log Rank test - for estimating the influence of the tested factors on the survival; ROC (Receiver operating characteristic) curve analysis - to determine the cut-off of the quantitative variables.

The study was approved by Regional Ethic Committee in the University Hospital „Queen Joanna", Sofia.

4. Results

4.1 Doppler endosonography

The average peak systolic velocity (PSV) of the tumour vessels was 23.1 ± 13.7 cm/s (from 6 to 88.9 cm/s). The average resistance index (RI) was 0.67 ± 0.12 (from 0.36 to 0.89). Cut-off values for PSV and RI were set based on a ROC analysis - 17.5 cm/s and 0.7, respectively. In 55 % (76/94) of the tumours, a high peak systolic velocity (above 17.5 cm/s) was observed (Fig. 7.).

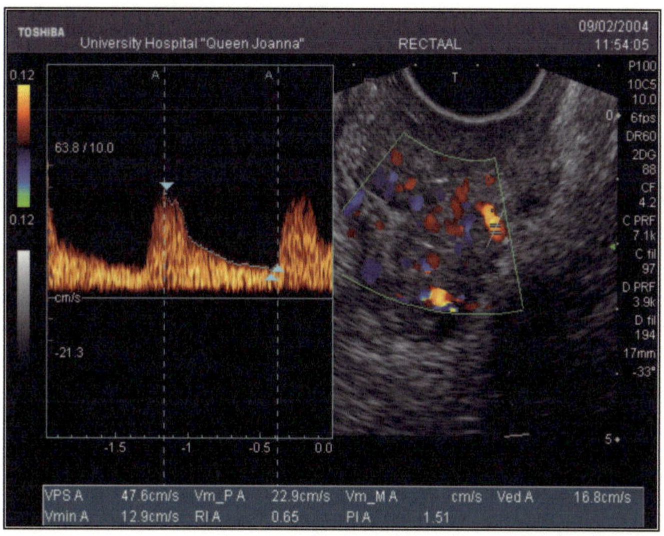

Fig. 7. Pulse colour Doppler endosonography of rectal cancer (high PSV - 47.6 cm/s and low RI - 0.65).

The power Doppler endosonographic evaluation determined poor vascularisation in 102 patients and abundant vascularisation in 93 patients (Fig. 8., Fig. 9.).
The mean PDVI measured in 195 patients was 8.9±6.0% (from 0 to 27.3%). According to ROC analysis the cut-off of PDVI was 8%. PDVI correlated with the tumour stage ($p<0.05$). The index value was higher in the advanced stages than in the initial ones.
The computer-assisted estimation of vascularisation, measured with a Power Doppler, correlated moderately inversely proportionally with the RI ($r=-0.45$, $p<0,001$) and moderately proportionally with the peak systolic velocity of the blood flow in the tumour vessels ($r = 0.39$, $p<0,001$).

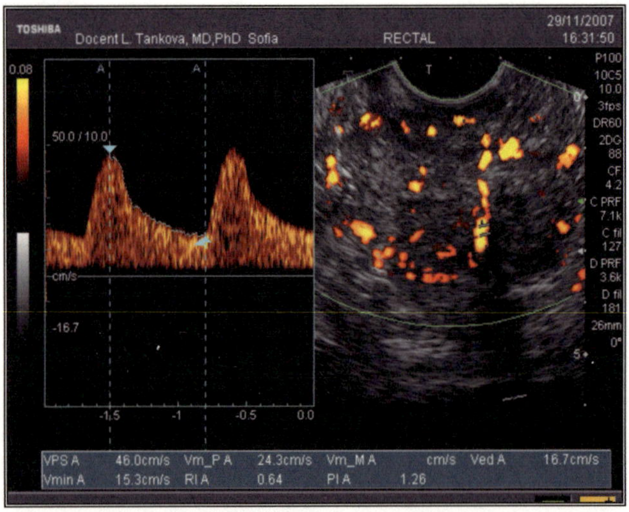

Fig. 8. Power Doppler endosonography of rectal cancer with high vascularisation - abundant chaotic vascularisation in the centre and periphery of the tumour (high PSV - 46 cm/s and low RI - 0.64)

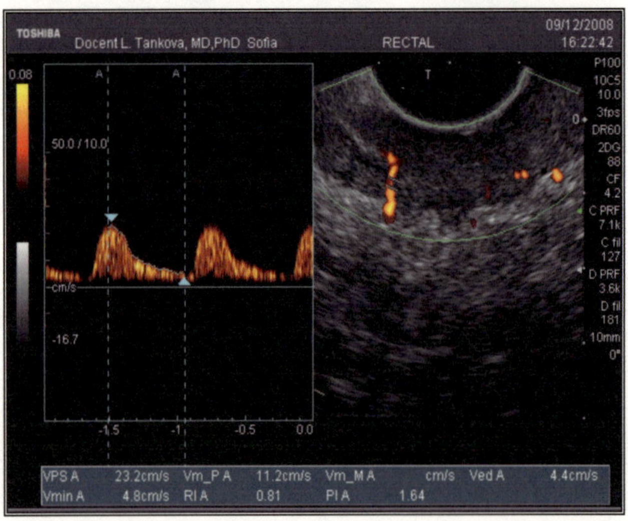

Fig. 9. Power Doppler endosonography of rectal cancer with poor vascularisation (high RI - 0.81)

4.2 Immunohistochemistry

4.2.1 Determination of the microvessel density and the coefficient of vascularisation

The average microvessel density per square millimetre in the examined 110 tumour samples was 163±69 microvessels/mm^2 (from 50 to 328). The agreement between the two observers was good. In cases of disagreement, a final score was determined by consensus. The cut-off values of MVD determined by the ROC curve allowed us to discriminate the hypervascularised tumours (≥ 160) from the hypovascularised ones (MVD < 160).

No correlations were found between the microvessel density and the patient age, gender or tumour size. There was a significant correlation between the microvessel density and the histological differentiation of the tumour. The MVD values for the low differentiation subset were significantly higher than these for the high differentiation subset. MVD correlated significantly with the tumour stage (Table 1.).

Stage	MVD		
	n	$\overline{X}$	SD
I	20	103.68[a]	39.83
II	29	137.41[b]	48.91
III	47	180.34[c]	64.84
IV	14	236.07[d]	66.22

*different letters (a, b, c, d) show a significant difference (p < 0.05).

Table 1. The correlation between microvessel density (MVD) and the rectal cancer stage

The digital assessment of the endothelial area by calculation of the coefficient vascularisation (CV) showed a mean CV of 5.8±3.9% (from 1.1 to 24.6%). According to the ROC curve analysis the hypervascularised group (CV ≤3.25%) was discriminated from the hypovascularised tumours (CV >3.25%) (Fig. 10.).

The coefficient of vascularisation was significantly higher in tumour stages III and IV compared to the stages I and II (Table 2.).

There was a close correlation between microvessel density, calculated by the traditional method and the coefficient of vascularisation determined by the computer-assisted method (r=0.536, p<0.001). There was a linear correlation between PDVI calculated using power Doppler examination and MVD (r=0.41, p<0.001) as well as between PDVI and the coefficient of vascularisation determined by the immunohistochemical examination (r=0.31, p<0.01).

Positive VEGF tumour expression was estimated in 59 tumours (54%) (Fig. 11.). No significant interobserver variability has been noticed between two pathologists.

There was a statistically significant correlation with the MVD values. The MVD value was higher in the VEGF positive group than in the negative group (P <0.05). In tumour samples with positive VEGF expression the mean microvessel density was 188/mm^2 and in the cases of negative VEGF expression, the mean MVD was 136/mm^2 (Table 3.).

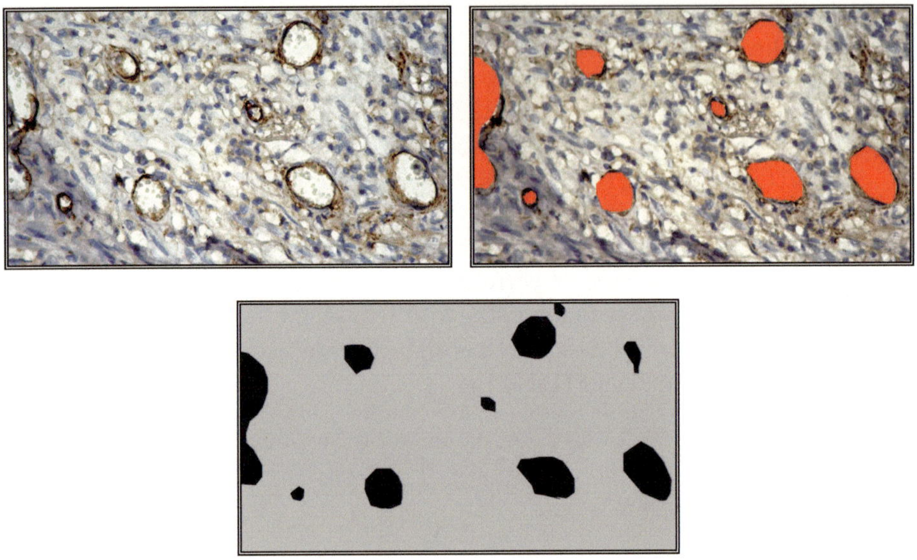

Fig. 10. Steps in the coefficient of vascularisation calculation. High coefficient of vascularisation - 9.2% (original magnification x100)

Stage	CV		
	n	$\overline{X}$ (%)	SD
I	20	3.59a	2.67
II	29	4.69a	4.33
III	47	6.56b	3.35
IV	14	8.30b	4.33

*the different letters (a, b) show a significant difference ($p<0.05$); the same letters show no significant difference ($p>0.05$).

Table 2. The correlation between the coefficient of vascularisation and the rectal cancer stage

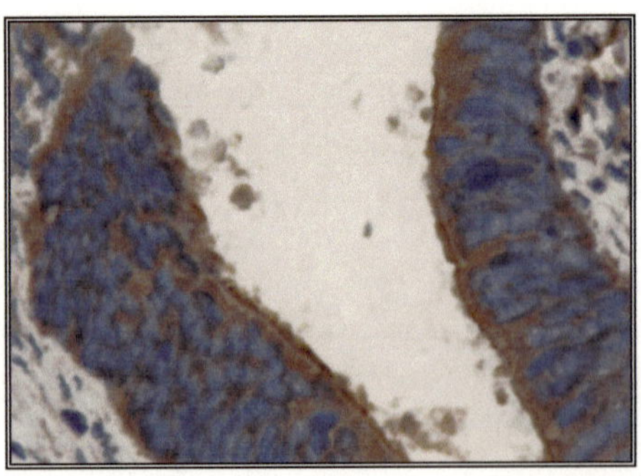

Fig. 11. VEGF expression showing a strong cytoplasmic immunostaining (original magnification x250).

VEGF	MVD		
	n	$\overline{X}$	SD
Negative expression	51	136.08a	66.53
Positive expression	59	187.92b	61.84

* the different letters (a, b) show a significant difference ($p < 0.05$).

Table 3. The correlation between VEGF and MVD

The conducted Kaplan-Meier analysis showed 21 months longer overall survival ($p<0.05$) of the patients with RI below 0.70 than those with higher values. As for the Power Doppler Vascularisation Index (PDVI), the overall survival of patients with PDVI lower than 8% was about 25 months longer than that of patients with PDVI above 8%, and the difference was significant. The survival curve showed a statistically significant relationship between microvessel density and the survival period. The overall survival of the patients with MVD tumours up to 160/mm² tended to be 36 months longer than that in the patients with elevated values of the microvessel density. The overall survival of patients with MVD above 160/mm² decreased very rapidly to circa 30 % within 30 months. A significantly better survival was observed in patients with MVD below 160/mm² (Fig. 12).

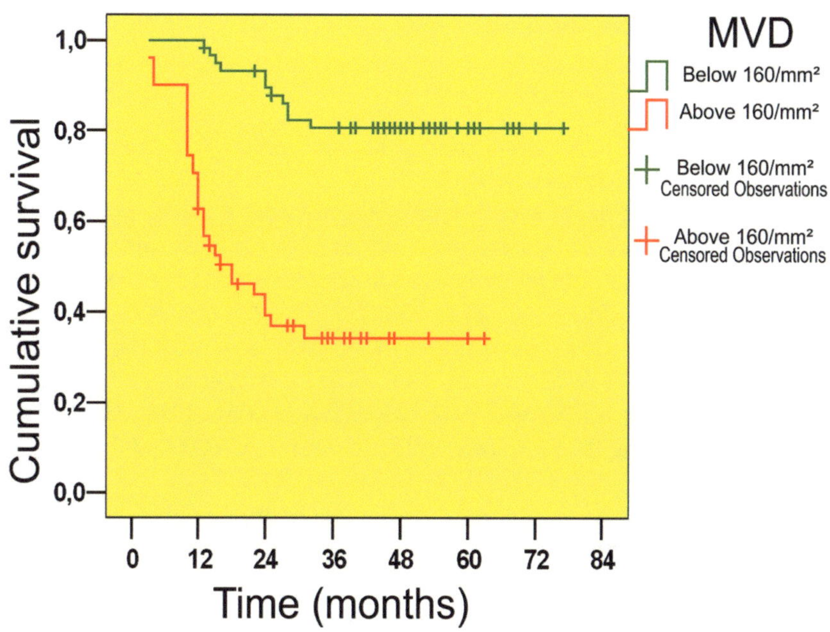

Fig. 12. Kaplan-Meier's curve, based on the MVD

We could establish a statistically significant higher survival period (with about 33.5 months) for patients with negative VEGF than for positive patients. The overall survival of patients with CV above 3.25% decreased very rapidly to circa 45% within 30 months. A significantly better survival was observed in patients with CV below 3.25% (Fig. 13).

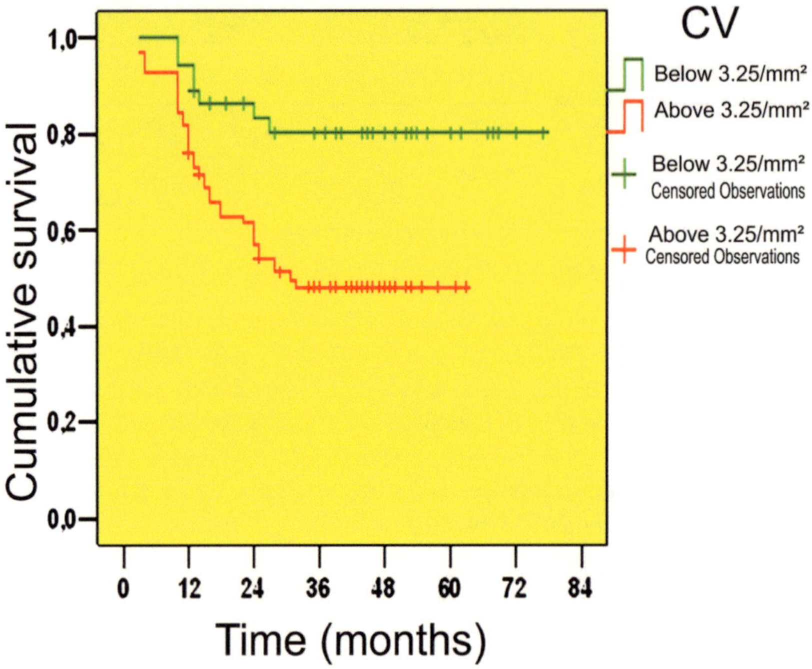

Fig. 13. Kaplan-Meier's curve, based on the CV.

5. Discussion

The determination of the microvessel density is a morphological "golden standard" for assessing the tumour neovascularisation.

Angiogenesis measured by microvessel density determination correlates with the tumour behaviour. There are a lot of reports showing that the higher microvessel density is associated with the metastases development, poor prognosis and life expectancy shortage in colorectal cancer patients (Choi et al., 1998; Engel et al., 1996; Frank et al., 1995; Galindo, 2000; Giatromanolaki et al., 2006 Koukourakis et al., 2005 Li et al., 2003; Rasheeda S. et al, 2009; Sternfeld et al., 1999, Takahashi et al., 1997; Takebayashi et al., 1996; Tanigawa et al., 1997; Tomisaki et al., 1996; Uribarrena et al., 2009; White et al., 2002). However, there are conflicting results regarding the prognostic value of tumour MVD (Abdala et al., 1999, Bossi et al., 1995; Ellis at al., 1998; Pietra et al., 2000; Tarta et al., 2002).

In the current study the microvessel counts are high (163/mm^2 on average), which confirms the assumption that the rectal carcinoma is strongly dependent on angiogenesis. Significant correlations between the microvessel density values, tumour differentiation and clinical stage are observed. MVD is significantly higher in more advanced tumour stages and may be used as a determinant of survival in patients with rectal cancers.

The high average values of microvessel densities in the present study probably are due to the dominance of advanced tumour stages in the clinical material (55% of the tumours were in Stages III and IV) and the use of CD31 as endothelial cell marker. CD31 marks the pre-existent mature vessels and neoformed vessels, the thrombocytes, plasmocytes and megakaryocytes.

There are considerable differences in microvessel counts of carcinoma tissue. The different results may be related to the lack of a standardized and an objective method of the tumour angiogenesis assessment (Vermeulen et al., 1995). The type of antibody used to label the endothelium is a possible cause for the large variation in microvessel counts among studies. Platelet endothelial cell adhesion molecule-1 (PECAM-1) also known as cluster of differentiation 31 (CD31) is a transmembrane glycoprotein involved in cell adhesion. Other commonly used antibodies to highlight tumour blood vessels are those against Factor VIII related antigen, CD34, CD105. Factor VIII related antigen is a part of the von Willebrand factor complex and plays a role in the coagulation cascade. Tissue slices stained with CD34 have been reported to give 1.8-fold higher microvessel counts than slices stained with factor VIII (Tomisaki et al., 1996). The criteria used for identification of microvessels (single endothelium or clusters of endothelium with or without lumen) may be another cause for the considerable differences.

The quantification of angiogenesis was made in the majority of studies with the classical "hot-spot" Weidner's method, which supposes the counting of positive microvessels with and without vascular lumen (Engel et al., 1996; Frank et al., 1995; Galindo, 2000; Pietra et al., 2000; Sternfeld et al., 1999; Takahashi et al., 1997; Takebayashi et al., 1996; Vermeulen et al., 1999).

Some authors use Chalkey count to minimize the subjectivity in the quantification of MVD (Li et al., 2003; White et al., 2002). The Chalkey count consists of applying a 25-point eyepiece graticule on several hot spots (usually 3) (Chalkey, 1943). The graticule is oriented to allow the maximum number of points to hit on or within the areas of stained microvessel profiles (Chalkey grid area: 0.196 mm^2).

Other possibility to assess tumour angiogenesis is to determine the endothelial area which is defined as the percentage area occupied by the positive endothelial cells in the microscope field (Leme et al., 2006; Uribarrena et al., 2009). The measurement of endothelial area by the computerized method is particularly useful in the evaluation of tumors with high vessel density, in which the presence of microvessels very close to each other makes manual counting difficult and laborious. Since measurement of the endothelial area represents the total quantity of vascular endothelium on the histological thin section, there is no need to separately identify each vessel. Automated computerized image analysis for quantifying the MVD may reduce subjective bias during the counting process (Goddard et al., 2002; Poon et al., 2003; Sprindzuk et al., 2009). In a study of breast cancer, tumor microvessel density obtained by automated computerized image analysis, but not the MVD obtained by manual counting, is an independent prognostic factor (Acenero et al., 1998).

We believe that the computerized method is more accurate than conventional MVD determination because the latter counts the vessels, but does not take into account other information such as vessel size or lumen size. The computer-assisted method overcomes some of the disadvantages of traditional microvessel counting. The researcher variations are decreased, because the measurements are done partly by the computer. Another advantage of the computer-assisted method is the faster assessment of the tumour angiogenesis, which makes it suitable for wider application in clinical practice.

A potential drawback of the computerized measurement of tumour vascularisation is the inclusion of non-endothelial structures, unspecifically stained with anti-CD31. However, this can easily be corrected by the pathologist.

The evaluation of expression of angiogenic factors in tumour specimens provides an alternative to MVD in assessing tumour angiogenic activity. This method may potentially reduce the bias associated with the selection of hot spots for MVD evaluation, and may provide more functional information on the tumour angiogenic activity than MVD.

The vascular endothelial growth factor is one of the most important angiogenesis regulators and is intimately involved in the progressing and metastasising of the colorectal cancer. VEGF/VPF (now termed VEGF-A) was first identified in 1983 by Senger and colleagues in ascites fluid of tumours in rodents (Senger et al., 1983). VEGF is a heparin binding glycoprotein that occurs in at least four molecular isoforms as the result of alternative VEGF mRNA splicing.

Numerous studies have demonstrated that tumour over expression of VEGF correlates with high tumour MVD and with the tumor invasiveness in various common human cancers (Des Guetz et al., 2006; Jacobson, 2000; Kaio et al., 2003; Lee et al., 2000; Seo et al., 2000; White et al., 2002). In some studies, VEGF expression in the tumour has been shown as a prognostic factor independent of conventional prognostic factors (Cascinu et al., 2000; Ferroni et al., 2005).

Our results also show a statistically significant relation between the VEGF expression level and the overall survival of rectal cancer patients.

MVD provides direct assessment of angiogenesis and requires tumour tissue, mainly from resection specimens. This process is, however, limited by the inability to provide information about vascular functionality, particularly in response to treatment. Indirect methods of assessing angiogenesis include determination of serum angiogenic cytokines and circulating endothelial cells as well as imaging methods. Several commonly available imaging techniques are able to assess human tumours in vivo with respect to the functional status of the vasculature. Both CT and MRI have the advantage of good spatial resolution, which is often equal to that of corresponding morphological images. Ultrasound, Perfusion CT, also called functional multi-detector row CT (f-MDCT), Dynamic contrast-enhanced MRI (DCE-MRI) are currently the favoured techniques for evaluating tumours with respect to their functional microcirculation (Cosgrove, 2003; McDonald & Choyke 2003). The introduction of ultrasound contrast agents (gas-encapsulated microbubbles of less than 10 μm in diameter) is a recent development in the imaging technology. Since microbubbles are confined to the vascular space, this makes them ideal for the perfusion imaging techniques. Microbubble-specific techniques allow imaging of vessels down to 50–100 μm in diameter (Cosgrove, 2003; McDonald & Choyke 2003; Turkbey et al. 2009).

Endorectal sonography is proven to be the most exact method for rectal cancer staging, but less attention was paid to the pulse colour and power Doppler evaluation. The color Doppler signals seen within the tumour represent the larger vessels (approximately 100 μm or more in diameter), possibly intratumoral arterioles, venules, and arteriole-venule shunts. The tumour vascularisation is usually chaotically distributed and heterogeneous. The microvessel numbers in a small part of the tumour is not enough to represent the global tumour angiogenesis, or to depict the functional properties of tumour blood supply. The colour Doppler allows visualization of the vessels via the colour coding. With the pulse Doppler one can assess the blood flow speed and the resistance of a particular vessel at a certain time point.

Several studies have suggested that color Doppler ultrasonography may provide a reliable preoperative quantitation of tumor angiogenesis and prognostic information in cancer patients (Ogura et al., 2001; Chen et al., 2002).

We hypothesized that the amount of detected supplying intratumoral arterioles and draining venules correlates positively with the degree of the microvascularisation in the tumour. Thus, the Power Doppler Vascularisation Index, by quantitatively depicting the larger supplying arterioles and draining venules, can reflect the extent of global neovascularisation of a tumour.

In the present study the patients with poor vascularisation, determined by the subjective Doppler assessment tend to live longer. Higher resistance index and lower peak systolic velocity (below 17.5 cm/sec) are favourable prognostic signs.

Our results show that the intensity of the intratumour angiogenesis, estimated with endorectal Doppler as well as with immunohistochemical methods, correlates to the tumour stage and tumour aggressiveness.

6. Conclusions

Endorectal pulse colour and power Doppler sonography is useful non-invasive method of preoperative in vivo evaluating the extent of angiogenesis.

In this study the determination of tumour angiogenic activity through endorectal Doppler evaluation, is well correlated with the conventional and computer-assisted immunohistochemical methods. The computer-assisted endosonographic Doppler and immunohistochemical based methods represent rapid, reliable and reproducible means for quantitative assessment of the tumour vascularisation.

7. References

Abdalla, S. A.; Behzad, F.; Bsharah, S.; Kumar, S.; Amini, S. K.; O'dwyer, S. T. & Haboubi, N. Y. (1999). Prognostic relevance of microvessel density in colorectal tumours. Oncol Rep, Vol. 6, No. 4, pp. 839-842, ISSN 1021-335X.

Acenero, M. J.; Gonzalez, J. F.; Gallego, M. G. & Ballesteros, P. A. (1998). Vascular enumeration as a significant prognosticator for invasive breast carcinoma. *J Clin Oncol*, Vol. 16, No. 5, pp. 1684-1688, ISSN 0732-183X.

Bossi, P.; Viale, G.; Lee, A. K.; Alfano, R.; Coggi, G. & Bosari, S. (1995). Angiogenesis in colorectal tumors: Microvessel quantitation in adenomas and carcinomas with clinicopathological correlations. *Cancer Res*, Vol. 55, No. 21, pp. 5049-5053, ISSN 0008-5472.

Cascinu, S.; Staccioli, M. P.; Gasparini, G.; Giordani, P.; Catalano, V.; Ghiselli, R.; Rossi, C.; Baldelli, A. M.; Graziano, F.; Saba, V.; Muretto, P. & Catalano, G. (2000). Expression of vascular endothelial growth factor can predict event-free survival in stage ii colon cancer. *Clin Cancer Res*, Vol. 6, No. 7, pp. 2803-2807, ISSN 1078-0432.

Chalkley H. W. (1943). Method for the quantitative morphologic analysis of tissues. *J Natl Cancer Inst*, Vol. 4, pp. 47-53, ISSN 0027-8874.

Chen, C. N.; Cheng, Y. M.; Lin, M. T.; Hsieh, F. J.; Lee, P. H. & Chang, K. J. (2002). Association of color doppler vascularity index and microvessel density with survival in patients with gastric cancer. *Ann Surg*, Vol. 235, No. 4, pp. 512-518, ISSN 0003-4932.

Choi, H. J.; Hyun, M. S.; Jung, G. J.; Kim, S. S. & Hong, S. H. (1998). Tumor angiogenesis as a prognostic predictor in colorectal carcinoma with special reference to mode of metastasis and recurrence. *Oncology*, Vol. 55, No. 6, pp. 575-581, ISSN 0030-2414.

Cosgrove, D. (2003). Angiogenesis imaging--ultrasound. Br J Radiol, Vol. 76 Spec No 1, pp. S43-49, ISSN 0007-1285.

Des Guetz, G.; Uzzan, B.; Nicolas, P.; Cucherat, M.; Morere, J. F.; Benamouzig, R.; Breau, J. L. & Perret, G. Y. (2006). Microvessel density and vegf expression are prognostic factors in colorectal cancer. Meta-analysis of the literature. *Br J Cancer*, Vol. 94, No. 12, pp. 1823-1832, ISSN 0007-0920.

Ellis, L. M.; Takahashi, Y.; Liu, W. & Shaheen, R. M. (2000). Vascular endothelial growth factor in human colon cancer: Biology and therapeutic implications. *Oncologist*, Vol. 5 Suppl 1, pp. 11-15, ISSN 1083-7159.

Engel, C. J.; Bennett, S. T.; Chambers, A. F.; Doig, G. S.; Kerkvliet, N. & O'malley, F. P. (1996). Tumor angiogenesis predicts recurrence in invasive colorectal cancer when controlled for dukes staging. *Am J Surg Pathol*, Vol. 20, No. 10, pp. 1260-1265, ISSN 0147-5185.

Ferroni, P.; Spila, A.; Martini, F.; D'alessandro, R.; Mariotti, S.; Del Monte, G.; Graziano, P.; Buonomo, O.; Guadagni, F. & Roselli, M. (2005). Prognostic value of vascular endothelial growth factor tumor tissue content of colorectal cancer. *Oncology*, Vol. 69, No. 2, pp. 145-153, ISSN 0030-2414.

Frank, R. E.; Saclarides, T. J.; Leurgans, S.; Speziale, N. J.; Drab, E. A. & Rubin, D. B. (1995). Tumor angiogenesis as a predictor of recurrence and survival in patients with node-negative colon cancer. *Ann Surg*, Vol. 222, No. 6, pp. 695-699, ISSN 0003-4932.

Galindo G. M.; Fernandez Acenero, M. J.; Sanz Ortega, J. & Aljama, A. (2000). Vascular enumeration as a prognosticator for colorectal carcinoma. *Eur J Cancer*, Vol. 36, No. 1, pp. 55-60, ISSN 0959-8049.

Giatromanolaki, A.; Sivridis, E. & Koukourakis, M. I. (2006). Angiogenesis in colorectal cancer: Prognostic and therapeutic implications. *Am J Clin Oncol*, Vol. 29, No. 4, pp. 408-417, ISSN 1537-453X.

Goddard, J. C.; Sutton, C. D.; Furness, P. N.; Kockelbergh, R. C. & O'byrne, K. J. (2002). A computer image analysis system for microvessel density measurement in solid tumours. *Angiogenesis*, Vol. 5, No. 1-2, pp. 15-20, ISSN 0969-6970.

Hamilton, S.; Vogelstein, B.; Kudo, S.; Riboli, S.; Nakamura, D.; Hainaut, J.; Rubio, C.; Sobin, L.; Fogt, F.; Winawer, S.; Goldgar, D. & Jass J. (2000). Tumours of the colon and rectum. In: *World Health Organization Classification of Tumours: Pathology and genetics of tumours of the digestive system*, Hamilton, S. & Aaltonen, L. (eds), pp. 104–143, IARC Press, ISBN 92 832 2410 8 Lyon, France.

Jacobsen, J.; Rasmuson, T.; Grankvist, K. & Ljungberg, B. (2000). Vascular endothelial growth factor as prognostic factor in renal cell carcinoma. *J Urol*, Vol. 163, No. 1, pp. 343-347, ISSN 0022-5347.

Kaio, E.; Tanaka, S.; Kitadai, Y.; Sumii, M.; Yoshihara, M.; Haruma, K. & Chayama, K. (2003). Clinical significance of angiogenic factor expression at the deepest invasive site of advanced colorectal carcinoma. *Oncology*, Vol. 64, No. 1, pp. 61-73, ISSN 0030-2414.

Koukourakis, M. I.; Giatromanolaki, A.; Sivridis, E.; Gatter, K. C. & Harris, A. L. (2005). Inclusion of vasculature-related variables in the dukes staging system of colon cancer. *Clin Cancer Res*, Vol. 11, No. 24 Pt 1, pp. 8653-8660, ISSN 1078-0432.

Lee, J. C.; Chow, N. H.; Wang, S. T. & Huang, S. M. (2000). Prognostic value of vascular endothelial growth factor expression in colorectal cancer patients. *Eur J Cancer*, Vol. 36, No. 6, pp. 748-753, ISSN 0959-8049.

Leme, M. B.; Waitzberg, A. F.; Artigiani Neto, R.; Linhares, M. M. & Matos, D. (2006). Assessment of angiogenesis expression and its relationship with prognosis of colorectal cancer by conventional and computer-assisted histopathological image analysis. *Acta Cir Bras*, Vol. 21, No. 6, pp. 392-397, ISSN 0102-8650.

Li, C.; Gardy, R.; Seon, B. K.; Duff, S. E.; Abdalla, S.; Renehan, A.; O'dwyer, S. T.; Haboubi, N. & Kumar, S. (2003). Both high intratumoral microvessel density determined using cd105 antibody and elevated plasma levels of cd105 in colorectal cancer patients correlate with poor prognosis. *Br J Cancer*, Vol. 88, No. 9, pp. 1424-1431, ISSN 0007-0920.

Mcdonald, D. M. & Choyke, P. L. (2003). Imaging of angiogenesis: From microscope to clinic. *Nat Med*, Vol. 9, No. 6, pp. 713-725, ISSN 1078-8956.

Ogura, O.; Takebayashi, Y.; Sameshima, T.; Maeda, S.; Yamada, K.; Hata, K.; Akiba, S. & Aikou, T. (2001). Preoperative assessment of vascularity by color doppler ultrasonography in human rectal carcinoma. *Dis Colon Rectum*, Vol. 44, No. 4, pp. 538-546; ISSN 0012-3706.

Pietra, N.; Sarli, L.; Caruana, P.; Cabras, A.; Costi, R.; Gobbi, S.; Bordi, C. & Peracchia, A. (2000). Is tumour angiogenesis a prognostic factor in patients with colorectal cancer and no involved nodes? *Eur J Surg*, Vol. 166, No. 7, pp. 552-556, ISSN 1102-4151.

Poon, R. T.; Fan, S. T. & Wong, J. (2003). Clinical significance of angiogenesis in gastrointestinal cancers: A target for novel prognostic and therapeutic approaches. *Ann Surg*, Vol. 238, No. 1, pp. 9-28, ISSN 0003-4932.

Rasheed, S.; Harris, A. L.; Tekkis, P. P.; Turley, H.; Silver, A.; Mcdonald, P. J.; Talbot, I. C.; Glynne-Jones, R.; Northover, J. M. & Guenther, T. (2009). Assessment of microvessel density and carbonic anhydrase-9 (ca-9) expression in rectal cancer. *Pathol Res Pract*, Vol. 205, No. 1, pp. 1-9, ISSN 0344-0338.

Senger, D. R.; Galli, S. J.; Dvorak, A. M.; Perruzzi, C. A.; Harvey, V. S. & Dvorak, H. F. (1983). Tumor cells secrete a vascular permeability factor that promotes accumulation of ascites fluid. *Science*, Vol. 219, No. 4587, pp. 983-985, ISSN 0036-8075.

Seo, Y.; Baba, H.; Fukuda, T.; Takashima, M. & Sugimachi, K. (2000). High expression of vascular endothelial growth factor is associated with liver metastasis and a poor prognosis for patients with ductal pancreatic adenocarcinoma. *Cancer*, Vol. 88, No. 10, pp. 2239-2245, ISSN 0008-543X.

Sprindzuk, M.; Dmitruk, A.; Kovalev, V.; Bogush, A.; Tuzikov, A.; Liakhovski, V. & Fridman. M. (2009). Computer-aided Image Processing of Angiogenic Histological Samples in Ovarian Cancer. *J Clin Med Res*, Vol. 1, No. 5, pp. 249-261, ISSN 1918-3003.

Sternfeld, T.; Foss, H. D.; Kruschewski, M. & Runkel, N. (1999). The prognostic significance of tumor vascularization in patients with localized colorectal cancer. *Int J Colorectal Dis*, Vol. 14, No. 6, pp. 272-276, ISSN 0179-1958.

Takahashi, Y.; Tucker, S. L.; Kitadai, Y.; Koura, A. N.; Bucana, C. D.; Cleary, K. R. & Ellis, L. M. (1997). Vessel counts and expression of vascular endothelial growth factor as prognostic factors in node-negative colon cancer. *Arch Surg*, Vol. 132, No. 5, pp. 541-546, ISSN 0004-0010.

Takebayashi, Y.; Aklyama, S.; Yamada, K.; Akiba, S. & Aikou, T. (1996). Angiogenesis as an unfavorable prognostic factor in human colorectal carcinoma. *Cancer*, Vol. 78, No. 2, pp. 226-231, ISSN 0008-543X.

Tanigawa, N.; Amaya, H.; Matsumura, M.; Lu, C.; Kitaoka, A.; Matsuyama, K. & Muraoka, R. (1997). Tumor angiogenesis and mode of metastasis in patients with colorectal cancer. *Cancer Res*, Vol. 57, No. 6, pp. 1043-1046, ISSN 0008-5472.

Tarta, C.; Teixeira, C. R.; Tanaka, S.; Haruma, K.; Chiele-Neto, C. & Da Silva, V. D. (2002). Angiogenesis in advanced colorectal adenocarcinoma with special reference to tumoral invasion. *Arq Gastroenterol*, Vol. 39, No. 1, pp. 32-38, ISSN 0004-2803.

Tomisaki, S.; Ohno, S.; Ichiyoshi, Y.; Kuwano, H.; Maehara, Y. & Sugimachi, K. (1996). Microvessel quantification and its possible relation with liver metastasis in colorectal cancer. *Cancer*, Vol. 77, No. 8 Suppl, pp. 1722-1728, ISSN 0008-543X.

Turkbey, B.; Kobayashi, H.; Ogawa, M.; Bernardo, M. & Choyke, P. L. (2009). Imaging of tumor angiogenesis: Functional or targeted? *AJR Am J Roentgenol*, Vol. 193, No. 2, pp. 304-313, ISSN 1546-3141.

Uribarrena, A. R.; Ortego, J.; Fuentes, J.; Raventos, N.; Parra, P. & Uribarrena, E. R. (2009). Prognostic value of microvascular density in dukes a and b (t1-t4, n0, m0) colorectal carcinomas. *Gastroenterol Res Pract*, Vol. 2009, No. 2009), pp. 679830, ISSN 1687-630X.

Vermeulen, P. B.; Gasparini, G.; Fox, S. B.; Toi, M.; Martin, L.; Mcculloch, P.; Pezzella, F.; Viale, G.; Weidner, N.; Harris, A. L. & Dirix, L. Y. (1996). Quantification of angiogenesis in solid human tumours: An international consensus on the methodology and criteria of evaluation. *Eur J Cancer*, Vol. 32A, No. 14, pp. 2474-2484, ISSN 0959-8049.

Vermeulen, P. B.; Verhoeven, D.; Fierens, H.; Hubens, G.; Goovaerts, G.; Van Marck, E.; De Bruijn, E. A.; Van Oosterom, A. T. & Dirix, L. Y. (1995). Microvessel quantification in primary colorectal carcinoma: An immunohistochemical study. *Br J Cancer*, Vol. 71, No. 2, pp. 340-343, ISSN 0007-0920.

Weidner, N.; Semple, J. P.; Welch, W. R. & Folkman, J. (1991). Tumor angiogenesis and metastasis-correlation in invasive breast carcinoma. *N Engl J Med*, Vol. 324, No. 1, pp. 1-8, ISSN 0028-4793.

White, J. D.; Hewett, P. W.; Kosuge, D.; Mcculloch, T.; Enholm, B. C.; Carmichael, J. & Murray, J. C. (2002). Vascular endothelial growth factor-d expression is an independent prognostic marker for survival in colorectal carcinoma. *Cancer Res*, Vol. 62, No. 6, pp. 1669-1675, ISSN 0008-5472.

Yang, W. T.; Tse, G. M.; Lam, P. K.; Metreweli, C. & Chang, J. (2002). Correlation between color power doppler sonographic measurement of breast tumor vasculature and immunohistochemical analysis of microvessel density for the quantitation of angiogenesis. *J Ultrasound Med*, Vol. 21, No. 11, pp. 1227-1235, ISSN 0278-4297

Part 3

Surgical Treatment

7

Rectal Carcinoma: Multi-Modality Approach in Curative Local Treatment of Early Rectal Carcinoma

S. H. Kho[1], S. P. Govilkar[1], A. S. Myint[2] and M. J. Hershman[1]
[1]Mid Staffordshire NHS Foundation Trust, Stafford;
[2]Clatterbridge Centre for Oncology NHS Foundation Trust, Wirral;
UK

1. Introduction

Rectal carcinoma is currently the fifth most common cancer in the United Kingdom, accounting for approximately 5800 deaths in the UK and 700,000 deaths worldwide annually (UK Cancer Research). The UK Co-ordinating Committee on cancer research defines rectal cancer as any tumour within 15cm of the anal verge on rigid sigmoidoscopy. The implementation of bowel screening programme has led to the identification of increasing numbers of early rectal cancer. An increasing elderly population associated with multiple co-morbidities has highlighted the importance of early diagnosis and local treatment options. It remains the leading cause of deaths in the over 75 year's age group.

Early rectal cancer is defined as invasive adenocarcinoma spreading into the submucosa or muscularis propria; T1 or T2 tumours in the tumour node metastasis (TNM) classification (Sobin & Wittekind, 2002) or Dukes' A in the Dukes' staging. These tumours have a smaller chance to metastasize to local lymph nodes compared to those invading deeper than the muscularis due to the scarce lymphatic system within colorectal mucosa (Day et al 2003).

2. Epidemiology

Colorectal cancer is the third most common cancer worldwide and the most common gastrointestinal malignancy in Western countries. From these, almost 30% arise in the rectum. The incidence of rectal cancer is higher in men (57.9%) when compared to women (42.1%), with women also showing an improved survival compared to men, 51.0% to 48.5% at 5 years. There has been a steady improvement in the mortality of rectal cancer but 5 year survival in Europe still falls short of American rates. Data collected from the 9 areas in USA over a 4 year period showed 5 year survival rates of 59-66% (Jeffreys et al., 2006; Sant et al., 2003).

3. Screening

A population-based national screening programme was initiated in 2006 based on results of a pilot study of faecal occult blood testing (FOBT) in the UK. A number of countries have recommended and now implemented FOBT into their health schemes. In the USA, the American College of Gastroenterology guidelines published in 1997 have stated asymptomatic individuals above the age of 50 years should have a FOBT +/- flexible sigmoidoscopy every 5 years, a double-contrast barium enema or colonoscopy every 10 years.

Colorectal cancer screening guidelines in high risk individuals are based on case-control studies comparing the incidence and the stage of the disease screened and control groups. About 10% of colorectal cancers run in family due to genetic predispositions (Lynch syndromes). All current evidence predicts that surveillance will improve disease specific survival in these patients. It has been established that screening the average risk population for colorectal cancer reduces cancer specific mortality by 15% with the FOBT and by 50-80% post flexible sigmoidoscopy (Rex, 2004; Sant et al., 2003). The international agreement and introduction of the FOBT will improve the prognosis of rectal cancer by improved early diagnosis. Further indirect benefits will also be seen due to increase endoscopic services and quality of endoscopic examinations.

However the colorectal cancer screening programme with FOBT has limitations due to its inability to detect adenomas. The future will see a change from guaiac testing to the use of computed tomography scanning, flexible sigmoidoscopy and faecal DNA testing for selecting patients that need further colonoscopy and polypectomy (Rex, 2000).

4. Investigations

Before a management strategy is determined, preoperative imaging is essential in order to determine the stage of the tumour and, therefore, prognostic factors in a patient.

Endorectal ultrasound (ERUS) is a diagnostic technique that allows the stage of both tumour invasion and lymph node metastatic involvement to be determined. Not only it is safe,it also plays a significant role in deciding the most adequate surgical strategy in patients with rectal carcinoma (Bhutani, 2009; Siddiqui et al., 2006). This diagnostic procedure has been used successfully in clinical practice since 1985 as a tool to stage rectal cancer and is most widely used in the United Kingdom.

In order to perform ERUS, the rectum must be empty to ensure that there is no distortion of images due to the presence of faecal matter. Laxative enemas are sufficient for rectal lesions and a preparation is required for colonic lesions. Pre-examination sigmoidoscopy is performed to ensure the lumen is free of debris. ERUS is a well-tolerated procedure and usually does not require sedation.

Carcinomas are hypoechoic, and the stage is determined by the scale to which they affect the rectal wall layers (Karantanas et al., 2007). The prefix "u" is used to represent stage and it corresponds to the TNM classification (Smith & Brown, 2008).

- uT1 - tumour does not penetrate the muscularis propria.
- uT2 - tumour penetrates the muscularis propria but not beyond it.
- uT3 - tumour proceeds beyond the muscularis propria, infiltrating the perirectal fat to a variable degree.
- uT4 - tumour infiltrates surrounding organ (Giovannini & Ardizzone, 2009).

There have been meta-analyses carried out to determine the value of ERUS. It has been found to be very accurate for the staging of superficial rectal tumours, with accuracy in evaluating tumour ingrowths into rectal wall layers ranging from 69% to 97% (Gualdi et al.,

2000). Furthermore, the sensitivity and specificity of ERUS to diagnose stage T1 cancer were 87.8% and 98.3%, respectively; for stage T2 the sensitivity and specificity were 80.5% and 95.6% respectively; for stage T3 the sensitivity and specificity were 96.4% and 90.6% respectively; for stage T4 the sensitivity and specificity were 95.4% and 98.3% respectively (Puli et al., 2009). ERUS is also good for differentiating early and advanced rectal lesions with a sensitivity of 96%, a specificity of 85% and an accuracy of 94% (Zorcolo et al., 2009). Also, there are data to suggest that ERUS is 62% to 92% accurate for T-staging and 64% to 88% accurate for N-staging (Geibel & Longo, 2006).

High-resolution three-dimensional ERUS is useful for assessing the depth of submucosal invasion in early rectal cancer and for selecting therapeutic options. Santoro et al. (2009) evaluated the accuracy of this modality in distinguishing slight from massive submucosal invasion of early rectal tumours in a prospective study. The depth of invasion was correctly determined in 87.2% of both pT1-slight and pT1-massive lesions. It also had an accuracy of 95.2% in selecting appropriate management. A meta-analysis by Puli et al. (2010) also showed that ERUS had a sensitivity of 97.3% (95% CI: 93.7–99.1) and specificity of 96.3% (95% CI: 95.3–97.2) in diagnosing T0. Such excellent sensitivity can help physicians offer endoscopic treatment to patients with T0 stage rectal cancers.

Through various research and clinical practice, ERUS has been found to be a safe and accurate method for staging rectal carcinoma, although it is operator-dependent. For this reason, adequate training and skill-development is essential.

Other imaging modalities used for preoperative staging of rectal carcinoma include computed tomography (CT) scan, magnetic resonance imaging (MRI) and positron emission tomography (PET) scan (Geibel & Longo, 2006).

An abdominopelvic CT scan is performed on the majority of patients with clinically localised rectal cancer in order to identify any intra-abdominal metastasis prior to curative or radical resection. However, its role in preoperative staging is much more limited with accuracy of T-staging being 53% to 94% and for N-staging 54% to 70%, which are substantially lower than ERUS (Schaffzin & Wond, 2004).

MRI is also less accurate than ERUS for staging rectal cancer, with an accuracy of 52% in T-stage and 68% in N-stage (Chen et al., 2000). Most of the inaccuracy is due to overstaging caused by inability of MRI to differentiate treatment-induced fibrosis from viable tumours.

Genetic and molecular research has also been performed by Zlobec, et al (2008), which aimed to determine an immunohistochemical protein profile to complement preoperative staging and identify rectal carcinoma patients at a high risk of an adverse outcome. Eight protein markers were selected for use in the investigation, based on their correspondence to various cellular processes and their prognostic value. These protein markers were APAF-1, EphB2, MSTI, Ki67, p53, RHAMM, RKIP and CD8+ tumour infiltrating lymphocytes (TL). 482 patients were retrospectively collected from three different centres in Switzerland. The inclusion criteria comprised of those patients with primary colorectal cancer who received treatment between 1987 and 1996. Patients were excluded from the study if their tumours were located in the colon or if the rectal carcinoma had been treated preoperatively. Clinicopathological features recorded for each participant included gender, pT and pN stage, tumour grade, vascular invasion, invasive margin, mismatch repair, recurrence, metastasis, postoperative therapy and 5-year survival. Follow-up reached 150 months.

Initial univariate survival analysis (Cox proportional hazards regression) for each protein marker showed that four markers were linked to survival time, including negative expression of Ki67, positivity for RHAMM, absence of RKIP and loss of CD8+ TILs. Further multivariable analysis found that only RHAMM ($p<0.001$; HR= 1.94 (1.44-2.61)) and loss of CD8+ TILs ($p=0.006$; HR= 0.63 (0.45-0.88)) were independent prognostic factors.
Therefore, this study proposes that the immunohistochemical protein profile of RHAMM and $CD8^+$ TILs can identify patients with adverse prognosis independent of the extent of the disease and. Collectively, they could aid in selecting early stage rectal cancer patients who are predominantly more likely to have poorer prognosis and thus will benefit the most from preoperative treatment.

5. Management

Radical surgery with total mesorectal excision (anterior resection and abdominoperineal excision) remains the 'gold standard' treatment for rectal cancer. Through this operation, both the primary tumour and the draining lymph nodes are removed which, in turn, leads to a reduction in recurrence. Although it gives the best chance of cure but have a significant risk of death (30-day mortality rate < 7%), morbidity (35%) and poor functional outcome (Association of Coloproctology of Great Britain and Ireland, 2007). One retrospective study evaluated 168 patients with T1-stage rectal cancer and found radical resection to have a local recurrence, distant recurrence and estimated 5-year overall recurrence of 3%, 3% and 6%, respectively (Bentrem et al., 2005).
On the other hand, local treatment in the management of early rectal cancer aims to minimize morbidity and mortality but at the same time to offer cure. The importance of early diagnosis and local treatment options has been highlighted by the increasing numbers of early rectal cancer detected through the introduction of bowel screening programme, an increasing elderly population associated with multiple co-morbidities and the significant number of patients who are 'stoma phobic' and refuse conventional major surgery. The decision to offer local treatment for early rectal cancer must involve all members of the multidisciplinary team.
Staging of the early rectal cancer is critical. Clinical staging of rectal cancer is based on TNM classification (Table 1). Histological assessment plays the most important factor in predicting the risk of lymphatic spread.
When selecting patient for local treatment, the aim is to choose those with tumours confined to rectal wall with a low probability of lymph node metastases. Patients can be assessed by digital rectal examination supplemented by endoscopy and radiology [endorectal ultrasound or endorectal magnetic resonance imaging (MRI)]. Selection criteria and exclusion criteria for local treatment are summarized in table 3 and 4 (Hershman et al., 2003).
Various local treatment options available will be discussed in the following paragraphs. However, combinations of local treatment options i.e. combined modality approach have been used successfully in treating early rectal cancer.

5.1 Local surgical options

5.1.1 Endoscopic Mucosal Resection (EMR)

EMR is usually reserved for benign pedunculated or flat polyps. In the treatment of rectal cancer, it is suitable for very early malignant T1 tumours (sm1 or selected sm2) (Table 2)

(Kikuchi et al., 1995). It is performed under sedation without the requirement of general anaesthesia. Hence, it is a major advantage for very unfit patients.

T - Primary tumour
Tx Primary tumour cannot be assessed
T0 No evidence of primary tumour
Tis Carcinoma *in situ*
T1 Tumour invades submucosa (sm)
T2 Tumour invades muscularis propria (MP)
T3 Tumour invades through MP into subserosa or into non-peritonealised pericolic or perirectal tissues
pT3a Minimal invasion <1mm beyond MP
pT3b Slight invasion 1-5mm beyond MP
pT3c Moderate invasion >5 -15mm beyond MP
pT3d Extensive invasion >15mm beyond MP
T4 Tumour directly invades other organs or structures (T4a)
Tumour perforates the visceral peritoneum (T4b)

N - Regional lymph nodes
Nx Regional lymph nodes cannot be assessed
N0 No regional lymph node metastasis
N1 Metastasis in 1 to 3 pericolic or perirectal lymph nodes
N2 Metastasis in 4 or more pericolic or perirectal lymph nodes
M - Distant metastasis
Mx Presence of distance metastasis cannot be assessed
M0 No distant metastases
M1 Distant metastases

Table 1. TNM Staging.

Classification of submucosal invasion by early colorectal cancer		
Sm1	a	< ¼ of the width of the tumour invading the submucosa
	b	¼ or ½ the width of the tumour invading the submucosa
	c	> ½ the width of the tumour invading the submucosa
Sm2		Intermediate between Sm1 and Sm3
Sm3		Carcinoma invasion near to the muscularis propria

Table 2. Classification of submucosal invasion by early colorectal cancer according to Kikuchi et al. (1995).

Selection criteria for suitability of local treatment	
1.	Mobile non-ulcerative exophytic tumours <10cm from anal verge (clinical assessment: digital rectal examination)
2.	Tumour <3cm or occupying less than 1/3 of the circumference (endoscopic assessment)
3.	cT1/Tx/cN0/cM0 (radiological assessment: endorectal ultrasound/ MRI
4.	Well to moderately well differentiated tumours (histological assessment)
5.	No lymphovascular or venous invasion (histological assessment)
6.	Patient must agree on long-term follow up

Table 3. Selection criteria for local treatment based on clinical practice of Dr. S Myint and Mr. M J Hershman.

Exclusion criteria for local treatment	
1.	Poorly differentiated tumour.
2.	T3/T4 tumour
3.	Clinically tethered or fixed tumour of any radiological T stage
4.	Deeply infiltrative ulcerative tumour

Table 4. Exclusion criteria for local treatment based on clinical practice of Dr. S Myint and Mr. M J Hershman.

During EMR, the polyp is assessed endoscopically, its base is then infiltrated by normal saline or gel to raise it away from the underlying muscle before it is resected using a diathermy or a hot loop. The specimen is then pinned and oriented for histological submission. EMR may not be appropriate if the polyp's base cannot be raised suggesting the tumour is probably more advanced.

The selection criteria for EMR in early rectal cancer are controversial, but generally include (Onozato et al., 2007):

- Well or moderately differentiated adenocarcinoma
- The mucosal or minute submucosal type
- No lymphatic or vascular invasion

No large studies have compared the effectiveness of EMR with transanal excision. A small retrospective study suggested that EMR was a safe and effective method for the treatment of early rectal cancer and its outcomes were comparable to those of transanal excision procedures (Lee et al., 2009) (complete resection was 93.8% for EMR vs. 87.5% for transanal excision; mean length of hospital-stay was 2.7 for EMR vs. 8.9 for transanal excision; no recurrence disease in either group at median follow up of 15 months). There were no significant differences between the two study groups with regard to rectal cancer size, location from the anal verge and histological differentiation.

A prospective study in Sheffield, UK suggested extended EMR for rectal neoplastic lesions can achieve superior results to those of per-anal excision and trans-anal microsurgery with regard to complications and recurrence rates (Hurlstone et al., 2005). The 30-day readmission and death rate was 0%, bleeding 8%; no procedural related complications or perforation with overall 'cure' rate of 98% at a median follow-up of 16 months.

5.1.2 Transanal Resection (TAR) / Transanal Endoscopic Microsurgery (TEM)

Locoregional treatment for early rectal cancer is gaining popularity compared with standard treatment of radical surgery (anterior or abdominoperineal resection). Local procedures for strictly selected patients should lead to similar oncological results and even better outcomes in terms of morbidity, mortality and quality of life (Moore & Guillem, 2002).
Conventional TAR allows the excision of tumours in the lower rectum using anal retractors. Preoperative staging is very important in determining TAR as an option for treating early rectal cancer. It is generally agreed that the criteria for TAR are (Stamos & Murrell, 2007):

- Mobile, non ulcerated T1 or T2 tumour
- Nodes negative on ultrasound
- < 8cm from anal verge
- Occupying < 1/3 of the circumference
- Low grade tumours (well or moderately differentiated)
- Favourable histology on biopsy without lymphovascular invasion

It should be performed as a full thickness resection down to perirectal fat, along with a 1cm radial margin. The defect is usually closed but it can be left open. The specimen should then be pinned and oriented for histology submission.
TAR is associated with relatively low morbidity and mortality, decreased hospital stay and has minimal effect on sphincter function. However, this technique is associated with relatively high rates of local recurrence when compared with standard excision (11.0%vs. 1.6% ; 13.2% vs. 2.7%) especially in patients with a high-grade tumour, or perineural or lymphovascular invasion (Nash et al., 2009; Peng et al., 2011).
If there are unfavourable pathological features like positive resection margins, lymphovascular invasion, lymph node metastasis, perineural invasions and recurrent lesion at follow-up; salvage surgery must be considered.
In summary, TAR has low morbidity and mortality, rapid recovery times and allows preservation of sphincter function but is associated with higher rate of recurrence especially high grade tumour and those with perineural or lymphovascular invasion. Therefore, it is essential to have strict selection criteria when considering this technique and patients should be informed of the risk of local recurrence and the need of frequent follow up.
TEM was first described by Buess in 1984 (Buess et al., 1983, 1984). A resectoscope is used to give stereoscopic view of the rectum and distal sigmoid colon. The rectum is distended with insufflated carbon dioxide to allow the passage of dissecting instruments. It has an exceptionally clear magnified view of the mucosa allows precise removal of mucosal lesions and avoiding the need for radical surgery. TEM is theoretically suitable for tumours lying up to 25cm from the anal verge, unlike TAR which only offers overview of the lower rectum. However, the procedure is usually used for tumours below the peritoneal reflection due to risk of intraperitoneal perforation, technical difficulty and unavailability of preoperative staging with endorectal ultrasonography for proximally sited tumours (Sharma et al., 2003).
TEM represents an effective curative treatment for pT1 sm1 rectal malignancies. A prospective study included 107 patients who had adenocarcinoma: 48 pT1, 43 pT2, and 16 pT3; the 5-year disease-free survival rate was 85.9%, 78.4%, and 49.4% respectively

($p = 0.006$). Recurrence rate was 0% (0/26) in pT1sm1 cancers and 22.7% (5/22) in sm2-3 ($p < 0.05$) (Morino et al., 2011). A submucosal infiltration represented a significant risk factor for recurrences: 0% sm1, 16.7% sm2, and 30% sm3.

Another prospective study (Ramirez et al., 2011) also supports transanal endoscopic microsurgery as an adequate treatment for T1 low-risk tumour and no additional measures are required. The five-year overall survival was 94% and cancer-specific survival was 96%. In addition, the quality of resection is better with TEMS than with TAR as shown in a retrospective study with 42 TEM and 129 TAR patients (Christoforidis et al., 2009).

The reasons for the superiority of TEM over TAR include:

- The use of an optical system with 3D-view
- 6-fold magnification
- The creation of a stable pneumorectum
- Specially designed instruments allow full-thickness excision under direct observation in the lower, middle and even upper parts of rectum
- Full thickness excision allows proper histological examinations

There are no large head to head studies comparing TEM with conventional radical surgery. There is 1 small prospective randomized trial and 2 retrospective cohort studies comparing TEM with radical surgery (Heintz et al., 1998; Lee et l., 2003; Winde et al., 1996) (Table 5). According to study by Winde et al, there was no significant difference in the local recurrence rate or the survival rate for patients treated with TEM or anterior resection. However, the power of the study was inadequate. Lee et al also reported similar outcomes for patients with T1 and T2 rectal cancers underwent TEM or radical surgery. Study by Heintz et al is difficult to interpret due to inclusion of patients who had inadequate local surgery.

TEM is a safe technique with low morbidity and recurrence rates (Koebrugge et al., 2009). Experience over times has led to a reduction in operation time, length of patients' hospital stay and complication rate. TEM remains the treatment of choice for stage T1 low risk rectal carcinomas. Patient with pT1 sm2-3 and T2 low risk lesions should be considered high-risk cases if treated only by TEM (Morino et al., 2011; Ramirez et al., 2011).

5.2 Contact radiotherapy

Rectal adenocarcinoma is radio-resistant. Doses above 80Gy are necessary and need to be delivered by endocavitary irradiation (contact x-ray therapy, brachytherapy) with high doses targeting the tumour but low doses to normal tissue.

Contact radiotherapy or known as Papillon's technique was developed in the 1950s and is performed with a 50kV hand held tube which is capable of delivering a dose of 20 Gy per minute. The percentage dose is 100% at 0mm, about 50% at 5mm depth and 20% at 10mm. The scatter from the tube is negligible.

For a T1N0 tumour, treatment is divided into 4 sessions:

- 35 Gy on day 1
- 30 Gy on day 7
- 20 - 25 Gy on day 21
- 10 - 20 Gy on day 35

The total dose may range from 80 - 110 Gy in four to five fractions depending on the initial size of the tumour and the shrinkage of the tumour which is measured on day 21. If a complete response is achieved at this stage, the chance of control with radiotherapy alone is very high. However, if there is still a visible lesion, patient should be referred for surgery or the dose increased to 100 - 120 Gy and combined with external-beam radiotherapy and a brachytherapy boost if inoperable.

Transanal Endoscopic Microsurgery Versus Radical Surgery for T1 and T2 Rectal Cancer						
Study	T Stage	TEM / Radical surgery (RS)	Number of patients	Local recurrence rate (%)	Overall survival rate (%)	Follow-up (Months)
Winde et al (1996)	1	TEM	24	4.2	96	46
		RS	26	0	96	
Lee et al (2003)	1	TEM	52	4.1	100	31-35
		RS	17	0	93	
	2	TEM	17	19.5 ($p<0.05$)	95	
		RS	83	9.4	96	
Heintz et al (1998)	1 (Low risk)	TEM	46	4.4	79	42-52
		RS	34	2.9	81	
	1 (High risk)	TEM	12	33	62	
		RS	11	18.2	69	

Table 5. Summary of results for TEM vs. Radical surgery studies.

Gerald et al (2002) reported contact radiotherapy can achieve local control in 85 - 90% of patients with T1N0 tumours, good tolerability in most with preservation of good anorectal function and no severe late toxic effects.

Sun Myint et al (2007) at Clatterbridge, UK reported their experience of treating patients with early rectal cancer using multimodality approach including contact radiotherapy. Clatterbridge uses the Therapax 50kV machine with a 0.5mm Al filter as opposed to the Philips machine. At Clatterbridge, patients who do not respond well to initial contact radiotherapy are offered external-beam radiotherapy alone, delivering 45Gy in 20 fractions over 4 weeks or chemoradiotherapy with 45Gy in 25 fractions over 5 weeks with 5-fluorouracil infusion 750-1000mg/m2 in weeks 1 and 5. 5-fluorouracil has been changed to oral capecitabine 825mg/m2 on the days of radiotherapy. From their experience, 124 out of 220 patients had Papillon's contact radiotherapy as part of the multimodality treatment. There were 24/220 (11%) with residual disease after initial radiotherapy. 71% of patients were still alive at a median follow-up of 4.6 years. The cancer specific survival was 93%.

Therefore, contact therapy is an efficient treatment for T1N0 rectal adenocarcinoma. It has the advantage of not needing general anaesthesia, can be performed on an outpatient basis, can be used to treat frail elderly patients and no risk of fistula.

For T2-3N0-1 tumours, the standard treatment is radical surgery. However, this may not be suitable if the patient has high co-morbidity or patient refuses to have permanent colostomy.

In these situations, a combination of contact radiotherapy and external-beam radiotherapy, brachytherapy or both may be considered. The combination treatment is essential as contact therapy alone is insufficient to penetrate the deeper layers of the rectal wall and no irradiation reaches the perirectal lymph nodes which are at high risk of involvement.

5.3 Local excision and adjuvant therapy

Postoperative radiation and chemotherapy have been used as an alternative to radical surgery to reduce the risk of local recurrence for patients. There are studies to suggest lower trends of local recurrence rates and higher disease free survival (DFS) rates with adjuvant therapy compared with local excision alone, especially in T2 tumours or in higher grade tumours.

Retrospective study by Chakravarti et al (1999) compared patients with T1/T2 rectal cancer treated by local excision alone with those treated by local excision plus adjuvant radiation therapy. There was no difference in the 5-year local recurrence and DFS between the 2 groups even though there were significantly higher proportions of T2 tumours and T1 tumours with unfavourable histological features in the radiation therapy group. However, subgroup analysis of high-risk patients showed substantially better local control rate with the addition of postoperative radiation (85% vs. 37% local excision alone).

A prospective multi-institutional trial by The Cancer and Leukaemia Group B comparing the outcomes of 59 patients with T1 lesions treated with local excision alone with those 51 patients with T2 lesions treated with local excision and postoperative chemoradiation (Greenberg et al., 2008). The recurrence rates were 7% for the T1 and 14% for T2 at a median follow-up of 7 years.

The Radiation Oncology Therapy Group study evaluating adjuvant chemoradiation therapy after local excision reported a 16% (8 out of 65) locoregional recurrence rate (Russell et al., 2000). The risk of recurrence correlated with T stage (T1 4%, T2 16%, T3 23%).

Despite the lack of randomized control trials, there are data to support benefit of adjuvant chemoradiation or radiation therapy after local excision for patients with T2 or in higher-grades tumours. More studies are still required before this can be adopted to routine clinical practice.

5.4 Local excision after neoadjuvant therapy

Local excision after neoadjuvant therapy may be considered for patients who refuse radical surgery or candidates who are at high risk of surgery due to significant medical co-morbidities.

Lezoche et al (2005) reported 2.8% (1 out of 106) recurrence rate in T2 rectal cancer patients treated with preoperative chemoradiotherapy followed by TEM at a median follow up of 38 months. This group has further conducted a randomised trial of preoperative chemoradiotherapy followed by TEM vs. radical surgery alone. This trial showed equivalent local control and survival at a median follow-up of 4-years however this study did not have adequate study power.

Although robust evidence is still lacking to support the routine use of neoadjuvant therapy with local excision, the tumoricidal effect of neoadjuvant chemoradiation is well documented in patients with advanced rectal cancer treated with radical surgery. Hence, it is reasonable to project the benefits of neoadjuvant therapy in treating patients with early rectal cancer by local excision especially in T2 tumours.

5.5 Salvage surgery after local excision

Salvage surgery can be offered to patients who have failed local treatment of early rectal cancer. There are two types available:

- Immediate salvage (rescue surgery)
  - This is performed within 6 months of the completion of local treatment.
  - This includes patients with inadequate resection margins of local surgery, unfavourable pathology and failure to eradicate tumour with local treatment.
- Delayed salvage
  - This is carried out for local recurrence after an apparent cure of cancer that has been sustained for a minimum of 3 months.

Hershman and Sun Myint (2007) reported that salvage surgery was an effective management after fail local treatment with an overall salvage rate of 68% (30/44) and a salvage cure rate of 87% (26/30). Mellgren et al (2000) reported a 5-year disease-free survival rate of 50% in 24 out of 25 patients with local recurrence treated with radical salvage surgery.

Therefore, intensive follow-up after initial local treatment in the first 3 years is important in order to identify patients who are suitable for salvage surgery and to enable prompt treatment.

Treatment Algorithm for Patients with Early Rectal Cancer are summarised in Table 6.

6. Complications

6.1 EMR

EMR is usually tolerated without many side effects. However, bleeding and recurrence has been reported especially for those with submucosal cancer. A retrospective study by Kim et al (2011) reported that 7 out of the 65 patients with submucosal cancer who underwent EMR showed adverse outcomes within 3 years: recurrence or residual of primary cancer or lymph node metastasis.

Metz et al (2011) reported 7% (21 out of 288 patients) experienced clinically significant delayed bleeding after undergoing EMR for laterally spreading tumours of 20mm or greater. 10 underwent colonoscopy, 1 required angiography and 1 required surgery after perforation following hemostatic clip placement. These were data analysed from two large prospective intention-to-treat studies of EMR. Their data have shown that proximal lesion location is a highly significant risk for clinically significant delayed bleeding following colonic EMR. Recent aspirin use also increases bleeding risk. Surprisingly, larger lesion size ($P = 0.2$), multiple excisions rather than en bloc resection ($P = 0.1$), polyp morphology ($P = 0.2$), and previous attempts ($P = 0.5$) are not associated with increased risk of bleeding.

6.2 TAR

TAR has been reported to be associated with local recurrence in the treatment for early rectal cancer. Taylor et al (1998) report a 30% recurrence rate for T1 and T2 tumours treated by local excision alone, Grarcia-Anguilar et al (2000) reported 18% recurrence with T1 tumours and 37% with T2 tumours at 54 months of follow up, Madbouley et al (2005) reported overall recurrence rate of a 28.8% in T1 rectal cancer and Huh et al (2009) reported similar recurrence rate of 28.5% in early rectal tumours with favourable pathologic features at median follow-up of 66 months

Local excision does not remove lymph nodes in the mesorectum, therefore, when considering patients for local excision, strict selection criteria are essential to give more favourable outcomes. Risk of lymph nodes involvement is 0-12% for T1 cancer and 12-28% for T2 cancers (Sengupta & Tjandra, 2001). Features associated with a significantly increased risk of lymph node metastases include poor differentiation, lymphovascular invasion and size greater than 3cm (Chambers et al., 2004; Nascimbeni et al., 2002).

6.3 TEM

Although TEM represents an effective curative treatment for pT1 sm1 rectal cancer, it can be associated with recurrence in pT1 sm2-3 patients. Study by Morino et al (2011) showed that recurrence rate was 0% (0/26) in pT1sm1 cancers and 22.7% (5/22) in sm2-3 ($p < 0.05$). In addition, other risk factors associated with recurrence include pT2 leisons and lesions larger than 3cm. Acording to a retrospective study by Yu et al (2011) involving 60 patients who underwent TEM, there was a significant difference in local recurrence rate between pT1 and pT2(2.6% vs. 40.0%, $P<0.05$). The recurrence rate was higher in lesions larger than 3 cm compared to those lesions smaller than 3cm(19.0%, 4/21 vs. 2.6%, 1/39, $P<0.05$) (Yu et al., 2011).

6.4 Contact radiotherapy

The main side effect of endocavitary irradiation (contact radiotherapy with or without iridium brachytherapy) combined with external-beam radiotherapy is rectal bleeding, which may require argon laser treatment. Other side effects include bowel urgency and frequency in the morning which do not generally affect normal life (Gerald et al., 2002). Late toxic effects include rectal fibrosis or stenosis and rectal ulcers with persistent bleeding leading to chronic anaemia have been reported (Birnbaum et al., 1994; Cho et al., 1995; Letschert, 1995).

7. Conclusion

Local treatment of early rectal cancer remains an attractive alternative to radical surgery in the current climate of increasing ageing population and the numbers of early rectal cancer detected through colorectal screening programme. This option is suitable for elderly patients, those patients with significant medical co-morbidities who are at increased operative risk and those who are stoma averse. Unlike radical surgery, it is associated with relatively low morbidity and mortality, decreased hospital stay and has minimal effect on sphincter functions. Although this treatment option is still debated, local excision alone should be used for selected patients with T1 tumours or low risk T2 tumours and patients should be informed of the risk of local recurrence and the need of frequent follow up. Contact radiotherapy is an efficient treatment for T1N0 rectal adenocarcinoma. It has the advantage of not needing general anaesthesia, can be performed on an outpatient basis, can be used to treat frail elderly patients and no risk of fistula. A combination of contact radiotherapy and external-beam radiotherapy, brachytherapy or both may be considered for patients with T2-3N0-1 tumours. Salvage surgery can be offered to patients with recurrences. Combination of local excision with adjuvant and neoadjuvant therapies may play a role in the treatment of early rectal cancer but more trials are needed. Patients and relatives should be informed fully regarding treatment options available and the side effects associated with each treatment. Careful selection of patient and preoperative staging are paramount for the successful outcome of multimodality approach and all multidisciplinary team members must be involved in order to deliver high quality of care to patients.

Clinical Stage	Primary Treatment	Pathology After Local Excision	Additional Treatment
<3cm T1N0M0/ T2N0M0	Local Excision (TEM/TAR)	T1 Negative CRM	Low risk -close follow up High risk (sm3, vascular / lymphatic invasion, G3, positive CRM) - additional treatment as T2 tumour
		T2 Negative CRM	Postoperative radiotherapy or chemoradiotherapy Possibility of conventional radical surgery
		T1 Positive / Uncertain CRM	Immediate conventional radical surgery If unfit or refuse surgery, then postoperative radiotherapy or chemoradiotherapy
		T2 Positive CRM	
	Endocavity radiotherapy / Papillon's technique: for unfit patients at presentation (ASAIII or above), patients refuse surgery		
>3cm T1N0M0/ T2N0M0	External beam radiotherapy / chemoradiotherap y followed by local resection	Negative CRM	Close Follow up
		Positive CRM	Immediate conventional radical surgery
	Intracavity boost (Papillon's) for patients unfit for surgery		

Table 6. Treatment Algorithm for Patients with Early Rectal Cancer.

8. Acknowledgment

Very grateful to Dr. Caroline Angit for her help in preparing and formatting the manuscripts.

9. References

Association of Coloproctology of Great Britain and Ireland. *Guidelines for the Management of Colorectal Cancer* (3rd edn). 2007. http://www.library.nhs.uk/theatres/Viewresource.aspx?res ID=31479.

Bentrem, D.J.; Okabe, S.; Wond, D. & et al. (2005). T1 adenocarcinoma of the rectum. Transanal excision or radical surgery? *Ann Surg,* Vol. 242, pp. 472-477.

Bhutani, M.S. (2009). Colorectal endoscopic ultrasound, In: *Gress FG, Savides TJ, editors. Endoscopic ultrasonography* (2nd ed), 160-171. West Sussex: Wiley-Blackwell.

Birnbaum, E.H.; Myerson, R.J. & Fry, R.D. et al. (1994). Chronic effects of pelvic radiation therapy on anorectal function. *Dis Colon Rectum,*Vol.37, pp.909–915.

Buess, G.; Theiss, R.; Hutterer, F.; Pichlmaier, H.; Pelz, C.; Holfeld, T. et al. (1983). Transanal endoscopic surgery of the rectum - testing a new method in animal experiments. *Leber Magen Darm,* vol.13, pp.73–77.

Buess, G.; Hutterer, F.; Theiss, J.; Bobel, M.; Isselhard, W. & Pichlmaier, H. (1984). A system for a transanal endoscopic rectum operation. *Chirurg,* Vol.55, pp. 677–680.

Chakravarti, A.; Compton, C.C.; Shellito, P.C.; Wood, W.C.; Landry, J.; Machuta, S.R.; Kaufman, D.; Ancukiewicz, M. & Willett, C.G. (1999). Long-term follow-up of patients with rectal cancer managed by local excision with and without adjuvant irradiation. *Ann Surg,* Vol.230, No.1, pp. 49-54.

Chambers, W.M.; Khan, U.; Gagliano, A.; Smith, R.D.; Sheffield, J. & Nicholls, R.J. (2004). Tumour morphology as a predictor of outcome after local excision of rectal cancer. *Br J Surg,* Vol.91, No.4, pp.457-459.

Chen, C.C.; Lee, R.C. ; Lin, J.K. & et al. (2000). How accurate is magnetic resonance imaging in restaging rectal cancer in patients receiving preoperative combined chemoradiotherapy? *Dis Colon Rectum,* Vol.82, pp. 967-981.

Cho, K.H.; Lee, C.K.K. & Levit, S.H. (1995). Proctitis after conventional external radiation therapy for prostate cancer: importance of minimizing posterior rectal dose. *Radiology,* Vol.3, pp.699–703.

Christoforidis, D.; Cho, H.M.; Dixon, M.R.; Mellgren, A.F.; Madoff, R.D. & Finne, C.O. (2009). Transanal endoscopic microsurgery versus conventional transanal excision for patients with early rectal cancer. *Ann Surg,* Vol.249, No.5, pp.776-782.

Day, D.W.; Jass, J.R,; Price, A.B.; Shepherd, N.A.; Sloan, J.M.; Talbot, I.C. & et al. (2003). Epithelial tumours of the large intestine, In: *Morson and Dawson's Gastrointestinal Pathology* (4th edn), 551-609. Blackwell Science: Oxford.

Garcia-Aguilar, J.; Mellgren, A.; Sirivongs, P.; Buie, D.; Madoff, R.D. & Rothenberger, D.A. (2000). Local excision of rectal cancer without adjuvant therapy: a word of caution. *Ann Surg,* Vol.231, pp.345–351.

Geibel, J. & Longo, W. (2006). Modern management of rectal cancer: A 2006 update. *World J Gastroenterol,* Vol.12, No.20, pp.3186-3195.

Gerald, J.P.; Chapet, O. & Ramaioli, A. (2002). Long term control of T2 - T3 rectal adenocarcinoma with radiotherapy alone. *Int J radiol Oncol Biol Phys,* Vol.54, pp.142-149.

Giovannini, M. & Ardizzone, S. (2009). Anorectal ultrasound for neoplastic and inflammatory lesions. *Best Prac Res Clin Gastroenterol,* Vol.44, pp.100-107.

Greenberg, J.A.; Shibata, D.; Herndon, J.E.; Steele, G.D.Jr.; Mayer, R. & Bleday, R. (2008). Local excision of distal rectal cancer: an update of cancer and leukemia group B 8984. *Dis Colon Rectum,* Vol.51, No.8, pp.1185-1191.

Gualdi, G.F.; Casciani, E.; Guadalaxara, A. & et al. (2000). Local staging of rectal cancer with transrectal ultrasound and endorectal magnetic resonance imaging: comparison with histologic findings. *Dis Colon Rectum,* Vol.43, pp. 338-345.

Heintz, A.; Mörschel, M. & Junginger, T. (1998). Comparison of results after transanal endoscopic microsurgery and radical resection for T1 carcinoma of the rectum. *Surg Endosc,* Vol.12, pp. 1145-1148.

Hershman, M.J.; Sun Myint, A. & Makin, C.A. (2003). Multi-modality approach in curative local treatment of early rectal carcinomas. *Colorectal Dis,* Vol.5, pp. 445-450.

Hershman, M.J. & Sun Myint, A. (2007). Salvage surgery after inadequate combined local treatment for early rectal cancer. *Clinc Onc,* Vol.19, pp.720-723.

Huh, J.W.; Park, Y.A.; Lee, K.Y.; Kim, S.A. & Sohn, S.K. (2009). Recurrences after local excision for early rectal adenocarcinoma. *Yonsei Med J,* Vol.31, No.50, pp.704-708.

Hurlstone, D.P.; Sanders, D.S.; Cross, S.S; George, R.; Shorthouse, A.J. & Brown, S. (2005). A prospective analysis of extended endoscopic mucosal resection for large rectal villous adenomas: an alternative technique to transanal endoscopic microsurgery. *Colorectal Dis,* Vol.7, No.4, pp. 339-344.

Jeffreys, M.; Rachet, B.; McDowell, S. & et al. (2006). Survival from rectal and anal cancers in England and Wales, 1986-2001. *Eur J Cancer,* Vol.42, pp.1434-1440.

Karantanas, A.H.; Yarmenitis, S.; & Papanikolaou, N. & et al. (2007). Preoperative imaging staging of rectal cancer. *Dig Dis,* Vol.25, pp.20-32.

Kikuchi, R.; Takano, M.; Takagi, K.; Fujimoto, N.; Nozaki, R.; Fujiyoshi, T. & Uchida, Y. (1995). Management of early invasive colorectal cancer. Risk of recurrence and clinical guidelines. *Dis Colon Rectum,* Vol.38, No.12, pp.1286-1295.

Kim, M.N.; Kang, J.M.; Yang, J.I.; Kim, B.K.; Im, J.P.; Kim, S.G.; Jung, H.C. & Song, I.S.; Kim, J.S. (2011). Clinical Features and Prognosis of Early Colorectal Cancer Treated by Endoscopic Mucosal Resection. *J Gastroenterol Hepatol,* Vol.22, (April 2011), pp. 1440-1746. [Epub ahead of print]

Koebrugge, B.; Bosscha, K. & Ernst, M.F. (2009). Transanal endoscopic microsurgery for local excision of rectal lesions: is there a learning curve? *Dig Surg,* Vol.26, No.5, pp.372-7.

Lee, S.H.; Jeon, S.W.; Jung, M.K.; Kim, S.K. & Choi, G.S. (2009). A comparison of transanal excision and endoscopic resection for early rectal cancer. *World J Gastrointest Endosc,* Vol.15, No.1, (Oct 2009), pp. 56-60.

Lee, W.; Lee, D.; Choi, S. & et al. (2003.) Transanal endoscopic microsurgery and radical surgery for T1 and T2 rectal cancer. *Surg Endosc,* Vol.17, pp.:1283-1287.

Letschert, J.G. (1995). The prevention of radio-induced small bowel complications. *Eur J Cancer*, Vol.31, pp. 1361– 1365.

Lezoche, E.; Guerrieri, M.; Paganini, A.M.; Baldarelli, M.; De Sanctis, A. & Lezoche, G. (2005). Long-term results in patients with T2-3 N0 distal rectal cancer undergoing radiotherapy before transanal endoscopic microsurgery. *Br J Surg*, Vol.92, No.12, (Dec 2005), pp.1546-1552.

Madbouly, K.M.; Remzi, F.H.; Erkek, B.A.; Senagore, A.J.; Baeslach, C.M.; Khandwala, F. & et al. (2005). Recurrence after transanal excision of T1 rectal cancer: should we be concerned? *Dis Colon Rectum*, Vol.48, pp.711–719.

Mellgren, A.; Sirivongs, P.; Rothenberger, D.A.; Madoff, R.D. & García-Aguilar, J. (2000). Is local excision adequate therapy for early rectal cancer? *Dis Colon Rectum*, Vol.43, No.8, (Aug 2000), pp.1064-1071.

Metz, A.J.; Bourke, M.J.; Moss, A.; Williams, S.J.; Swan, M.P. & Byth, K. (2011). Factors that predict bleeding following endoscopic mucosal resection of large colonic lesions. *Endoscopy*, Vol.43, No.6, (Jun 2011), pp.506-511.

Morino, M.; Allaix, M.E.; Caldart, M.; Scozzari, G. & Arezzo, A. (2011). Risk factors for recurrence after transanal endoscopic microsurgery for rectal malignant neoplasm. *Surg Endosc*, (June 2011). [Epub ahead of print].

Moore, H.G. & Guillem, J.G. (2002). Local therapy for rectal cancer. *Surg Clin North Am*, Vol.82, pp. 967-981.

Nascimbeni, R.; Burgart, L.J.; Nivatvongs, S. & Larson, D.R. (2002). Risk of lymph node metastasis in T1 carcinoma of the colon and rectum. *Dis Colon Rectum*, Vol.45, No.2, pp. 200-206.

Nash, G.M.; Weiser, M.R.; Guillem, J.G.; Temple, L.K.; Shia, J.; Gonen, M.; Wong, W.D.& Paty, P.B. (2009). Long-term survival after transanal excision of T1 rectal cancer. *Dis Colon Rectum*, Vol.52, No.4, pp. 577-582.

Onozato, Y.; Kakizaki, S.; Ishihara, H.; Iizuka, H.; Sohara, N.; Okamura, S.; Mori, M. & Itoh, H. (2007). Endoscopic submucosal dissection for rectal tumours. *Endoscopy*, Vol.39, No.5, pp. 423-427.

Peng, J.; Chen, W.; Sheng, W.; Xu, Y.; Cai, G.; Huang, D. & Cai, S. (2011). Oncological outcome of T1 rectal cancer undergoing standard resection and local excision. *Colorectal Dis*, Vol.13, No.2, pp. :e14-19.

Puli, S.R.; Bechtold, M.L.; Reddy, J.B.; Choudhary, A. & Antillon, M.R. (2010). Can endoscopic ultrasound predict early rectal cancers that can be resected endoscopically? A meta-analysis and systematic review. *Dig Dis Sci*, Vol.55, No.5, pp.1221-1229.

Puli, S.R.; Bechtold, M.L.; Reddy, J.B. & et al. (2009). How good is endoscopic ultrasound in differentiating various T stages of rectal cancer? Meta-analysis and systematic review. *Ann Surg Oncol* Vol.16, pp. 254-265.

Smith, N. & Brown, G. Preoperative staging of rectal cancer. *Acta Oncol* Vol. 47, pp.20-31.

Ramirez, J.M.; Aguilella, V.; Valencia, J.; Ortego, J.; Gracia, J.A.; Escudero, P.; Esco, R. & Martinez, M. (2011). Transanal endoscopic microsurgery for rectal cancer. Long-term oncologic results. *Int J Colorectal Dis*, Vol.26, No.4, pp. 437-443.

Rex, D.K. (2000) American College of Gastroenterology Action Plan for Colorectal Cancer Prevention 2000: screening recommendations. *Am J Gastroenterol* Vol.95, pp.868-877.

Rex, D.K. (2004). Americal College of Gastroenterology Action Plan for Colorectal Cancer Prevention. *Am J Gastroenterol*, Vol.99, pp. 574-577.

Russell, A.H.; Harris, J.; Rosenberg, P.J.; Sause, W.T.; Fisher, B.J.; Hoffman, J.P.; Kraybill, W.G. & Byhardt, R.W. (2000). Anal sphincter conservation for patients with adenocarcinoma of the distal rectum: long-term results of radiation therapy oncology group protocol 89-02. *Int J Radiat Oncol Biol Phys*, Vol.15, No.46, pp.313-322.

Sant, M.; Aareleid, T.; Berrino, F. & et al. (2003). EUROCARE-3: survival of cancer patients diagnosed 1990-94 - results and commentary. *Ann Oncol*, Vol.14, No.5, pp. v61-v118.

Santoro, G.A.; Gizzi, G.; Pellegrini, L.; Battistella, G. & Di Falco, G. (2009). The value of high-resolution three-dimensional endorectal ultrasonography in the management of submucosal invasive rectal tumours. *Dis Colon Rectum*, Vol.52, No.11, pp.1837-1843.

Schaffzin, D.M. & Wond, W.D. (2004). Endorectal ultrasound in the preoperative evaluation of rectal cancer. *Clin colorectal Cancer*, Vol.4, pp.124-132.

Sengupta, S.& Tjandra, J.J. (2001). Local excision for rectal cancer: what is the evidence? *Dis Colon Rectum*, Vol.44, pp. 1345-1536.

Sharma, A.; Hartley, J. & Monson, J.R. (2003). Local excision of rectal tumours. *Surg Oncol*, Vol.12, pp.51-61.

Siddiqui, A.A.; Fayiga, Y. & Huerta, S. (2006). The role of endoscopic ultrasound in the evaluation of rectal cancer. *Int Semin Surg Oncol*, Vol.3 pp. 36.

Sobin, L.; Wittekind C (eds). (2002). *TNM Classification of Malignant Tumours* (6th edn). Wiley-Liss: New York.

Stamos, M.J. & Murrell, Z. (2007). Management of early rectal T1 and T2 cancers. *Clin Cancer Res*, Vol.15, No.13, (November 2007), pp.6885s-6889s.

Sun Myint, A.; Griev, R.J.; McDonald, A.C.; Levine, E.L.; Ramani, S.; Perkins, K.; Wong, H.; Makin, C.A. & Hershman, M.J. (2007). Combined modality treatment of early rectal cancer: the UK experience. *Clin Oncol (R Coll Radiol)*, Vol.19, No.9, pp.674-681.

Taylor, R.H.; Hay, J.H. & Larsson, S.N. (1998). Transanal local excision of selected low rectal cancers. *Am J Surg*, Vol.175, pp. 360-363.

UK Cancer Research. http://infocancerresearchukorg/cancerstats/types/bowel/.

Winde, G.; Nottberg, H.; Keller, R. & et al. (1996). Surgical cure for early rectal carcinomas (T1). Transanal endoscopic microsurgery vs. anterior resection. *Dis Colon Rectum*, Vol.39, pp.969-976.

Yu, H.H.; Liu, B.; Xia, L.J.; Liu, A.W.; Yang,M.Y. & Li, K. (2011). Outcomes after transanal endoscopic microsurgery for early rectal cancer and risk factors associated with recurrence. *Zhonghua Wei Chang Wai Ke Za Zhi*, Vol.14, No.1, pp. 37-39.

Zlobec, I.; Baker, K.& Terracciano, L. & et al. (2008). Two-marker protein profile predicts poor prognosis in patients with early rectal cancer. *British J Canc*, Vol.99, pp.1712-1717.

Zorcolo, L.; Fantola, G.; Cabras, F. & et al. (2009). Preoperative staging of patients with rectal tumours suitable for transanal endoscopic microsurgery (TEM): comparison of endorectal ultrasound and histopathologic findings. *Surg Endosc,* Vol.23, pp.1384-1389.

8

Single – Incision Laparoscopic Surgery for Rectal Cancer

Orhan Bulut
University of Copenhagen
Dept. of Gastrointestinal Surgery, Section of Colon and Rectal surgery
Hvidovre University Hospital, Copenhagen
Denmark

1. Introduction

There have been major advances in the treatment of rectal cancer in the last two decades. Improvements in surgical instrumentation has dramatically impacted the surgical approach to rectal cancer. Particularly laparoscopic procedures have been assumed a central role in the management of benign and malignant colorectal diseases as a result of a recent paradigm shift toward minimally invasive surgery. The reasons include faster recovery times with reduced hospital stay, fewer wound-related complications, better cosmesis and oncological outcomes identical to the open traditional procedures (1,2). Although conventional laparoscopic surgery (CLS) is less traumatic than open surgery, it still continues to be associated with tissue trauma due to the size and the number of ports, each at least 1-2 cm in length (3,4). Each incision carries potential morbidity risks of bleeding, visceral organ damage, pain and formation of incisional hernia. Morover the small incisions performed for trocar placement may results in multiple scar formation and compromised cosmetic outcome (5). Single-port access (SPA) or single-incision (SILS) laparoscopic surgery has been developed as a new alternative to conventional laparoscopy. SILS technique uses a solitary incision with a specialised multilumen (3-4) port and curved or articulated instruments. This surgical innovation obviates the need for triangulation, a fundemantal requirement of conventional laparoscopy, thus minimising the number of ports. SILS surgery is emerging as a method to help decrease morbidity, optimize the cosmetic benefits of CLS and minimize the surgical trauma. Early clinical series with various procedures have demonstrated not only the feasibility but also the safety of the SILS surgery (6,7). Recently, there is an increasing trend toward the application of SILS surgery in complex abdominal operations (8). Although there has been published accounts of SILS laparoscopic colon resections and some cases of proctocolectomy and total colectomy (9-16) the literature regarding SILS laparoscopic surgery for rectal cancer is currently very rare (17,18). This is probably due to the technical challenges of the rectal dissection and to the fact that the evidence for the use of CLS in the setting of rectal cancer is limited when compared with colon cancer.

This chapter will outline the current evidence for SILS as a treatment option for patients with rectal cancer and highlight the technical details of different procedures in rectal surgery.

2. Limitations and patient selection

Absolute contraindications to SILS for rectal surgery are the same as for laparoscopic colorectal procedures. Patients with serious underlying cardiovascular or pulmonary diseases, patients with peritonitis or gross fecal contamination of the peritoneal cavity, extensive adhesions in the operative field, patients with a high body mass index (BMI), and patients suspected of harbouring large intra-abdominal abscesses should not undergo SILS at the present.

Patient selection is crucial. There are several criterias for the selection of patient including the level and the size of rectal tumor, BMI, T-staging, previous intestinal surgery, evidence of tumor infiltration of adjacent organs, uncertinity of the clearance margins etc. Big midrectal tumors in male patients and bulky tumors are not suitable for SILS for rectum cancer at present. Intraoperative complications as uncontrollable bleeding, fecal contamination, inability to visualise critical anatomic landmarks or prolonged operative time without obvious progress in procedure should immediately result in conversion to multiport or conventional open surgery.

3. Recommended equipment

A single-incision port that provides access for several instruments is used. The range of available equipment and instrumentation applicable to SILS is currently undergoing a rapid innovative development. There are several commercial ports available on the market . In addition, there is also a possibility to use a self-constructed "home-made" multichannel port system using a surgical glove and a medium size of Alexis ™ wound retractor (Applied Medical, Santa Margarita, CA, USA) (Fig. 1a and 1b).

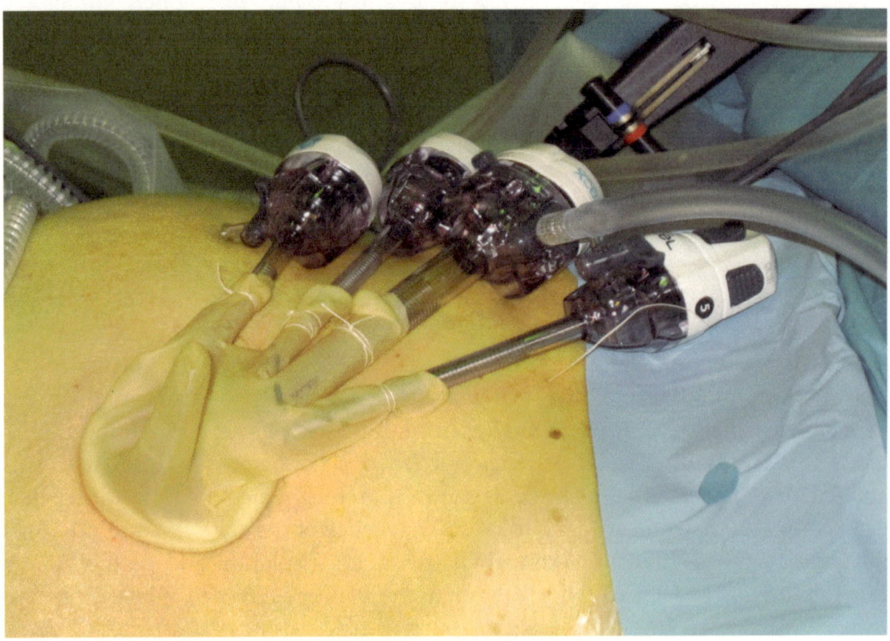

Fig. 1a. Self-constructed port with multiple trochars before establishment of the pneumoperitoneum

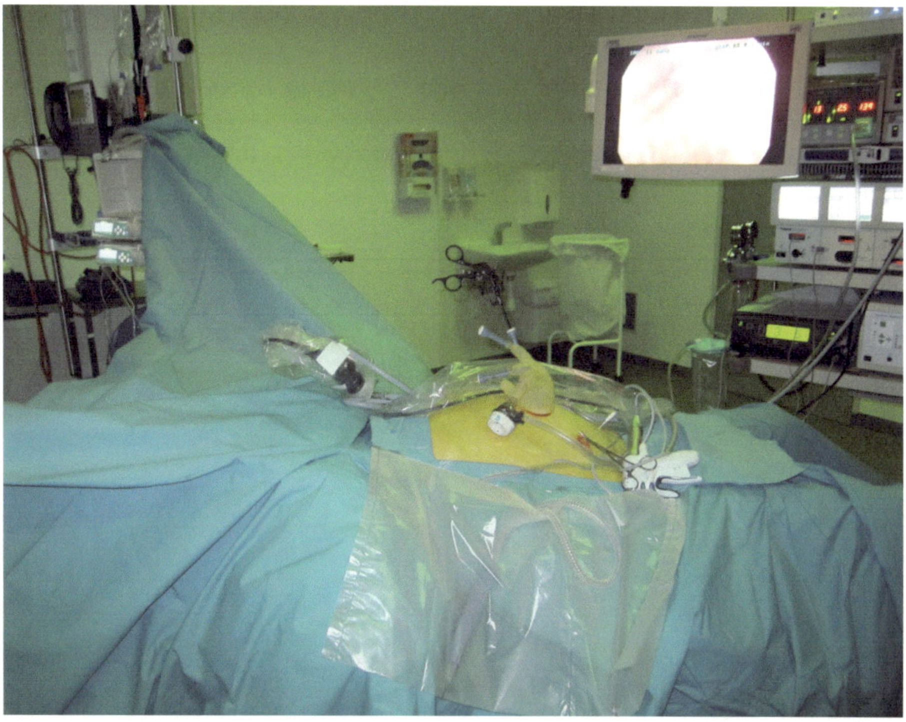

Fig. 1b. Operative photograph showing self-consructed port and external view of transabdominal suture.

A 30^0 high-definition laparoscopic camera with 5-mm diameter provides optimal visualization, for SILS for rectal surgery, especially when working in the deep pelvis. The basic hardware of laparoscopic instruments required include a tissue grasper for retraction of the intestine or applying the necessary traction on the mesentery and peritoneal attachments and an energi-based device for haemostasis and dissection (Fig. 2). Although some surgeons favour the use of atraumatic 5-mm flexible graspers, they are not essential for the performance of SILS for rectal surgery. We are now using standard straight graspers. Dissection can successfully be performed by energi-based devices as Harmonic scalpel or Ligasure in general. Endoscopic staplers are applied for ligation and division of the large vascular pedicles and for bowel transection and stapling. Multifired clip appliers are used for ligation of dissected vessels as well.

4. Patient preparation

Preoperative preparation of the patients for SILS of rectum is identical to that used in conventional multiport laparoscopic or open procedures. Preoperative preparation should include pathological examination, endoscopy, computed tomography (CT), liver ultrasound, chest x-ray and magnetic resonance imaging (MR) for diagnosis and staging in all patients with rectal cancer. Informed written consent must be obtained from all patients following discussion of risks and potential benefits with the operating surgeon. Patients should also be counselled that additional incisions and/or conversion to open surgery may be necessary as warranted during the operation. The routine anti-thrombotic precautions should be taken with low-dosis heparin and TED stockings. Stoma sites are marked preoperatively. The patients may undergo a standard bowel preparation the day before operation or a phosphate enema is given as bowel preparation prior to surgery. All patients receive standard antibiotic prophylaxis at the induction of anethesia in our institution. An urinary catheter is placed to monitor urinary output and a nasogastric tube is placed to decompess the stomach temprorarily, if it is necessary.

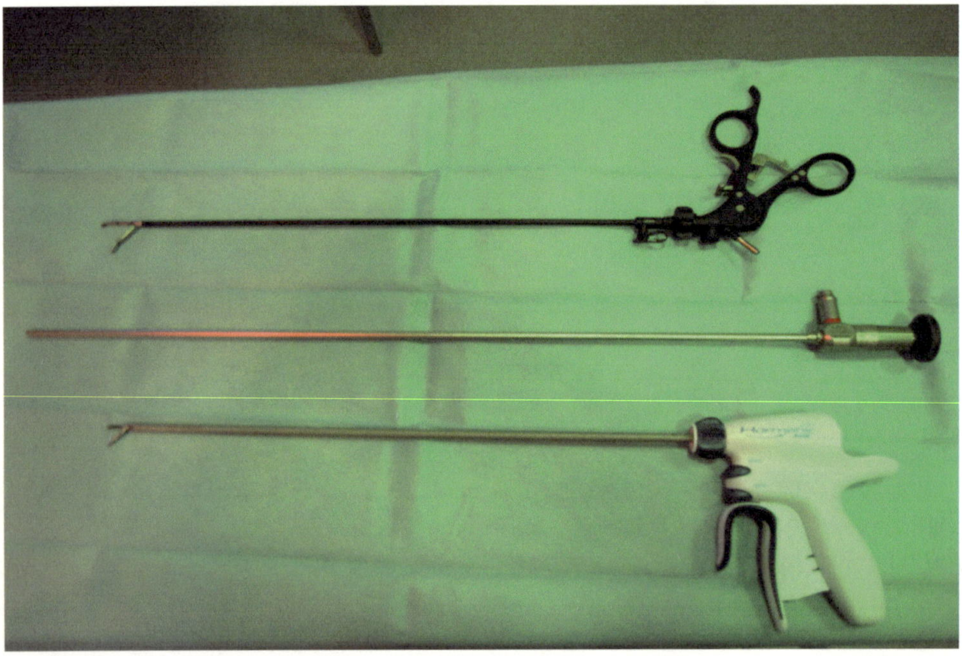

Fig. 2. Basic instruments for SILS.

5. Operative setup and patient positioning

After anaesthesia induction, the patient is placed into Lloyd-Davis position. A right or left lower quadrant possible stoma site and/or umbilical site, depending on operative procedure and the location of rectal tumor, is used to access the abdomen. An open skin and fascial incision of 2,5 cm is used to access the abdominal cavity. The abdomen is entered under direct vision and the SILS port is placed. The abdomen is insufflated with CO2 to a pressure of 12 mmHg. We use a 5 mm straight long laparoscope with a 30^0 optic to image abdominal cavity. A 5 mm ultrasound dissector and a 5 mm endoscopic grasper, are introduced via two other 5 mm ports. The camera operator is located on the right side of the patient together with the surgeon in all patients operated with transumblical access and/or chosen stoma site in the right side of abdomen (Fig. 3). The surgeon stands with the camera assistant on the left side of the patient, when the chosen stoma and extraction site is located in the left lower quadrant.

6. Operative techniques

The techniques developed during early clinical reports and case series including our personal experience are described below as stepwise procedure.

6.1 Low anterior resection

6.1.1 Position of the patient

After anaesthesia induction, the patient is placed into Lloyd-Davis position with padded leg stirrups (in Dan Allen). The shoulders and legs should be securely strapped to prevent any possible sliding of the patient on the operating table during the procedure, as the table will be tilted through several different directions during surgery to keep small intestine away from the dissecting field. There should be a free access to the patient´s perineum so that a stapler may be inserted for anastomosis and an endoscopic examination may be performed, if necessary. The arms are tucked to the patient´s side in general. However, for cases in which the anaesthesiologist needs access, left arm may be kept out for low anterior resection and right arm out for Hartmann´s operation and abdominoperineal resection (Fig. 3-4). This is because the assistant needs space to stand beside the surgeon during the whole procedure.

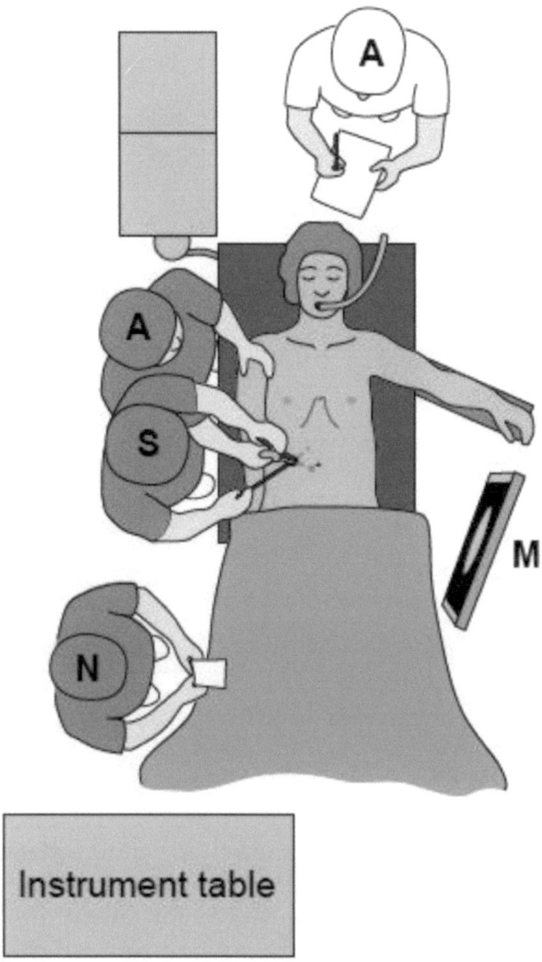

S: surgeon, A: camera assistant, N: nurse, A: anesthesiologist

Fig. 3. Schematic view of operating room setup for low anterior resection.

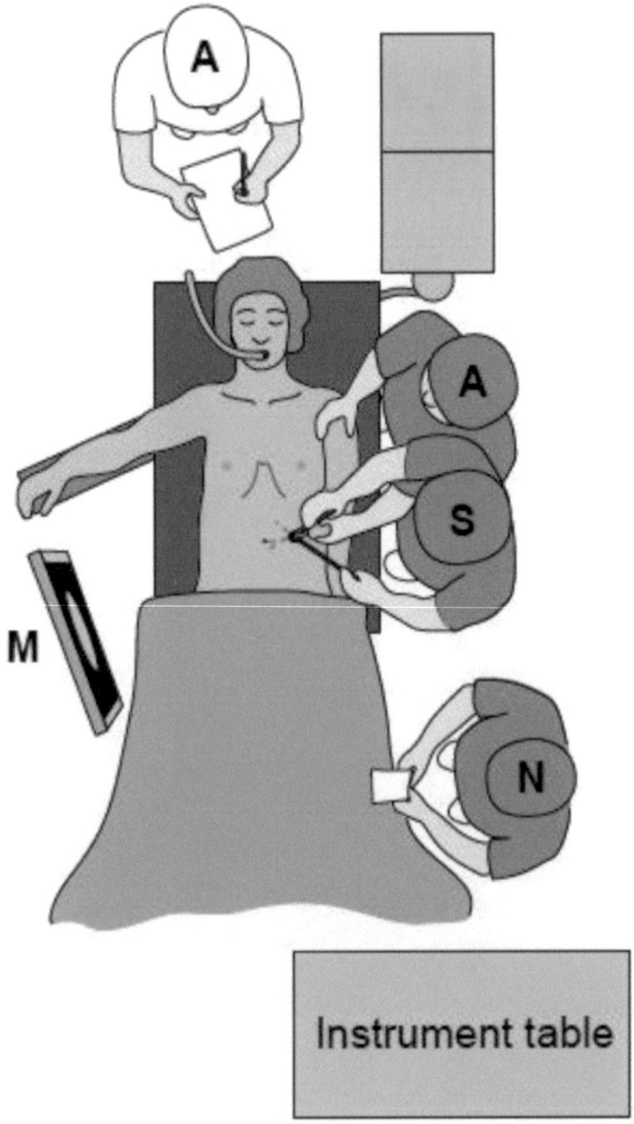

Fig. 4. Patient positioning and the surgical team for Hartmann´s operation and abdominoperineal resection.

6.1.2 Position of video monitor

The operative monitor should be located on the left side of the patient at approximately the level of the left knee for low anterior resection and the right knee for Hartmann´s operation and abdominoperineal resection. If there is a need for takedown of splenic flexure, the patient is placed in a reverse Trandelenburg position with left side elevated slightly as needed to assist with small bowel retraction and the monitor is now located near the left shoulder of the patient. The surgeon can also stand between the legs of the patient to get a better exposure of operative field as an option (Fig. 5).

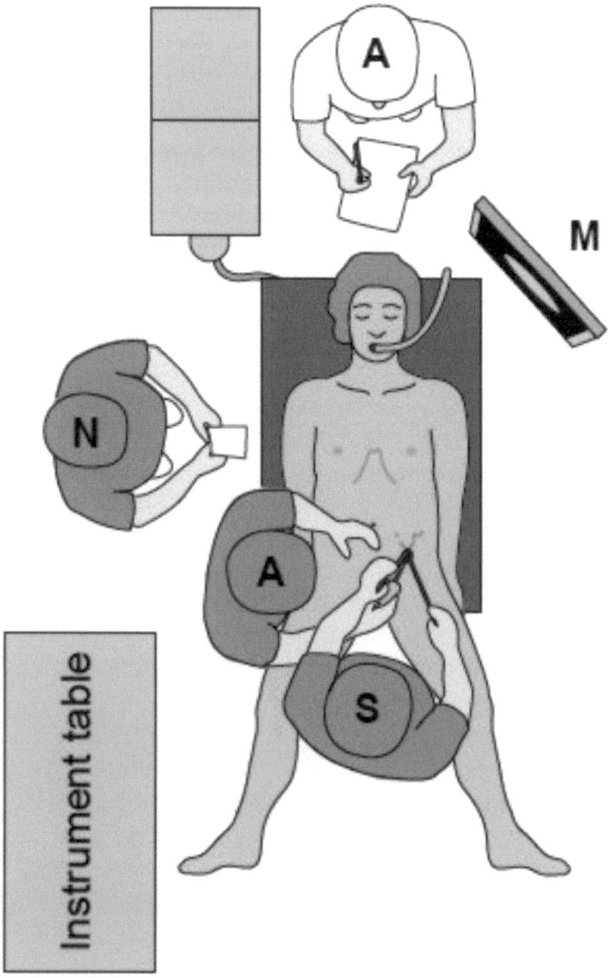

Fig. 5. Optional positioning of the surgical team for the takedown of splenic flexure.

6.1.3 SILS port placement

A right or left lower quadrant possible stoma site and/or umbilical site, depending on operative procedure and the location of rectal tumor, is used to access the abdomen. An open skin and fascial incision of 2,5 cm is done to access the abdominal cavity. The underlying fasciae is divided in a transverse fashion exposing the rectus abdominus muscle and the peritoneum is entered through the rectus muscle under direct vision and a SILS port is placed. The abdomen is insufflated with CO2 to a pressure of 12 mmHg. A 5 mm straight laparoscope with a 30° optic is used to image abdominal cavity. A 5 mm ultrasonic dissector and a 5 mm curved or straight endoscopic grasper, are introduced via two other 5 mm ports. The camera operator is located on the right side of the patient together with the surgeon in all patients, operated with transumblical access and/or chosen stoma site in the right side of abdomen. The surgeon stands on the left side of the patient, when the chosen stoma and extraction site is located in the left lower quadrant. The patient is then placed in steep

Trendelenburgs position and the operating table is rotated towards the right side for the pelvic portion of the procedure.

6.1.4 Technique

The surgeon and assistant are positioned on the right side of the patient (Fig. 6). The small bowel is gently swept out of the pelvis after performing initial laparoscopy. Subsequently the sigmoid colon is suspended towards the abdominal wall with transparietel sutures through the mesentery (Fig. 7). The peritoneum is incised along the groove between the right side of the inferior mesenteric pedicle at the level of the sacral promontory, opening the plane cranially up to the origin of the inferior mesenteric artery (Fig. 8). Blunt dissection is then used to lift the vessels away from the retroperitoneum and presacral autonomic nerves. Mesocolic dissection and inferior mesenteric pedicle isolation is achieved with medial approach and the inferior mesenteric artery is divided appoximately 1 cm. from the aorta after application of 5 mm clips (Endo Clip™ III 5 mm, Covidien, Norwalk, Connecticut, USA) or sometimes with Endo-GIA (vascular cartridge). The left ureter is then recognized and subsequently, with the patient placed supine and rotated left side up, medial-to-lateral dissection is continued cranially up until the left colon is mobilised. We do not routinely mobilize the splenic flexure in rectal surgery. If there is a need to take down the splenic flexure, the inferior mesenteric vein can be divided just inferior to the pancreas with medial dissection. The surgical team then repositions itself with the surgeon standing between the legs of the patients and the assistant on the right side of the patient (Fig. 5).

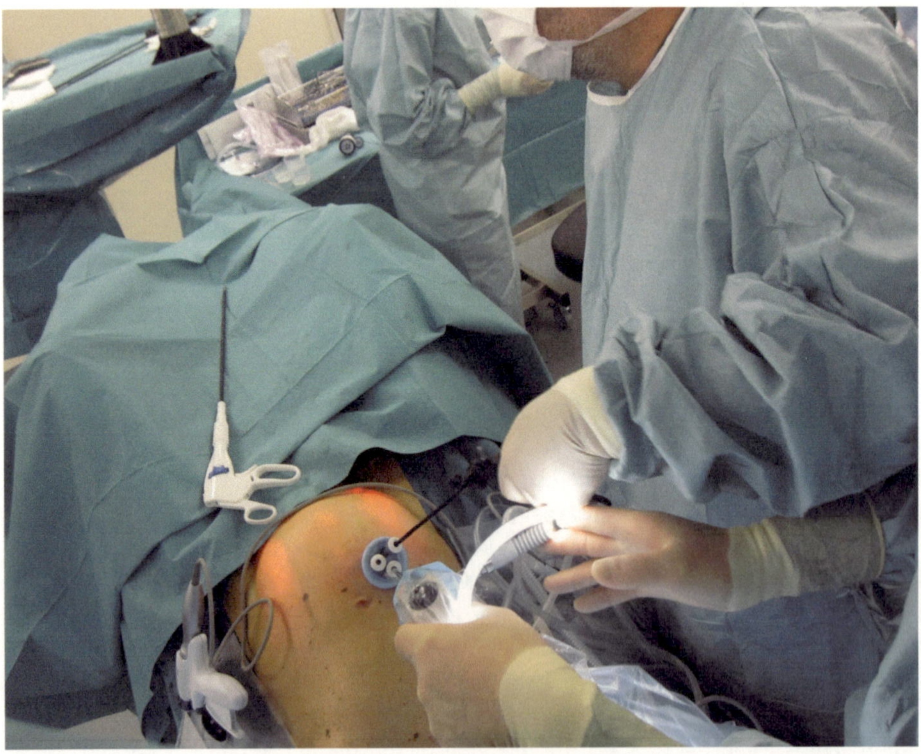

Fig. 6. Positioning of SILS port at proposed right-sided ileostomy site.

The divided pedicle is elevated, and the avascular retroperitoneal plane is dissected bluntly with medial approach entering into the lesser sac. If the splenic flexure is difficult to mobilize, the dissection can be commenced at the distal tranverse colon. The vascular plane between the greater omentum and the transverse colon is dissected close to the colon edge entering into the lesser sac. This dissection is continued going from the left side of the transverse colon toward the splenic flexure. The connection to the lateral dissection allows the left flexure to be fully mobilized.

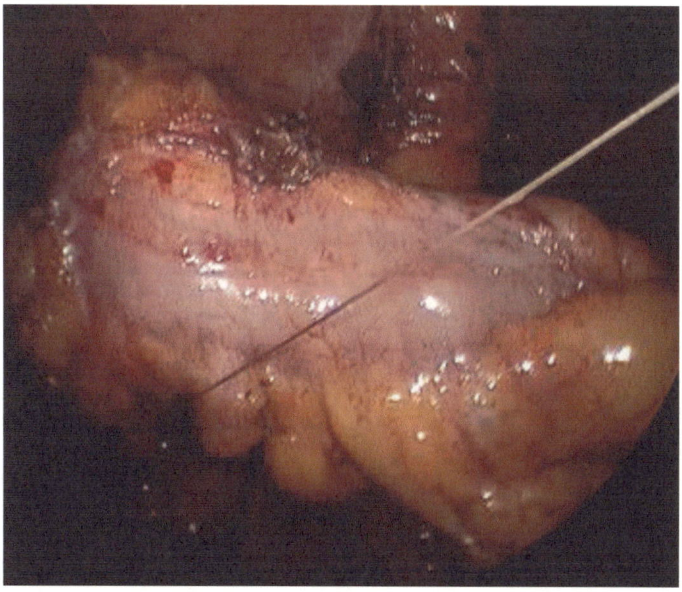

Fig. 7. The suspension of sigmoid colon with a transparietal suture.

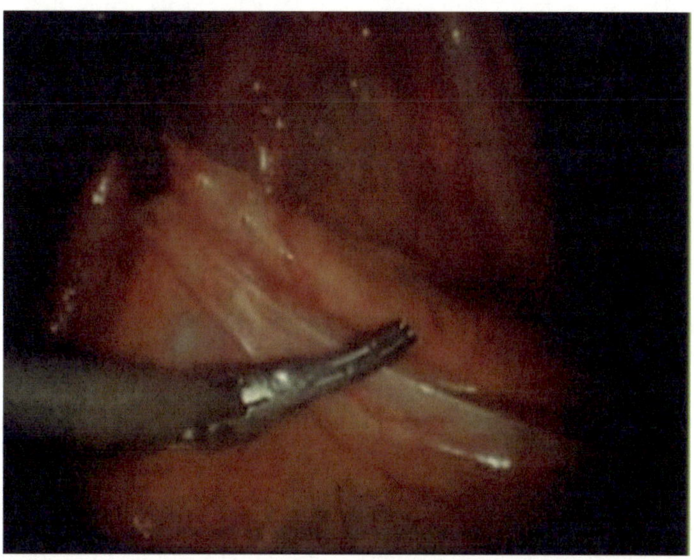

Fig. 8. Starting to open the medial peritoneum at the level of sacral promontory

The patient is returned to the Trendelenburgs position, and the small bowel is reflected cranially after the completion of full mobilisation of the left colon. The surgical team rearranges itself once again back to its original position. The grasper and previously inserted transabdominal sutures are used to elevate the rectosigmoid colon out of the pelvis and away from the retroperitoneum and sacral promontory, to enable entry into the presacral space. The posterior aspect of the mesorectum is easily identified and the mesorectal plane dissected with ultrasonic scissors or electrocautery-based, intruments preserving the hypogastric nerves. Dissection is continued down to the presacral space in this avascular plane toward the pelvic floor. Elevation of the upper rectum by transabdominal sutures facilitates further posterior dissection along the back of mesorectum to the pelvic floor. The anterior dissection between the rectum and the posterior vaginal wall (in females) and the seminal vesicles and prostate (in men) is performed by decreasing tension of the transabdominal sutures and retracting the peritoneal fold anterior to the rectum. Dissection is proceeded laterally on both sides of rectum until circumferential mobilisation of lower rectum is accomplished. Digital examination is performed to verify the distance between tumors inferior margin and the line of resection and the adequacy of distal margin is marked with a clip. One 5 mm port is now replaced with a 10 mm port. A blue EndoGIA roticulator stapler (Covidien Ltd., Norwalk, Conn. USA) 45-mm is fired twice from this port to divide the lower rectum safely. The abdomen is then deflated and a wound protector (Alexis O ™, Applied Medical Rancho Santo Margarita, CA) placed at the aperture of SILS port. The specimen is extracted through the SILS aperture and resected. Extracorporal preparation of the proximale colon is completed with placement of the anvil of a 29-mm circular stapler in position to perform a side-to-end or end-to-end colorectal anastomosis.

After pneumoperitoneum reestablishment, a conventional intracorporeal colorectal anastomosis is made with transanal insertion of a circular stapler (Proximate ILS circular stapler, Ethicon, Endo-surgery, Puerto Rico USA) under direct vision. Testing for anastomosis is performed by insufflating air into the rectum while having the pelvic cavity filled with water. If there is a small leak it can be located by using methylene blue and eliminated by inserting a stitch that is tied intracorporally. This procedure often needs the insertion of an additional port. Drainage is not indicated routinely. As in open or CLS it is always imperative to check the resected tissue doughnuts to make sure they are complete. An incomplete doughnut should prompt a laparoscopic suture repair of the anastomosis. If the area of the defect is not recognised, the whole anastomosis should be revised and if necessary, interrupted sutures placed around the whole circumference. This is a challenging procedure with SILS technique at present. Therefore the procedure should be converted to either a CLS or an open operation. If the transumblical access is used, the fascia is closed with PDS sutures continuously and the skin is first trimmed to adapt the incision and is then closed with interrupted 3/0 nylon sutures (Fig. 9). In the cases needing a proximal diverting ileostomy, the diversion loop ilostomy is brought out through the SILS aperture approximately 20 cm proximate to the ileocoecal valve. The loop ileostomy is created using 3/0 vicryl sutures (Fig. 10). Intraabdominal smoke formation is drained via the insertion of a intravenous cannula working as a separate venting channel at the suprapubic site.

6.2 Hartmann´s operation

The procedure is similar to that of low anterior resection except that the splenic flexure need not be taken down routinely, there is no anastomosis and the mobilised colon is exteriorized through the left premarked colostomy site which is used as the placement of a SILS port as well.

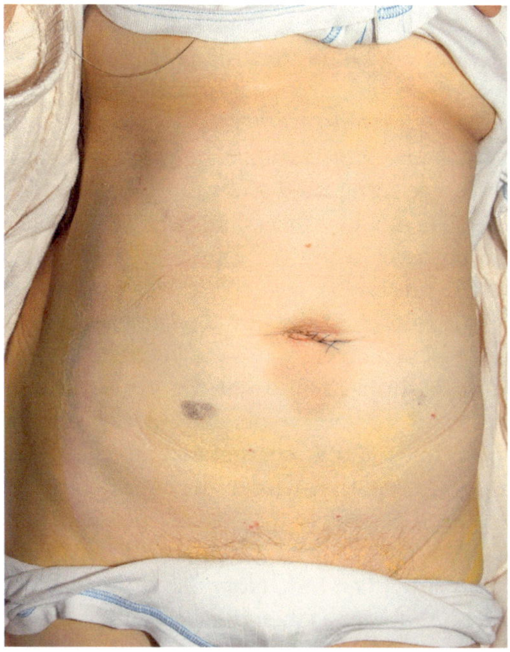

Fig. 9. Umblical wound after low anterior resection with transumblical access

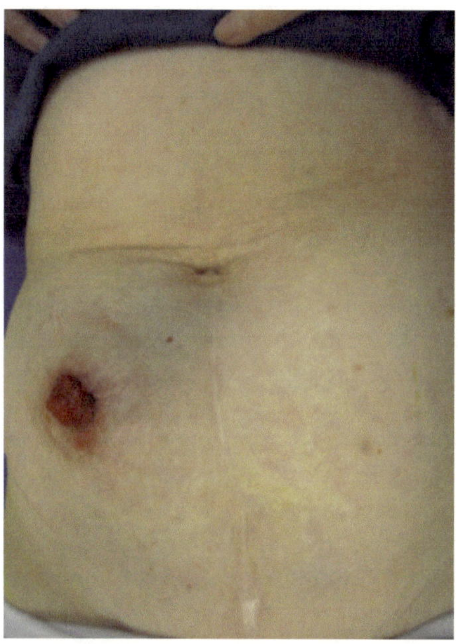

Fig. 10. Appereance at six days following low anterior resection with protective ileostomy performed with SILS technique.

An incision of 2,5 cm located at the marked stoma site on the left side is used to access the abdomen and the SILS port is placed. A 5 mm straight laparoscope with a 30 degree optic is used to image abdominal cavity. The surgeon and the camera assistant is located on the left side of the patient (Fig. 4). The patient is then placed in steep Trendelenburg position. Transabdominal sutures are used and rectosigmoid colon is suspended towards the abdominal wall. Mesocolic dissection and inferior mesenteric pedicle isolation is achieved with lateral approach by using 5 mm instruments. The superior rectal artery is divided just below the inferior mesenteric artery after application of 5 mm clips or Endo-GIA (vascular cartridge). The left ureter is then recognized and subsequently lateral-to-medial dissection is continued until the left colon is mobilised so that it may be brought up comfortably through the stoma site. Then the posterior aspect of the mesorectum is easily identified and the mesorectal plane dissected, preserving the pelvic nerves. The total mesorectal excision (TME) dissection is continued down to the presacral space in the avascular space towards the pelvic floor untill the level of os coccygis in the posterior level. At the anterior level the dissection is continued till the upper margin of the vagina. By decreasing tension of the transabdominal sutures to the sigmoid colon the anterior dissection can be performed. Lateral dissection is performed until circumferential mobilisation of the rectum is accomplished. A 5 mm port is replaced with a 10 mm port inside the device (SILS port). Digital examination is performed to verify the distance between tumors inferior margin and the line of resection and the adequacy of distal margin is marked with a clip. A blue EndoGIA roticulator stapler (Covidien Ltd., Norwalk, Conn. USA) 45-mm is fired to divide the lower rectum safely. The abdomen is then deflated and a wound protector (Alexis O ™, Applied Medical Rancho Santo Margarita, CA) placed at the aperture of SILS port. The specimen is extracted through the SILS aperture and resected. The divided left colon is brought out to form a colostomy in the SILS aperture and then the colostomy is fashioned with interrupted 3/0 vicryl sutures and a colostomy bag is attached to the skin.

There are some potential technical difficulties with operating from the left side of the patient:

1. Most of the laparoscopic colorectal surgeons, have not been familiar with left side approach and exposure to abdominal cavity through a left-sided port, although we have previously used traditional approach of the lateral-to-medial dissection sequence from the right side of abdomen. There is an adaptation process for laparoscopic surgeons to this approach.
2. The distance between left-sided single-port and anatomical landmarks as inferior mesenteric artery or left ureter are relatively short and this condition can limit the free manoeuvre possibilities of laparoscopic instruments and the facility of proper mesenteric dissection.
3. In some rare conditions in which the tumor coexists with a colonic inflammatory process (e.g., diverticulitis), the initial divisions of the sigmoid lateral attachments may be difficult and dangereous because the lateral dissection plane is blurred. There is an increased risk of inadvertent injury of left ureter and gonadal vessels.
4. If there is a need of early division of the white line of Toldt before vessel ligation increases the sigmoid redundancy and sometimes hinders the upcoming procedures (e.g. dissection of inferior mesenteric artery) during the operation. On the other hand, tilting of the patient to the right side allows gravity to aid in the retraction of the colon and makes identification of the ureter extremely simple.

6.3 Abdominoperineal resection

6.3.1 Abdominal approach

The abdominal part of the procedure is similar to that of low anterior resection except that the splenic flexure need not be taken down routinely and no distal rectal transection is required. The left lower quadrant premarked colostomy site is used as the placement of SILS port. The patient and surgical team positions are similar to those in Hartmann´s operation. An incision of 2,5 cm located at the marked stoma site on the left side is used to access the abdomen and the SILS port is placed. The surgeon and the camera operator is located on the left side of the patient (Fig. 11). The patient is then placed in steep Trendelenburg position.

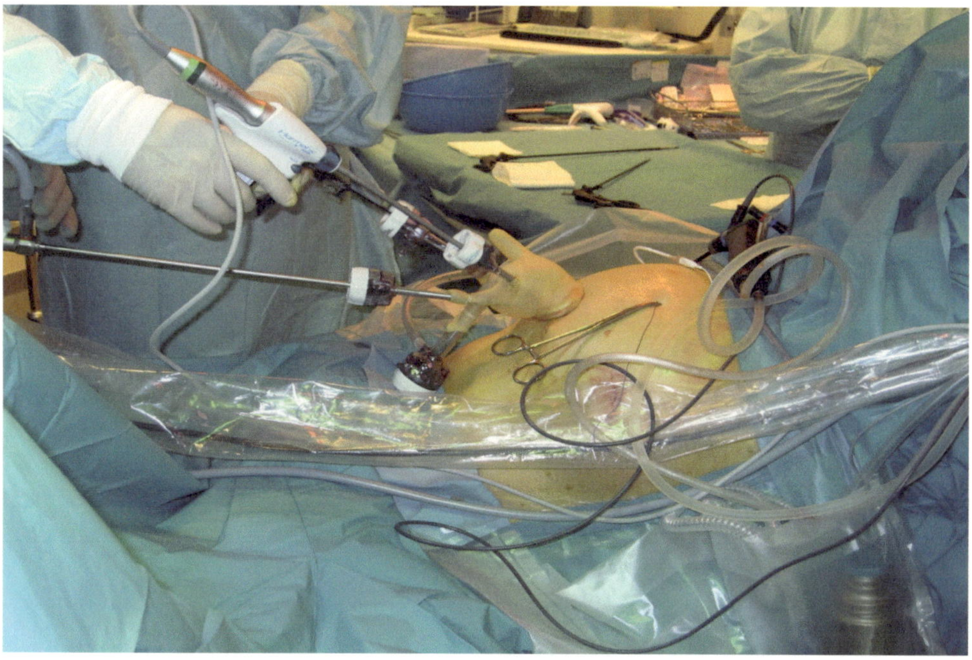

Fig. 11. Operative view of self-constructed port position at proposed left-sided colostomy site.

Mesocolic dissection and inferior mesenteric pedicle isolation is achieved with lateral approach by using 5 mm instruments and rectosigmoid colon is suspended towards the abdominal wall with transabdominal sutures. The superior rectal artery is divided just below the inferior mesenteric artery. The left ureter is then recognized and subsequently lateral-to-medial dissection is continued until the left colon is mobilised so that it may be brought up comfortably through the stoma site.Then, the posterior aspect of the mesorectum is easily identified and the mesorectal plane dissected with harmonic scalpel, preserving the pelvic nerves. The total mesorectal excision (TME) dissection is continued down to the presacral space in the avascular space towards the pelvic floor untill the level of os coccygis in the posterior level. At the anterior level the dissection is continued till the upper margin of the vagina. By decreasing tension of the transabdominal sutures to the sigmoid colon the anterior dissection can be performed. Lateral dissection is performed until circumferential mobilisation of the rectum is accomplished as mentioned the above. A 5 mm ports is replaced with a 10 mm port inside the device (SILS port). The sigmoid colon is divided with a blue EndoGIA 60 stapler (Covidien Ltd., Norwalk, Conn. USA). The abdomen is deflated and the divided left colon is brought out to form a colostomy in the SILS aperture and then the left-sided colostomy is fashioned with interrupted 3/0 vicryl sutures.

6.3.2 Perineal dissection

The patient is then turned into jack-knife position with legs spread to enable the surgeon to stand between the legs with one assistant on each side (Fig. 12a). A purse-string suture is tied tightly to close the anus. After the skin is prepared, a drop formed incision around the anus is made and extended cranially to the coccyx (Fig. 1b). The dissection continues in the subcutaneous fat around the subcutaneous part of the external anal sphincter. The perineal incision is deepened into ischiorectal fossa on both sides and the outer side of the levator muscle is identified all around. A small transverse incision is made immediately proximal of the tip of os coccyx, which is disarticulated from the sacrum and Waldeyer´s fasciae divided (19). The pelvic or presacral cavity is entered and the incision into it enlarged by cutting the levator ani muscles on both sides, from posterior to anterior. The specimen is gently withdrawn and dissected off the prostate or posterior vaginal wall.

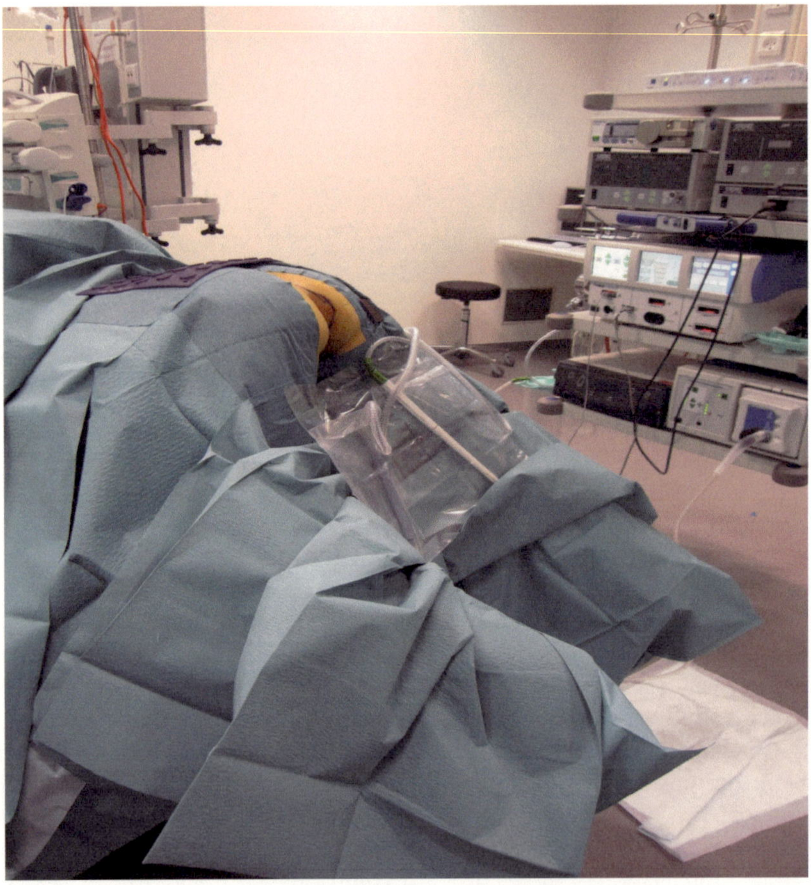

Fig. 12a. Patient in the prone jack-knife position (lateral view)

The anterior dissection is carried out immediately behind and to the upper level of the transversus perineal muscles and the dissection is completed with the division of the puborectalis muscle on both sides. In cases of anterior tumours with local invasion, a portion of the prostate or the posterior vaginal wall may be resected en bloc with the anorectum. In some cases, venous bleeding from the posterior and posterolateral aspect of the prostate or vagina can be troublesome. Meticulous haemostasis by diathermy or stitching can control this bleeding. When the specimen is removed and hemostasis is secured, the perineal wound is closed in layers using interrupted sutures with vicryl 2/0 and vicryl rapid 3/0 in the skin.

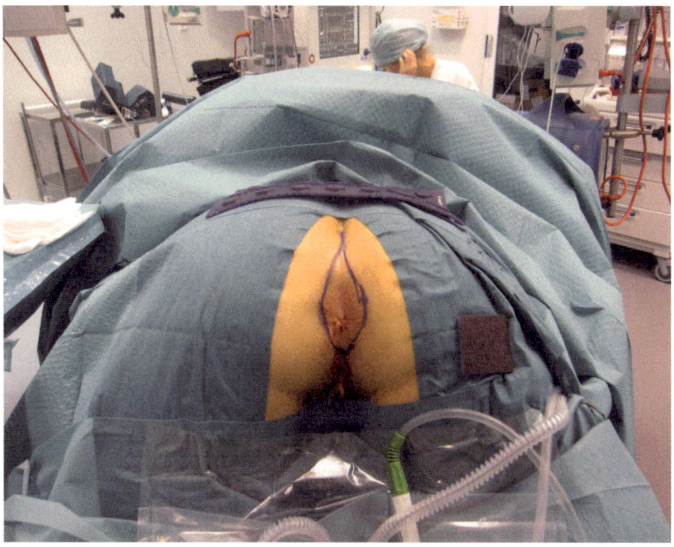

Fig. 12b. Patient in the prone jack-knife position (perineal view)

7. Complications

We have seen no specific complications following SILS for rectal cancer compared to conventional multiport laparoscopic surgery or conventional open surgery. There is no report about visceral or vascular injuries in the literature at present. We believe that there is a theoretical risk for unrecognized injury to viscera caused by the use of laparoscopic instruments away from the surgical field as in laparoscopic surgery. Wound complications will probably be shown to be decreased. However, complications with stoma and the perineal wound should remain unchanged.

8. Discussion

The SILS technique for rectal surgery is still in its infancy and the published studies are highly inhomogeneous. To date, a total of ten articles as single case reports and small case series have been available in the English literature on single-access laparoscopic rectal surgery. Table 1. summarizes the technical aspects and operative outcomes of SILS for rectal surgery. Operative outcomes are comparable with CLS in these very limited preliminary data. The data reviewed in this chapter shows the safety and feasibility of the procedure.

Authors	No. of Pts. (TCR/RS) (n)	Procedure (n)	Age (years) (range)	BMI (kg/m2) (range)	PAS (%)	Port type	Indication for RS (n)	OT(min) (range)	Incision length (cm) initial/final/range	C	Complications (n)	HLN (range)	LOS (days) (range)
Chambers et al. (25)	7/1	AR (1)	44	24	none	Triport	Benign	75	2.5/2.5/	0	0	NS	1
Bulut&Nielsen (17,18)	2/2	LAR (2)	(64-83)[c]	(20-24)[c]	50	SILS	Malignant (2)	(244-315)[c]	2.5/NS/2.5-3	0	0	(3-13)[c]	7
Gash et al. (26)	20/6	AR (2) LAR (3) APR (1)	(44-72)[c]	(24-26)[c]	*40	TriPort	Malignant (4#) Benign(2#)	(75-210)[c]	2.5/NS/NS	#1 to CLS	(5)* NS for rectal procedures	(14-19)[c]	(1-6)[c]
Law et al. (13)	8/1	AR (1)	76[#](*49-88)	*22.7[b](17.7-27)	NS	TriPort	Malignant (1[#])	*175[b](103-260)	3[#]/NS/*3-5	0[#]	None[#]	*13.5[b] (9-36)	3[#]
Hamzaoglu et al. (27)	4/4	AR (2) LAR (2)	(51-68)[c]	(22-35)[c]	NS	SILS and TriPort	Malignant (4)	347[a](240-480)	3.5/NS/3-4	0	None	15[a] (8-28)	(4-5)[c]
Ramos-Valades et al. (28)	35/6	AR (6)	*54.3±10.9[a] (29-78)	*28.1±6.3[a] (17.7-49)	*42.9	SILS and GelPornt	NS	158.8±31.8[b,#] (119-192)	¤2-2.5/4.0±1.2[b] /2.5-6	*2 to HALS *1 to CLS	(4)* NS for rectal procedures	¤23.5±12[b]	*2.9±1[b] (2-6)
Uematsu et al. (29)	7/7	LAR (7)	73[b] (52-88)	NS (20-24)	NS	SCP	Malignant (7)	205[b] 8175-245)	3/NS/NS	0	AL (1)	18[b] (13-27)	7[b] (7-21)
Katsuno et al. (30)	31/2	AR (2)	*66.5±5[a]. (58-79)	*22.5±2.3[a] (19-25)	NS	SILS and SCP	Malignant (2#)	*156±45[a] (101-263)	*2.72±0.79[a]/ NS /3-5	0	WI(1)	*18±2.1[a] (NS)	*9.2±1.2[a] (NS)
Bulut et al. (31)	10/10	AR (2) LAR (6) HO (1) APR (1)	67[b] (49-83)	23.5[b] (20-24)	60	SILS	Malignant (10)	229[b] (185-318)	NS	0	PC (1), CS (1)	14[b](3-20)	7[b] (4-14)

TCR total colorectal procedures, RS rectal surgery, AR anterior resection, LAR low anterior resection, APR abdominoperineal resection, HO Hartmanns operation, BMI body mass index, CLS conventional laparoscopic surgery, HALS hand-assisted laparoscopic surgery, HLN harvested lymph nodes, LOS lenght of hospital stay, OT operative time, PAS previous abdominal surgery, C conversion, NS not specified, SCP self-constructed port, WI wound infection, PC pelvic collection, UTI urinary tract infection, CS compartment syndrome, AL anastomotic leakage

* all patients
[#] only for rectal surgery
¤ all malign cases
[a] mean data
[b] median data
[c] range

Table 1. Studies showing outcomes of single-incision laparoscopic rectal surgery

Although operative times seems to be longer in some series, nevertheless the results are in general comparable with conventional multiport laparoscopic rectal procedures. Another issue is the adequacy of oncological results of SILS for rectal cancer.

The adequacy of lymph node retrieval plays an important role in tumor staging and prognosis. A minimum number of 12 lymph nodes have been endorsed as a consensus standard of performance in colorectal resections (20). However, many factors affect the number of lymph nodes examined, including extent of surgical resection, patient age, tumor location, pathologist, surgeon and the method of specimen preparation. The data shows that the number of harvested lymph nodes in malignant cases appears oncologically satisfactory. The reported number of median or mean lymph nodes extraction in these cases are comparable to multiport laparoscopic series and population based studies (21-24). However, the given data regarding pathological examination and the shortness of follow-up are inadequate to evaluate the oncological outcome. A more detailed pathological report including margin clearance and the quality of mesorectal fasciae would be important to make long-term comparisons.

The potential advantages of a small skin incision include, not only better cosmetic appereance, but decreasing rate of port-site related complications. The final length of the skin and fasciae incision depends on specimen size. This is particularly important in rectal surgery due to relatively fast mesorectum. Extraction difficulties may often be encountered for the patients with large rectal tumors or thickened mesorectum. In addition, when the colon is full of stool in the case of distal stenosis, it is also difficult to bring the rectosigmoid colon out. The length of skin and fascia incision is often enlarged to permit the intact extraction of the specimen. Another expected advantage of a small incision is the reduction of postoperative pain. None of the published reports assessed the postoperative pain or analgesic requirements (32-35). Technical difficulties of single-access as the lack of triangulation and exposure, the inaxis view and conflicts between instruments are the most important challenges. The handling of both a grasper and an energi-based device in parallel with the laparoscope through the single port decreases the possibility of the surgeons manoeuvre and result in inadequate exposure and difficult dissection in the surgical field (Fig. 13).

To ensure an adequate and timely traction and to have a better surgical view and dissection, transparietal sutures are applied through abdominal wall. A 30^0 laparoscope and articulating or curved graspers are also helpful to improve view and dissection. The possibility of using a planned ileostomy or sigmoidostomy site as the port placement and extraction of the specimen reduced parietal trauma and improved cosmesis as a real no-scar procedure in some cases. The case studies in literature have shown that the length of stay did not appear to be decreased using SILS in rectal cancer. Health care systems have the duty to offer the citizen the best available medical care, taking economic cost and priority into consideration. SILS colorectal procedures stands now where conventional laparoscopic surgery stood in the early 1990s. Today, SILS for rectal cancer is under trial. Larger comparative studies to conventional laparoscopic surgery with oncologic outcomes, cost analysis and long-term results are necessary to determine patient benefits. Another important issue is the education of surgeons in the future. SILS for rectal procedures presents a challenge for teaching residents and surgeons. There are some similarities between SILS and Transanal Endoscopic Microsurgery (TEM). The colorectal surgical community should use the experiences in training of surgeons in TEM for teaching SILS in the procedure.

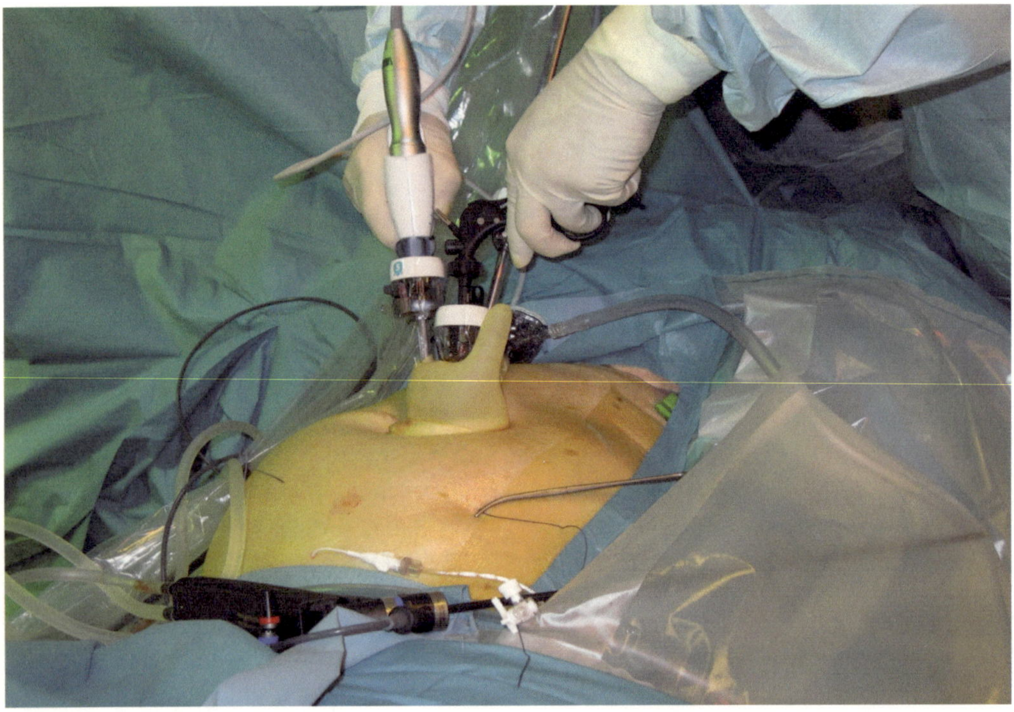

Fig. 13. External view of the instruments working in parallel position through a self-constructed single port.

9. Conclusions

SILS for rectal cancer is a challenging procedure that seems to be feasible. These technical challenges could explain why the operating time may be considerably lengthened. When using SPA for complex procedures such as rectal cancer surgery, advanced laparoscopic experience is mandatory. In addition to this a significant learning curve must be expected. It can be performed safely on slim patients with no bulky tumour using one incision, either through the patient´s umbilicus or through a chosen stoma site which may become the diversion ileostomy or end-sigmoidostomy aperture. SILS has a potential of reducing postoperative pain. The decrease in incision number may decrease the development of wound infection or hernias and the formation of intra-abdominal adhesions as well as improve cosmetic results. However, the existing clinical evidence is limited, and potential benefits or disadvantages of SILS procedures require further evaluation. There is a need to standardize the technique and carefully evaluate its oncological outcomes. Prospective comparative studies between SILS and conventional laparoscopic colorectal surgery are needed to clearly determine its short- and long-term outcome

10. The future

SILS is a major step after CLS and represents the crossing link between robotic surgery and NOTES (Fig. 14). The huge developments in the fields of imaging, data processing, simulation and virtual reality in the future have the potential to help SILS mature as computer-assisted single-access surgery through a single transabdominal incision or a natural orifice. It is believed that the future of minimally invasive surgery will be a hybrid form of SILS, NOTES and robotic surgery.

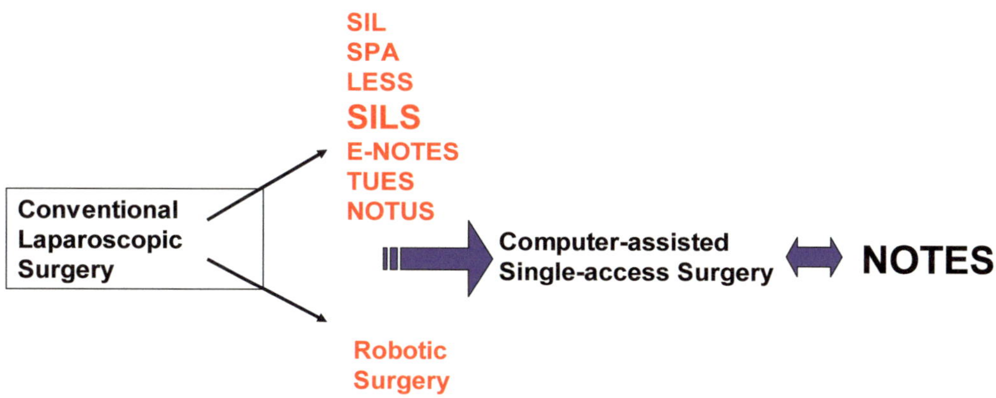

Fig. 14. The development of minimally invasive surgery in the future.

11. References

[1] Bonjer H.J., Hop W.C., Nelson H., et al.(2005). Laparoscopically assisted vs open colectomy for colon cancer: a metaanalysis. Arch Surg, 142, 298-303.

[2] Schwenk W., Haase O., Neudecker J., Muller J.M. (2008). Short term benefits for laparoscopic colorectal resection. Cochrane Database of Systematic Reviews. CD003145.

[3] Lowry P.S., Moon T.D., D'Alessandro A., Nakada S.Y. (2003). Symptomatic port-site hernia associated with a non-bladed trocar after laparoscopic live-donor nephrectomy. J Endouro, 117,493-49413.

[4] Marcovici I. (2003). Significant abdominal wall hematoma from an umbilical port insertion. JSLS, 5, 293-295.

[5] Dunker M.S., Stiggelbout A.M., van Hogezend R.A., Ringers J., Griffioen G., Bemelman W.A. (1998). Cosmesis and body image after laparoscopicaly-assisted and open ileocolic resection for Crohn's disease. Surg.Endosc,12,1334-1340.

[6] Raman J.D., Bagrodia A., Cadeddu J.A. (2009). Single-incision, umbilical laparoscopic versus conventional laparoscopic nephrectomy: a comparison of perioperative outcomes and short-term measures of convalescence. Eur Urol, 55, 1198-1204.

[7] Podolsky E.R., Curcillo P.G. 2nd. (2010). Single Port Access (SPA) Surgery-a 24-Month Experience. J Gastrointest Surg, 14, 759-767.

[8] Ahmed K., Wang T.T., Patel V.M., et al. (2011). The role of single-incision laparoscopic surgery in abdominal and pelvic surgery: a systematic review, 25, 378-396.

[9] Remzi F.H., Kirat H.T., Kaouk J.H., Geisler D.P. (2008). Single port laparoscopy in colorectal surgery. Colorectal Dis, 10, 823-826.

[10] Remzi F.H., Kirat H.T., Geisler D.P. (2010). Laparoscopic single-port colectomy for sigmoid cancer. Tech Coloproctol, 14, 253-255.

[11] Bucher P., Pugin F., Morel P. (2008). Single port access laparoscopic right hemicolectomy. Int J Colorectal Dis, 23, 1013– 1016.

[12] Bucher P., Pugin F., Morel P. (2009). Single-port access laparoscopic radical left colectomy in humans. Dis Colon Rectum, 52,1797- 1801.

[13] Law W, Fan J.K.M., Poon J.T.C. (2010). Single-incision laparoscopic colectomy: early experience. Dis Colon Rectum, 53, 284-288.

[14] Wong M.T.C., Ng K.H. , Ho K.S., Eu K.W. (2010). Single-incision laparoscopic surgery for right hemicolectomy: our initial experience with 10 cases. Tech Coloproctol, 14, 225-228.

[15] Geisler D.P., Condon E.T., Remzi F.H. (2010). Single incision laparoscopic total proctocolectomy with ileopouch anal anastomosis. Colorectal Dis, 12, 941-943.

[16] Ramos-Valadez D.I., Chirag B. Patel, M.R., Pickron T.B., Haas E.M. (Published online ahead of print 2010).Single-incision laparoscopic right hemicolectomy: safety and feasibility in a series of consecutive cases. Surg. Endosc, DOI: 10.1007/s00464-010-1017-y.

[17] Bulut O. and Nielsen C.B.(2010). Single-incision laparoscopic low anterior resection for rectal cancer. Int J Colorectal Dis, 25,1261-1263.

[18] Bulut O. and Nielsen C.B. (2011). Single-incision laparoscopic low anterior resection combined with salpingooferectomy. Ugeskrif for Læger (in press)

[19] Holm T., Ljung A., Haggmark T., Jurell G. and Lagergren J.(2007). Extended abdominoperineal resection with gluteus maximus flap rekonstroction of the pelvic floor for rectal cancer. Br. J Surg, 94, 232-238.

[20] Nelson H., Petrelli N., Carlin A., et al. (2001). Guidelines 2000 for colon and rectal cancer surgery. J Natl Cancer Inst, 93, 583-596.

[21] Guillou P.J., Quirke P., Thorpe H., et al.(2005). MCR CLASICC trial group. Short-term endpoints of conventional versus laparoscopic-assisted surgery in patients with colorectal cancer (MCR CLASICC trial):multicentre, randomised controlled trial. Lancet, 364, 1718-1726.

[22] Park J.S., Kang S.B., Kim D.W., Lee K.H., Kim Y.H.(2009). Laparoscopic versus open resection without splenic flexure mobilization for the treatment of rectum and sigmoid cancer: a study from a single institution that selectively used splenic flexure mobilization. Surg Laparosc Endosc Percutan Tech, 19, 62–68.
[23] Kang S.B., Park J.W., Jeong S.Y., et al.(1010). Open versus laparoscopic surgery for mid or low rectal cancer after neoadjuvant chemoradiotherapy (COREAN trial): short-term outcomes of an open-label randomised controlled trial. Lancet Oncol, 11, 37-645.
[24] Baxter N.N., Virnig D.J., Rothenberger D.A., Morris A.M., Jessurun J, Virnig BA. (2005). Lymph node evaluation in colorectal cancer patients: a population-based study. J Natl Cancer Inst, 97, 219-225.
[25] Chambers W., Bicsak M., Lamparelli M., Dixon A. (2011). Single-incision laparoscopic surgery (SILS) in complex colorectal surgery: a technique offering potential and not just cosmesis. Colorectal Dis, 13, 393-398.
[26] Gash K.J., Goede A.C., Chambers W., Greenslade G.L., Dixon A.R. (Published on line 24 august 2010). Laparoendoscopic single site surgery is feasible in complex colorectal resections and could enable day case colectomy. Surg Endosc, DOI 10.1007/s00464-010-1275-8.
[27] Hamzaoglu I., Karahasanoglu T.; Baca B., et al. (2011). Single-port laparoscopic sphincter-saving mesorectal excision for rectal cancer. Report of the first 4 human cases. Arch Surg, 146,75-81.
[28] Ramos-Valadez D.I., Chirag B. Patel, M.R., Pickron T.B., Haas E.M. (Published on line: 29 march 2011). Single-incision laparoscopic colectomy: outcomes of an emerging minimally invasive technique. Int J Colorectal Dis, DOI10.1007/s00384-011-1185-9.
[29] Uematsu D., Akiyama G., Narita M., Magishi A. (2011). Single-access laparoscopic low anterior resection with vertical suspension of the rectum. Dis Colon Rectum, 54, 632-637.
[30] Katsuno G., Fukunaga M., Nagakari K., Yoshikawa S., Ouchi M., Hirasaki Y. (2011). Single-incision laparoscopic colectomy for colon cancer: Early experience with 31 cases. Dis Colon Rectum, 54,705-710.
[31] Bulut O., Nielsen C.B. and Jespersen N. (2011). Single-port access laparoscopic surgery for rectal cancer: Initial experience with 10 cases. Dis Colon Rectum, 54, 803-809.
[32] Adair J., Gromski M.A., Lim R.B., Nagle D. (2010). Single-incision laparoscopic right colectomy: Experience with 17 consecutive cases and comparison with multiport laparoscopic right hemicolectomy. Dis Colon Rectum, 53,1549-1554.
[33] Waters J.A., Guzman M.J., Fajardo A.D., et al. (2010). Single-port laparoscopic right hemicolectomy: A safe alternative to conventional laparoscopy. Dis Colon Rectum, 53, 1467-1472.
[34] Chen W.T.L., Chang S.C., Chiang H.C. et al. (Published on line 27 february 2011). Single-incision laparoscopic versus conventional laparoscopic right hemicolectomy: a comparison of short-term surgical results. Surg Endosc. DOI 10.1007/s00464-010-1481-4.

[35] Champagne B.J., Lee E.C., Leblanc .F, Stein S.L. and Delaney C.P. (2011). Single-incision vs straight laparoscopic segmental colectomy: A case-controlled study. Dis Colon Rectum, 54,183-186.

9

Intraoperative Sentinel Lymph Node Mapping in Patients with Colorectal Cancer

Krasimir Ivanov, Nikola Kolev and Anton Tonev
Medical University "Prof. Dr. Paraskev Stoyanov"
Bulgaria

1. Introduction

The sentinel lymph node (SLN) is defined as the first lymph node/nodes receiving direct drainage from the tumor and consequently possessing the greatest metastatic potential. (Nieweg OE. et al., 2001; Tanis PJ. Et al, 2002; Saha S et al, 2004; Bilchik A et al., 2001; Wood Th. F. et al, 2001; Bertagnolli M. et al, 2001; Dahl K. Et al, 2005; Feig BW et al, 2001; Patten LC et al, 2001) Sentinel lymph node mapping in colorectal cancer (CRC) is related to two questions that are important for the surgeon:

1. Is the extending of the lymph dissection necessary in certain patients and which are these patients?
2. Is the staging of the disease correct?

Additional questions that may be answered in the future are:

1. Can the volume of the visceral resection and lymph dissection be decreased (economy resections) in the aspect of implantation of laparoscopic surgery or local tumor excision - endoscopic or transanal?
2. Can the method help in deciding for sphincter preservation and nerve preservation in rectal surgery?
3. What is the impact on survival rates?
4. Is PET-CT a comparable method?
5. Will sentinel lymph node mapping have clinical application?

To answer these questions well-designed trials are needed.

The most important factor affecting the outcomes of the surgical treatment and the survival rate is the presence of metastases. (Bertoglio S et. Al, 2004; Wood Th. F. et al, 2001; Bertagnolli M. et al, 2001; Saha S. et al, 2000; Paramo JC. Et al, 2001; Trocha SD. et al, 2003; Wood TF et al, 2001) The presence of lymph metastases places the patients from first and second stage into third stage and significantly deteriorates the prognosis and the survival rate. (Bilchik AJ et al., 2002; Philips RKS. et al., 1984; O'Connell MJ. et al., 1997; Saha S. et al.,2000) The atypical lymph-drainage occurs in about 8-14% of the patients. (Saha S. et al., 2001; Saha S. et al., 2001; Wood TF et al, 2001; Kitagawa Y. et al., 2002; Bilchik AJ et al., 2001) The failure to detect the atypical drainage is one of the reasons for recurrences due to incorrect staging and adjuvant therapy. (Bilchik AJ et al., 2001; Paramo JC. et al., 2001; Martinez SR et al., 2005) It results from specific anatomical features of the lymph flow. The atypical lymph metastases are observed in terms of the localization level of the metastatic lymph nodes (jumping or "skip" metastases and also in affecting the atypical lymph basin

(aberrant lymph drainage) for the given localization of the primary tumor. (Kitagawa Y. et al., 2000; Bilchik AJ et al., 2002; Wood TF et al., 2002)
In CRC the resection volume and the lymph dissection are determined by the tumor localization and they have been standardized to a great extent. (Schlag PM et al., 2004) The metastatic lymph nodes in the presence of aberrant lymph drainage can be found beyond the lines of the standard lymph dissection. In these cases the radicality of the surgery requires extension of the lines of lymph dissection. (Paramo JC et al., 2001; Tsioulias G. et al., 2002; Kitajima M. et al., 2004) It is important to apply a method for lymph metastases detection. The possibilities of the intraoperative examination and palpation as well as the existing methods for imaging diagnostics of the lymph basin in CRC are not sufficiently reliable. Their sensitivity varies between 20% and 50%, only lymph nodes with size over 5mm are detected and the metastatic potential is determined based on the increased size. (Kitagawa Y. et al., 2000) According to literary data 50% to 78% of the metastatic lymph nodes are sized under 5 mm. (Saha S. et al., 2004; Rodriguez-Bigas MA et al., 1996; Haboubi NY et al., 1992; Paramo JC et al., 2002). This is a reason for the unsatisfactory capability of the preoperative and intraoperative diagnostics of the lymph metastases. Lymph node mapping with dye visualizes the lymph vessels and the SLN very well in the surgical field even if they are very small in size less than 5mm, otherwise undetectable. (Saha S. et al., 2004; Rodriguez-Bigas MA et al., 1996; Haboubi NY et al., 1992; Paramo JC et al., 2002).
The direct tumor drainage in the SLN is demonstrated by means of blue stained lymph vessel linking the tumor to the SLN, when marked with dye (Fig.1.a), b), c))
Recurrences are observed in 20 – 40% of the operated patients in the first and second stage. (Martinez SR & AJ Bilchik , 2005; Rodriguez-Bigas MA et al., 1996; Wolmark N. et al., 1986) In half of the patients with recurrences it was established that they were due to metastatic lymph nodes, which have not been detected and remove during the surgery. (Dimitrov V. et al., 2003; Macintosh E., 1997; Makela J.& Kiviniemi H., 2000; Morson BC et al., 1963; Pietra N. et al., 1998) For these patients the following was true: adequate lymph dissection was not performed; the disease has not been correctly staged; no indications have been given for adjuvant therapy (Saha S. et al., 2000; Cohen AM et al., 1998).
According to the TNM system the micrometastases are designated with the index "mi" and their presence stages the disease as third stage, determining a relevant treatment and prognosis. (Bilchik AJ et al., 2003; Sobin LH, 2002)
For the assessment of the lymph status it is obligatory to investigate morphologically at least 12 lymph nodes. (Martinez SR& Bilchik AJ, 2005; Rodriguez-Bigas MA et al., 1996). If lymph metastases are not detected, it is advisable to search for micrometastases (MM) A great number of authors in the literature suggest that the presence of MM is a poor prognostic factor and therefore are indicative for adjuvant therapy which would improve the prognosis in these "troublesome" 30% of the patients "without metastases". The prognostic value of the metastases in CRC requires further investigations in the future. In their studies a number of authors confirm the prognostic value of MM (Broll R. et al., 1997; Greenson JK et al., 1994; Isaka N. et al., 1999; Palma RT et al., 2003; Yasuda K. et al., 2001; Liefers GJ et al., 1998), others aren't support this suggestion. (Adell G. et al., 1996; Choi HJ et al., 2002; Lindmark G. et al., 1994). If the all LNs are to be investigated, the methods for micrometastases detection are costly, expensive and time consuming. (Tsioulias G. et al., 2002; Martinez SR& Bilchik AJ, 2005; Bilchik AJ et al., 2003; Doekhie FS et al., 2005)

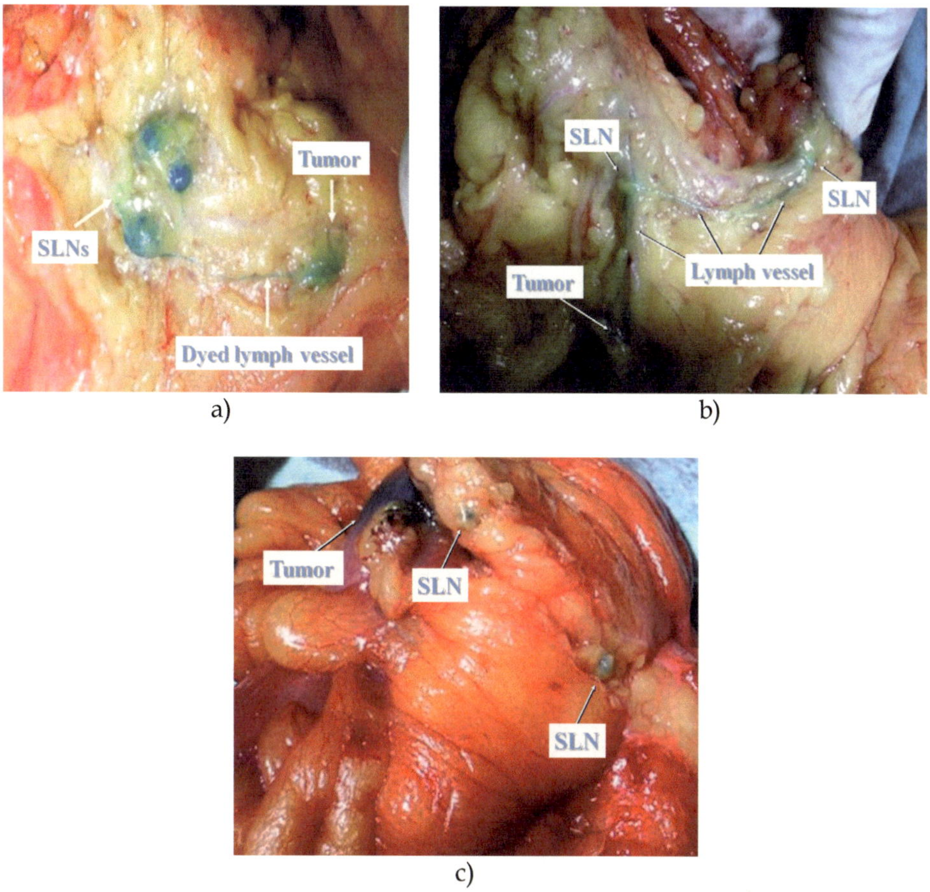

Fig. 1. Intraoperative view of stained lymph nodes and lymph vessels with Patent Blue V.

2. Methodology

2.1 Intraoperative procedure

We performed intraoperative sentinel mapping in 103 consecutive patients operated for colon or rectal cancer. An algorithm was worked out for sentinel mapping in colorectal cancer. The dying method with Patent Blue V was used.

a. Indications or inclusion criteria:
- Patients with invasive colorectal cancer
- Histological diagnosis and preoperative staging performed not later than 3 months before the surgery;
- Life expectancy over 5 years (age up to 80 years);
- Class after ASA I–III.

b. Contraindications and exclusion criteria:
- Presence of distant metastases;
- Preceding Previous local excision of the primary tumor;
- Metachronous colorectal cancer (with some exceptions);
- Recurrent colorectal cancer;

- Presence of cancer in another organ localization during the past 5 years, especially in the cases when the colorectal cancer is difficult to be differentiated histologically;
- Preceding Previous surgical interventions affecting the anatomy of the lymph basin;
- Complicated colorectal cancer (emergency operation);
- Class ASA IV–V.

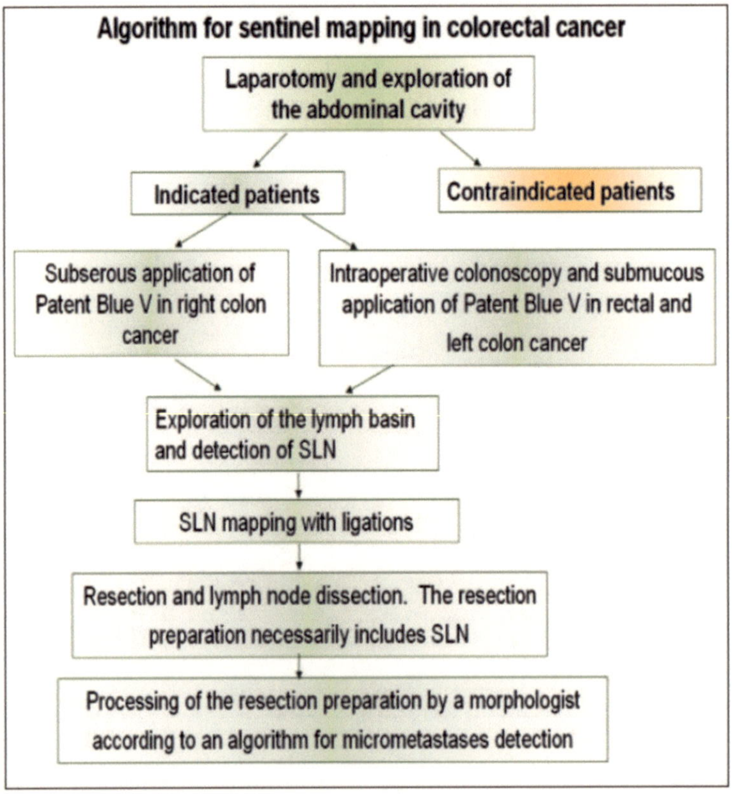

Fig. 2. Algorithm for sentinel mapping in colorectal cancer.

After the laparotomy and the exploration of the abdominal cavity in the absence of distant metastases and no palpatory data for the presence of lymph metastases in patients with cancer of the rectum and the left colon, we performed intraoperative colonoscopy. By means of an endoscopic injector we applied submucosally 0,5-2 cc of Patent Blue V peritumorally on 2 to 4 locations. Since in right colon cancer the intraoperative colonoscopy to the caecum is technically difficult and is time-consuming, we injected the dye subserously in these tumor localizations by means of a needle and a syringe (0,5-2cc) peritumorally on 2 to 4 locations. In 1 to 10 minutes time the blue-stained lymph node(s) is visualized, connecting the primary tumor with blue-dyed sentinel lymph node(s). We assume the first 1-4 blue-dyed lymph nodes to be sentinel and we mark them with ligatures. It is important that the procedure is performed accurately and precisely timed after the gradually coloring of the whole lymph basin, because the SLN can lose their color with time.

According to the tumor localization we perform thorough exploration of the regional lymph basin, the whole mesocolon, the stem of the mesenterial root of mesentery vessels and

paraaortically, the obturatory fosses and along the course of the iliac vessels in order to detect SLN and the presence of atypical lymph drainage.
We applied the method of the sentinel mapping in five patients with CRC who had been operated laparoscopically - figure 3.

2.2 Morphological investigations

The SLN tagged by the surgeon are sent to the morphological laboratory together with the specimen where a routine processing to a paraffin block is performed with 10 resections in every 20-25μm. Immunohistochemistry with cytokeratin20 is performed per one resection (usually the fifth one). The remaining resections together with the preparations from the case are dyed with Hematoxilin-Eosin. Micrometastases are defined as a focus of tumor cells sized under 2 mm or a focus detected only by means of immunohistochemistry. (Feezor RJ et al., 2002)

2.3 Statistical analysis

The statistical results were reported as detection rate of the sentinel lymph node, accuracy and sensitivity of the test, and false negative rate; formulas, for the assessment of these parameters were as follows: The staging benefit was calculated by comparison between *pN* staging in the sentinel lymph node group and *pN* staging in the non-sentinel lymph node group. The comparison between groups was performed using the *chi-square* test; the significance was assumed for$p<0.05$ (95% confidence interval). The statistics were performed using XLSTAT 2010 (Addinsoft 1995-2010).

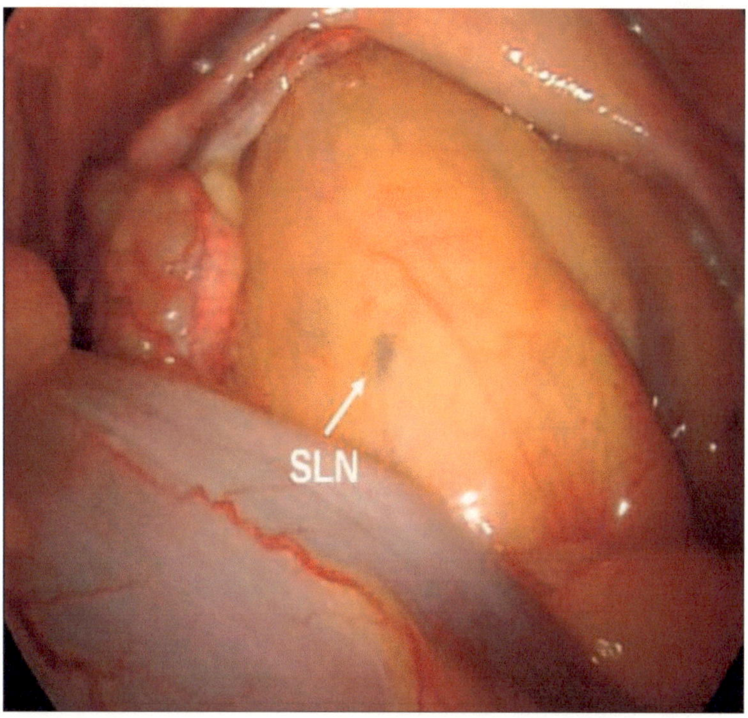

Fig. 3. Laparoscopic view of a SLN.

3. Results

The distribution of the patients is shown on Table 1. The relation between the T stage of the primary tumor and the presence of lymph metastases after sentinel mapping is shown on Table 2. Metastases were detected in 57% of the SLN (105 out of 184) as compared to 9% metastases incidence in the nonsentinel LN (198 out of 2208). In the absence of metastases in SLN the likelihood for metastases occurrence in the nonsentinel LN is only 0,6% (4 out of 657 nonsentinel LN). (Table 3)

TABLE 1

	Colon Cancer	Rectal Cancer
Patients	48	55
Male	22 (46%)	25 (45%)
Female	26 (54%)	30 (55%)
Average age (years)	63	66

Table 1. Distribution of patients according to cancer localization.

TABLE 2

	T3 n(%)	T4 n(%)
Patients	44 (43)	11 (10)
Presence of lymph node metastases	40 (90)	11 (100)
Micrometastases	3 (7)	0 (0)

Table 2. Relation between tumor stage and metastases, including micrometastases.

TABLE 3

	Colon cancer n (%)	Rectal cancer n (%)
Patients	48	55
Successful mapping	48 (100)	55 (100)
Presence of lymph node metastases	24 (50)	27 (49)
False negative rate	0 (0)	3 (5)
Metastases only in SLN	8 (17)	9 (16)
Detected MM	5 (19)	6 (21)

Table 3. SLN in colorectal cancer – rate of success, rate of detection, false negative rate, rate of metastases only in SLN, rate of detected micrometastases (MM).

The mean number of the lymph nodes in the specimen is 14.7 in cancer of the colon vs. 13.2 in cancer of the rectum. The average number of SLN in cancer of the colon is 1.9 vs. 1.6 in cancer of the rectum. False negative results were reported in the presence of metastases, not detected in the SLN. We observed false negative results in 3 patients. All of them had large T4 tumors infiltrating adjacent organs. Therefore, we suggest that such patients are relatively contraindicated for sentinel mapping. In most cases the SLN were located in proximally to the primary tumor. One, two, three and four SLN were detected in 40%, 39%, 19% and 2% of the patients, respectively.
In spite of this we detected a presence of atypical lymph drainage with positive SLN outside the limits of the standard resection in 10 (10%) of the patients. In 3 out of these 10 patients the aberrant SLN were the only site of lymph metastases. In 5 patients we performed extended right hemicolectomy with the inclusion of the lineal flexure and its mesocolon because we detected SLN in the region of the flexure (Fig. 4.).

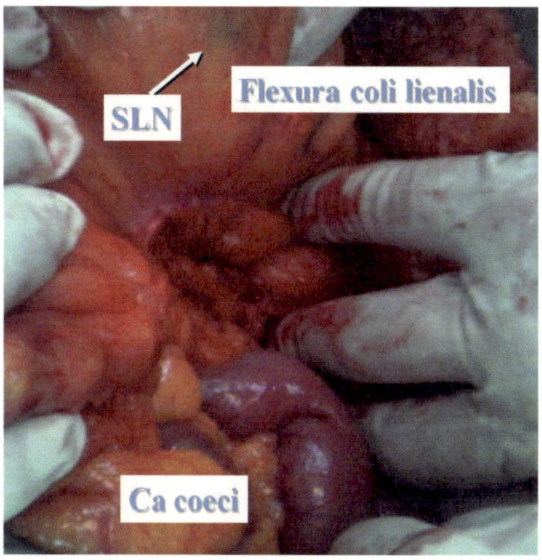

Fig. 4. SLN in the region of flexura coli lienalis.

We extended the size of the lymph dissection in 5 patients with rectal cancer. In one of them we detected SLN in the root of inferior mesenteric atrery artery, which necessitated its high ligation with additional dissection around the root. In the remaining 4 cases we detected SLN in the left or right iliac region and we performed lateral lymph node dissection (Fig. 5). In the rest of the cases when no SLN or enlarged lymph nodes were detected in the lateral ligaments, obturatorialy fosses or along the iliac vessels, we did not consider appropriate to perform lateral lymph node dissection in patients with rectal cancer.
On Figure 6, it is shown the visualization of direct lymph drainage from cancer of the rectum T2 to SLN from the IIIrd level in the root of inferior mesenteric artery. In the same patient the morphological investigation did not reveal metastases in any of the LN in the surgical preparation. The immunohistochemical study of the only SLN revealed MM, i.e. skip metastasing. In nine of the ten patients with extended resections were found metastases in the lymph nodes, and in one - no metastases. The analysis of the results shows that in 9 of 10 patients with extended resection, based on the results from the intraoperative sentinel lymph node mapping, were dissected metastatic sentinel lymph nodes located beyond the lines of the standard resection, by which we achieved surgical radicalism. In 7 patients with

rectal cancer intraoperative visual detection of SLN during mobilization of the rectum was impeded even after additional introduction of the colonoscope in the mobilized rectum and transilumination, probably due to the fatty tissue and insufficient staining of the SLN.

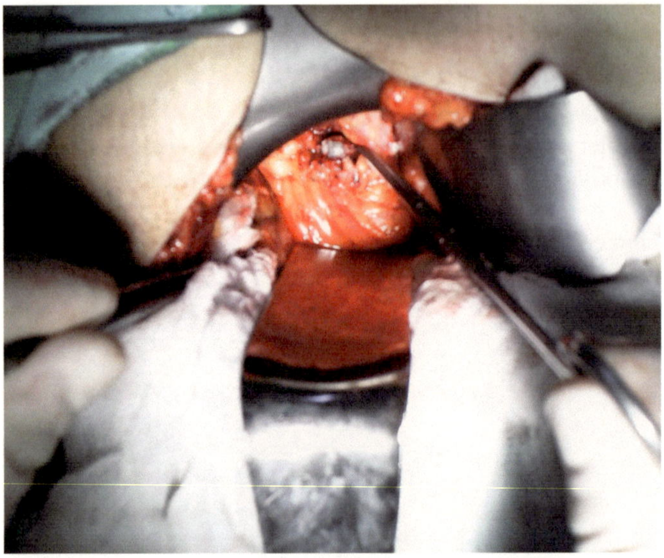

Fig. 5. SLN in the left ilac region - lateral lymph node dissection.

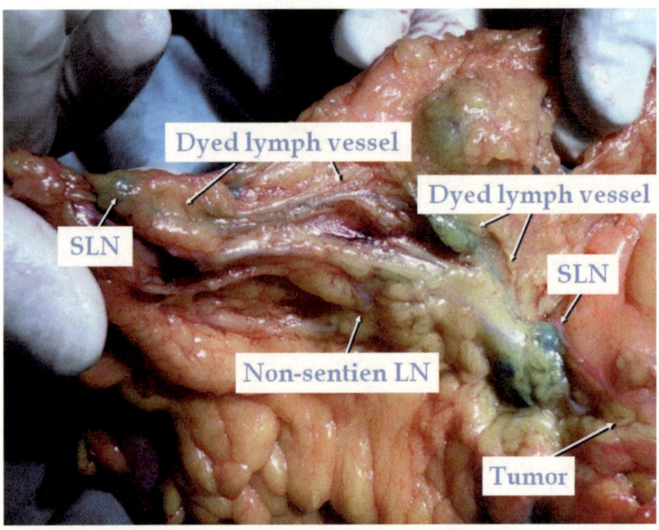

Fig. 6. Direct lymph drainage from the tumor to the root of inferior mesenteric artery. Case of SLN with micrometastasis - example of skip metastasing.

In the same patients we performed detection of the SLN in the mesorectum after destruction of the fascial layers in the presence of pathologist immediately after the resection of the rectum in the operation room. The detection of the SLN was preceded by making biopsy of the circumferential margin, which is an important predictive factor for the disease. In these 7 cases we followed the protocol on Fig. 7. 100% success rate without false-negative results was achieved by adherence to the protocol of procedure in the cases with immediate postoperative detection (Fig. 8). The only disadvantage in these 7 patients is the presence of higher number SLN (3-5) average 3.6 vs. 1.6 in the patients with intraoperative detection, which is explained with delay in the detection with average 20 minutes, during which time the dye has spread to more lymph nodes.

4. Additional methods of sentinel lymph node mapping

The practical application of the method is facilitated with the following additional methods:

4.1 Method for immediate ex vivo detection of mesorectal SLN after failure of the intraoperative detection.

The intraoperative detection of SLN in rectal cancer is easy, because the blue-stained SLN are in contrast with the yellowish fatty tissue and gain distinction during exploration of the pelvis and are visible through the mesorectal fascia. The visualization of SLN in the mesorectum is helped by transilumination of the mesorectum with halogen light from the fibrocolonoscope. The first stained SLN in the mesorectum are easily found.

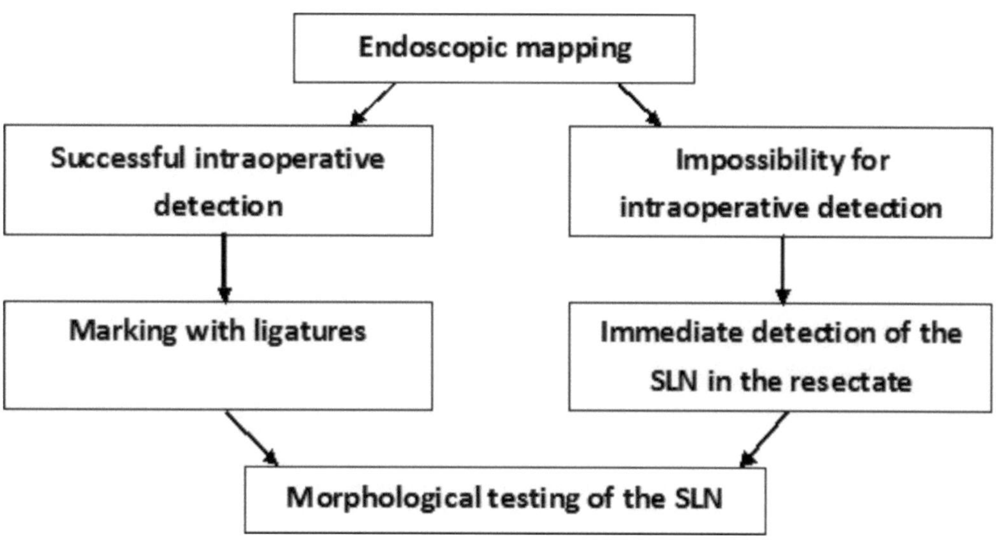

Fig. 7. Algorithm for immediate detection of SLN in the specimen.

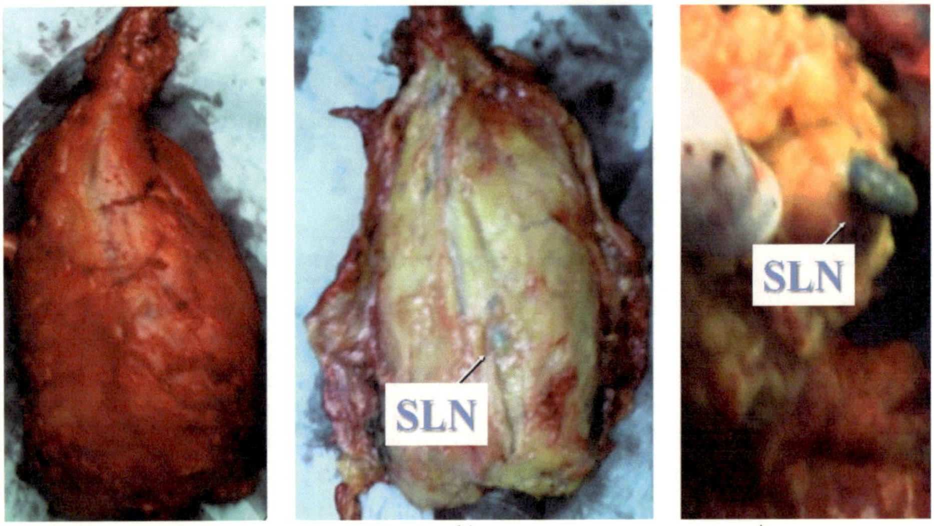

a) b) c)

Fig. 8. Method of immediate postoperative detection. a) the SLN are not visible through fascia propria recti; b)after removal of fascia propria recti one SLN was visualized in the mesorectum; c) the visualized SLN - close view.

4.2 Application of the method of additional lymph node mapping

An existing problem remains the examination of insufficient number of lymph nodes in patients with colorectal cancer. This leads to decreased probability for discovery of metastatic lymph nodes and inaccurate staging. The main reason is the small size of the lymph nodes, which are not found by palpation in the fatty tissue of the specimen. Aiming maximal increase in the number of discovered and examined lymph nodes we developed method for additional lymph mapping of the specimen and we evaluated the results together with a pathologist. The method of additional lymph mapping was applied in 103 patients with colorectal cancer and SLN mapping. The method was applied on fresh specimen immediately in the operating room. Intraoperative SLN mapping has been performed and the SLN were identified and marked with ligatures. Additionally 2-3cc Patent Blue V was applied subserosally and submucosally. This method vastly stains the whole lymph node basin. Fig 9. (a,b,c)

4.3 Results from the additional methods

The results we achieved show that the lymphatic system of the specimen facilitates the spread of the dye. In postoperative lymph node mapping the dye stains vastly the lymph nodes and the lymphatic vessels. The evaluation of the lymphatic status in colorectal cancer relies not only on quantitative criteria, e.g. number of examined lymph nodes, but also on qualitative characteristics on the lymph nodes: their size, distance from the primary tumor, sentinel or non-sentinel lymph nodes.

After analyzing the data from the morphological examination after application of the intraoperative SLN mapping and the additional lymph nodes mapping of the specimen we achieved the following results. The number and the average number of examined lymph nodes in relation to pT and pN is shown on Table 4.

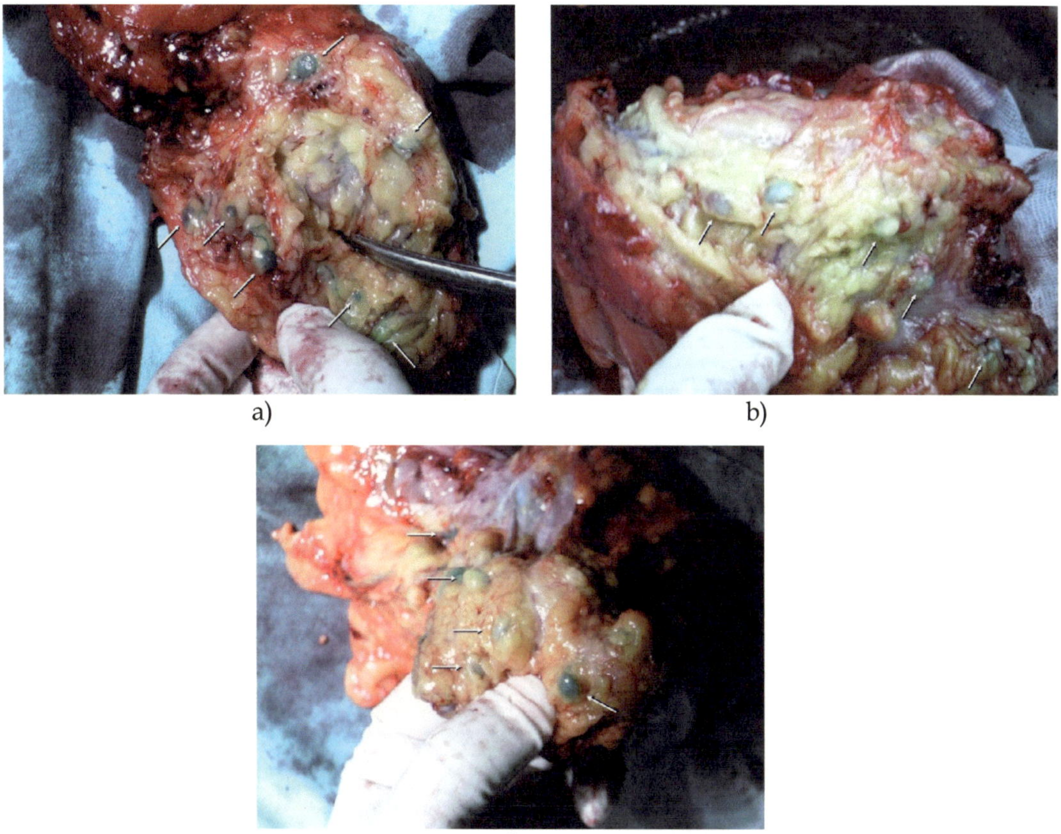

a) b) c)

Fig. 9. a),b),c) Intraoperative view of the additional lymph node mapping.

pT \ pN	pN0 (n)	pN1 (n)	pN2 (n)
pT1	18,3 (n = 10)	17,2 (n = 4)	-
pT2	17,2 (n = 35)	14,2 (n = 11)	16,1 (n = 5)
pT3	17,6 (n = 19)	16,5 (n = 16)	16,8 (n = 22)
pT4	-	12,1 (n = 7)	12,4 (n = 7)

Table 4. Relation of number patients to pT and pN

From these data it is understood, that no clear relation between the tumor infiltration (pT) and the number of metastatic lymph nodes (pN). In pN0 the largest and the least number of examined lymph nodes was established in pT1 and pT2 tumors. A larger number of examined lymph nodes are found in patients with pT3 pN2 tumors, comparable to the number of examined lymph nodes in pT3 pN0 and pT3 pN1 tumors. The data for the number of patients, average number of examined lymph nodes and the length of the specimen in relation to the tumor localization are shown on Table 5.

pN / pT	pN0	pN1	pN2	**Total**
pT1	10	4	0	**14**
pT2	35	11	5	**51**
pT3	19	16	22	**57**
pT4	0	7	7	**14**
Total	**64**	**38**	**34**	**136**

Table 5. Relation of the average number of examined LN in relation to T/N

We analyzed the data in relation to the size of the examined lymph nodes, the distance from the primary tumor and the localization of the lymph nodes in relation to the rest of the lymph nodes and the primary tumor. The average size of the examined lymph nodes was 4.5mm. The average size of the lymph nodes in colorectal cancer with presence of lymph metastases was larger - 4.7mm in comparison to 4.3mm without presence of lymph metastases, as 53% of the metastatic lymph nodes are less than 5mm.

Along with the size of the examined lymph nodes the distance of the lymph node from the primary tumor and its localization in the mesocolon or the mesorectum also have relationship to the metastatic potential of the lymph node. We analyzed the results in relation to the localization of the sentinel lymph nodes in patients with colorectal cancer. The results for the localization of the SLN are shown on Figure 10.

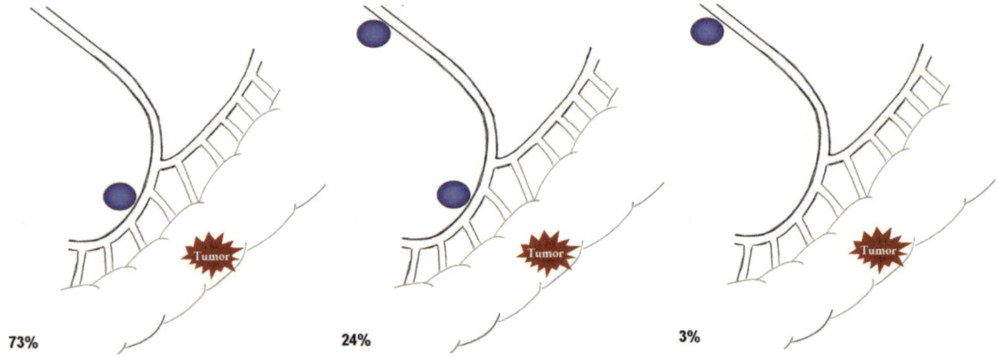

Fig. 10. a) in 73% of the cases the SLN are localized solely in the pericolic or the perirectal fatty tissue. b) in 24% of the cases the SLN are localized simultaneously on the first and upper levels. c) in 3% of the cases the SLN are localized on the second level.

We established that the average size of the metastatic lymph nodes was larger than that of the non-metastatic lymph nodes. As in 53% of the metastatic lymph nodes their size is less than 5mm, the size is not a certain criteria for evaluating its metastatic potential.

Significantly promising criteria is the result after application of diagnostic method for evaluation of the lymphatic status - intraoperative SLN mapping, which discovers

metastatic lymph nodes in 98% of the cases. The data show that the closer the lymph node to the tumor is, the higher its metastatic potential is.
The examination of higher number of lymph nodes is connected with increased possibility for more accurate evaluation of the lymphatic status. The application of the method made it possible to detect more than 12 lymph nodes in the specimen and to shorten the time for detecting of maximal number lymph nodes in examination of the specimen. Fig. 11

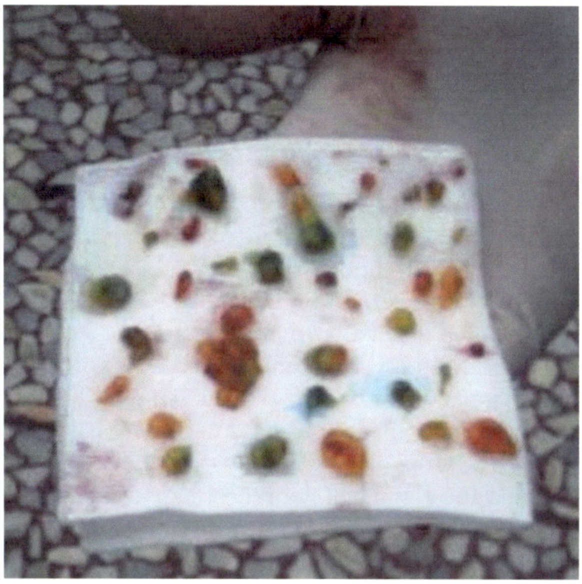

Fig. 11. Thirty-eight stained lymph nodes subject to morphological evaluation from a rectal cancer specimen.

Localization	Number of patients	Average number of lymph nodes	Average length of the specimen
Coecum	12	17,1	27,5
Ascendens	6	16,2	22,1
Hepatic	4	19,7	27,2
Transversum	5	17,3	23,4
Lienalis	1	13,2	15,8
Descendens	9	15,4	25
Sigma	28	12,8	21,2
Rectum	71	14,7	15,7
Total	**136**	**17**	**22,2**

Table 6. Number of patients, average number of lymph nodes and average length of the specimen in relation to the tumor localization.

5. Discussion

Surgical treatment is the basis of the complex therapeutic approach aimed at a lasting cure for patients with colorectal cancers. The quality of surgery is determined apart from the choice of appropriate operating method, but also the characteristics of the tumor in his lymph drainage and possibilities of preoperative and intraoperative staging.

Carrying out an operation with adequate volume fulfils the oncologic criteria and is a prerequisite for precise morphological staging of cancer, which determines the postoperative treatment. Treatment of colorectal cancer is the most successful in stages I and II of the disease before the tumor is metastatic.

The consequences of inaccurate assessment of lymph status lead to development of recurrence in one third of operated patients with "nonmetastatic" colorectal cancers.

The lymph node status is the most important prognostic factor in colorectal cancer. Not always and everywhere can be done accurate preoperative assessment of the lymph status. Clinical examination and intraoperative exploration are only indicative and have relatively low sensitivity and specificity. Prompt intraoperative histological examination has low sensitivity and cannot detect the presence of lymph node micrometastases.

Leaving metastatic lymph nodes located beyond the standard lymph dissection is the cause for recurrence after the radical surgery. The problem is the lack of method for intraoperative assessment of atypical lymphatic drainage. (Bilchik AJ et al., 2001) According to the literature metastatic lymph nodes in the presence of aberrant lymphatic drainage can be found beyond the standard volume of lymph node dissection. In these cases the oncologic principles require to expand the volume of lymph node dissection. (Kitagawa Y. et al., 2004) SLN mapping changes the volume of resection in 8% of cases. Aberrant drainage is not uncommon in patients with tumors of the digestive tract (Cohen, AM et al., 1993). Some authors (Yamamoto, Y. et al., 1998) shows metastasis in 10% of 452 patients with colorectal cancers. Aberrant lymphatic drainage is found in 29% of cases (Bilchik, A J,& Trocha SD, 2003) and may later expand the volume of resection (Bilchik AJ et al., 2001), therefore all the blue stained lymph nodes must be accurately located and marked. Regional lymphatic basin of the colon is removed and sent for morphological examination. Reported values for the successful SLN localization ranged from 58 to 100%. (Bilchik AJ et al., 2001; Bilchik AJ et al., 2003; Tsioulias GJ et al., 2002) Applying this method we achieved success in about 94% of cases. Another important advantage of in vivo SLN mapping in colorectal cancer is detection of patients with aberrant lymphatic drainage occuring in 14% of the cases leading to a change in the initial operational plan (Wood TF et al., 2001). The reccurence in nodal-negative patients is attributed to residual nodal disease after inadequate lymphadenectomy or aberrant lymphatic drainage. (Prandi M. e al., 2002; Schrag, D. et al. 2002) Aberrant lymphatic drainage can be due to anatomical variations or due to altered lymph drainage caused by metastatic involvement of the lymphatic system (Bilchik AJ et al., 2001; Bilchik AJ et al., 2003; Saha S. et al., 2001). In colorectal cancer the standard oncological resection is recommended regardless of the status of SLN. Sometimes, however, it appears that aberrant drainage continues beyond the normal lines of resection. This unusual pattern of lymph drainage was observed in 8% of patients with CRC, where the lines of the lymphatic and organ resection should be extended beyond the conventional (Saha, S. et al. 2004).

The method of intraoperative SLN mapping achieves better intraoperative visualization of the lymph nodes with the highest metastatic potential even if they are very small and detects the presence of aberrant lymphatic drainage and skip metastases. Our study found aberrant lymphatic drainage in 2% of patients and skip metastases in 3% of patients with lymph mapping. We expanded the volume of surgical procedure in 7% of the patients in which positive lymph nodes were detected beyond standard lymphatic dissection. In three of them skip metastases were observed and in other three patients was observed aberrant lymphatic drainage. All the patients' sentinel lymph nodes revealed the presence of metastases or micrometastases after ultrastaging.

The examination of insufficient number of lymph nodes is the reason leading to a reduced chance of detection of metastatic lymph nodes and inaccurate staging of the disease. The cause is the small size of lymph nodes that are not detected by palpation in adipose tissue of the specimen. Our results from the application of the method of additional lymph node mapping indicate that it allows quickly discovering and exploring the maximum number of lymph nodes and contributes to the precise staging of colorectal cancer. We found that the average size of metastatic lymph nodes was 4.7 mm. Our results show that the lymphatic system of the specimen has potential for diffusion of the dye. The postoperative lymph node mapping stains the lymphatic vessels and the lymph nodes.

We found that in case of right colon cancer it is appropriate to apply the method of intraoperative subserosal SLN mapping. The rectal cancer and the left colon cancer are more suitable to perform intraoperative colonoscopy and to apply the method of intraoperative endoscopic submucous sentinel marking. The analysis of the results from the application of the methods of intraoperative endoscopic submucous SLN mapping and intraoperative subserous SLN mapping indicates that both methods are equally reliable and highly sensitive. Additionally the method of intraoperative SLN mapping is equally applicable to patients with colon and rectal cancer.

The ultrastaging of sentinel lymph nodes aids the accurate staging and treatment of patients with colorectal cancer. By application of the method of intraoperative sentinel marking and the ultrastaging of lymph nodes is achieved upstaging of the disease and determination of exact definitive diagnosis in 20% of patients.

The method is convenient because it is not related to the need for expensive equipment and supplies and does not require a complex organization, the training of the surgeons is easy and the staff readily agrees for application of the method.

Our own results and literature data show that intraoperative SLN mapping is a method with high success rate and sensitivity for intraoperative diagnosis of the lymph status.

The surgical approach and the volume of lymphatic dissection should respond to the state of the lymphatic basin, estimated using an objective diagnostic method such as intraoperative SLN mapping. This leads to an increase of surgical radicalism in the treatment of colorectal cancer, which is proved in our study.

Surgeons and oncologists are aware that ensuring of optimal conditions for patients with colorectal cancer requires precise surgery, if necessary combined with adjuvant therapy. In order to provide quality treatment for colorectal cancer a multidisciplinary team including GPs, surgeons, imaging diagnostic specialists, gastroenterologists, oncologists and pathologist, etc is required.

SLN mapping increases the number of collected lymph nodes, as well as the sensitivity of nodal assessment. In addition, in cases with aberrant lymph drainage extensive resection is performed, containing remote SLN. A multidisciplinary approach is required to standardize the detection and assessment of the SLN, contributing to colorectal cancer staging. Detection of micrometastases in the lymph nodes is generally recognized as pN1(mi), but the risk of recurrence is unknown. Large prospective studies are essential to determine the clinical significance of nodal micrometastases. The introduction of coordinated screening programs for low-risk patients or tracking of high-risk patients, the application of more sensitive methods for preoperative staging, the advance in treatment and methods of morphological evaluation create opportunities for improving the survival and the quality of life of patients with colorectal cancers. (Bilchik A. et al., 2001; Bilchik, A J,& Trocha SD, 2003; Esser, S. et al., 2001; Feinstein, AR et al., 1985; Merrie, AE et al., 2001; Paramo JC et al., 2001; Tsopelas, C.& Sutton R., 2002; Wood, TF et al., 2001).

The accuracy may increase with the increasing of the number of lymph nodes sectioned, and with involving of immunohistochemistry or molecular markers' panels as demonstrated in many studies, but will also increase the cost and the workload for pathologists (Bilchik AJ et al., 2006; Bembenek A. et al., 2007; Kelder W. et al., 2007). Even though the accuracy was good for colon and rectal cancer, the sensitivity of the method somewhere is reported very low (66.66% for colon and 50% for rectal cancer), and the false-negative rate was high (23.07% for colon cancer and 18.18% for rectal cancer). The sensitivity of the method varies in the literature between 54% in the study of the Bembenek , and 88.2–89% in the study of Bilchik AJ *et al.*, and Kelder W *et al.* (Bilchik AJ et al., 2006; Bembenek A. et al., 2007; Kelder W. et al., 2007). The smallest false-negative rate was achieved by Bilchick AJ *et al.* (7.4%), but other authors reported a significantly higher rate of false-negative results (46% for colon cancer in the study of Bembenek AE *et al.* and 43% in rectal cancer in the study of Baton O *et al.*) (Bilchik AJ et al., 2006; Bembenek A. et al., 2007; Baton O. et al., 2005). Thus, with such high risk of failure (lower detection rate, low sensitivity and high false-negativity rate), the technique of sentinel lymph node in rectal cancer is obviously not feasible; in colon cancer, the method may be improved by increasing the number of the examined lymph nodes, and using specific immunohistochemical staining methods. However, doing so, it will not represent a relief for pathologist, but probably will increase the quality of the *pN* staging. In this matter, our study has shown an increase in the detection of the positive lymph nodes (37.2% *N+* in sentinel lymph node group *vs.* 26.67% in the control group), but statistical significance was not reached. Moreover, the quality of the upstaging was not determined by the examination technique itself (micrometastases were detected in only two cases - 9.37% upstaging rate), but probably by the increased number of the identified and examined lymph nodes in the studied group *vs.* comparison group (the blue staining of the lymph node in the study group made it easy to identify them, and probably an increasing awareness and close collaboration between the surgeon and pathologist) (Bilchik AJ&Compton C., 2007). In literature, there are better results in upstaging the *pN* category, using the sentinel lymph node technique, varying from 15% for rectal cancer (Baton O *et al., 2005*) to 18–23.6% in colon cancer (Bilchik AJ et al., 2006; Bembenek A. et al., 2007; Kelder W. et al., 2007).

The high incidence of distant metastasis of CRC in patients whose nodes are negative may be due to insufficient numbers or sections of lymph nodes. Bilchik A.&Compton C., 2007 Because multiple sectioning and IHC staining cannot be routinely used to examine all lymph nodes in a CRC specimen, we focused on the first regional node(s) to receive lymphatic drainage from a primary tumor. In melanoma and breast cancer, lymphatic mapping and excision of the SN is used to determine the tumor status of the entire nodal basin and avoid complete lymph node dissection in node-negative patients. The application of the SN technique in CRC is different because all regional lymph nodes are routinely removed en bloc with the primary tumor. However, as in melanoma and breast cancer, examination of the SN allows the pathologist to focus on the regional node(s) most likely to contain tumor cells and thus improve tumor cell detection and accuracy of staging. The tumor occludes the lymphatic vessels resulting in drainage to another (nonsentinel) node. Because these nodes are large and solid, it is unlikely that SN and lymphatic mapping will be of value in this group of patients. The prognostic significance of nodal micrometastases by either CK-IHC or RT-PCR in CRC remains unclear. In a recent study in patients initially reported as node negative, re-examination using CK-IHC and carcinoembryonic antigen (CEA)-IHC demonstrated evidence of micrometastases in 26% of the node negative patients (Bilchik et al., 2001). However, the presence of nodal micrometastases did not significantly affect 5-year survival. Similarly, Jeffers (Jeffers MD et al., 1994) detected CK-IHC micrometastases in 25% of 77 patients who's CRCs were initially staged as Duke's B. Again, the presence of nodal micrometastases had no significant effect on survival; however, random micro sectioning may have missed tumor cells, thereby causing insignificant survival differences between the two groups. More recently, Greenson (Greenson JK et al., 1994) demonstrated that micrometastatic disease missed by routine HE staining but identified by CK-IHC had an adverse effect on survival. The lack of consensus in the literature in part reflects the absence of standard antibody titers and staining techniques; there are considerable interinstitutional variations in the analysis of CRC lymph nodes by CK-IHC. Although to date no randomized study has demonstrated significance for the detection of micrometastases by CKIHC, the American College of Surgeons Oncology Group currently is conducting a multicenter trial (Z-0010) to assess the utility of CK-IHC in detecting micrometastases, of SNs draining primary breast carcinoma. Clinical outcome studies of marker expression in CRC are also limited. Hayashi (Hayashi N. et al., 1995) demonstrated decreased survival in patients with p53 or K-ras mutations in colonic lymph nodes. In another study of patients whose CRC was staged Duke's B by conventional techniques, Liefers (Liefers GJ et al., 1998) reported a 5-year survival rate of 50% for patients whose nodes expressed CEA, versus 91% for those whose nodes did not express CEA. Several other investigators have reported that histologically negative lymph nodes contained evidence of occult metastases by RT-PCR using CK20 30 or guanylyl cyclase C 31 in qualitative assay systems. However, guanylyl cyclase C, CEA, and cytokeratin are expressed by normal tissues and therefore may introduce false-positive results. Our group and others have questioned their utility for the detection of micrometastatic CRC. Our approach has been to use a combination of mRNA markers in a semi-quantitative assay to detect occult micrometastases. Focused analysis of multiple sections of the SN by CK-IHC and RT-PCR provides a unique tool for accurate staging of CRC. As demonstrated in our study, lymphatic mapping of the SN also can identify unexpected nodal drainage patterns that alter the margins of surgical resection. Focused examination of SN diagnoses micrometastatic disease missed by conventional techniques. Although the significance of micrometastatic disease is yet to be defined in CRC, it is likely to be an important stratifying factor in choosing those who may benefit from adjuvant chemotherapy

6. Conclusions

The method of intraoperative SLN mapping using Patent Blue V is an accurate and objective diagnostic method for assessment of the lymphatic status in patients with colorectal cancer. The method is an objective criterion for intraoperative surgical behavior

The method of intraoperative SLN mapping is applied with high success in patients with colon and rectal cancer. The method has 100% success rate and 98% sensitivity.

The analysis of the results from the application of methods of intraoperative endoscopic submucous SLN mapping and intraoperative subserous SLN mapping indicates that both methods are equally reliable and highly sensitive.

The method of intraoperative SLN mapping achieves better intraoperative visualization of lymph nodes with the highest metastatic potential, even if they are very small. It was found that the average size of metastatic lymph nodes was 4.7 mm. The method can detect the presence of aberrant lymphatic drainage and lymphatic skip metastases.

The sentinel lymph node reflects with high reliability the status of the entire lymphatic basin. Metastatic lymph nodes beyond the standard volume of lymphatic dissection are detected by intraoperative SLN mapping. By increasing the surgical volume was achieved greater radicalism in 7% of patients with colorectal cancers. It does not increase the postoperative morbidity.

Our study demonstrates that metastases in sentinel lymph nodes are found 6 times more frequently than in other lymph nodes. In 98% of cases the metastases are found in the sentinel lymph nodes.

In the absence of metastases in sentinel lymph nodes, the likelihood of metastases in other lymph nodes is only 0.6%.

Only through the application of the method of intraoperative SLN mapping and the ultrastaging of the lymph nodes it is liable to achieve more precise clinical staging of disease and determining of exact definitive diagnosis in 20% of patients.

The method of additional lymph node mapping allows quick discovery and exploration of maximum number lymph nodes, which contributes to the accurate staging of colorectal cancer.

The endoscopic submucous application of the lymphatic marker is the only appropriate method for intraoperative SLN mapping in case of subperitoneal localization of rectal cancer.

We conclude that SLN mapping in colorectal cancer is a convenient diagnostic method allowing the surgeon to individualize the approach to every single patient. Further studies are needed to validate if routine use of this method will increase the survival rates of patients operated for colorectal cancer.

We can conclude that the operational approach and the volume of the conducted lymphatic dissection must comply with the status of the lymphatic basin, assessed by an objective diagnostic method such as the intraoperative sentinel lymph node mapping. This leads to increased surgical radicalism in the surgical treatment of colorectal cancers. Our recommendation is that the method should be promoted and clinical trials should follow.

7. References

Adell, G, Boeryd, B, Franlund, B, Sjodahl, R, Hakansson, L: Occurrence and prognostic importance of micrometastases in regional lymph nodes in Dukes B colorectal carcinoma: an immunohistochemical study. Eur J Surg 1996; 162:637-642.

Baton O, Lasser P, Sabourin Jc, Boige V, Duvillard P, Elias D, Malka D, Ducreux M, Pocard M, Ex vivo sentinel lymph node study for rectal adenocarcinoma: preliminary study, World J Surg, 2005, 29(9):1166–1170; discussion 1171.

Bembenek A, Rosenberg R, Wagler E, Gretschel S, Sendler A, Siewert Jr, Nährig J, Witzigmann H, Hauss J, Knorr C, Dimmler A, Gröne J, Buhr Hj, Haier J, Herbst H, Tepel J, Siphos B, Kleespies A, Koenigsrainer A, Stoecklein Nh, Horstmann O, Grützmann R, Imdahl A, Svoboda D, Wittekind C, Schneider W, Wernecke Kd, Schlag Pm, Sentinel lymph node biopsy in colon cancer: a prospective multicenter trial, Ann Surg, 2007, 245(6):858–863.

Bembenek A., Haensch W, Schneider U, Markwardt J, Schlag PM: Immunohistochemical detection of lymphnode metastases The Lancet 2000; 355:144-145.

Bertagnolli M, Miedema B, Redston M, Dowell J, Niedzwiecki D, Fleshman J, Bem J, Mayer R, Zinner M, Compton Carolyn: Sentinel Node Staging of Resectable Colon Cancer: Results of a Multicenter Study. Ann Surg Oncol 2004; 240:624-630.

Bertoglio S, Sandrucci S, Percivale P, Goss M, Gipponi M, Moresco L, Mussa B, Mussa A: Prognostic Value of Sentinel Lymph Node Biopsy in the Pathologic Staging of Colorectal Cancer Patients Journal of Surgical Oncology 2004; 85:166–170.

Bilchik A, Saha S, Wiese D, Stonecypher JA, Wood TF, Sostrin S, Turner RR, Wang HJ, Morton DL, Hoon D. SB. Molecular staging of early colon cancer on the basis of sentinel node analysis: a multicenter phase II trial. J. Clin. Oncol. 2001; 19:1128-1136.

Bilchik A: More(Nodes)+More(Analysis) = Less (Mortality): Challenging the Therapeutic Equation for Early-Stage Colon Cancer Annals of Surgical Oncology 2003; 10:203-205.

Bilchik AJ, Compton C, Close collaboration betweensurgeon and pathologist is essential for accurate staging of early colon cancer, Ann Surg, 2007, 245(6):864–866.

Bilchik AJ, Dinome M, Saha S, Turner RR, Wiese D, McCarter M, Hoon DS, Morton Dl, Prospective multicenter trial of staging adequacy in colon cancer: preliminary results, ARCH SURG, 2006, 141(6):527–533; DISCUSSION 533- 534.

Bilchik AJ, Giuliano A, Essner R, Bostick P, Kelemen P, Foshag LJ, Sostrin S, Turner RR, Morton DL: Universal application of intraoperative lymphatic mapping and sentinel lymphadenectomy in solid neoplasms. Cancer J Sci Am. 1998; 4:351-358.

Bilchik AJ, Nora D, Tollenaar R.A.E.M., van de Velde C.J.H., Wood T, Turner R, Morton DL, Hoon D.S.B: Ultrastaging of early colon cancer using lymphatic mapping and molecular analysisEuropean Journal of Cancer 2002; 38: 977–985.

Bilchik AJ, Nora DT, Sobin LH, Turner RR, Trocha S, Krasne D: Effect of lymphatic mapping on the new tumor-node-metastasis classification for colorectal cancer. J Clin Oncol 2003; 21:668–672.

Bilchik AJ, Nora DT: Lymphatic Mapping of Nodal Micrometastasis in Colon Cancer: Putting the Cart Before the Horse? Annals of Surgical Oncology 2002; 9:529-531.

Bilchik AJ, Saha S, Tsioulias GJ: Aberrant drainage and missed micrometastases: the value of lymphatic mapping and focused analysis of sentinel lymph nodes in gastrointestinal neoplasms. Ann Surg Oncol 2001; 8:82–5S.

Bilchik, A. J., S. D. Trocha. Lymphatic mapping and sentinel node analysis to optimize laparoscopic resection and staging of colorectal cancer: an update. - Cancer Control, 10, 2003, 219–223.

Broll R, Schauer V, Schimmelpenning H: Prognostic relevance of occult tumor cells in lymph nodes of colorectal carcinomas: an immunohistochemical study. Dis ColonRectum 1997; 40:1465-1471.

Choi, HJ, Choi, YY, Hong, SH: Incidence and prognostic implications of isolated tumor cells in lymph nodes from patients with Dukes B colorectal carcinoma. Dis Colon Rectum. 2002 Jun;45(6):750-5; discussion755-6.

Cohen AM, Kelsen D, Saltz L, Minsky BD, Nelson H, Farouk R, et al: Adjuvant therapy for colorectal cancer. Curr Probl Cancer 1998; 22:5–65.

Cohen AM, Kelsen D, Saltz L: Adjuvant therapy for colorectal cancer. Curr Prob Cancer 1998; 22:5–65.

Cohen, A. M., B. D. Minsky, R. L. Schilsky. Rectal cancer. - In: Cancer Principles&Practice. Eds: Helman De Vita Jr., S. Rosenberg, Philadelphia, Lippinkott Co., 1993. p. 929–966.

Cutait, R, Alves, VA, Lopes, LC: Restaging of colorectal cancer based on the identification of lymph node micrometastases through immunoperoxidase staining of CEA and cytokeratins. Dis Colon Rectum 1991 34:917-20.

Dimitrov V, Delijski T: Lymph Node Dissection in anorectal and intestinal tumors. In: Lymph node dissection in breast, gastrointestinal and urogenital carcinomas. Pleven, 2003.

Doekhie FS, Peeters K.C.M.J., Kuppen P.J.K., Mesker W.E., Tanke H.J., Morreau H., van de Velde C.J.H., Tollenaar

Esser, S. et al. The role of sentinel lymph node mapping in staging of colon and rectal cancer. - Dis Colon Rectum, 44, 2001, 850–854.

Feezor RJ, Copeland Edward M. III, Hochwald Steven N: Significance of Micrometastases in Colorectal Cancer Ann Surg Oncol 2002; 9:944-953.

Feig BW, Curley S, Lucci A, Hunt K, Vauthey JN, Mansfield PF, Cleary K, Hamilton St, Ellisa V, Brame M, Berger DH: A caution regarding lymphatic mapping in patients with colon cancer The American Journal of Surgery 2001;182: 707–712.

Feinstein, A. R., D. M. Sosin, C. K. Wells. The Will Rogers phenomenon. Stage migration and new diagnostic techniques as a source of misleading statistics for survival in cancer. - N Engl J Med, 312, 1985, 1604–1608.

Fielding P: Staging systems. In Cohen A, Winawer S, eds. Cancer of the Colon, Rectum and Anus. New York, McGraw-Hill, 1995, 207.

Giuliano AE, Kirgan DM, Guenter JM: Lymphatic mappingand sentinel lymphadenectomy for breast cancer. Ann Surg 1994; 3:391-401.

Greenlee RT, Murray T, Bolden S, Wingo PA: Cancer statistics. CA Cancer J Clin 2000; 50:7–33.

Greenson JK, Isenhart CE, Rice R, Mojzisik C, Houchens D, Martin EW, Jr: Identification of occult micrometastases in pericolic lymph nodes of Duke s B colorectal cancer patients using monoclonal antibodies against cytokeratin and CC49. Correlation with long-term survival. Cancer 1994; 73:563-569.

Haboubi NY, Clark P, Kaftan SM: The importance of combining xylene clearance and immunohistochemistry in the accurate staging of colorectal carcinoma. J Royal Soc Med 1992; 85:386–388.

Hayashi N, Ito I, Yanagisawa A, et al: Genetic diagnosis of lymph-node metastasis in colorectal cancer. Lancet 1995;345:1257-1259.

Herrera-Ornelas L: Metastasis in small lymph nodes from colon cancer. Arch Surg 1987; 122:1253–1256.

Hiroya T, Bilchik A, Saha S, Turner R, Wiese D, Tanaka M, Kuo Ch, Wang He-Jing and Hoon D: c-MET Expression Level in Primary Colon Cancer Clinical Cancer Research 2003; 9:1480-1488.

Isaka N, Nozue M, Doy M, Fukao K: Prognostic significance of perirectal lymph node micrometastases in Dukes B rectal carcinoma: an immunohistochemical study by CAM5.2. Clin Cancer Res 1999; 5:2065-2068.

Jeffers MD, O'Dowd GM, Mulcahy H, Stagg M, O'Donoghue DP, Toner M. The prognostic significance of immunohistochemically detected lymph node micrometastases in colorectal carcinoma. J Pathol. 1994 Feb;172(2):183-7.

K. Dahl, J. Westlin, W. Kraaz, O. Winqvist, L. Bergkvist and M: Thurn Identification of sentinel nodes in patients with colon cancer European Journal of Surgical Oncology 2005; 31:381-385.

Kelder W, Braat Ae, Karrenbeld A, Grond Ja, De Vries Je, Oosterhuis Jw, Baas Pc, Plukker Jt, The sentinel node procedure in colon carcinoma: a multicenter study in The Netherlands, Int J Colorectal Dis, 2007, 22(12):1509–1514.

Kitagawa Y, Fujii H, Mukai M, Kubota T, Ando N, Watanabe M, Ohgami M, Otani Y, Ozawa S, Hasegawa H, Furukawa T, Kumai K, Ikeda T, Nakahara T, Kubo A, Kitajima M: The role of the sentinel lymph node in gastrointestinal cancer. Surg Clin North Am. 2000; 80:1799-809.

Kitagawa Y, Fujii H, Mukai M: Current Status and Future Perspectives of Sentinel Node Navigation for Gastrointestinal Cancer. Proceedings of the 3rd International Sentinel Lymph Node Congress 2002; 2:136.

Kitagawa Y, Kitajima M: Gastrointestinal cancer and sentinel node navigation surgery, J. Surg. Oncol. 2002; 79:188-193.

Kitagawa Y, Watanabe M, Hasegawa H, Yamamoto S, Fujii H, Yamamoto K, Matsuda J, Mukai M, Kubo A, Kitajima M: Sentinel Node Mapping for Colorectal Cancer With Radioactive Tracer Dis Colon Rectum, 2002 Nov;45(11):1476-0.

Kitagawa, Y. et al. Current Status and Future Prospects of Sentinel Node Navigational Surgery for Gastrointestinal Cancers. - Ann Surg Oncol, 11, 2004, 3, 242S–244S.

Kitajima M, Kitagawa Y: Universal Applications of Sentinel Node Technology Annals of Surgical Oncology 2004; 11(Supplement):144S-146S.

Liefers GJ, Cleton-Jansen AM, van de Velde CJ, Hermans J, van Krieken JH, Cornelisse CJ: Micrometastases and survival in stage II colorectal cancer. N Engl J Med 1998; 339:223–228.

Lindmark G, Gerdin B, Pahlman L, Bergstrom R, Glimelius B: Prognostic predictors in colorectal cancer. Dis Colon Rectum 1994; 37:1219-1227.

Macintosh, E.: Colorectal carcinoma. In: Cancer patients follow-up by F. Johnson and R. Virgo. St. Louis, Mosby-

Makela, J., H. Kiviniemi: Survival after operation for colorectal cancer. Eur. J Surg. 2000.

Martinez SR, AJ Bilchik: Quality control issues in the management of colon cancer patients Eur J Surg Oncol. 2005; 31:616-629.

Merrie A.E. H, Phillips LV, Yun K, McCall J: Skip metastases in colon cancer: Assessment by lymph node mapping using molecular detection Surgery 2001; 129:684-691.

Merrie, A. E. et al. Diagnostic use of the sentinel node in colon cancer. - Dis Colon Rectum, 44, 2001, 410–417.

Morson BC, Vaughon, EG, Bussey HIR: Pelvic recurrence after excision of rectum for carcinoma. BMJ 1963; 2:13-17.

Morton DL, Chan AD: The concept of sentinel node localization: how it started. Semin Nucl Med 2000; 30:4–10.

Morton DL, Wen DR, Wong JH, et al: Technical details of intraoperative lymphatic mapping for early stage melanoma. Arch Surg 1992; 127:392–399.

Morton, D: Sentinel Node Mapping and an International Sentinel Node Society: Current Issues and Future Directions Annals of Surgical Oncology 2004; 11(Supplement): 137S-142S.

Nieweg OE, Estourgie SH: What is a Sentinel Node and What is a False-Negative Sentinel Node? Ann Surg Oncol 2004; 11(Supplement):169S-173S.

Nieweg OE, Tanis PJ, Kroon BBR: The Definition of a Sentinel Node Ann Surg Oncol 2001; 8:538-541.

O'Connell MJ, Mailliard JA, Kahn MJ: Controlled trial of fluorouracil and low-dose lecucovorin given for 6 months as postoperative adjuvant therapy for colon cancer. J Clin Oncol 1997; 15:246–250.

Oberg A, Stenling R, Tavelin B, Lindmark G: Are lymph node micrometastases of any clinical significance in Dukes stages A and B colorectal cancer? Dis Colon Rectum 1998; 41:1244–1249.

Ota D. M.: Is Intraoperative Lymph Node Mapping and Sentinel LymphNode Biopsy for Colorectal Carcinoma Necessary? Annals of Surgical Oncology Ann Surg Oncol. 2000 Mar;7(2):82-4

Ota D. M: Is Intraoperative Lymph Node Mapping and Sentinel Lymph Node Biopsy for Colorectal Carcinoma Necessary? Annals of Surgical Oncology, 7:82–84.

Palma RT, Waisberg J, Bromberg SH, Simao AB, Godoy AC: Micrometastasis in regional lymph nodes of extirpated colorectal carcinoma: immunohistochemical study using anti-cytokeratin antibodies AE1/AE3. Colorectal Dis 2003; 5:164-168.

Paramo JC, Summerall J, Poppiti R, Mesko ThW: Validation of Sentinel Node Mapping in Patients With Colon Cancer Annals of Surgical Oncology 2002; 9:550-554.

Paramo JC, Summerall J, Wilson Ch, Cabral A, Willis I, Wodnicki H, Poppiti R, Mesko Th W: Intraoperative sentinel lymph node mapping in patients with colon cancer The American Journal of Surgery 2001; 182:40–43.

Patten LC, Berger DH, Rodriguez-Bigas M, Mansfield P, Delpassand Eb, Cleary KR, Fagan ShP, Curley StA, Hunt KK, Feig BW: A Prospective Evaluation of Radiocolloid and Immunohistochemical Staining in Colon Carcinoma Lymphatic Mapping Cancer 2004; 100:2104-2109.

Philips RKS, Hittinger R, Blesovsky L: Large bowel cancer: Surgical pathology and its relationship to survival. Br J Surg 1984; 71:604–610.

Pietra N, Sarli L et al: Role of follow-up in management of local recurrence of colorectal cancer. Dis. Colon Rectum,

Prandi, M. et al. Prognostic evaluation of stage B colon cancer patients is improved by an adequate lymphadenectomy: results of a secondary analysis of a large scale adjuvant trial. - Ann Surg, 235, 2002, 4, 458–463.

R.A.E.M.: The feasibility and reliability of sentinel node mapping in colorectal cancer EJSO 2005; 31:854–862.

Rodriguez-Bigas MA, Maamoun S, Weber TK, Penetrante RB, Blumenson LE, Petrelli NJ: Clinical significance of colorectal cancer: metastases in lymph nodes 5 mm in size. Ann Surg Oncol 1996; 3:124–130.

Saha S, Bilchik A, Wiese D, Espinosa M, Badin J, Ganatra BK, Desai D, Kaushal S, Singh T, Arora M: Ultrastaging of Colorectal Cancer by Sentinel Lymph Node Mapping Technique—A Multicenter Trial. Ann Surg Oncol 2001; 8(Supplement):94S-98S.

Saha S, Dan AG, Bilchik A, Kitagawa Schochet, E, Choudhri Sh, Saha L, Wiese D, Morton D, Kitajima M: Historical Review of Lymphatic Mapping in Gastrointestinal Malignancies Ann Surg Oncol 2004; 11(Supplement):245S-249S.

Saha S, Ganatra BK, Gauthier J: Localization of sentinel lymph node in colon cancer. A feasibility study. SSO 50th Annual Cancer Symposium 1997; 80:54.

Saha S, Monson KM, Bilchik A, Beutler Th, Dan AG, Schochet E, Wiese D, Kaushal S, Ganatra B, Desai D: Comparative Analysis of Nodal Upstaging Between Colon and Rectal Cancers by Sentinel Lymph Node Mapping: A Prospective Trial The American Society of Colon and Rectal Surgeons 200410.1007/s10350-004-0661-5.

Saha S, Nora D, Wong JH, Weise D: Sentinel lymph node mapping in colorectal cancer—a review. Surg Clin North Am 2000; 80:1811–1819.

Saha S, Weise D, Badin J, et al: Technical details of sentinel lymph node mapping in colorectal cancer and its impact on staging. Ann Surg Oncol 2000; 7:120–124.

Schlag PM, Bembenek A, Schulze T: Sentinel node biopsy in gastrointestinal-tract cancer European Journal of Cancer 2004; 40:2022–2032.

Schrag, D. et al. Adjuvant chemotherapy use for Medicare beneficiaries with stage II colon cancer. - J Clin Oncol, 20, 2002, 3999–4005.

Sobin LH, Wittekind C (eds): TNM Classification of Malignant Tumors (ed 6). New York: Wiley, 2002.

Taback B, Bilchik AJ, Saha S, Nakayama T, Wiese DA, Turner RR, Kuo CT, Hoon DS. Peptide nucleic acid clamp PCR: a novel K-ras mutation detection assay for colorectal cancer micrometastases in lymph nodes. Int J Cancer. 2004; 111:409-414.

Tang R, Wang JY, Chen JS: Survival impact of lymph node metastasis in TNM stage III carcinoma of the colon and rectum. J Am Coll Surg 1995; 180:705-712.

Tanis PJ, Nieweg OE, Hart A.A. M and Kroon B.B. R: The Illusion of the Learning Phase for Lymphatic Mapping Annals of Surgical Oncology 2002; 9:142-147.

Thompson JF, Uren RF: What is a 'sentinel' lymph node? Eur J Surg Oncol 2000; 26:103–104.

Trocha SD, Nora DT, Saha SS, Morton DL, Wiese D, Bilchik AJ: Combination probe and dye-directed lymphatic mapping detects micrometastases in early colorectal cancer. J Gastrointest Surg. 2003; 7:340-5; discussion 345-6.

Tsioulias G, Wood T, Morton D: Lymphatic mapping and focused analysis of sentinel lymph nodes upstage gastrointestinal neoplasms. Arch Surg 2000; 135:926–932.

Tsioulias GJ, Wood TF, Spirt M, Morton DL, Bilchik AJ: A novel lymphatic mapping technique to improve localization and staging of early colon cancer during laparoscopic colectomy. Am Surg. 2002; 68(7):561-565.

Tsopelas, C., R. Sutton. Why certain dyes are useful for localizing the sentinel lymph node. - J Nucl Med, 43, 2002, 1377–1382.

Williams NS: Surgical Treatment in Rectal Cancer. In: Surgery of the Anus, rectum and colon, WB Saunders 1993, 939.

Wolmark N, Fisher B, Wieand HS: The prognostic value of the modifications of the Dukes' C class of colorectal cancer. An analysis of the NSABP clinical trials. Ann Surg 1986; 203:115–122.

Wong JH, Bowles BJ, Bueno R, Shimizu D: Impact of the number of negative nodes on disease free survival in colorectal cancer patients. Dis Colon Rectum 2002; 45: 1341–1348.

Wood TF, Nora DT, Morton DL, Turner RR, Rangel D, Hutchinson W, Bilchik AJ: One hundred consecutive cases of sentinel lymph node mapping in early colorectal carcinoma: detection of missed micrometastases. J Gastrointest Surg. 2002; 6:322-329; discussion 229-30.

Wood TF, Tsioulias GJ, Morton DL: Focused examination of sentinel lymph nodes upstages early colorectal carcinoma. Am Surg 2001; 66:998-1003.

Wood Thomas F, Saha S, Morton Donald L, Tsioulias George J., Rangel Decio, Hutchinson William Jr., Foshag Leland J., Bilchik Anton J: Validation of Lymphatic Mapping in Colorectal Cancer: In Vivo, Ex Vivo, and Laparoscopic Techniques. Ann Surg Oncol 2001; 8:150-157.

Wood, T. F. et al. Lymphatic mapping improves staging during laparoscopic colectomy for cancer. - Surg Endosc, 15, 2001, 715–719.

Yamamoto, Y. et al. Clinicopathological characteristics of skipping lymph node metastases in patients with colorectal cancer. - Jpn J Clin Oncol, 28, 1998, 6, 378–382.

Yasuda K, Adachi Y, Shiraishi N, Yamaguchi K, Hirabayashi Y, Kitano S: Pattern of lymph node micrometastasis and prognosis of patients with colorectal cancer. Ann Surg Oncol 2001; 8:300–304. Year Book, 1997, 118-47.

10

Is Neo-Rectum a Better Option for Low Rectal Cancers?

Fazl Q. Parray, Umar Farouqi and Nisar A. Chowdri
Department of Surgery, Sher-I-Kashmir Institute of Medical Sciences, Srinagar India

1. Introduction

Distances have been traveled on foot, by boat, carts, bus, car, trains, or by aero planes but what maters ultimately after the travel is "Time & Quality". Same logic applies to surgical treatment. Orthodox surgeons criticize technology, question new procedures and are reluctant to accept new modalities. They may not be wrong but may neither be "right."What they believe in is a typical Cooperian thought.

- "If you are too fond of new remedies, first you will not cure your patients; Secondly, you will have no patients to cure " (A Cooper, 1768-1841) But we believe in guiding the technology rather than vice versa and we should question new procedures till evidence based. We should accept and try evidence based modalities, be technology friendly, or get outdated. Our belief is;
- "If you are not too fond of new remedies you will have no patients to cure"

Colorectal Carcinomas lead to 655,000 deaths per year. It is the third most common form of cancer and second leading cause of cancer- related death .Cancer rectum continues to be a dreadful malignancy. 5 year survival inspite of aggressive modalities has improved only from 50% to 75%.

2. Historical aspects

Czerny is credited with abdominoperineal excision for rectal carcinoma in 1884.Krate gave the concept of trans sacral approach for rectal resection in 1885. Sir Ernest Miles the British surgeon in 1908 improved on the concept of abdominoperineal excision (APR) for rectal carcinoma on basis of "Anatomic rectal carcinoma" studies and introduced the concept of "Zone Of Upward Spread" and stressed on Wide Perineal Excision. (Lancet 1908; 2:1812-3)
In recent times pathological studies of Dukes and Westhues demonstrated "Central lymphogenic spreading" in early developing carcinoma rectum hence the era of sphincter preserving procedures started. (Br. J. Surg 1930; 17:643-8, Arch Klin Chir 1930; 161:582-91)
Dixon (Mayo Clinic, 1930) devised low anterior resection (LAR) for treatment of favorable tumors of mid-rectum and it became the procedure of choice and after comparison of results viz-a-viz morbidity, mortality or local recurrence no difference was found by several studies. (Goliger et al Br. J Surg 1951; 39:199-211, Parks AG. Proc R Soc Med 1972; 69:975-6, Goliger JC. Adv Surg 1979; 13:1-31)

Until 1970s most thought that 5cm distal margin from the tumor is a must for achieving distal tumor free margin but Williams et al(1983) described that distal spread of tumor >2cm in less than 2.5% of excised tumors after extensive pathological & clinical studies of sphincter saving procedures and concluded that a distal margin of 2 cm is safe. (Pollet WG, Nichollas RJ. Ann Surg 1963; 198:159-63; Fain SN et al. Arch Surg 1975; 110:1079-82)
Studies also confirmed 2cm distal margin did not compromise survival and overall results were similar for LAR vs. APR.

3. Treatment modalities

Various surgical treatment modalities which can be offered to the patient with cancer rectum at present are:

- Colostomy / Ileostomy
- APR
- Neoadjuvant to downstage
- Anterior resection; LAR; ultra low anterior resection (ULAR) +/- followed by adjuvant treatment
- Trans anal local resection
- Trans anal endoscopic microsurgery (TEMS)
- Trans sacral resection

In recent times LAR got more popular because it is a sphincter saving procedure and distal resection margin (DRM) needs to be only 2 cms. Use of staplers popularized the procedure because staplers reached more than the hand. The resection is followed by end to side anastamosis or end to end anastamosis .Then came the era of Oncological concern. The embryology predicates that cancer spread will remain within the mesorectum and fascia. This fascia provides the surgeon with a "navigation system" on which the efficient performance of total mesorectal excision (TME) is based.
Oncologically correct surgical treatment for carcinoma middle and lower third of rectum is total mesorectal excision (TME) and it was William Heald who gave this concept based on "Zone Of Downward Spread". (Quirke P et al. Lancet 1986; 2:996-9; Malloy RG et al. Dis Colon Rectum 1992; 35:462-4)
But most the new surgical procedures always come with a price and that is what proved exactly true even for LAR; it lead to loss of "rectal reservoir function". This new entity was named as "Anterior Resection Syndrome" (ARS). It comprises of

- Functional disorders
- Difficulty in postoperative stool evacuation
- High stool frequency
- Decreased continence for gas and liquid
- Increased stool urge, clustering
- Feel of incomplete evacuation

Hence, a complex mixture of anal and neo-rectal dysfunction is common during the phase of adaptation in the first postoperative year.(Predersen IK et al. Ann Surg 1986; 204:133-5; Lewis WG et al. Dis Colon Rectum 1995; 38:259-63; Miller S et al. Br J Surg 1995; 82:1327-30)

4. Reservoir

A need for a neo-rectal reservoir was felt to overcome the problem of ARS. Lazorthes et al and Parc et al in 1986 designed a "Colonic J Pouch" (CJP) to address these problems. Even though nothing can replace a natural reservoir but this type of pouch is aimed at achieving at least an artificial reservoir to improve the overall quality of life (QOL). (Parc R et al Br J Surg 1986; 73:139-41, Hida J et al Dis Colon Rectum 1996; 39:986-91)

5. Preoperative assessment

It comprises of

- General physical examination(GPE)
- Digital rectal examination(DRE)
- Proctoscopic examination(PE), Sigmoidoscoy, Colonoscopy with biopsy
- Baseline hematology and biochemistry
- Carcino embryonic antigen(CEA) levels
- Ultrasonography(USG),Multidetector computerized tomogram(MDCT),Endorectal Coil magnetic resonance imaging(Ec MRI),Trans rectal ultrasonography (TRUS)
- Neoadjuvant for locally advanced tumors

6. Indications

T2, T3 lesions 4 - 12 cm. from anal verge
T3 +/-T4 lesions down staged after neo-adjuvant

7. Contraindications

- Narrow pelvis
- Bulky sphincters
- Pregnancy
- Locally advanced cancers
- Sphincter tone is already lost or low
- Mucinous or poorly differentiated carcinoma

8. Preoperative counseling

- Consent for surgical procedure with possibility of permanent or temporary stoma to be explained, stoma sites to be discussed and marked preoperatively
- Stoma therapist involvement encouraged in the preoperative period for marking the sites and psychologically preparing the patient
- Possibility of inoperability also to be explained
- Bowel preparation done one day prior to surgery
- Intra venous antibiotics (3rd generation cephalosporin) used at the time of induction after test dose
- J pouch pros and cons explained to the patient and his attendants
- Staplers use to be discussed because of the cost factor and the complications associated with their use

9. Intra operative management

All such procedures should be planned under general anesthesia (GA) supplemented with epidural analgesia. A provision for ureteral stents intraoperatively has to be kept in mind in case of surrounding desmoplasia or a recurrent cancer. A Foley's catheter should always be put in the bladder to keep it deflated during the procedure. Patient should be placed in modified lithotomy position with legs in stirrups. A pneumatic compression stocking with use of low molecular weight heparin will always be an added guard against deep venous thrombosis. Always remember to do a DRE under GA to reassess the tumor with a special emphasis on degree of involvement of anal sphincters, the level of distal edge of the tumor and response of the tumor to neo-adjuvant treatment if at all that was used.

Proper operation theatre headlights and lighted retractors will always be a great help to facilitate the procedure. Other gadgets of immense importance in pelvic surgery would be Balfour or Bookwalter retractors, Saint Mark pelvic retractor, long instruments, highly trained assistant, presence of an experienced 2nd surgeon and a regular team.

10. Intra operative decision

Intraoperative findings may necessitate a change in plan. Never try to be egoistic about sphincter saving procedures in case there arise some technical difficulties on table. Use midline incision, head down position for performing laparotomy. Proper packing of small gut, use of self retaining retractors and proper mobilization of rectosigmoid area is a must. A decision about sphincter saving or sphincter sacrificing after mobilizing rectum should be revised.

11. Mobilization of colon

Rectosigmoid is retracted to right. Peritoneal attachment on left incised along avascular plane, left ureter and gonadal vessels are isolated. Transilluminate to identify avascular plane (Holy plane) adjacent to inferior mesenteric artery (IMA). Peritoneum is incised on either side(fig 1). High ligation of IMA may provide a complete nodal harvest but at the cost of autonomic nerve plexus injury. Low ligation is done distal to left colic artery(LCA) it ensures better supply to proximal colon and saves nerve injury at base of IMA but at the cost of complete nodal harvest. Ligate IMA and start posterior dissection in holy avascular plane .Aim at total mesorectal excision (TME) with nerve preservation. The key to posterior dissection is sharp dissection of avascular plane and allow air to enter areolar tissue. Follow the air for dissection. Preserve superior hypogastric plexus at sacral promontry, pre aortic and inferior mesentric plexus at the base of IMA. Hypogastric nerves can be identified at sacral promontory. These nerves descend in presacral space in a "wishbone shape". Preserve them for postoperative sexual and urinary function. Attention to "Nerve preservation" will retain sexual function in males > 60%; in females up to 86 %.(Havenga K et al. J Am Coll Surg: 1996; 182:495)

Rectrosacral fascia is divided under vision to the level of coccyx (fig 2). Dissect in posterior to lateral direction. Nervi erigentes should be preserved on lateral pelvic sidewalls. Middle rectal artery (MRA) which may or may not be a content of lateral ligaments should be fulgrated or ligated. Final attachments are divided anterolaterally. Nerve sparing resection improves QOL in patients of rectal carcinoma. The lateral ligament of the rectum is a definite anatomic entity. Some studies suggest that the ligament contains a few nerve fibers but no significant blood vessels. (Pak-art DCR 2005)

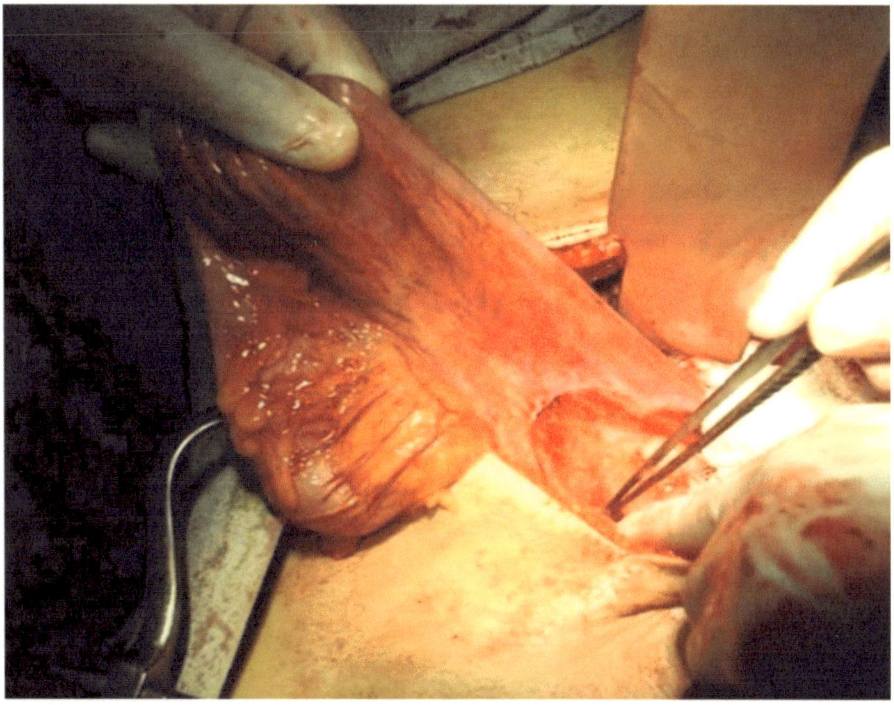

Fig. 1. Operative photograph showing mobilization of rectosigmoid

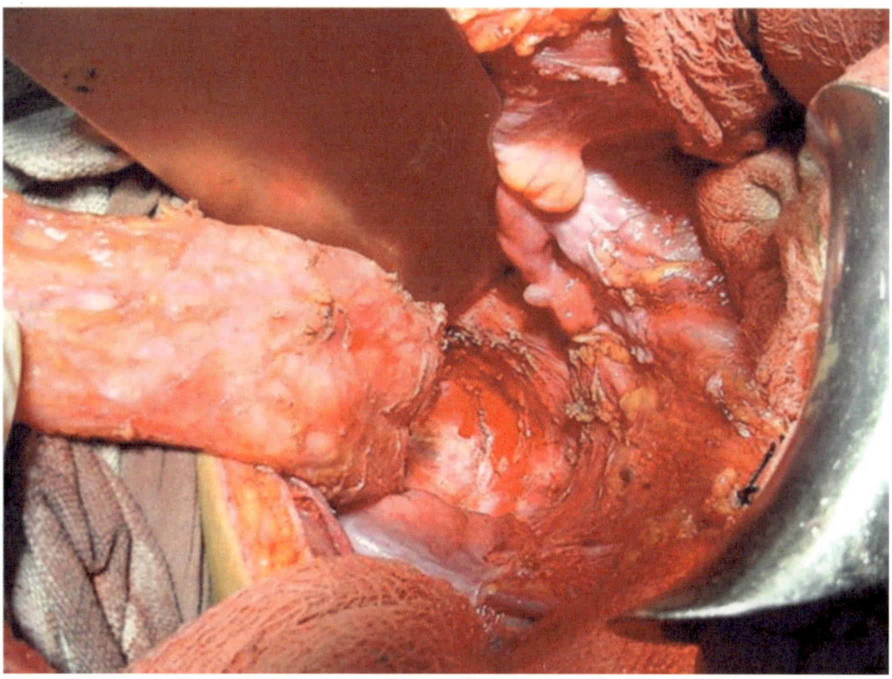

Fig. 2. Operative photograph showing posterior dissection

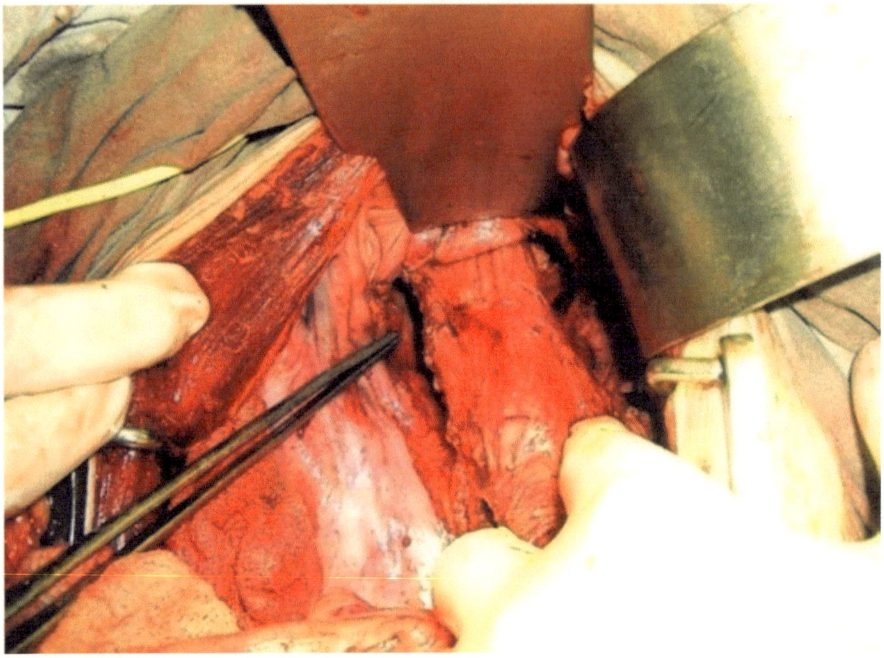

Fig. 3. Operative photograph showing anterior dissection

Mesorectum appears to be adherent to inferior hypogastric plexus at 11 and 2 o'clock position so one needs to be careful and meticulous while dissecting at these positions. Anterior Dissection should be done last of all. Exposure is facilitated by reverse trendlenburg position. Open cul de sac and incise Denonviller's fascia. Use deep pelvic retractors to protect seminal vesicles and prostate in males and posterior wall of vagina in females (Fig 3).

- Cut well, see well and your patient will get well (Charles Aubrey Pannet)

Proximal end is usually cut at junction of descending and sigmoid colon. Cut with a linear cutter 55 mm /75mm(Ethicon); 60 mm/80mm (auto suture).Proximal limb is arranged in J configuration with 2 or 3 sutures (seromuscular).A 2 cm hole is made at base of J pouch. Linear cutter is disengaged and put in 2 limbs of J pouch. Length recommended for each limb is 5 - 10 cm. Linear cutter is fired after approximating the two limbs.

12. Assessment of distal margin

Revise your decision again at this juncture about sphincter saving or sphincter sacrificing surgery. Two components to distal margin should be taken into consideration. Intramural where 2.0 cm margin is adequate and mesorectal where a margin of 5 cm is considered to be adequate .Stanskey clamp should be applied on proximal side for staplers to avoid any spillage of contents. Linear articulating stapler (access 55), contour or roticulator is used for dividing rectum leaving a closed rectal cuff for anastamosis (fig 4). Specimen is removed.Washes given with cetrimide / saline.

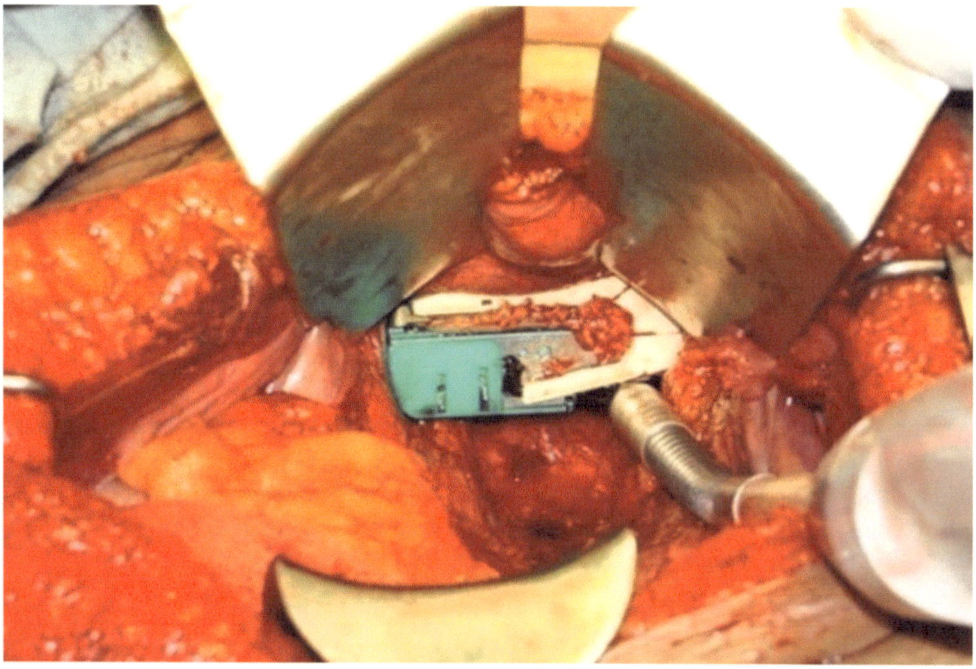

Fig. 4. Stapler "Access 55" used for distal end

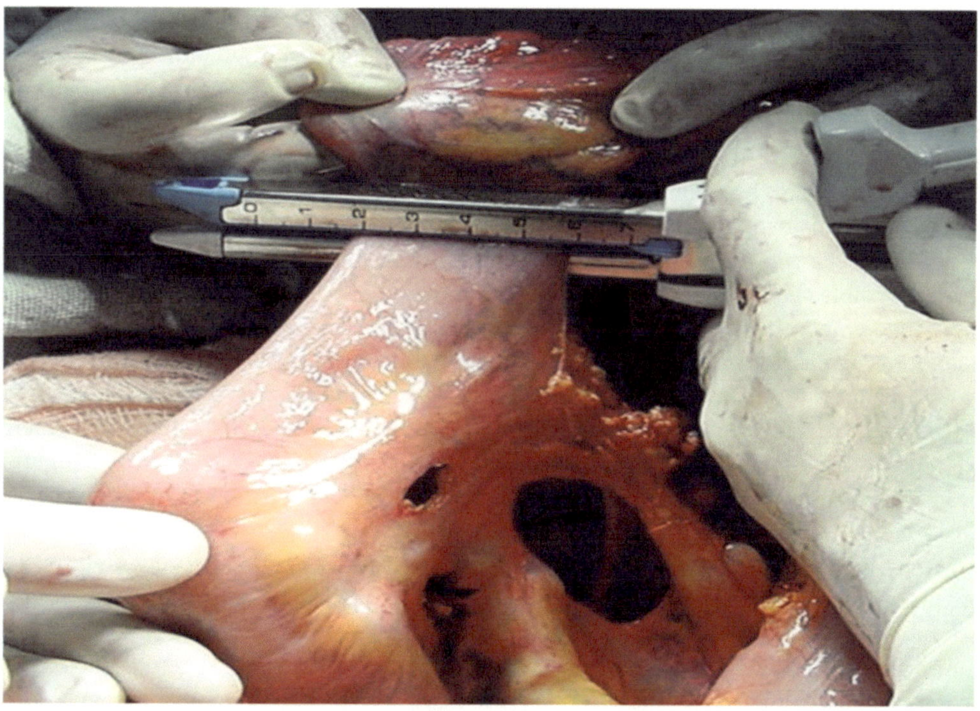

Fig. 5. Mesentric windows made to gain length

13. How to gain length

First assess the mobility of the colon apex of J should be 6 cm down the symphysis pubis. If not, then skeletonize the vessels. Make windows in the mesentery (Fig 5). Mobilize the left lateral peritoneal attachments. Mobilize the splenic flexure of the colon. Cut any withholding vessels after using a vascular clamp for 5 minutes. Ensure good vascularity of the segment to be used for construction of J pouch .In case of any doubts about the vascularity give up the idea.

14. Creation of anastamosis

In J pouch the anastamosis is always end to side (Baker technique).Hand sewn anastamosis is technically difficult in low rectal cancers. Ideal is to use a circular stapler CDH (circular detachable head) or CEEA (circular end to end anastamosis) for completion of anastamosis. Functional results are good for proximal anastamosis and suboptimal for low anastamosis .Hence, J pouch or coloplasty is carried out to serve the function of a neo-rectum and improve the overall functional results. Use Staplers only after formal training.

- "A fool with a tool is still a fool"

15. J pouch

We prefer 6 - 8 cm. limbs. Engage the two limbs of stapler in two limbs of colon. Maintain proper orientation. Push down the mesentery before locking the staplers. Fire and hold the instruments for 2 minutes to achieve a good hemostasis (fig 6).Examine the staple line, if there are any oozers ligate them with absorbable sutures. Use the same hole of "J" to engage the anvil of CDH /CEEA. Hold the anvil with an artery forceps. Put a purse string stitch of 1^0 Prolene around the anvil (fig 7).Close CDH/CEEA with rotating knob. Dilate anal canal gently using 2% xylocaine. Then push "CDH" gently till you can see the circular head abutting against stapled line. Select the appropriate place of entry of the knob which may be anterior or posterior. Keep on opening the rotator head till the knob makes an entry into the perineum till main operator sees the orange cuff. Engage the assembly of anvil spring loaded self locking shaft into the trocar projecting out of staple housing of rectal side till you hear an audible click (Fig 8). Keep on rotating the knob of CDH till the tissues of two sides approximate and on the instrument you can see a green line appearing in the gap setting scale of the stapler indicating the proper approximation of tissues. Fire the stapler and wait for two minutes for complete hemostasis (Fig 9). Unlock the knob and make two complete 180 degree turns. Remove the stapler from the anorectum with fishtailing movements. Examine for 2 complete doughnuts. Send the excised specimen and two labeled doughnuts for histopathological examination (HPE) .Fill the pelvis with saline. Inject air per rectum and look for any air leaks. If you have any doubts, cover it with an ileostomy. Covering ileostomy is preferred in cases of very low anastamosis as leak rates are quite high for very low anastamosis. Even though the covering ileostomy has been found not to decrease the leak rates but saves the patient from the catastrophe of fecal peritonitis in case of any leaks from the anastamosis. Patients in the post operative or follow up period can be subjected to a contrast study using water soluble contrast to demonstrate the anatomy and angulation of pouch(Fig-10,Pouchogram).

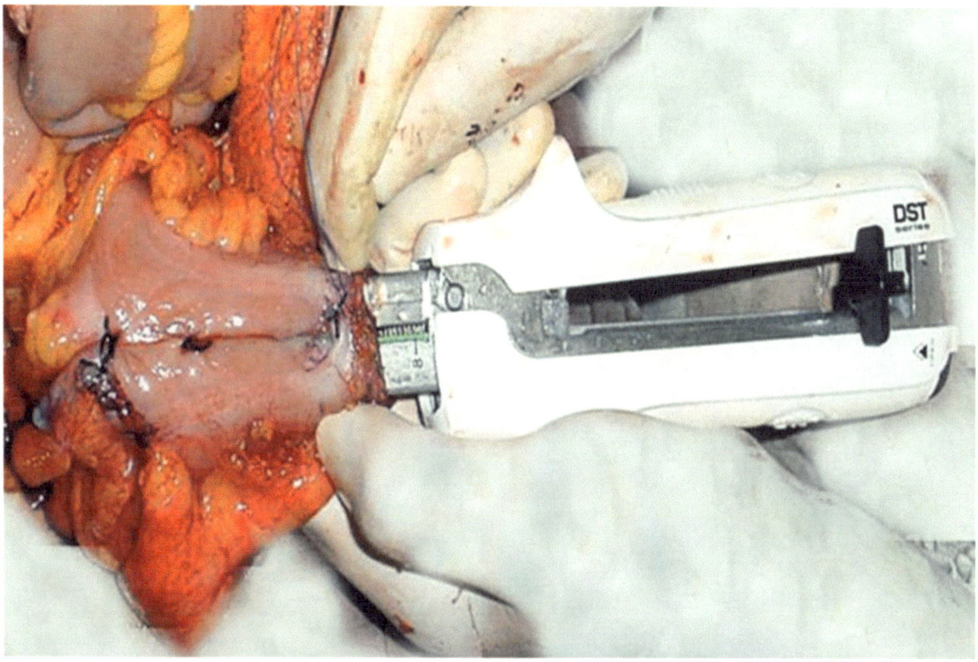

Fig. 6. Linear Stapler for J Pouch

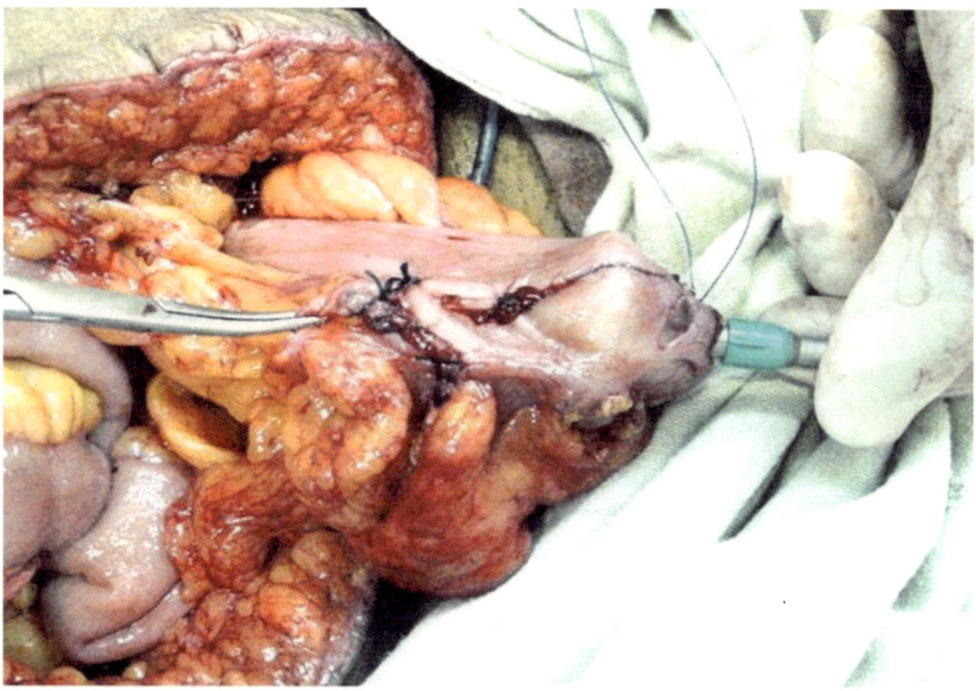

Fig. 7. Anvil fixation in base of J Pouch

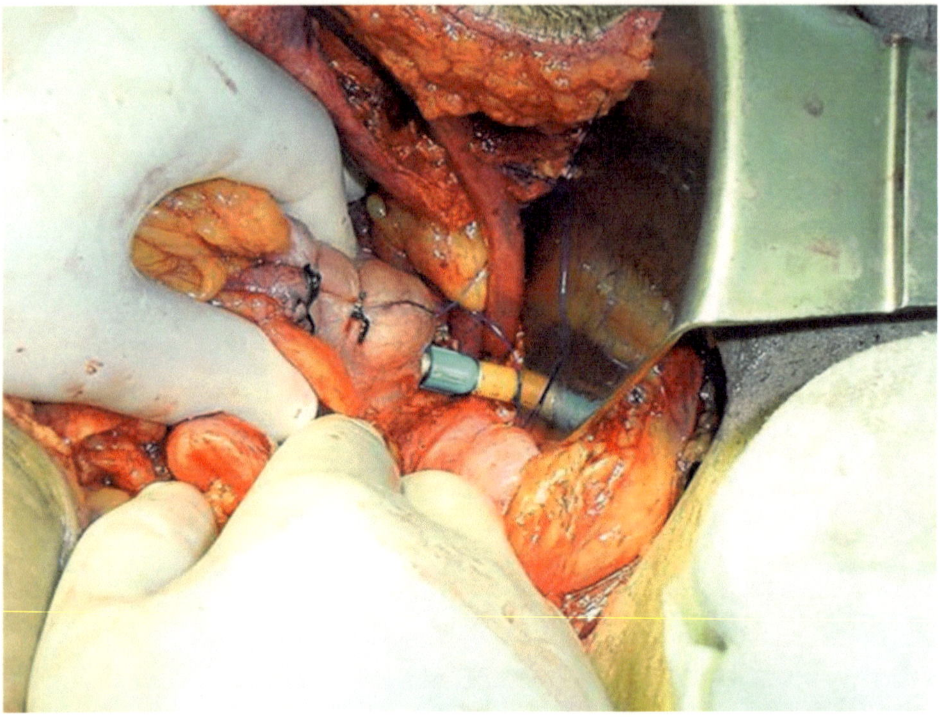

Fig. 8. Fixation of anvil into the trocar projecting out of staple housing of rectal side.

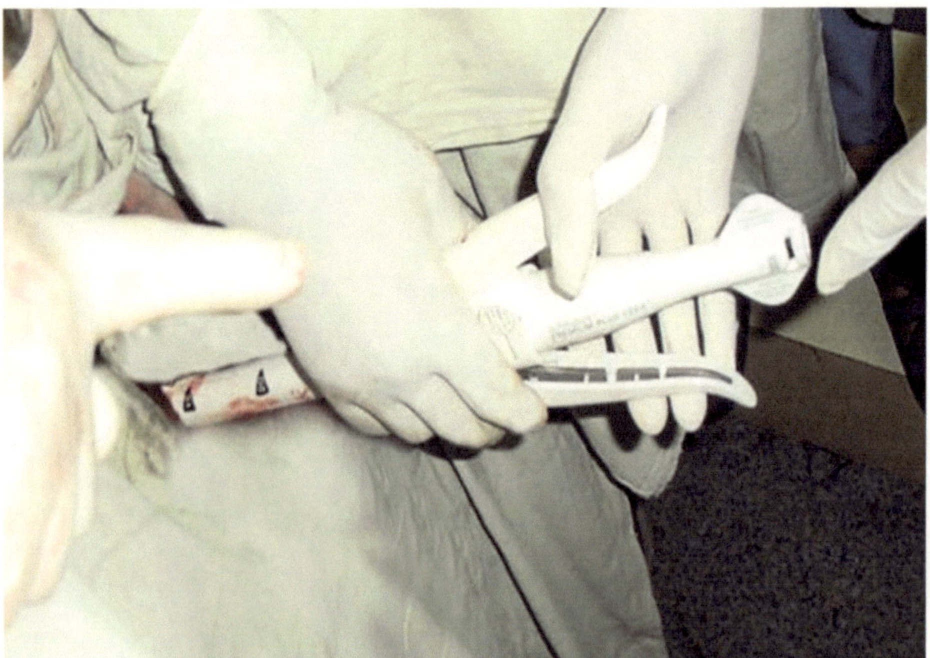

Fig. 9. Firing CDH/CEEA

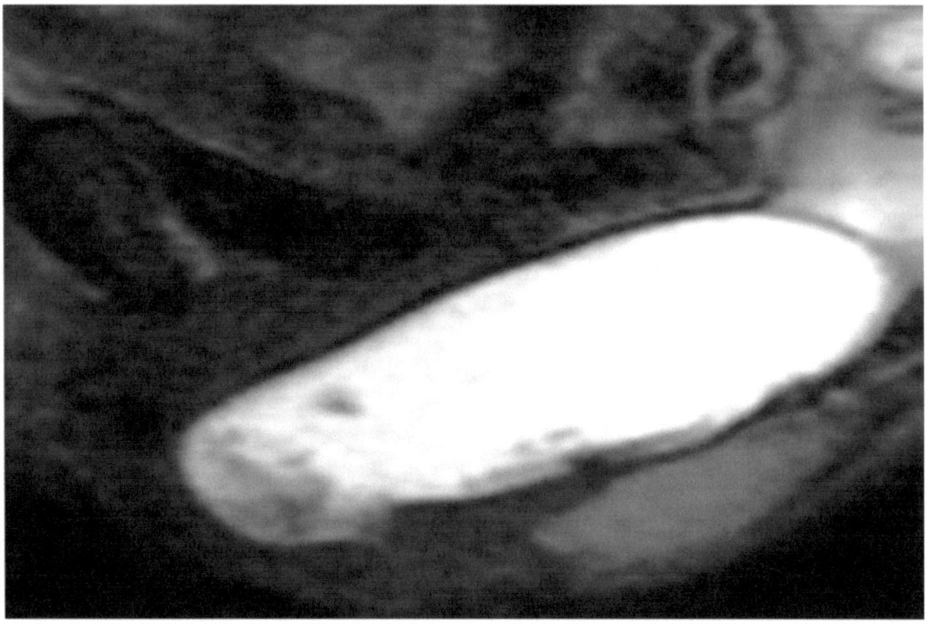

Fig. 10. Contrast study of the Pouch on follow up(Pouchogram)

16. Our experience at SKIMS

We conducted a Prospective randomized study in our tertiary care hospital.22 patients were assigned to Colonic J Pouch(CJP) group and 20 patients to Straight anastamosis (SA) group and the two groups were compared on basis of:

- Functional outcome
- Composite incontinence score
- QOL
- Anastamotic leak was 3.3 times more common in the SA group.
- Anastamotic strictures were 2.3 times more common in the SA group.
- The frequency of bowel movement per 24 hours was less in the CJP group.
- CJP group had no nocturnal bowel movements at six months.
- CJP was able to defer defecation better than the SA group.
- Retarding medication use more common in SA group.
- Bulking medication use more common in CJP group.
- CJP patients were better able to differentiate between gas and stool.
- There was an increased ability to evacuate bowel within 15 minutes in SA group
- The CJP patients were more continent to gases, liquids and solids at 2 and 6 months duration.
- All these findings were statistically significant
- Stastical methods used were Fischers exact test, Chi square using SPSS 15

17. Laparoscopic TME

Laparoscopic ultralow anterior resection could be offered routinely and completed safely in Western populations, where obesity and adhesions from previous abdominal surgery is common. A laparoscopic technique readily allowed visual identification of the autonomic nerves in the abdomen over the aorta, which could then be followed down into the pelvis. If the pelvis was deep, inversion of the 30° laparoscope in the "upside down" position facilitated incision of Waldeyer's fascia.. Further randomized, controlled studies that include assessing five-year cancer survival/recurrence, pelvic nerve dysfunction, and bowel function are needed before laparoscopic ultralow anterior resection becomes widely accepted.

(Selvindos PB & HO YK.DCR 2008;51(11))

Laparoscopic assisted surgery for colorectal cancer has been widely adopted without data from large scale randomized trials to support its use. MRC CLASICC trial -a multicentre, randomized controlled trial compared short term end points of conventional versus laparoscopic assisted surgery in patients with colorectal cancer to predict long term outcomes. They found that the conversion rate for rectal cancer after laparoscopy is 34% in patients undergoing anterior resection, circumferential resection margin(CRM) positivity was greater in the laparoscopic than in the open surgery group 16 [12%] of 129 Individuals versus four [6%] of 64, respectively but this difference was not significant (95% CI -2.1 to 14.4%, p=0.19).They concluded that there are 'impaired short-term outcomes after laparoscopic assisted anterior resection for cancer of the rectum and still do not yet justify its routine use'. (Lancet 2005; 365:1718-26)

What we believe in is that don't run before being able to walk.

18. Discussion

APR was once the operation of choice for a low rectal cancer but the development of LAR and circular stapler increasingly allowed restorative surgery with preservation of anal sphincters but unfortunately many patients pay the price for avoidance of a permanent stoma by developing ARS as already described. Various studies were undertaken to understand the real cause of this syndrome. The majority used anorectal manometry as an investigative tool to investigate these patients. The three features appearing most frequently are reduced anal tone, loss of rectoanal inhibitory reflex (RAIR) (Iwai N etal.DCR 1982; 25:652-9), and reduced rectal compliance. (Batignani G.DCR 1991; 34:329-35).Rectal compliance seems to be the only feature susceptible to change by alteration of rectal volume. In 1986 Lazorthes et al and Parc and colleagues (Parc etal;BJS 1986;73:139-141)described that formation of a CJP fashioned from sigmoid or descending colon would obviate much of the dysfunction associated with the low straight anastamosis by increasing neorectal volume. In recent times the CJP is becoming the operation of choice for the cancers of low rectum. Despite its increasing popularity still some misconceptions exist about its routine use outcome and evacuation problems. But the evidence in literature suggests that CJP is safer because of the reduction in the incidence of anastamotic leaks, better functional outcome with reduced frequency and better continence. (Dennet ER and Parry BR; DCR 1999 June, vol 42).Since the colonic pouch reduces the incidence of leaks so automatically the incidence of strictures is decreased. As all of us know that anastamotic integrity and healing is dependant mainly on good vascularity, technique and avoiding tension on anastamosis. Tension can be decreased by adequate mobilization which most of the times needs complete mobilization of the splenic flexure of colon and blood supply is improved by use of colonic J pouch as was proved by the use of laser doppler flowmetry during surgery. (Hallbook O et al;BJS 1996;83:389-92).

Evidence also suggests that if sigmoid colon is used for pouch construction it is presumed to cause excessive functional problems. The reasons for these functional problems can be that sigmoid colon is a high pressure segment and is more prone to develop severe motility dysfunction as compared to descending colon pouches. (Seow-Choen F,Goh HS;BJS 1995;82:608-10).Sigmoid colon is also more prone to develop diverticulosis which makes it more thickened and rigid and not suitable for the construction of J pouch. Besides high ligation of inferior mesenteric artery may render the sigmoid colon ischemic and not fit for use.

One of the main advantages cited in literature for colonic J pouch is the decreased daytime and nocturnal frequency of bowel as compared to straight anastamosis. This has been proved time and again by the comparative studies done from time to time. Lazorthes etal found that after one year, 86% patients with colonic J pouch had a bowel frequency less than 3 stools per day compared to only 33% of patients with a straight anastamosis. Parc etal described a mean of 1-6 bowel movements per day after I month and 1.1 per day after 3 months in a group of 31 patients with a CJP. This was further substantiated by studies of Ho etal, Seon Choen etal and Nicholls etal. Harris etal in their study found that the median frequency of bowel movements at night time was zero in the CJP patients compared to SA group. This was at 0-4 years and 5-9 years duration on follow up. Routine work schedule in the busy life makes it imperative for the person to be able to hold his stools for some time till he finds a toilet to ease out. Inability to do so has its own social and psychological stigmas. According to Dennet and Parry(DCR 1999;42:804-811) 14 studies report on post operative urgency after CJP but in only 10 of them it is compared to a SA group. From this comparison it appears that CJP is almost a near perfect solution to post operative urgency but Ho etal reports no significant improvement. Incontinence is one of the major determinants of functional outcome after low anterior resection and it was found from most of the studies that continence to gases, liquids and solids improves significantly after the construction of colonic J pouch especially in very low rectal cancers. It was further substantiated by observing a significant difference in their composite incontinence score at 2 months and one year.(Hallbook etal;Ann Surg 1996;224:58-65).Most of the studies definitely are in favor of a better functional outcome with CJP as compared to SA especially when the rectal cancer is of low variety and post resection the anastamotic line is below 8 cms on DRE. For higher lesions usually the lower or some part of midrectum may be preserved hence the reservoir is not needed and the functional outcome may not show any advantage over SA. (Table-1)

Colonic reservoir: Meta analysis (BJS-2006): The conclusion of meta analysis was that CJP after anterior resection has significant functional advantages over SA and this persisted over time and seems to be the procedure of choice.

Another study on **Colonic J-pouch anal anastomosis** after ultralow anterior resection proved that Colonic J-pouch anal anastomosis decreases the severity of fecal incontinence and improves the quality of life. (World J Gastroenterol 2005 May;11(17):2570-2573)

One study compared Colonic J Pouch versus Coloplasty following resection of distal rectal cancer and found similar functional results in the coloplasty group compared to the J-pouch group.(Dis Colon Rectum. 2003 Sep;46(9))

Colonic J-Pouch, Coloplasty, Side-to-End Anastomosis: Meta-Analysis proved that CJP is able to obviate some of the functional problems of SA, it comes with an additional problem of pouch evacuation. Therefore, alternatives techniques, such as transverse coloplasty pouch and side-to-end coloanal anastomosis, have been adopted. (Seminars in Colon and Rectal Surgery.Aug 2009; Volume 20, Issue 2, Pages 69-72)

18.1 Remaining surgical issues in rectal cancer

We have to improve outcome in very low cancer, improve sphincter preservation technique sentinel node technique which is still questionable in colorectal cancers and needs to be assessed in future studies and at the same time ascertain the validity of laparoscopic resection which at present as per the latest studies based on randomized trials is still inferior to open surgery.

Laparoscopic Colorectal Surgery is still associated with a higher intraoperative complication rate than Open Surgery. (Tarik S et al Annals of Surgery: January 2011; 253 (1): 35–43)

Author		Number	Stool frequency Per 24 hours	Continent no.(%)
Lazorthes et al	Pouch	15	1.7±0.67*	12 (80)
	Control	36	3 ± 1.25	28 (78)
Cohen	Pouch	23	1- 4	19 (83)
Hallbook et al	Pouch	42	2 (1.3-2.3)	^
	Control	47	Median (Interquartile range) 3.5(2.4 - 4.50	^
Hida et al				
(5 cm)	Pouch	20	^	^
(10 cm)	Pouch	20	^	^
Lazorthes et al				
(6 cm)	Pouch	14	1.8±1.1	8 (57)
(10 cm)	Pouch	17	2 ± 1.6	12 (70)
Joo et al	Pouch	26	2.4 ± 1.3	^
	Control	30	4 ± 2	^

^ = a functional score is given for continence is given rather than raw data.
Unless otherwise stated the stool frequency is mean (range) or ± standard deviation.
* Values that are statistically significant

Table 1. Functional outcome after coloanal J-Pouch anastomosis (Dennet and Parry; DCR, 1999 June, Vol 42)

18.2 Problems with CJP

- Surgeons need proper training to use staples. Many a times surgeons try new procedures in technology boom without properly learning them in animal laboratories which is a dangerous trend and puts their patient at a greater risk which may at times be life threatening.
- Learning curve - Rectal cancer surgeries as such are technically demanding procedures.The problems are further compounded in presence of obesity, narrow pelvis, redosurgery and low rectal cancers. Hence all surgeons go through a long learning curve to master these procedures and then only they should think of going for any further advances like CJP or coloplasty.
- Patient selection - This is very important from technical point of view.In case you have selected a very obese patient,patient with previous adhesions , narrow pelvis , bulky sphincters or patients with diverticulosis ;you will definitely get discouraged to adopt

the procedure,hence a proper patient selection especially in the initial days is very important.

- Volume of the centre - This is one of the biggest contributory factors which can make you to master a particular surgery but in case the volume of the centre for a particular disease is quite less then it is not worthwhile trying these technically demanding procedures.
- Ideal pouch size to be decided - Initially most of the surgeons who adopted this procedure would prefer a 10 cm limb of the J pouch but with the rising number of evacuation problems the recent trend is to go for 5 cm limb.We believe this size compromises with the neorectal volume,hence we prefer a limb of 6-8cms which balances between the volume and evacuation.
- Evacuation problems - arise because of the peristaltic wave travelling in its natural direction, so the wave travels to other limb of J rather than going in the direction of anal canal. The problem gets further aggravated by the long size of a limb,so the remedial measures are already discussed in the proceeding paragraph.Besides these patients may many a time need the support of a bulk laxative to facilitate the evacuation.Horizontal angling of the pouch during the act of defecation can become another contributory factor in failure of pouch evacuation, however, this problem can be overcome by fixation of the pouch with presacral fascia.
- Technically not possible in all - Many factors like thick mesocolon, adhesions, failure to gain adequate length, narrow pelvis, poor vascularity may pose some technical difficulties to construct a pouch.
- Pouch failure - Some pouches inspite of a good construction may fail to evacuate and inspite of the support of enemas and laxatives may not be helped so may need a revision surgery in the form of APR.
- Cost factor - This continues to be a concern in resource poor countries. The staplers cost a good bit of money which still is out of reach of the most in this part of globe.
- It is just the beginning.

18.3 Is CJP a gold standard?

We believe that it is too early probably to say that, it will need larger trials, long term follow up to really label it as a gold standard. Even though there is so much of evidence in its favor but still the evidence is not enough to establish its supremacy and justify its routine use in all cases of low cancer rectum but it is an evidence based option so needs to be tried on larger series.

19. Acknowledgement

Prof G Q Peer who always trusted and believed in me and infused confidence in me at critical junctures. Prof Nazir A Wani Ex Dean Faculty,Chairman Surgical division at SKIMS my guide,teacher who always persuaded and inculcated the craft of writing in me and always encouraged me to do better in life.
Prof Khursheed Alam Wani -Head Dept of Surgery at SKIMS who always encouraged and facilitated my research work and kept on appreciating my good work at all junctures.
Dr Sameer H Naqash,Dr Ajaz A Malik and Dr Rouf A Wani my dearest colleagues in the department who always stood by me morally and professionally during the study period.

My revered parents for their love, affection and blessing.
My beloved wife Nighat who is a big psychological, emotional and moral support for my all academic work and my sweet kids Shaheem and Liqa who always bear with me in my hours of toil at the cost of their time. My dearest students who always gave me lots of love and respect and made me to do better.
Mr. Farooq A Nadaf for the computer execution and the proper design of this book chapter with utmost commitment, sincerity and dedication.

20. References

Alois Fürst, Silvia Suttner, Ayman Agha, Alexander Beham and Karl-Walter Jauch. Colonic J- Pouch vs. Coloplasty Following Resection of Distal Rectal Cancer Early Results of a Prospective, Randomized, Pilot Study. Dis Colon Rectum. 2003 Sep; 46(9).

Batignani G, Monaci I, Ficari F, Tonelli F. What affects continence after anterior resection of the rectum?Dis colon rectum 1991; 34:329-35.

Dukes CE. The spread of cancer of the rectum. Br J Surg 1930; 17:643–8.

Dennett ER, Parry BR. Misconceptions about the colonic J pouch.Dis colon rectum 1999.42:804-811.

Fain SN, Patin CS, Morgenstern L. Use of a mechanical suturing apparatus in low colorectal anastomosis. Arch Surg. 1975 Sep; 110(9):1079-82.

Golihrt JC, Dukes CE, Bussey HJ. Local recurrences after sphincter saving excisions for carcinoma of the rectum and Rectosigmoid Br J Surg. 1951 Nov; 39(155):199-211.

Goligher JC. Recent trends in the practice of sphincter-saving excision for carcinoma of the rectum. Adv Surg.1979; 13:1-31.

Guillou PJ, Quirke P, Thorpe H, Walker J, Jayne DG, Smith AM, Heath RM, Brown JM. MRC CLASICC trial group. Short-term endpoints of conventional versus laparoscopic-assisted surgery in patients with colorectal cancer (MRC CLASICC trial): multicentre, randomised controlled trial. Lancet 2005 May; 365 (9472): 1718-26.

Hallbook O, Pahlman L, Krog M, Wexner SD, Sjodahl R. Randomized comparison of straight and colonic J pouch anastamosis after low anterior resection.Ann Surg 1996; 224:58-65.

Hallbook O, Johansson K, Sydahl R. Laser Doppler blood flow measurement in rectal resection for carcinoma; Comparison between straight and colonic J pouch reconstruction.Br J Surg 1996; 83:389-92.

Hida J, Yasutomi M, Fujimoto K, Okuno K, Ieda S, Machidera N, Kubo R, Shindo K, Koh K. Functional outcome after low anterior resection with low anastomosis for rectal cancer using the colonic J-pouch. Prospective randomized study for determination of optimum pouch size. Dis Colon Rectum. 1996 Sep; 39(9):986-91.

Ho YH, Tan M, Seow Cheon F. Prospective randomized controlled study of clinical functionand anorectal physiology after low anterior resection.Comparision of straight and colonic J pouch anastamosis. Br J Surg 1996; 83:978-980

Harris GJ, Lavery IC, Fazio VW. Function of a colonic J pouch continues to improve with time.Br J Surg 2001; 88:1623-27.

Iwai N, Hashimoto K, Yamne T, Kojima O, Nishioka B, Fujita Y, etal. Physiologic states of anorectum following sphincter saving resection for carcinoma of the rectum. Dis colon rectum 1982; 25:625-9.

Lazorthes F, Fages P, Chiotasso P, Lemozy J, Bloom E. Resection of the rectum with construction of a colonic reservoir and coloanal anastamosis for carcinoma of the rectum.Br J Surg 1986; 73:136-138

Lewis WG, Martin IG, Williamson ME, Stephenson BM, Holdsworth PJ, Finan PJ, Johnston D. Why do some patients experience poor functional results after anterior resection of the rectum for carcinoma? Dis Colon Rectum. 1995 Mar; 38(3):259-63.

Miles WE. A method for performing abdomino-perineal excision for carcinoma of the rectum and the terminal portion of the pelvic colon. Lancet. 1908; 1812-1813.

Molloy RG, Moran KT, Coulter J, Waldron R, Kirwan WO. Mechanism of sphincter impairment following low anterior resection. Dis Colon Rectum. 1992 May; 35(5):462-4.

Miller AS, Lewis WG, Williamson ME, Holdsworth PJ, Johnston D, Finan PJ. Factors that influence functional outcome after coloanal anastomosis for carcinoma of the rectum. Br J Surg. 1995 Oct; 82(10):1327-30.

Nicholls RJ, Lubowoski DZ, Donalson DR. Comparision of colonic reservoir and straight coloanal reconstruction after rectal excision.Br J Surg 1988; 75:318-320

Ooi BS , Lai JH. Colonic J-Pouch, Coloplasty, Side-to-End Anastomosis: Meta-Analysis and Comparison of Outcomes. Seminars in Colon and Rectal Surgery 2009 June; 20(2):69-72.

Parks AG. Transanal technique in low rectal anastomosis. Proc R Soc Med. 1972 Nov; 65(11):975-6.

Pollett WG, Nicholls RJ. The relationship between the extent of distal clearance and survival and local recurrence rates after curative anterior resection for carcinoma of the rectum. Ann Surg. 1983 Aug; 198(2):159-63.

Parc R, Tiret E, Frileux P, Moszkowski E, Loygue J. Resection and colo-anal anastomosis with colonic reservoir for rectal carcinoma. Br J Surg. 1986 Feb; 73(2):139-41.

Pedersen IK, Christiansen J, Hint K, Jensen P, Olsen J, Mortensen PE. Anorectal function after low anterior resection for carcinoma. Ann Surg. 1986 Aug; 204(2):133-5.

Park JG, Lee MR, Lim SB, Hong CW, Yoon SN, Kang SB, Heo SC, Jeong SY, Park KJ. Colonic Jpouch anal anastomosis after ultralow anterior resection with upper sphincter excision for low-lying rectal cancer. World J Gastroenterol. 2005 May; 11(17):2570-3.

P. Wille-Jørgensen. Meta-analysis of colonic reservoirs versus straight coloanal anastomosis after anterior resection. Br J Surg 2006; 93: 19–32.

Quirke P, Dixon MF, Durdey P, Williams NS. Local recurrence of rectal adenocarcinoma due to inadequate surgical resection. Lancet 1986; 2: 996-9.

Seon Choen F, Goh HS. Prospective randomized trial comparing J colonic pouch anal anastamosis and straight coloanal reconstruction.Br J Surg 1995; 82:608-610

Selvindos PB, Ho YH. Laparoscopic ultralow resection with colonic J pouch analanastamosis. Dis colon rectum 2008; 51(11):1710-1711

Tarik S, Arman K, Sanket S, Ian B P, Hill, Andrew G. Laparoscopic colorectal surgery is associated with a higher intraoperative complication rate than open surgery. Annals of Surgery: 2011 January; 253 (1): 35–43.

Westhues H. Uber die Entstehung und Vermeidung des lokalen Rektumkarzinom-Rezidivs. Arch Klin Chir 1930; 161:582–91.

11

Experimental Evaluation of the Mechanical Strength of the Stapling Techniques: Experimental Study on Animal Model

Kentaro Kawasaki[1], Kiyonori Kanemitsu[2],
Tadahiro Goto[2], Yasuhiro Fujino[1] and Yoshikazu Kuroda[2]
[1]*Division of Gastroenterological Surgery, Hyogo Cancer Center, Akashi, Hyogo*
[2]*Division of Gastroenterological Surgery*
Kobe University Graduate School of Medicine, Kobe
Japan

1. Introduction

The creation of a gastrointestinal tract anastomosis is a fundamental and important surgical procedure. The mean incidence of clinically apparent leakage after gastrointestinal tract anastomosis ranges from 2.1% to 14.9%. Although many techniques for successfully producing such anastomoses have been described, the goal of these techniques to be technically feasible and safe.

In the 1960s, Steichen and Ravitch introduced stapling instruments. During the subsequent years, automatic stapling instruments have continued to be refined, and many automatic anastomotic techniques have been applied to gastrointestinal surgery. In addition, various instruments and techniques for stapling intestinal anastomoses have been applied to colorectal surgery. Functional end-to-end anastomosis (FETEA), stapled end-to-end anastomosis (ETEA), and stapled side-to-end anastomosis (STEA) are the most common techniques. Moreover, there are two types of stapled ETEA, the single stapling technique (SST) and the double stapling technique (DST).

Although these methods have been shown to be reliable and safe, anastomosis leakage remains a major problem. Major leakages affect the long-term quality of life (QOL) of patients. In addition, leakage can cause significant morbidity. Studies have reported that the frequency of leakage ranges from 2.9 to 23%, and that the shorter the distance from the anal verge to the anastomosis the greater the risk of leakage.

As mentioned above, automatic stapling instruments have been refined over the years, and many automatic anastomotic techniques have been applied to colorectal surgery; however, the optimal instrument and method remain unclear. Since the mechanical strength of an anastomosis is an important factor affecting leakage during the initial postoperative phase, experimental evaluation of this factor would be useful for clarifying these issues.

In this chapter, we examined the pressure required to induce failure (bursting pressure) in various kinds of stapled anastomosis and investigated which stapling technique is most suitable.

2. Materials and methods

2.1 Materials

All animal experiments were carried out according to the "Guidelines for Animal Experimentation at COVIDIEN, Japan". Young domestic pigs (10-12 weeks) weighing 30 to 40 kg were used in this study. After the induction of general anesthesia using intramuscular ketamine (15 mg/kg) and intravenous pentobarbital (30 mg/kg), the pig was intubated and maintained on mechanical ventilation. An intravenous catheter was then placed in the right external jugular vein, and the animal was given approximately 500 ml isotonic intravenous fluid. After making a midline incision, segments of the small intestine were isolated and transected. All specimens were maintained in warm natural saline and randomly allocated to the following anastomotic techniques.

After the experiments, the animals were sacrificed under anesthesia using intravenous potassium chloride.

2.2 Surgical procedure

The stapled anastomoses were created using the EndoGIA 60 blue, EndoGIA60 green, GIA 60 blue, or PCEEA 21 (COVIDIEN, Japan). The characteristics of each device are summarized in Table 1. All anastomoses were performed by an expert surgeon.

Instrument	Staple	Thickness (mm)
EndoGIA blue®	3 lines	1.5
EndoGIA green®	3 lines	2
GIA Blue®	2 lines	1.5

Table 1. Comparison of instruments

2.3 Examination of bursting points and pressure

A 16-Fr Foley catheter was placed into the lumen of the transected small intestine, and a balloon was inflated to close the lumen (Figure 1). The schema was described as Figure 2.

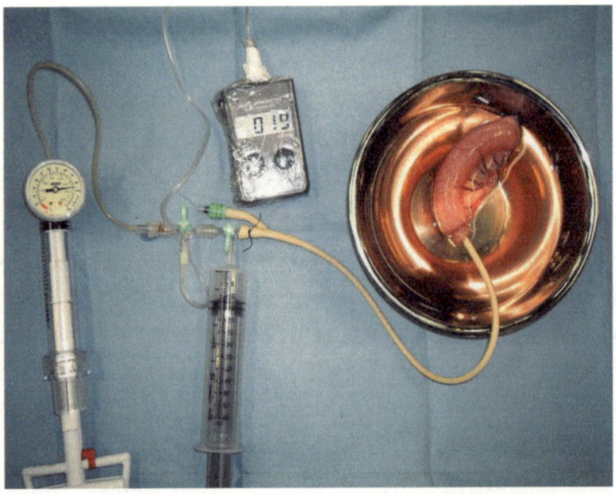

Fig. 1. System used in this chapter

The balloon catheter was then connected to an infusion pump and a pressure recorder (Pressure Sensors PG-100, COPAL ELECTRONICS) via a pressure transducer. Each anastomosis was immersed in water, and air was infused into the intestine at a rate of 30mL/min. The intraluminal pressure was continuously recorded. The bursting pressure was defined as the pressure at which air leakage from the anastomosis was initially observed (Figure 3). The location of the bursting point was also recorded.

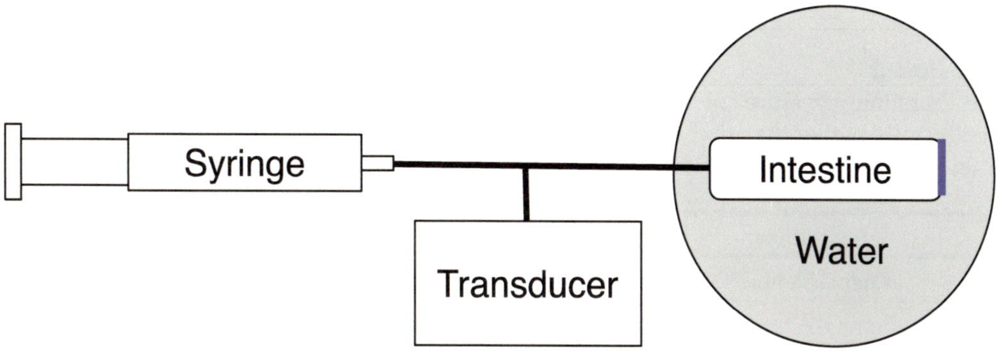

Fig. 2. Measurement of Bursting Pressure and Bursting Point

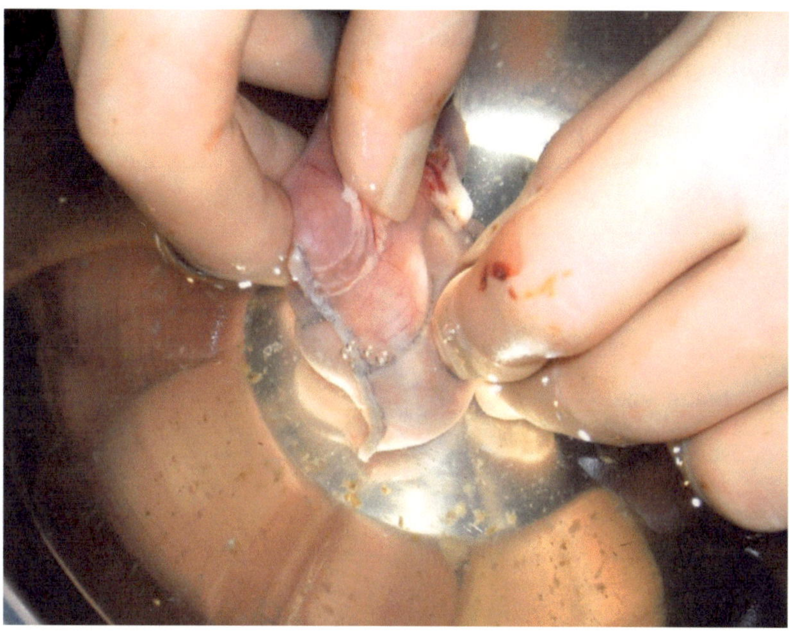

Fig. 3. The moment air leakage was seen

2.4 Statistical analysis

Discrete variables were analyzed using the Mann-Whitney test, Factorial Analysis of Variance (ANOVA), and Scheffe's test. Statistical significance was indicated at $P<0.05$. All statistical computations were carried out using StatView5.0 software.

3. Experiment

3.1 Experiment 1: Comparison of the bursting pressure of anastomoses produced using various instruments

3.1.1 Method

A segment of the intestine was isolated using the EndoGIA 60 blue, EndoGIA 60 green, or GIA 60 blue. Then, the bursting pressures of the staple lines produced using each instrument were examined. Three sets of each staple line were examined.

3.1.2 Result

The bursting pressure of anastomoses produced using the EndoGIA 60 blue was significantly higher than that of those produced using the EndoGIA 60 green or GIA 60 blue (Table 2).

Instrument	Pressure (mmHG)	*p*
EndoGIA blue®	80.3 *S.D.* 10.5	
EndoGIA green®	37.3 *S.D.* 4.2	<0.01 VS EndoGIA blue®
GIA blue®	31.7 *S.D.* 4.5	<0.01 VS EndoGIA blue®

Table 2. Comparison of bursting pressure of instruments

3.2 Experiment 2: Comparison of the bursting pressure of buttressed and non-buttressed cutting sites

3.2.1 Method

After isolating the intestine with the EndoGIA 60 blue, the cut end of the staple line was buttressed with 3-0 silk serosa-muscular sutures (Figure 4). Then, the bursting pressure of each type of anastomosis was measured.

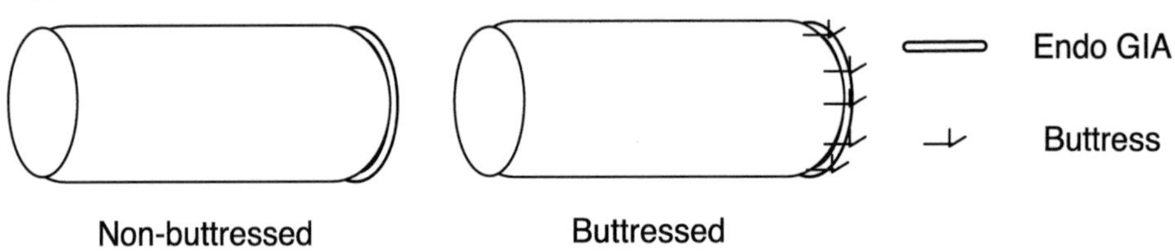

Fig. 4. Comparison of buttressed and non-buttressed cutting sites

3.2.2 Result

Comparison of the bursting pressures of buttressed and non-buttressed cutting sites
The bursting pressure of the buttressed group was significantly higher than that of the non-buttressed group (Table 3).

Groups	Pressure (mmHG)	*p*
buttressed	149.6 *S.D.* 37.6	< 0.01
non-buttressed	75.3 *S.D.* 25.1	

Table 3. Comparison of bursting pressure of buttressed

3.3 Experiment 3: Comparison of the bursting pressures of the three kinds of the anastomosis (FETEA, STEA and ETEA).

3.3.1 Method

FETEA was performed using the EndoGIA 60 blue, ETEA was performed using the PCEEA circular stapler, and STEA was performed using the PCEEA circular stapler or the EndoGIA 60 blue. Then, the bursting pressure and points of each anastomosis were examined. Three or four sets of each anastomosis were examined.

3.3.2 Result

The bursting pressure was not significantly different between the three groups (Table 4). FETEA failed at the intersection of the stapled lines or the crotch of the anastomosis or both. All stapled ETEA failed along the staple line. All stapled STE anastomoses failed along the circular staple line (Figure. 5).

Anastomosis	Pressure (mmHG)	*p*
FETEA	28.3 *S.D.* 6.8	
STEA	17.3 S.D. 6.4	N. S.
ETEA	19.8 S.D. 7.4	

Table 4. Comparison of FETEA, ETEA and ETEA

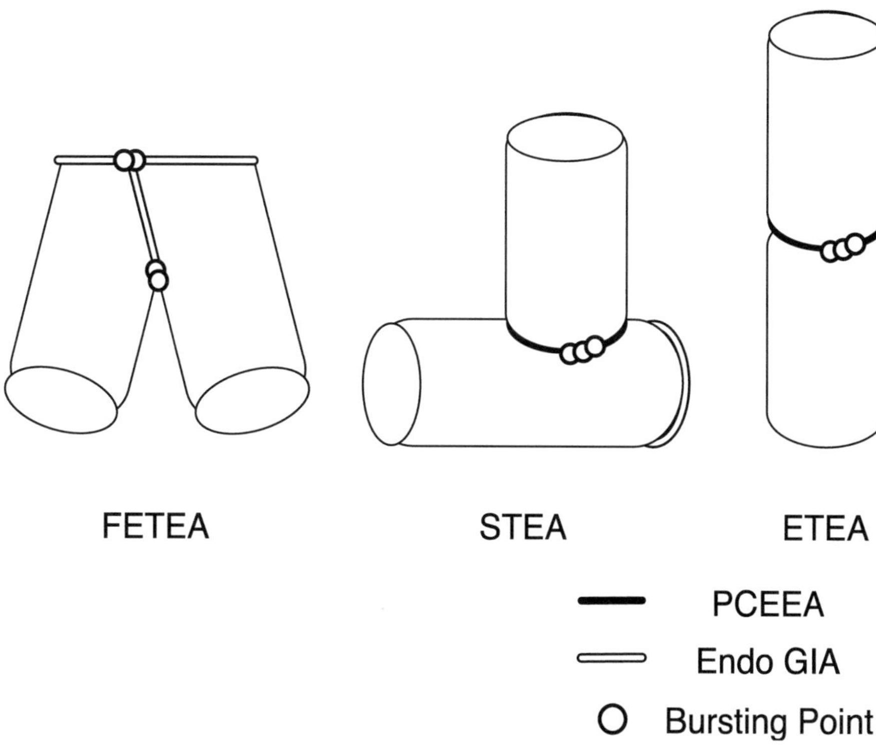

Fig. 5. Bursting points of FETEA, STEA and ETEA

3.4 Experiment 4: Comparison of the bursting points and the bursting pressure between the SST, DST, and DST with buttressing techniques

3.4.1 Method

SST was performed with the PCEEA21, and DST was performed with the EndoGIA 60 blue or PCEEA21. In addition, buttressing of the staple line with 3-0 silk sutures was performed in combination with DST (DST + buttressing). Then, the bursting pressure and bursting points of each anastomosis were measured.

3.4.2 Result

The bursting points of the anastomoses are shown in Figure 3a. Eight bursting points were located at staple line intersections in the anastomoses created using the PCEEA, while only one bursting point was located at a staple line intersection in the anastomoses created using the PCEEA and EndoGIA (black circle). Bursting pressure was not significantly different between the three groups (Table 5). However, the bursting pressure of the staple line intersection (black circle) was much lower than those of the others (Figure 3b).

Anastomosis	Pressure (mmHG)	*p*
SST	34.0 *S.D.* 3.6	
DST	30.7 *S.D.* 14.5	N. S.
DST with buttressing	39.3 *S.D.* 11.9	

Table 5. Comparison of SST, DST, and DST with buttressing

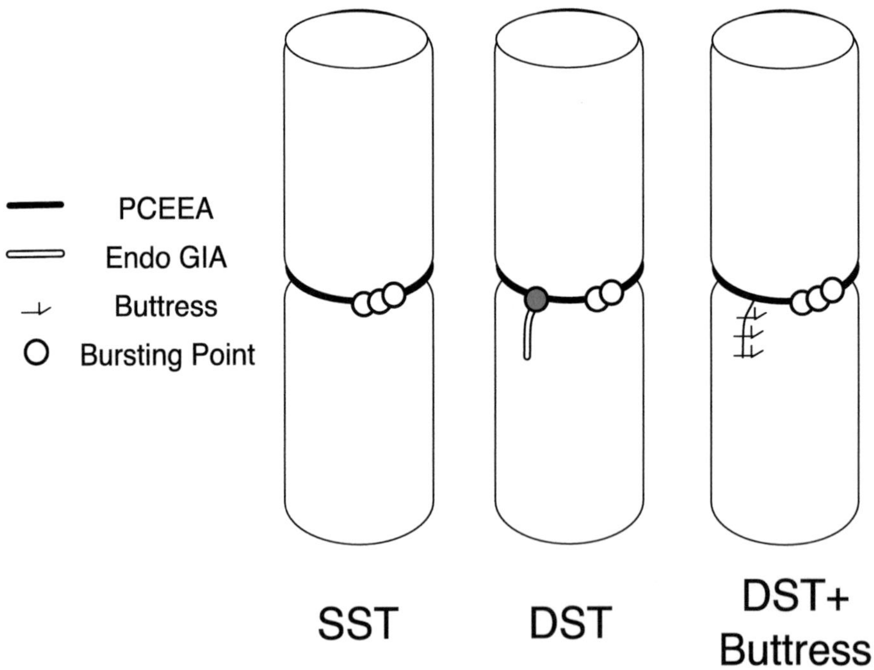

Fig. 6a. Bursting Point

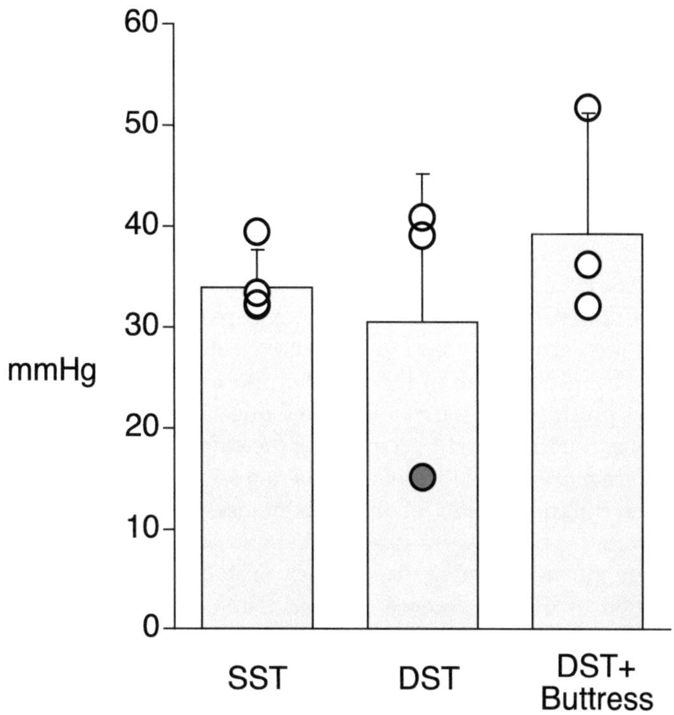

Fig. 6b. Bursting Pressure

4. Discussion

In choosing the best anastomotic technique, surgeons should consider the features and limitations of each technique, rather than their experience or preference. Unfortunately, no matter how safe stapling instruments have become, they are unlikely to ever become risk-free. The consequences of these instruments misfiring can be significant. In addition, complications can occur even when the instruments function normally. Anastomotic failure depends on various parameters, including tissue thickness, collagen content, blood flow, improper selection of staple cartridges, ischemia, and tension.

The most common problem associated with intestinal anastomoses is leakage. The bursting pressure of an anastomosis reflects its strength, and higher bursting pressure correlates to a stronger anastomosis at less than one week after surgery. Leakage also appears to be closely connected with the strength of a freshly completed intestinal anastomosis. Therefore, bursting pressure is considered to be the most important factor for assessing the quality of an intestinal suture line.

In experiment 1, the EndoGIA blue produced the strongest anastomoses. The bursting pressure of the anastomoses produced using this device was approximately twice as high as that of those produced using the EndoGIA green and GIA blue. This suggests that anastomotic strength is regulated by the number of staple lines and the relationship between the device and tissue thickness. Thus, experiment 2 was performed using the EndoGIA blue.

Experiment 2 demonstrated that buttressing the cutting site significantly increased the strength of the anastomosis. Therefore, buttressing the staple line to strengthen it seems to be effective.

In experiment 3, the FETEA, STEA and SSTA techniques were compared. The results of the present study demonstrate that none of the anastomotic techniques was superior to the others as far as bursting pressure was concerned. The bursting point was located along the staple line in anastomoses created using the PCEEA and at the intersection of the stapled lines or the crotch of the anastomosis in those produced using the EndoGIA, which could have caused leakage to occur. In our experiments, when the anastomotic crotch was buttressed, the bursting pressure was significantly increased. In particular, in automatic anastomoses, the locations where staple lines cross might be weak points.

In experiment 4, the SST, DST, and DST with buttressing techniques were compared. There were no significant differences between these three groups with regard to bursting pressure. However, the staple lines created by the PCEEA were weaker than those produced using the EndoGIA. This may have been due to the fact that the EndoGIA creates 3 staple lines, in contrast to the 2 lines produced by the PCEEA. If a 2-line stapler (e.g. the GIA or TA) is used to isolate the intestine, bursting might occur along the staple line. Therefore, 3-line staplers (e.g., the EndoGIA) are more useful for isolating the intestine.

In experiment 4, the bursting points of the anastomoses were also examined. In 8 of 9 PCEEA cases, the bursting points were located at staple line intersections, and all bursting pressure values were above 30mmHg. In contrast, only one bursting point occurred at a staple line intersection in the anastomoses created using both the PCEEA and EndoGIA; moreover, its bursting pressure was only 14mmHg. While bursting may be a rare event, it can cause leakage or infection during the initial postoperative phase because intra-anal pressure has been reported to reach 24-73 mmHg. Therefore, the SST technique, which does not create staple line intersections, may be the safest method. Although the DST with buttressing is sometimes performed, it did not significantly increase the strength of the anastomosis. Therefore, this technique may be fairly useless. In this experiment, the buttressing of anastomoses produced using the PCEEA was not examined since buttressing a PCEEA produced anastomosis is impossible during lower rectal cancer surgery.

The above stapling techniques have been accepted widely for the treatment of rectal cancer. However, complications can occur, and when they do, they reduce the patient's QOL. These data are relevant to acute phase conditions and were derived from an animal model so they may not completely reflect human clinical data. However, animal experimental evaluations are often found to be useful by gastroenterological surgeons. Although many factors influence anastomotic healing, our results may help to decrease the incidence of postoperative complications after the creation of a gastrointestinal tract anastomosis.

5. Conclusion

The EndoGIA blue is the most suitable device for stapling intestinal anastomoses. Buttressing the stapling line may increase the strength of the anastomosis. The stapling line intersection might be a weak point, especially when the DST technique is used. Although our findings relate to acute phase conditions and were derived from a small number of anastomoses in an animal model, we believe that gastro-enterological surgeons will find our results useful.

6. Acknowledgment

We thank COVIDIEN Japan for the technical support.

7. References

Rullier E, Laurent C, Garrelon JL & Michel P. (1998). Risk factors for anastomotic leakage after resection of rectal cancer. Br J Surg 85: 355–358, ISSN 1365-2168

Schwab R, Wesendorf S, Gutcke A & Becker HP. (2002). Early bursting strength of human colon anastomoses: an in vitro study comparing current anastomotic techniques. Langenbeck Arch Surg 386: 507–511, ISSN 0272-5533

Steichen FM. (1968). The use of staplers in anatomical side-to-side and functional end-to-end enteroanastomoses. Surgery 64: 948- 953, ISSN 0039-6060

Hardcare JM, Mendoza-Sagaon M, Murata K & Talamini MA. (2000). Use of a cauterizing laparoscopic linear stapler in intes- tinal anastomosis. Surg Laparosc Endosc Percutan Tech 10: 128–132, ISSN 1530-4515

Ravitch MM & Steichen FM. (1979). A stapling instrument for end to end inverting anastomosis in the gastrointestinal tract. Ann Surg 189: 791–797, ISSN 0003-4932

Ritchey ML, Lally KP & Ostericher R. (1993). Comparison of dif- ferent techniques of stapled bowel anastomoses in a canine model. Arch Surg 128: 1365–1367, ISSN 0272-5533

Steichen FM & Ravitch MM. (1973). Mechanical sutures in surgery. Br J Surg 60: 191–197, ISSN 1365-2168

Knight CD & Griffen FD. (1980). An improved technique for low anterior resection of the rectum using the EEA stapler. Surgery 88:710-714 , ISSN 0039-6060

Stericher R, Lally KP, Barrett DM & Ritchey ML. (1991). Anastomotic obstruction after stapled enteroanastomosis. Surgery 109:799-801, ISSN 0039-6060

Graf W, Glimelius B, Bergstrom R & Pahlman L. (1991). Complications after double and single stapling in rectal surgery. Eur J Surg 157:543-547, ISSN 1102-4151

Chiarugi M, Buccianti P, Sidoti F, Franceschi M, Goletti O & Cavina E. (1996). Single and double stapled anastomoses in rectal cancer surgery; a retrospective study on the safety of the technique and its indication. Acta Chir Belg 96:31-36, ISSN 0001-5458

Vignali A, Fazio VW, Lavery IC, Milsom JW, Church JM, Hull TL, Strong SA & Oakley JR. (1997). Factors associated with the occurrence of leaks in stapled rectal anastomoses: a review of 1,014 patients. J Am Coll Surg 185:105-113, ISSN, ISSN 1072-7515

Luna-Perez P & Rodriguez-Ramirez SE. (2002). Multivariate analysis of risk factors associated with dehiscence of colorectal anastomosis after anterior or lower anterior resection for sigmoid or rectal cancer. Rev Invest Clin 54:501-581, ISSN 0034-8376

Sato H, Maeda K, Hanai T, Matsumoto M, Aoyama H & Matsuoka H. (2006). Modified double-stapling technique in low anterior resection for lower rectal carcinoma. Surg Today 36:30-36, ISSN 0941-1291

Bardini R, Tosato SM & Termini B. (2003). Pursestring placement before transsection of the rectum for facilitating the stapled low colorectal anastomosis. Dis Colon Rectum 46:1712-1714, ISSN

Bluett MK, Healy DA, Kalemeris GC & O'Leary JP. (1986). Comparison of automatic staplers in small bowel anastomoses. South Med J 79:712-716, ISSN 0012-3706

Arnold W & Shikora SA .(2005). A comparison of burst pressure between buttressed versus non-buttressed staple-lines in an animal model. Obes Surg 15:164-171, ISSN 0960-8923

Hardacre JM, Mendoza-Sagaon M & Murata K. (2000). Use of a cauterizing laparoscopic linear stapler in intestinal anastomosis.Surg Laparosc Endosc Percutan Tech 10:128-132, ISSN

Roumen RM, Rahusen FT, Wijnen MH & Croiset van Uchelen FA. (2000). "Dog ear" formation after double-stapled low anterior resection as a risk factor for anastomotic disruption. Dis Colon Rectum 43:522-525, ISSN 0960-8923

Hendriks T & Mastboom WJ. (1990). Healing of experimental intestinal anastomoses. Parameters for repair. Dis Colon Rectum 33:891-901, ISSN 0960-8923

Alper D, Ram E, Stein GY & Dreznik Z. (2005). Resting anal pressure following hemorrhoidectomy and lateral sphincterotomy. Dis Colon Rectum 48:2080-2084, ISSN 0960-8923

Bittorf B, Stadelmaier U, Gohl J, Hohenberger W & Matzel KE. (2004). Functional outcome after intersphincteric resection of the rectum with coloanal anastomosis in low rectal cancer. Eur J Surg Oncol 30:260-265, ISSN 0748-7983

Kawasaki K, Fujino Y, Kanemitsu K, Goto T, Kamigaki T, Kuroda D & Kuroda Y. (2007). Experimental evaluation of the mechanical strength of stapling techniques. Surg Endosc. 2007 Oct;21(10):1796-9. , ISSN 0930-2794

Goto T, Kawasaki K, Fujino Y, Kanemitsu K, Kamigaki T, Kuroda D, Suzuki Y & Kuroda Y. (2007). Evaluation of the mechanical strength and patency of functional end-to-end anastomoses. Surg Endosc. 2007 Sep;21(9):1508-11. ISSN 0930-2794

Kanemitsu K, Kawasaki K, Goto T, Fujino Y, Kamigaki T, Kuroda D & Kuroda Y. (2009). Experimental comparison of the stapled intestinal anastomotic techniques. Surg Technol Int. 2009;18:98-102. , ISSN 1615-7591

12

Management of Locally Recurrent Rectal Cancer

Zoran Krivokapic and Ivan Dimitrijevic
First Surgical Clinic, Clinical Centre of Serbia
Serbia

1. Introduction

The treatment of colorectal cancer, that presents considerable health problem, still has a lot of space for improvement. The overall recurrence rate for this disease is between 8 and 50% according to literature data (Das, Skibber et al. 2006; Kaiser, Kang et al. 2006). The risk for recurrence is highest in the first two years postoperatively (Juhl G 1990; McCall JL 1995; Micev M 2000; Krivokapic Z 2004).
Local recurrence is defined as growth of adenocarcinoma in the pelvis after a previous resection for rectal cancer. Involvement of the ovaries is regarded as distant metastases, unless continuous overgrowth is noted.
For rectal cancer the risk of local recurrence is estimated to be somewhere between 5 and 40% (Kjeldsen, Kronborg et al. 1997). With the improvement of the surgical technique and use of neoadjuvant and adjuvant therapy the incidence of locally recurrent disease is expected to be around 10% (Rothenberger and Wong 1985).
Other, most common sites of metastatic disease are liver and lung (Tepper JE 2003). The best treatment results in the terms of surgery are achieved with solitary lesions. Radical surgery for liver and lung metastases is well accepted, on the other hand, aggressive surgery for local recurrence is often controversial despite the fact that median survival without treatment is usually 6-7 months not mentioning refractory pain, obstruction and other accompanying complications. Also, approximately 50% of local recurrences are restricted to the pelvis. However, the number of patients that can be resected for cure is less than 50 % (between 30 and 40 %) and median survival of these patients varies from 21 to 36 months (Gagliardi, Hawley et al. 1995).
In this chapter we`ll try to deal with different aspects of diagnosis and management of rectal cancer local recurrence, the most dangerous, difficult and unpleasant possible outcome of surgical treatment.

2. Risk factors associated with local recurrence

Many risk factors have been identified as predictors of rectal cancer local recurrence. Factors as tumor features, patient constitution and surgeons ability and knowledge often play a crucial role in genesis of local recurrence.
Tumor stage is, apparently extremely important risk factor (Kim, Kim et al. 2009). Poor differentiation, lymphovascular and perineural invasion are also associated with this phenomenon. Besides this, lower, bulkier, macroscopically infiltrating tumors as well as the presence of mucinous component are to be blamed for local recurrence (Choen AM 1990).

Patient constitution affects genesis of local recurrence in two ways.
First group of patient related factors is anatomical one; narrow, "male" pelvis and obesity can in some cases make surgery extremely demanding, thus compromising its oncological quality. As the evidence for this may serve the fact that tumor irresectability is earlier suspected and diagnosed in male patients (Law WL 2000).
Second group of factors contains all those which can negatively affect immunological status of a patient- immunodeficiency disorders, advanced age or any other non-related serious conditions.
Surgeons experience and caseload is tightly related to the percentage of local recurrence. Surgeons with more than 10-12 rectal cancer cases per year have significantly lower number of patients with local recurrence. We can find evidence for this in many published trials. In Stockholm trial, for example local recurrence was 4 versus 10% when comparing high and low-volume surgeons. Surgeons with proper training more frequently performed sphincter saving procedures and administered neoadjuvant therapy (Martling A 2002).
In terms of surgeons influence on local recurrence we`ll discuss some aspects including surgical management of rectal cancer as well as some quality measurements of operation itself.
Surgical options available for treatment of rectal cancer are anterior resection, abdominoperinal resection (APR), local excision along with transanal endoscopic microsurgery and in some cases Hartmann`s procedure.
All surgical modalities concerning abdominal approach have in the essence same basic rules, well proven in numerous studies published in the past twenty years. Those are total mesorectal excision (TME), with proper distal and lateral clearance (circumferential margin of resection-CRM), high ligation of inferior mesenteric artery, removal of the intact limfovascular "baring" segment and correct visualization and preservation of pelvic vegetative nerve structures.
There`s no doubt that TME is nowadays well established method of rectal cancer treatment. Principals postulated by Bill Heald in 1982. are very well known by all rectal cancer surgeons and include meticulous sharp dissection between mesorectal and endopelvic fascia following avascular, areolar "holy" plane under direct control of vision (Quirke P 1986; MacFarlane, Ryall et al. 1993).
CRM is proven to be one of the most important predictive factors for genesis of local recurrence. Many published studies proved that tumor involvement of CRM is a sole pathohistological variable that influences local recurrence and survival. Lateral clearance of less than 1mm (positive CRM) means significantly higher chance for recurrence (3,5 times greater risk) and doubles the risk of poor survival. CRM status is very accurate in predicting local recurrence. In 75% of cases with positive CRM local recurrence is inevitable. In 38,2% of patients with local recurrence CRM was positive, and in only 10% the situation was opposite. Following this, 5-year survival s also severally affected (72 versus 29% comparing positive and negative CRM) (Quirke and Dixon 1988; Birbeck KF 2002; Nagtegaall ID 2002).
CRM in the context of APR is being carefully evaluated, and as a consequence, more extensive APR with en-bloc resection of the levator muscles and mesorectum has been recently introduced (Holm, Ljung et al. 2007). This technique results in lower risk of involved CRM and fewer intra-operative bowel perforations (West, Finan et al. 2008).
Distal clearance has been a matter of debate in era of dramatically increased percentage of sphincter saving procedures. Old "5cm rule" is nowadays a part of surgical history. Papers by Madsen and Williams (Williams, Dixon et al. 1983; Madsen and Christiansen 1986)

initially showed that distal propagation of tumor deposits is infrequent. This evidence enabled significant increase of oncologically safe sphincter saving procedures. In favor of this goes a fact that cases were intersphincteric resection with complete or partial internal sphincter removal was performed local recurrence rates were similar to those achieved in patients were APR was the only solution (Heald RJ 1997).

The type of local recurrence considerably varies depending on the nature of original procedure.

After anterior resection, local recurrence can be anastomotic, or localized elsewhere in the pelvis.

It is very uncommon to find a recurrence originating from mucosal suture line, it almost always originates from the bowel wall or from a point within the pelvis when we call it perianastomotic one (Selvaggi, Cuocolo et al. 2003).

Favorable aspect of this recurrence type is that, contrary to the one seen after APR, it provides more options for follow-up (digital, endoscopical examination, biopsy). Additionally, this type of recurrence often becomes symptomatic earlier than one found after APR. Genesis of local recurrence in this case can be found in biology of the initial tumor, tumor stage, and most importantly in surgical technique. Concerning the tumor stage, for example, we can clearly demonstrate its impact on percentage of local recurrence-stage I of the disease, according to TNM classification has 5-year recurrence rate of around 10%, stage II, approximately 24% and stage III about 41% (Manfredi S 2001).

Concerning the impact of initial surgery on the type of local recurrence, it is interesting to note that recurrences after operations where proper TME was not conducted are much more amenable to salvage surgery, with notably better results (Williams, Dixon et al. 1983; Madsen and Christiansen 1986). This can be explained with longer period needed for recurrent tumor to infiltrate surrounding structures, because of still existing mesorectal "envelope". Infiltration of surrounding structures, especially pelvic sidewall makes salvage surgery much more difficult. Of course, another important fact is that local recurrence is more frequent and rapid in patients were incomplete TME was performed (Quirke P 1986; Bergamaschi R 2001; Krivokapic Z 2002).

Surgical treatment of local recurrence is much more difficult after APR (MacFarlane, Ryall et al. 1993) and more frequent (Friel CM 2002). Curative surgical treatment in these cases is possible in much lower percentage. Several factors contribute this. Usually, APR is conducted in patients with bulkier, more advanced tumors. Surgical options are limited in attempted salvage surgery; normal pelvic anatomy is much more violated. Additionally, follow-up of these patients is inadequate (MacFarlane, Ryall et al. 1993). Asymptomatic period is much longer (no apparent bleeding or obstruction) and physical examination is limited. In females, vaginal examination (especially endovaginal ultrasound) can be useful in detection of local recurrence. On the other hand, in males, we can only perform imaging methods (CT, NMR, and PET scan).

Local excision alone, for rectal cancer is oncologically insufficient operation. Local recurrence and salvage surgery for it are frequent. Authors report salvages surgery rates in these conditions of 22 up to 100% (Cuthbertson and Simpson 1986; Suzuki, Dozois et al. 1996; Lopez-Kostner, Fazio et al. 2001). For patients in stage I disease in carefully selected indications local excision can be a therapy of choice. In recent years, with the introduction of preoperative chemoradiotherapy, this approach gains ground in the treatment of T1 and T2 tumors. Several retrospective case series and a small prospective study suggest that chemoradiotherapy before local excision reduces recurrence to a level comparable with TME (Kim, Yeatman et al. 2001;

Borschitz, Wachtlin et al. 2008; Lezoche, Baldarelli et al. 2008). Yet complications induced by neoadjuvant therapy combined with complications from local excision itself cast certain doubt on this approach. More large, prospective, randomized studies are needed to justify this strategy. In the case of non radical local excision, immediate salvage surgery is an option. Results of this type of surgery are excellent, better than after surgery for existing recurrence, unfortunately still less favorable than after initial radical resection (Killingback M 2001).
In any way, after local excision, close follow-up is mandatory using endorectal ultrasound every two months for up to 4 years.
Neoadjuvant treatment of rectal cancer is therapeutic modality, now well proven and administered worldwide. Combined with TME further reduces the percentage of local recurrence. In the Dutch trial (Wiggers, Mannaerts et al. 2003) good results were achieved. After TME alone local recurrence was 8,2% and after TME combined with preoperative radiotherapy was 2,4%. Nevertheless, in a number of studies (Holm, Cedermark et al. 1994) interesting fact was noted, namely, survival in patients with local recurrence, after preoperative radiotherapy was reduced. It was explained with the fact that those recurrences were more frequently associated with distant metastases and with limited possibilities for further irradiation as a part of multimodality treatment. There is now solid evidence that preoperative chemoradiotherapy is able to downstage rectal tumours. In around 8–30% of cases, this can lead to complete response. Some data suggest that local control can be significantly improved and this may lead to improved long-term survival in this group of patients (Capirci, Valentini et al. 2008).

3. Follow-up

To justify the treatment of recurrent disease, including, of course local recurrence, there has to be a proof that all measures taken actually improve survival of these patients. Without proper follow-up the treatment of recurrence can`t be optimally effective.
The indiscriminate use of all tests available is expensive. In order to reduce costs, we have to have in mind specific patterns of recurrence and to stratify patients according to the risk groups. Parameters in stratification are stage of the disease, invasion of other structures, tumor fixation and grading, mucionus component of a tumor and adjuvant treatment. It would be very useful to include surgeon as a risk factor, but the extent of this influence is very difficult to assess (Seow-Choen 2002).
Additionally, follow-up is important for discovering metachronous tumors and other malignancies. Discovering early metachronous lesion is rewording and cost effective.
There are a number of studies that dealt with the problem how to administer a proper test at optimal moment.
It has been noted by some authors (Polk Jr and Spratt Jr 1971) that follow-up is appropriate if you tend to identify 2-3% of patients with recurrence per visit. They recommended this regimen for two years and to follow patients at 6 month intervals for additional 3 years. Over 90% of recurrences are discovered in first 5 years of follow-up.
Others state that patient should be followed-up for three years and divided into risk groups (Kraemer M 2001).

4. Detection of local recurrence

During follow-up, most relapses when discovered are locally advanced or combined with disseminated disease. Majority of patients with local recurrence is discovered in first two years of follow-up. Small number of these is fit enough, with resectable recurrence and no distant metastases.

Earliest possible detection of local recurrence is usually achieved by a set of tests that usually include physical examination, CEA and Ca 19-9 measurements, endoscopy and imaging (CT, NMR, ERUS and FGD-PET scan) (Beart RW 1983; Carlsson U 1983).

Usually, only one of these tests raises doubt that local recurrence may be present.

The first sensitive test to determine the presence of recurrence is to listen to the patient.

Symptoms of local recurrence usually are pelvic pain, with or without irradiation to lower extremities, rectal bleeding and change in bowel habits. Some authors tend to classify patient into groups, according to symptoms- S0 asymptomatic, S1 symptomatic, no pain, S2 symptomatic with pain (Hahnloser D 2003).

Significant number of patients (around 50%) is asymptomatic, despite existing local recurrence.

Physical examination may reveal palpable mass in the pelvis. Digital examination may reveal recurrence amenable to surgical treatment.

A list of symptoms, together with physical examination can detect recurrence in 21% of cases (Sugarbaker PH 1987).

CEA represents a glycoprotein oncofetal tumor associated antigen being expressed by more than 90% of colorectal adenocarcinomas, but it is not increased in the serum of more than 90% of patients (Cutait, Alves et al. 1991). As a marker, CEA is used to monitor treated patients for recurrent disease. The European Society for Medical Oncology (Van Cutsem and Kataja 2005; Van Cutsem, Oliveira et al. 2005) proposes CEA determination every 3-6 months for 3 years and every 6–12 months in year 4 and 5 after surgery, if initially elevated. Interestingly, it is stated that clinical, laboratory, and radiological examinations are of unconfirmed help and shall be limited to patients with suspicious symptoms. Sensitivity of this test ranges from 43 to 98% and specificity ranges from 70 to 90% (Sugarbaker PH 1987). It is difficult to ascertain what level of CEA assay should be considered as abnormal. Some define this as tree progressively rising CEA values, with at least one value over 10ng/ml (Sugarbaker PH 1987).

Currently CT scan is the preferred method for diagnosis of local recurrence (Abir, Alva et al. 2006). This examination may provide useful anatomical information. In some comparable studies CT correctly diagnosed recurrent rectal cancer in 76% of the cases (Blomqvist, Holm et al. 1996). Nevertheless, results of this examination should be taken with caution because of a significant percentage of false positive results (Sugarbaker PH 1987). In recent years, use of MSCT showed initial promising results, notably better than those achieved with regular CT scan (diagnosed pelvic recurrence in range between 82 and 97%) (Blomqvist, Holm et al. 1996).

Magnetic resonance imaging (MRI) is one of the leading imaging modalities for detection of pelvic recurrence. It is highly recommended method, due to its excellent soft-tissue resolution, providing detailed information. Compared to CT scan the distinction of recurrent cancer in presacral scar is more accurate, but still with limitations (Hughes K 1997). Routine use of MRI in follow-up is not justified (Titu, Nicholson et al. 2006). MRI should be reserved for selective patients, with suspicion rose using some other diagnostic modalities.

Fluoro-deoxy-glucose positron emission tomography (FDG-PET scan) is an accurate modality for detecting pelvic recurrence in rectal cancer patients (Fukunaga, Sekimoto et al.

2002) and may have advantages over CT and MRI scan in differentiating scar from viable tumor. The reported accuracy of FDG-PET for pelvic recurrence ranges from 74% to 96% (Gearhart, Frassica et al. 2006). Nevertheless, PET has certain limitations, inability to detect small lesions, mucionus tumors and positive lymph nodes. Radiochemotherapy is also shown to diminish sensitivity and specificity of this method (Moore, Akhurst et al. 2003; Kamel, Cohade et al. 2004; Von Schulthess, Steinert et al. 2006).

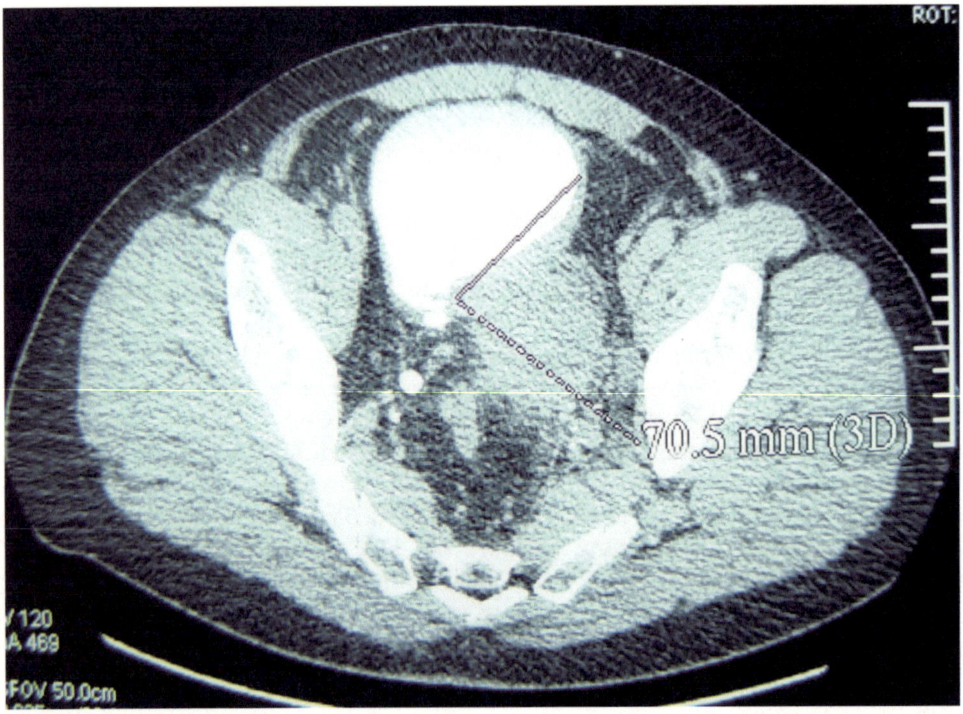

Fig. 1. Pelvic CT scan showing local recurrence with infiltration of urinary bladder

Other diagnostic methods are also available, and in some cases of crucial importance in deciding whether the patient is a candidate for curative procedure: barium enema, full lung tomography, intravenous pyelography (IVP), liver, spleen and bone scintigraphy.

Some new diagnostic tools are being evaluated, for example, carcinoembryonic antigen radioimmunodetection of colorectal cancer recurrence. It is a method compatible to CT scan and potentially can help in avoiding more invasive diagnostic methods (Hughes K 1997). Lechner et al. (Lechner, Lind et al. 1993) report an overall accuracy of 91,6% in detecting recurrent colorectal cancer, which is superior to the results that could be obtained by the means of CT scan and/or endoscopy. Also, immunoscintigraphy detected more lesions in extrahepatic areas, compared to CT scan (Lechner, Lind et al. 1993).

In ideal circumstances a diagnostic laparascopy could provide accurate information, and help in avoiding further, more invasive surgery. However, aside from its invasive nature, sometimes is very difficult to explore all areas of interest, without excessive manipulation.

When all other, non-invasive diagnostic methods fail to confirm the existence of highly possible existence of recurrent tumor, "second look" surgery is indicated.

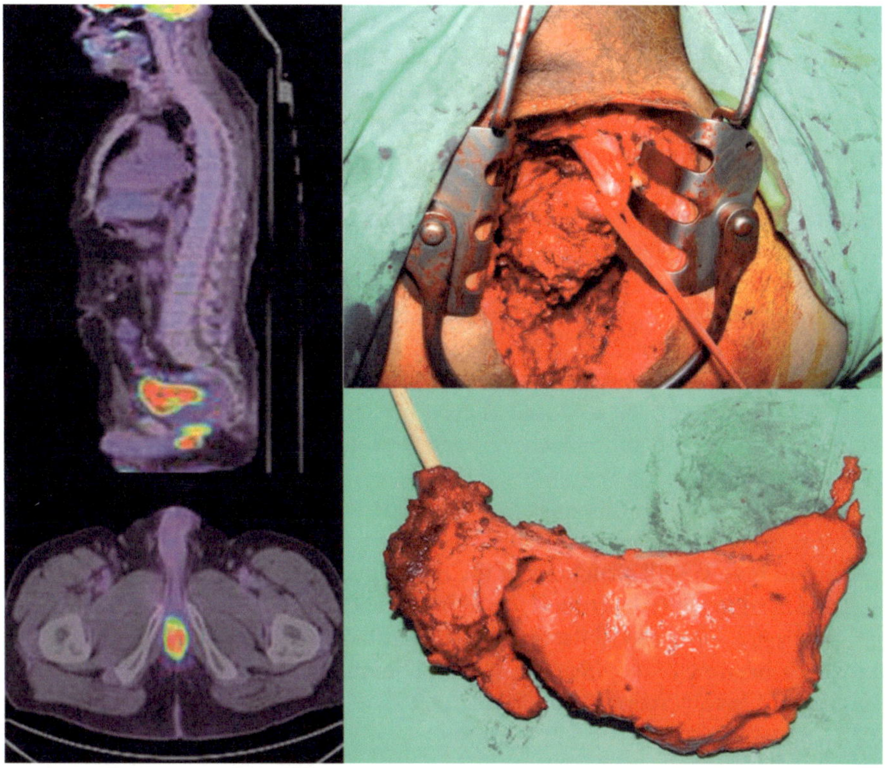

Fig. 2. PET/CT showing recurrent rectal cancer in the base of penis, imaging performed after CRT; intraoperative finding and specimen with visible recurrent tumor

5. Classification of local recurrence

Many authors have tried to classify local recurrence. The Mayo Clinic authors (Suzuki, Dozois et al. 1996) divided local recurrence in terms of level of fixation both in context of site (anterior, sacral, right, or left) and number of points of fixation (F0 non-fixed, F1 fixed to the one side, F2 two sides, and F3 three or more sides). Patients with more extensive fixation presented later and had more complications after salvage surgery and in our practice we tend to employ this classification. Others (Wanebo, Antoniuk et al. 1999) proposed a classification system based on the UICC TNM system (Sobin L (1997 5th edition)); TR 1 and2 -intraluminal local recurrence at the primary resection site; TR3-anastomotic recurrence with full thickness penetration beyond the bowel wall and into the perirectal fat tissue; TR4-invasion into adjacent organs including vagina, uterus, prostate, bladder, seminal vesicles or presacral tissues with tethering but not fixation and TR5-invasion in the bony ligamentous pelvis including sacrum, low pelvic/side walls, or sacrotuberous/ischial ligaments.
Of course, there are many other classifications, but the idea is similar to the mentioned ones.

6. Surgical management of local recurrence

Multimodal therapy is required when managing local recurrence of rectal cancer, a considerable challenge for a surgeon. Contrary to the majority of other locally recurrent tumors in the digestive system, it's possible to radically remove locally recurrent rectal cancer.

As different studies show (Tschmelitsch J 1994; Wiggers T 1996; Bozzeti F 1997) 5-year survival after reresection is 2-13 % of all patients with locally recurrent cancer, both alone and associated with distant metastases. We can say that the goals of this kind of surgery are respectively: palliation of symptoms, a good quality of life and, if possible, cure with low treatment-related complication rate.

The primary goal of surgical intervention is to achieve *en bloc* R0 resection, if it's technically feasible and safe. Radical R0 resection can be attained in 30-60% of cases.

Palliation can also be a very important goal of re-resection, preferably without extensive surgical procedures, unless disabling complications of sepsis or bleeding are an issue.

The decision for salvage surgery should be brought on the basis of:

- Patients general health-the patient should be fit enough for potentially extensive surgery.
- Necessary surgical expertise should also be available for these operations, which should be undertaken in the specialized centers were a multidisciplinary team is available (Carlsson U 1983).

The most important issue in this matter is to decide when to avoid surgical treatment. The first and most obvious contraindication for surgery is "frozen pelvis", the condition where recurrent tumor involves all structures of the minor pelvis, including the pelvic walls.

The next contraindication is clinical or CT evidence of invasion of the pelvic nerves, lymphatics or veins, or ureters bilaterally (as indicated by the presence of sciatic pattern of pain, unilateral swelling of the lower limb and bilateral hydronephosis, respectively).

Also, evidence of involvement of the lateral pelvic sidewalls and/or upper sacral marrow, above S2 level is an absolute contraindication for surgery (Bergamaschi R 2001).

Every surgical procedure begins with an explorative laparatomy. Peritoneal seeding, unexpected liver metastases and invasion of para-aoric lymph nodes are, in general, contraindications for continuing with a procedure. It is recommended to avoid injury of critical structures before the decision on resectability.

Pelvic recurrences are usually amenable to resection if they are strictly anterior or posterior. Lateral sidewall involvement diminishes a chance for R0 resection, as well as involvement of two pelvic walls simultaneously (fixation degree F2). Recurrent tumor that occurs below S2 level is amenable to resection by distal sacrectomy; unfortunately, the existence of tumor in this location usually excludes R0 resection. Similarly, unilateral tumor involvement of blood vessels distal to the aorta may be resectable, bilateral affection of these structures with the recurrent tumor is a contraindication for radical resection. When prostate or base of the bladder are minimally adherent to the recurrent tumor, and have good function it's preferable to attempt combined external-beam radio therapy (EBRT) with infusional 5-FU, followed by organ preserving resection and intra-operative radio therapy (IORT). The alternative to this is pelvic exenteration. In cases of more advanced disease and the existence of severe postoperative and postirradiational adhesions, this can't be avoided.

Another downside of surgery for recurrent rectal tumor is the problem of intestinal continuity. It's rarely possible or reasonable to create another anastomosis in that kind of surroundings which is at high risk of another relapse. In some series of patients treated for local recurrence (Salo JC 1999) even 93 % of them ended up with permanent colostomy. Nevertheless, sometimes, in highly motivated patients with favorable local findings (mucosal anastomotic recurrence), it's possible to perform a low coloanal anastomosis. To perform a low anterior resection with anastomosis, in these situations, moderate doses of preoperative EBRT and chemotherapy are needed. Unfortunately, usually, a previous low

AR is being converted to an APR, and previous APR to an abdominosacral resection or pelvic exenteration.

If at the end of resection if decided that postoperative EBRT in needed, vascular clips should be placed in the area of peritumoral fibrosis or residual tumor tissue (Gunderson LL 2002).

Extensive procedures employed in treatment of local recurrence carry significant risk. Patients suffer significant blood loss, morbidity, mortality, longer hospital stay and operative time. Postoperative complications also occur: infectious disease (sepsis, intrabdominal abscess, enteric fistula, wound infection), urinary disease (fistulous communications with other organs, stenosis, anastomotic leak), and bowel obstruction (Yamada K 2002). The incidence of complications after abdominosacral resection, for example, according to some authors, is higher than 80%. The commonest are: perineal wound complication (48%) and urinary retention/incontinence, followed by peritonitis, pneumonia, pyelonephritis, and different fistulous communications, respectively (Mannaerts G 2001).

Mortality rates after these complicated procedures are less than 5% (Bergamaschi R 2001).

7. Adjuvant therapy

It is very difficult to surgically achieve desired aim of the treatment for local recurrence i.e. clear margins of resection for reasons of non existing clear planes disrupted by previous surgery. Preoperative radiotherapy is often administered to patients with local recurrence in order to improve outcome. But since a lot of these patients already received radiotherapy prior to the initial operation; question arises on the matter of possible complications of re-irradiation of tissue within the pelvis. It is usually possible to give a further 30-40 Gy if we can exclude small bowel (Glimelius 2003). Reduction of pain and bleeding was achieved in majority of patients, whereas a response to other pelvic symptoms was not apparent. Unfortunately, the duration of effective palliation is achieved for only about one third of remaining life span of the patient (Wong, Cummings et al. 1998).

Also, complications of this mode of therapy are not to be disregarded.

In conclusion, EBRT and IORT when combined only with R0 resection improve results of therapy (Alektiar, Zelefsky et al. 2000).

Chemotherapy as a component of aggressive treatment approach is recommended, because a local relapse is a prelude of distant metastases in about 50 % of cases (Lybert Ml 1992).

8. Prognostic factors

A number of factor influence the outcome of local recurrence treatment.

Age, gender and the initial stage of primary tumor do not appear to change postresection survival rate (Salo JC 1999). Prior APR, presentation with pain, elevated CEA levels and unresectable disease are adverse factors. Completeness of resection strongly influences survival, which is significantly shorter in R2, than in R0 and R1 cases. R0 resection is, of course, in correlation with the best results.

Patients with prior APR have significantly worse prognosis than those with AR. They more frequently present with pain, elevated CEA levels, and experience longer period between primary and salvage operation. Longer period is explained with no possibility for digital examination, sigmoidoscopoy, or changes in bowel habits. Reported resectability rate after APR is 60% and after AR is 86 % (Salo JC 1999). But on the positive side, in case of resectable

disease, there is no statistically significant difference in postsalvage survival rates between APR and AR, though results after AR tend to be better (Bozzeti F 1997). As mentioned, the best results in salvage surgery are achieved after local excision when the indication for operation is unfavorable patohistological report.
In other cases, the most favorable outcome is achieved with patients who had recurrent disease within the bowel wall (Salo JC 1999).
Many attempts have been made to determine the value of prognostic predictors, for patients planned for curative salvage surgery (St. Marks group, Mayo Clinic group). So far, no consensus was made. The only predictive factor, for now, that appears to be valuable is the tumor diameter larger than 3 cm, and tumor fixation degree 2. However, it can be useful to follow the recommended tests, CEA level of 9 ng/ml, if reached in non-smokers, laparatomy is indicated even if all other tests are negative (Selvaggi, Cuocolo et al. 2003).

9. Conclusion

Recurrent rectal cancer remains considerable therapeutical problem. Without surgery acceptable quality of life or long survival are not to be expected. Salvage surgery for well selected patients is nowadays well established and offers a realistic hope for long survival and possibly cure. Even if no cure is possible, acceptable palliation of symptoms offers good quality of life for these patients.
Close follow-up and early detection of recurrence are conditions for curative salvage surgery. Advanced stage of disease may not always be a contraindication for operative treatment, providing a good surgical strategy and tactics.
Multidisciplinary approach and teamwork are ultimate conditions for success. Besides surgery, which is a dominant method of treatment other modalities of therapy, namely hemoradiotherapy, should be employed.

10. References

Abir, F., S. Alva, et al. (2006). "The postoperative surveillance of patients with colon cancer and rectal cancer." American Journal of Surgery 192(1): 100-108.

Alektiar, K. M., M. J. Zelefsky, et al. (2000). "High-dose-rate intraoperative brachytherapy for recurrent colorectal cancer." International Journal of Radiation Oncology Biology Physics 48(1): 219-226.

Beart RW, O. C. M. (1983). "Postoperative follow up of patients with carcinoma of the colon." Mayo Clin Proc 58: 361-363.

Bergamaschi R, P. P., Burtin P, Arnaud JP (2001). "Abdominoperineal resection for locally recurrent rectal cancer." Tech Coloproctol 5: 97-102.

Birbeck KF, M. C., Tiffin NJ, et al (2002). "Rates of circumferential resection margin involvement vary between surgeons and predict outcomes in rectal cancer surgery." Ann Surg 235: 449-457.

Blomqvist, L., T. Holm, et al. (1996). "MR imaging, CT and CEA scintigraphy in the diagnosis of local recurrence of rectal carcinoma." Acta Radiologica 37(5): 779-784.

Borschitz, T., D. Wachtlin, et al. (2008). "Neoadjuvant chemoradiation and local excision for T2-3 rectal cancer." Annals of Surgical Oncology 15(3): 712-720.

Bozzeti F, B. L., Rosseti C et al (1997). "Surgical treatment of locally recurrent rectal carcinoma." Dis Colon Rectum 40: 1421-1424.

Capirci, C., V. Valentini, et al. (2008). "Prognostic Value of Pathologic Complete Response After Neoadjuvant Therapy in Locally Advanced Rectal Cancer: Long-Term Analysis of 566 ypCR Patients." International Journal of Radiation Oncology Biology Physics 72(1): 99-107.

Carlsson U, S. J., Ekelund G, Leandoer L (1983). "Is CEA analysis of value in screening for recurrences after surgery for colorectal carcinoma?" Dis Colon Rectum 26: 369-373.

Choen AM, M. B. (1990). "Agrressive surgical management of locally advanced primary and recurrent rectal cancer. Current status and future directions." Dis Colon Rectum 33: 432-438.

Cutait, R., V. A. F. Alves, et al. (1991). "Restaging of colorectal cancer based on the identification of lymph node micrometastases through immunoperoxidase staining of CEA and cytokeratins." Diseases of the Colon and Rectum 34(10): 917-920.

Cuthbertson, A. M. and R. L. Simpson (1986). "Curative local excision of rectal adenocarcinoma." Australian and New Zealand Journal of Surgery 56(3): 229-231.

Das, P., J. M. Skibber, et al. (2006). "Clinical and pathologic predictors of locoregional recurrence, distant metastasis, and overall survival in patients treated with chemoradiation and mesorectal excision for rectal cancer." American Journal of Clinical Oncology: Cancer Clinical Trials 29(3): 219-224.

Friel CM, C. J., Marra C, Madoff RD (2002). "Salvage radical surgery after failed local excision for early rectal cancer." Dis Colon Rectum 45: 875-879.

Fukunaga, H., M. Sekimoto, et al. (2002). "Clinical relevance of fusion images using (18)F-2-fluoro-2-deoxy-D-glucose positron emission tomography in local recurrence of rectal cancer." International journal of oncology 20(4): 691-695.

Gagliardi, G., P. R. Hawley, et al. (1995). "Prognostic factors in surgery for local recurrence of rectal cancer." British Journal of Surgery 82(10): 1401-1405.

Gearhart, S. L., D. Frassica, et al. (2006). "Improved staging with pretreatment positron emission tomography/computed tomography in low rectal cancer." Annals of Surgical Oncology 13(3): 397-404.

Glimelius, B. (2003). "Recurrent rectal cancer. The pre-irradiated primary tumour: Can more radiotherapy be given?" Colorectal Disease 5(5): 501-503.

Gunderson LL, N. H., Martenson JA et al. (2002). "Treatment of localy advanced primary and locally recurrent colorectal cancer." IN: Bleiberg H (ed) Colorectal cancer, a clinical guide to therapy Martin Dunitz, London: 205-227.

Hahnloser D, N. H., Gunderson LL et al. (2003). "Curative potential of multimodality therapy for locally recurrent rectal cancer." Ann Surg 4: 502-508.

Heald RJ, S. R., Kald A, Sexton R, Moran BJ. (1997). "Abdominoperineal excision of the rectum - an endangered operation. Norman Nigro Lectureship." Dis Colon Rectum 40: 747-51.

Holm, T., B. Cedermark, et al. (1994). "Local recurrence of rectal adenocarcinoma after 'curative' surgery with and without preoperative radiotherapy." British Journal of Surgery 81(3): 452-455.

Holm, T., A. Ljung, et al. (2007). "Extended abdominoperineal resection with gluteus maximus flap reconstruction of the pelvic floor for rectal cancer." British Journal of Surgery 94(2): 232-238.

Hughes K, P. C., Petrelly NJ et al. (1997). "Use of carcinoemryonic antigen radioimmunodetection and computed tomography for predicting the resectability of recurrent colorectal cancer." Ann Surg 226: 621-631.

Juhl G, L. G., Mullins R, Bond S (1990). "Six-year results of annual colonoscopy after resection of colorectal cancer." World J Surg 14: 255.

Kaiser, A. M., J. C. Kang, et al. (2006). "The prognostic impact of the time interval to recurrence for the mortality in recurrent colorectal cancer." Colorectal Disease 8(8): 696-703.

Kamel, I. R., C. Cohade, et al. (2004). "Incremental value of CT in PET/CT of patients with colorectal carcinoma." Abdominal Imaging 29(6): 663-668.

Killingback M, B. P., Dent O (2001). "Local recurrence after curative resection of the rectum without total mesorectal excision." Dis Colon Rectum 44(4): 473-483.

Kim, C. J., T. J. Yeatman, et al. (2001). "Local excision of T2 and T3 rectal cancers after downstaging chemoradiation." Annals of Surgery 234(3): 352-359.

Kim, Y. W., N. K. Kim, et al. (2009). "Factors associated with anastomotic recurrence after total mesorectal excision in rectal cancer patients." Journal of Surgical Oncology 99(1): 58-64.

Kjeldsen, B. J., O. Kronborg, et al. (1997). "The pattern of recurrent colorectal cancer in a prospective randomised study and the characteristics of diagnostic tests." International Journal of Colorectal Disease 12(6): 329-334.

Kraemer M, W. S., Seow-Choen F et al (2001). "Stratifying risk factors for follow-up: a comparation of recurrent and nonrecurrent colorectal cancer." Dis Colon Rectum 44(6): 815-821.

Krivokapic Z, B. G., Markovic V, et al. (2004). "First thousand rectal cancer cases: local recurrence and survival." Acta Chir Iugosl 2: 133-137.

Krivokapic Z, B. G., Markovic V, et al. (2002). "Local recurrence and five year survival after abdominoperineal resection of the rectum due to rectal carcinoma." Acta Chir Iugosl 49(2): 19-22.

Law WL, C. K. (2000). "Resectio of local recurrence of rectal cancer: results." World J Surg 24: 486-490.

Lechner, P., P. Lind, et al. (1993). "Anticarcinoembryonic antigen immunoscintigraphy with a 99mTc-Fab' fragment (Immu 4(TM)) in primary and recurrent colorectal cancer: A prospective study." Diseases of the Colon and Rectum 36(10): 930-935.

Lezoche, G., M. Baldarelli, et al. (2008). "A prospective randomized study with a 5-year minimum follow-up evaluation of transanal endoscopic microsurgery versus laparoscopic total mesorectal excision after neoadjuvant therapy." Surgical Endoscopy and Other Interventional Techniques 22(2): 352-358.

Lopez-Kostner, F., V. W. Fazio, et al. (2001). "Locally recurrent rectal cancer: Predictors and success of salvage surgery." Diseases of the Colon and Rectum 44(2): 173-178.

Lybert Ml, M. H., de Neve W et al (1992). "Radiotherapy for locoregional relapses of rectal carcinoma after initial surgery: definite but limited influence of relapse free survival and survival." Int J Radiat Oncol Biol Phys 24: 241-246.

MacFarlane, J. K., R. D. H. Ryall, et al. (1993). "Mesorectal excision for rectal cancer." Lancet 341(8843): 457-460.

Madsen, P. M. and J. Christiansen (1986). "Distal intramural spread of rectal carcinomas." Diseases of the Colon and Rectum 29(4): 279-282.

Manfredi S, B. A., Meny B et al (2001). "Population-based study of factors influencing occurrence and prognosis of local recurrence after surgery for rectal cancer." Br J Surg 88: 1221-1227.

Mannaerts G, R. H., Martijn H et al. (2001). "Abdominosacral resection for primary irresectable and locally recurrent rectal cancer " Dis Colon Rectum 44: 806-814.

Martling A, C. B., Johansson H, et al. (2002). "The surgeon as a prognostic factor after the introduction of total mesorectal excision in the treatment of rectal cancer." Br J Surg 89(8): 1008-1013.

McCall JL, C. M., Wattchow DA (1995). "Analysis of local recurrence rates after surgery alone for rectal cancer." Int J Colorectal Dis 10: 126-132.

Micev M, K. Z., Popov I (2000). "Prognoza bolesnika sa potencijalno izlečivim karcinomom kolorektuma." Srp Arh Celok Lek 130: 1-6.

Moore, H. G., T. Akhurst, et al. (2003). "A case-controlled study of 18-fluorodeoxyglucose positron emission tomography in the detection of pelvic recurrence in previously irradiated rectal cancer patients." Journal of the American College of Surgeons 197(1): 22-28.

Nagtegaall ID, v. d. V. C., van der Worp E, et al (2002). "Macroscopic avaluation of rectal cancer resectio specimen: Clinical significance of the pathologist in quality control." J Clin Oncol 20: 1729-1734.

Polk Jr, H. C. and J. S. Spratt Jr (1971). "Recurrent colorectal carcinoma: Detection, treatment, and other considerations." Surgery 69(1): 9-23.

Quirke, P. and M. F. Dixon (1988). "The prediction of local recurrence in rectal adenocarcinoma by histopathological examination." International Journal of Colorectal Disease 3(2): 127-131.

Quirke P, D. P., Dixon MF, et al. (1986). "Local recurrence of rectal adenocarcinoma due to inadequate surgical resection: Histologic study of lateral tumour spread and surgical excision." Lancet 2: 996-999.

Rothenberger, D. A. and W. D. Wong (1985). "Rectal cancer--adequacy of surgical management." Surgery annual 17: 309-336.

Salo JC, P. P., Jose G, Minsky BD, harrison LB, Cohen AM (1999). "Surgical salvage of recurrent rectal carcinoma after currative resection: a 10-year experience." Ann Surg Oncol 6: 171-177.

Selvaggi, F., A. Cuocolo, et al. (2003). "FGD-PET in the follow-up of recurrent colorectal cancer." Colorectal Disease 5(5): 496-500.

Seow-Choen, F. (2002). "Adjuvant therapy for rectal cancer cannot be based on the results of other surgeons." British Journal of Surgery 89(8): 946-947.

Sobin L, W. C. ((1997 5th edition)). UICC International Union Against Cancer: TNM classification of malignant tumours. New York, John Wiley and Sons. Inc.

Sugarbaker PH, G. F., Dwyer A, Newman NR (1987). "A simplified plan for follow-up of patients with colon and rectal cancer supported by prospective studies of laboratory and radiologic test results." Surgery 1: 79-87.

Suzuki, K., R. R. Dozois, et al. (1996). "Curative reoperations for locally recurrent rectal cancer." Diseases of the Colon and Rectum 39(7): 730-736.

Tepper JE, O. C. M., Hollins D et al (2003). "Analysis of surgical salvage after failure of primary therapy in rectal cancer: results of intergroup study 0114." J Clin Oncol 21: 3623-3628.

Titu, L. V., A. A. Nicholson, et al. (2006). "Routine follow-up by magnetic resonance imaging does not improve detection of resectable local recurrences from colorectal cancer." Annals of Surgery 243(3): 348-352.

Tschmelitsch J, K. P., Glaser K et al. (1994). "Survival after surgical treatment of recurrent carcinoma of the rectum." J Am Coll Surg 179: 54-58.

Van Cutsem, E. J. D. and V. V. Kataja (2005). "ESMO minimum clinical recommendations for diagnosis, adjuvant treatment and follow-up of colon cancer." Annals of Oncology 16(SUPPL. 1): i16-i17.

Van Cutsem, E. J. D., J. Oliveira, et al. (2005). "ESMO minimum clinical recommendations for diagnosis, treatment and follow-up of advanced colorectal cancer." Annals of Oncology 16(SUPPL. 1): i18-i19.

Von Schulthess, G. K., H. C. Steinert, et al. (2006). "Integrated PET/CT: Current applications and future directions." Radiology 238(2): 405-422.

Wanebo, H. J., P. Antoniuk, et al. (1999). "Pelvic resection of recurrent rectal cancer: Technical considerations and outcomes." Diseases of the Colon and Rectum 42(11): 1438-1448.

West, N. P., P. J. Finan, et al. (2008). "Evidence of the oncologic superiority of cylindrical abdominoperineal excision for low rectal cancer." Journal of Clinical Oncology 26(21): 3517-3522.

Wiggers T, d. W. M., Veeze-Kuypers B (1996). "Surgery for local recurrence of rectal carcinoma." Dis Colon Rectum 39: 323-328.

Wiggers, T., G. H. H. Mannaerts, et al. (2003). "Surgery for locally recurrent rectal cancer." Colorectal Disease 5(5): 504-507.

Williams, N. S., M. F. Dixon, et al. (1983). "Reappraisal of the 5 centimetre rule of distal excision for carcinoma of the rectum: A study of distal intramural spread and of patients' survival." British Journal of Surgery 70(3): 150-154.

Wong, C. S., B. J. Cummings, et al. (1998). "Treatment of locally recurrent rectal carcinoma - Results and prognostic factors." International Journal of Radiation Oncology Biology Physics 40(2): 427-435.

Yamada K, I. T., Niwa K et al. (2002). "Pelvic exenteration and sacral resection for locally advanced primary and recurrent rectal cancer." Dis Colon Rectum 45: 1078-1084.

13

Causes and Prevention of Functional Disturbances Following Low Anterior Resection for Rectal Cancer

Eberhard Gross
Asklepios Medical School Hamburg
Germany

1. Introduction

Surgical therapy of a colon carcinoma does not usually affect the patient's quality of life in the medium or long term, if the tumor does not involve adjacent organs and there are no post-operative complications. In rectal cancer, however, dysfunctions such as anal continence disorders occur in quite a few patients following anterior resection, and particularly low anterior resection (LAR) with total mesorectal excisison (TME), as a result of the total or almost total loss of the rectum, and disorders of the bladder and sexual function can occur because the autonomic nerves, which regulate bladder and sexual function as well as anal continence, are often damaged due to their anatomical proximity. Not only have healing rates improved with the introduction and more general use of total mesorectal excision, the local recurrence rates have fallen below 10 %, in part below 5 %, with TME and neoadjuvant radiotherapy or radio chemotherapy, so that disorders which affect quality of life naturally take on more importance for the individual patient, especially if he has been healed, but are also considered to be increasingly important by the surgeon. In the past decade anal continence disturbance has become quantitatively more significant, since the majority of patients with a rectal tumor undergo anterior resection. Hence 70 - 90% of rectal tumors can currently be operated with sphincter-preserving surgery without violating oncological principles. Rectal cancer surgery thus aims both at preventing a local recurrence and at preserving anal continence and bladder and sexual function. The risk of injury to the autonomic nerves is naturally greater when the tumor is more advanced, when the surgery is more extensive and the cancer itself is closer to the autonomic nerves, as is the case when the tumor is localized in the lower or middle third of the ventral circumference of the rectum, so that bladder and sexual dysfunction occur most frequently in this tumor site or after abdomino-perineal excision (APE). Further risk factors for dysfunction are age , local postoperative complications and radio- or radio-chemotherapy, in particular adjuvant therapy.

If the appropriate surgical technique is applied, dysfunction can generally be avoided if the tumor is not so advanced that parts of the bladder, the prostate or the posterior vaginal wall and autonomic nerves also have to be resected. In such cases a preparation technique which causes no mechanical or thermal damage to the autonomic nerves is important.

With ever increasing knowledge of the complex function of anal continence and the causes of postoperative disorders, surgical techniques and post-operative measures have been adopted which do not completely rule out continence disorders, but with which they can be largely avoided, or at least reduced, so that they do not significantly affect quality of life.

2. Anal continence disorders

2.1 Anterior resection syndrome, diagnostics

Anal continence is a complex function and is made possible by different continence factors with their specific anatomical and physiological substrates (Tab. 1), including the visceral and somatic muscles, the rectum with its reservoir function and the extremely sensitive anoderm, which is capable of discrimination. The continence organ is controlled neurologically at the local spinal and cerebral level. Continence is affected if one of the continence factors, such as discrimination is deficient or the compliance of the remaining rectum or the replacement rectum is deminished. Depending on the cause, anal continence dysfunction, in addition to incontinence in the true sense, can manifest itself in various ways, including in evacuation disorders. This clinical picture is now known as anterior resection syndrome and includes the following symptoms: repetitive imperative urge to defecate post defecation, increased stool frequency, shortened warning period, incomplete bowel movements, fragmented defecation, increased stool frequency due to errors in diet, decreased stool consistency, nocturnal bowel movements, no formed stool, the need for increased abdominal pressure, and incontinence of varying degrees of severity (Tab2 (156). Continence disorders can be objectified with the different continence scores, although the most common ones, such as the Cleveland Clinic Continence Score and the Fecal Index Severity Score (Tab.3), only cover incontinence as such. Scores which also ask about other symptoms, such as discrimination, help to determine both the severity of the incontinence and to localize the causes of the continence disorders or the anterior resection syndrome. A proctologic examination is obligatory for diagnosing continence disorders. Whether further examinations, such as anal sonography, defecation radiography or a dynamic MRT of the pelvis are necessary, will depend on whether the findings have therapeutic consequences.

rectal distension	stretching receptors in the pelvic floor musculature and (?) lateral pelvic wall
sensory discrimination	free ending nerve fibers und org.nerve cells in the anoderm und transitional zone
anal high pressure zone	internal sphincter (70-80%)
	external sphincter (20 %) hemorrhoids (15 %)
sampling	rectoanal inhibitory reflex
reservoir function	compliance: 4-14 ml/cm H_2O,sensory volume: 10-70 ml maximal tolerable volume: 300 ml
voluntary contraction) (squeeze)	external sphincter
Reflectory increase of anal pressure	puborectal reflex, muscle spindles in external sphincter

Table 1. Factors of continence and their anatomical und physiological substrates

Fragmentationof stool
Frequent bowel movement
Repetitive urge to defecate
Shortened warning period
Disturbed discrimination
Incontinence of various degree of severity
Incomplete evacuation
Nocturnal bowel movement
Decreased stool consistency
Frequent bowel movement due to error in diet
Need for abdominal pressure

Table 2. Symptoms of the anterior rectum resection syndrome

	2 or more times a day	Once a day	2 or more times a week	Once a week	1 or 3 times a month	never
gas	O	O	O	O	O	O
mucus	O	O	O	O	O	O
liquid stool	O	O	O	O	O	O
solid stool	O	O	O	O	O	O

Table 3. Fecal Incontinence Severity Index (FISI)

3. Causes of anterior resection syndrome

3.1 Diminished reservoir function

Retrospective studies show that more than half the patients with straight coloanal anastomosis (26,27,73,127,162,163) and about 30 to 50 % of patients with straight low colorectal anastomosis (12,14,106,107,137) suffer from continence disorders after low anterior resection. The inevitable extensive or complete loss of the rectum after LAR and TME results in reduced compliance and a decrease in maximal tolerable volume (MTV) and sensory volume (SV). The reservoir function of the remaining rectum or the rectal replacement can be quantified with these parameters. A post-operative reduction in these parameters could be measured in patients compared with pre-operatively (5,25,89,115,123,161), as well as in patients compared with healthy controls (25,39,154,158). Compliance is also influenced by the height of the anastomosis and the length of the rectal stump. Anastomotic leakages (44,115) with consecutive scarring of the wall of the replacement rectum or the remaining rectum and late radiation reactions following adjuvant radio chemotherapy with the formation of a rigid wall in the neorectum naturally also result in reduced compliance, and thus to deterioration in the reservoir function

3.2 Reduction in resting anal pressure (RP) due to stretching trauma

Many manometric studies before and after low anterior resection have shown a reduction in resting anal pressure up to one year post-operatively compared with pre-operatively, regardless of whether the reconstruction had been made with a colon pouch or with a straight coloanal or colorectal anastomosis (5,25,30,37,66,69,72,71,89,158,161). As might be expected, these findings were also seen following intersphincteric resection (80.106,145). Several studies show that resting anal pressure in patients is significantly reduced for up to one year after surgery compared with healthy controls (161). Several studies have also shown that stretching trauma plays a significant role in reducing resting anal pressure: in a randomized (55) significantly reduced resting anal pressure was found after LAR with stapled anastomosis compared with the group with hand-sewn anastomosis from the abdomen according to HAR. The lesion on the internal sphincter caused by the stapler could also be verified endosonographically six months after the operation (38), and up to 2 years postoperatively (28). Intra-operative measurement of resting anal pressure at each step of the operation during a LAR, from the beginning of anesthesia through to anastomosis, showed that resting anal pressure levels decreased significantly only after stapler anastomosis (61). Intersphincteric resection is associated with considerable stretching trauma. Hence a significantly shorter functional length of anal canal was found measuring resting anal pressure in the group with intersphincteric resection compared with LAR with TME, LAR with PME and with HAR (53). With regard to the role of stretching trauma as the reason for reduced resting anal pressure, as expected no difference was found between patients with and without a pouch system (10.37,40), or between groups with different anastomotic heights (66,90,105).

3.3 Disorders of sphincter function due to lesions of the autonomic nervous system

The autonomic nerves at the pelvic plane of inlet and in the pelvis (Fig1.) can be damaged at various points in their course during anterior resection, particularly during LAR with TME. The inferior mesenteric plexus is formed at the level of the inferior mesenteric artery by taking up fibers from the sympathetic chain. After running the aorta the nerve fibers fuse at the level of the bifurcation and the promontory to the superior hypogastric plexus, a flat, plate-like structure, which branches below the promontory into the hypogastric nerves. These consist mainly of preganglionic sympathetic fibers from T8 to L2 and fuse with parasympathetic splanchnic nerves from S2 to S4, occasionally also from S5 (108) to the inferior hypogastric plexus. This is also a flat structure, which in women is more triangular with a posterior base. The plexus receives irregular afferents from the sacral sympathetic ganglia (108). It lies on the fascia pelvis parietalis interna and the pelvic wall. The postganglionic fibers then lead from the plexus in bundles of nerve fibers to the pelvic organs, the seminal vesicles and the prostate, the bladder and the anorectum and the internal sphincter. The cavernous nerve is formed periprostatic, passes through the pelvic floor and reaches the corpora cavernosa. Six nerve fiber bundles leading to the organs were identified in female corpses (109). Afferent fibers also lead from the pelvic organs into the inferior hypogastric plexus.

The external sphincter is supplied via the pudendal nerve, which is formed from the roots of S2 -S4, leaves the pelvis through the piriform foramen and, after emerging from the alcock's canal, runs along the outer side of the levator to the fascia pelvis parietalis externa. The pudendal nerve also consist of sensitive fibers. The levator muscle itself is supplied by the levator nerve, which are also formed from S2 to S4 and run under the fascia pelvis parietalis interna on the inside of the levator muscle. They also supply a portion of the external anal sphincter (150)

The aganglionic internal sphincter tone is generated by myogenic pacemakers, relaxation is regulated by nonadrenergic and noncholinergic fibers (NANC) which release NO ,VIP or

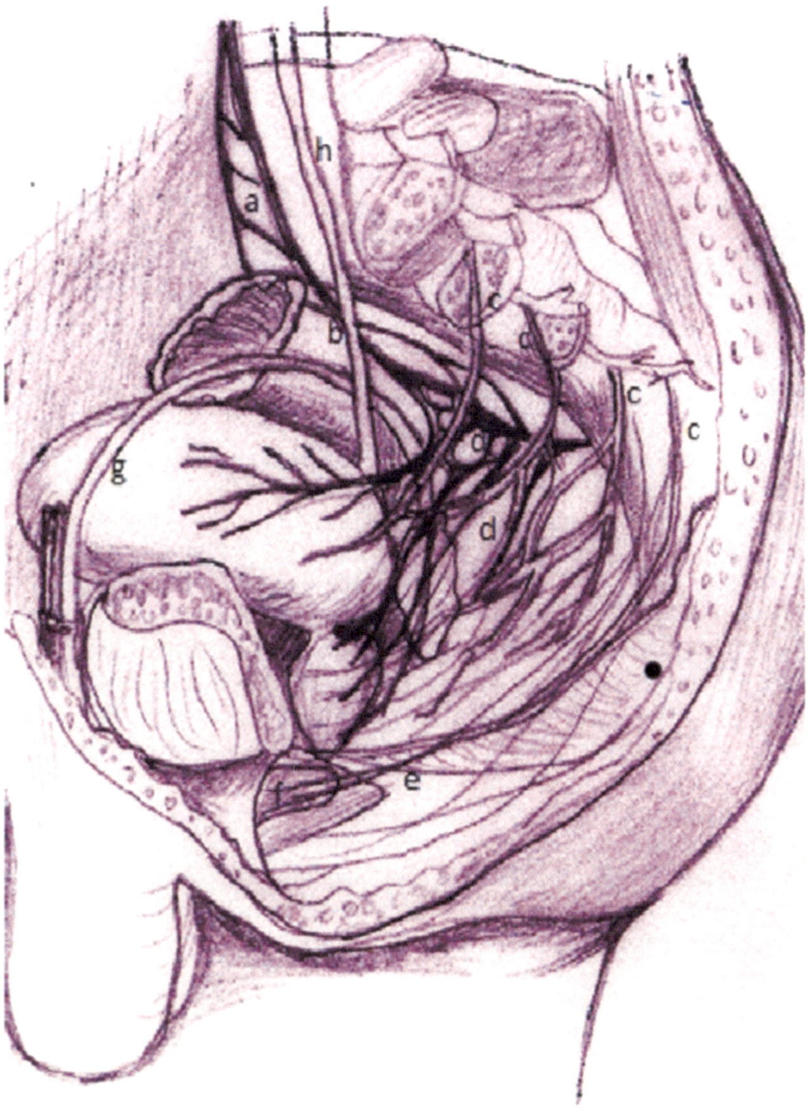

Fig. 1. Pelvic autonomic nerves left lateral aspect. a.superor hypogastric plexus b. splanchnic nerves (parasympathetic) c. hypogastric nerve d. inferior hypogastric plexus e. cavernosous nerve f. corpora cavernosa g. deferens duct h. ureter

ATP (120). The internal sphincter is controlled by the intrinsic and extrinsic nervous systems with their sympathetic and parasympathetic fibers, whereby stimulation of the sympathicus has an excitatory effect. Hence it was possible to trigger a contraction of the internal sphincter by stimulating the hypogastric nerve electrically during rectal resection (19). Blocking the sympathicus with high spinal anesthesia led to a significant reduction in resting anal pressure compared with a parasympathetic blockade using low spinal

anesthesia (31). The activity of the internal sphincter is controlled predominantly by the alpha adrenergic mechanism, as has been shown in in vitro studies using preparations from different species and from humans (34,104), as well as in in vivo studies (4).
The pelvic floor and the external and internal sphincters (164)) are controlled by special motor neurons, the Onuf nucleus, which lies between the spinal cord segments S2 and S3, medial to the ganglion cells in the anterior horn.
Long-term studies of anal continence disorders in the Dutch rectal cancer study patient collective showed that 41.4 % suffered from anal continence disorders preoperatively and 48.7% five years after surgery, and that in 38.8% anal incontinence had newly developed as a result of the treatment. Risk factors were preoperative continence disorders and radiotherapy (159). The greatest risk of injury to the autonomic nerves is at the level of the so-called "rectal stalk" or "rectal pillar", where the splanchnic nerves which are attached to the inferior hypogastric plexus are found. The rectal stalk is formed when the mesorectum is detached dorsally. If these are not detached from the fascia recti they will be unavoidably severed. A further risk of injury occurs if the rectal stalk is stretched and detached from the inferor hpogastric plexus as a result of strong contralateral tension on the mesorectum. The risk for a nerve damage, particularly to cause an erectile dysfunction (ED) may be also very high if the Denonvilliers` fascia is resected.It lies posterior to the prostate and the seminal vesicles and anterior to the thin rectal fascia.The Denonvilliers`fascia in men is regularly a leathery membrane. Immediately to the anterior lateral border of the fascia nerves run to supply the corpora cavernosa and govern the erectile function. When the tumour involves the anterior rectal quadrant ,the dissection should be conducted on the Denonvilliers fascia for oncological reason.Though the risk for a nerve damage is high with the special dissection technique these nerves can be preserved and the risk can be diminished. Damage may also be caused to the levator nerves (LAN) which supply the levator ani muscle (see above) and sometimes also parts of the external sphincter: The fascia recti and the endopelvic fascia fuse about 2- 3 cm cranially to the pelvic floor. The endopelvic fascia must be cleanly severed in order to further detach the mesorectum, in order to reach the pelvic floor along which the LAN run.
Damage to the autonomic nerves during TME has been recently described as a cause of anal continence disorders (79). The sphincter function in patients where the autonomic nerves (AN) were completely preserved was significantly better than in patients where there was some damage. To date, scant attention has been paid to the connection between damage to the AN and anal continence disorders compared with disorders of the bladder and sexual function; since anal incontinence may be due to other factors, a connection can be more difficult to establish. According to electromyographic (78) and manometric investigations of the internal sphincter on animals (4,34,53) and on humans (19) during an anterior resection while the AN is subjected to electro-stimulation, it can be assumed that lesions on the AN play a not insignificant role as a cause of anal incontinence. This is also supported by findings such as spontaneous relaxation of the internal sphincter (140) and high amplitude pressure oscillations in the anal canal, with a spontaneous marked drop in incontinent patients following coloanal reconstruction (46) and ileoanal pouch procedure(153).

3.4 Low anastomosis

Many studies show that the height of the anastomosis affects continence (105,111,116,141). High rates of incontinence have been described both for an anastomosis height below 6 cm (73) and below 4 cm (89,90,127), and after pouch anal anastomosis compared with pouch rectal anastomosis. According to Lewis (91), the height of anastomosis and the anal resting anal pressure are the continence-determining parameters. As with the influence of compliance on continence and the connection between compliance and remaining rectum, there is also a connection between the height of anastomosis and continence disorders. The fact that preservation of the distal rectum generally results in better continence, although it is only about 3 - 4 cm in length, is probably due to the particularly dense covering of rectospinal afferents, as has been seen in animals (117)

3.5 Disorders of the rectoanal inhibitory reflex

The rectoanal inhibitory reflex is important for fine continence based on the discrimination. Transient stretching of the rectum causes relaxation of the internal sphincter which triggers an involuntary decrease in resting anal pressure, whereby the amplitude and duration of relaxation until basal resting anal pressure is reached depend on the volume by which the rectum is distended. Bowel contents enter the upper anal canal while the rectum is filling as a result of this reflex, and can be perceived in the highly sensitive transitional zone and the upper anoderm. The reflex is communicated via the intrinsic nervous system, and is not triggered in patients with Hirschsprung disease as a result of the dysfunction of the intrinsic innervation. The reflex can also not be triggered initially after LAR (61,66,128), but is restored within a period of one year after the operation (25,26,83,89,121,124,141). In our own study the reflex was seen only in 40 % of patients at the first follow-up examination, and in 75 % six months later (26). An animal study has shown that restitution of the reflex is due to nerve growth which bridges the anastomosis (62).

3.6 Continence disorders following intersphincteric resection (ISR)

The entire rectum is resected during intersphincteric resection, including the mesorectum-free cloacogenic segment, to which a special sensory function is attributed (117,149). Different-sized portions of the internal sphincter are also removed during this process. In principle the ISR can also be performed from the pelvis. In our peranal approach the anoderm or the mucosa is incised circularly with the internal sphincter. After closing the rectum with a pursestring suture on the margin of the mucos and internal sphincter to avoid contamination, the actual dissection is performed in the intersphincteric plane to the level of the dissection in the pelvis. The intersphincteric resection is usually associated with poorer continence performance than LAR with colorectal anastomosis (9,12,13,14,53). In addition to the loss of the cloacogenic segment and the transitional zone with its sensory function, including the hemorrhoids with their contribution to continence, more frequent incontinence is due to the partial loss of the internal sphincter and to the greater stretching trauma involved in peranal access compared with stapler anastomosis.

3.7 Continence disorders and manometric findings

According to several studies, altered anorectal manometry parameters were detected in patients with continence disorders following LAR: a significant reduction in anal resting pressure in incontinent patients compared with continent patients (91,110,137) and an inverse correlation between functional anal canal length and stool frequency (57,) or degree of incontinence (53), significantly lower values of the volumetric parameters MTV, SV and of compliance in incontinent patients compared with continent patients (26,91,105,137), and a loss of the des recto-inhibitory reflex (26,64) or greater distension pressure to trigger the reflex (110). Saigusa(141) ascertained a deficient reflex in patients with nocturnal incontinence and an ileoanal pouch.

4. Restoration with colon pouch to improve continence

4.1 Colon J pouch (CJP)

Building on successful experience with the ileoanal pouch in familial adenomatous polyposis and ulcerative colitis following proctocolectomy, the colonic J pouch was introduced by Lazorthes and Parc (26,125)

The clinical results and manometric data have been compared with straight colorectal and coloanal anastomosis in controlled studies, including numerous randomized trials (29,33,41,54,56,63,88,100,122,123,143,146). According to a meta-analysis (49), the CJP has unique advantages compared with straight coloanal anastomosis: Bowel movement was significantly less up to 2 years after surgery, significantly fewer patients suffered from an imperative urge to defecate up to one year post-operatively and significantly fewer patients had to take antidiarrheals. According to the recent Cochrane review (15) in two out of six studies, or in two out of seven which examined the continence score, significantly fewer incontinent patients were found in the early post-operative phase (< 8 months post-operative) or in a period up to 18 months . In numerous controlled studies volumetric parameters of reservoir function, such as MTV, SV and compliance, were examined. In 13 out of 16 studies a significantly higher MTV was measured in the pouch group compared with the group without a pouch (5,32,43,52,54,64,69,82,86,102,118,122,123,160,162). In most studies the patients were examined one year post-operatively. In a randomized trial comparing 5cm and 10 cm long pouches, a significantly lower MTV was established with the smaller pouch, so that it can be assumed that the MTV is dependent on pouch volume (50). In 11 out of 12 controlled studies (5,40,43,52,54,64,49,102,143,160,162), compliance was higher in the pouch group than in the group with straight colorectal or coloanal anastomosis, in 9 studies significantly so. In 8 studies (32,50,64,82,88,123,160,162) SV was lower in the group without pouch, the majority significantly so compared with the pouch group. The studies on volumetric parameters confirm the better reservoir function of the pouch compared with straight coloanal or colorectal anastomosis.

4.2 Coloplasty v colon J pouch

The transverse coloplasty (165) consists of a plastic extension of the colon lumen about 4 cm proximal to the resection margin and similar to a pyloroplasty. It is easier to make and can be located in the pelvic floor even when there is a lot of fatty tissue in the mesocolon. In randomized studies (29,33,58,131 comparing coloplasty with the colon J pouch, no difference was found in the frequency of bowel movement in the early post-operative phase up to eight months, and the same result was seen in three studies up to 18 and 24 months respectively after surgery. In one of the studies (58) an advantage was seen with the colon J pouch with regard to imperative urge to defecate up to eight months post-operatively, however not after a longer period (29,33,131). In the studies the continence scores and use of antidiarrheals did not differ in the early post-operative period (29,33,58,131), nor in two studies covering a longer period after surgery (29,33,131). In a meta-analysis no differences were found in the SF or in the manometric and volumetric parameters (93).

4.3 Side to end anastomosis v colon J pouch

In 3 randomized studies side to end anastomosis was compared with the colon J pouch. One study showed a significantly lower SF in the colon J pouch group in the early phase after the operation (60), in two studies SF was the same in the period up to 18 months post-operatively and longer. In three studies no difference was found between the two methods with regard to imperative urge to defecate and continence score in the early post-operative phase (60,67,100), or in the medium and long term in two studies (67,101)

4.4 Von Flüe pouch

The interposition of an ileo ascending segment is more complex than the other pouch procedures and is not routine, especially as no advantages in terms of function could be shown in a randomized study compared with the CJP. It is an alternative procedure when the descending colon is missing, where the blood supply does not permit anastomosis with the left colon, or a left side nephrectomy has been performed, resulting in pronounced adhesions of the mesocolon transversum and descending colon

4.5 Clinical long-term results

90 % the 102 patients with a colon J pouch were continent in a study with a medium-term follow-up of 2.6 years (3). In a controlled study (10) comparing coloanal anastomosis and the colon J pouch no difference was found in the SF after a mean follow-up period of 10 years.

One study with a follow up period of 5 years showed a significantly less SF and imperative urge to defecate in the pouch group compared with straight colorectal anastomosis (52). In a retrospective study (45) with a follow-up of 5 years, imperative urge to defecate was less frequent in the pouch group compared with patients without a pouch. In a controlled study with a follow-up period of at least 3 years, the patients with a pouch showed significantly better results regarding SF, taking antidiarrheals and dietary restrictions (24).

5. Evacuation disorders

Evacuation disorders manifest with various symptoms: as a sensation of incomplete evacuation, as prolonged defecation time, fragmented stools, use of laxative suppositories or enemas. The first symptom is the one most frequently mentioned, as did 79% of patients after LAR with and without pouch (156). There are many reasons for evacuation disorders, and different factors may aggravate the problem.

5.1 Length of pouch

One reason for impaired evacuation following construction of a colon J-pouch is that the pouch is too long. Evacuation disturbances were observed in up to 60 % of patients when the colon J pouch was first introduced into clinical practice (11,4354,113,125,130), and this increased the more time passed after the operation (88)

The evacuation disorders were attributed to an overlong pouch, since such disorders occurred in particularly high numbers when the pouch was longer than 8 cm (11,41,113,125,130). Randomized trials with different lengths of pouch then showed a tendency to, or a significantly higher rate of evacuation disorders when the pouch was 10 cm long (30,87). Large pouches also have a tendency to dilate .In addition secondary changes which resulted in outlet obstruction, such as rectocele (51) and angulations have been described. In animal experiments it was not possible to pharmacologically stimulate the large pouch with cerelutid (142). In view of these studies, a pouch length of 5 - 6 cm is currently recommended.

5.2 Other reasons for evacuation disorders

Evacuation disorders also occur with a pouch length of 5 - 6 cm, as well as in patients without a pouch, so that the hypothesis that evacuation disorders are a side effect of the pouch, and particularly of the colon J-pouch, is not borne out. According to a meta-analysis (139), evacuation dysfunction also occurs after straight coloanal or colorectal anastomosis (SCA) and transverse coloplasty (TCP), which have indeed been recommended just in order to avoid this. According to one of the meta-analyses (139) evacuation disorders such as sensation of incomplete evacuation and fragmentation occur in the early post-operative phase in the SCA group more frequently than in patients with colon J-pouch. In the mid and long-term post-operative phase, 14.8 % and 7.7 % of patients with colon J-pouch suffer much less from either complaint than patients without pouch (29.5 % and 28.9 %). If randomized studies only are considered, significantly fewer patients suffered from prolonged defecation time. When compared with the colon J-pouch, the typical disorders do not occur less often with TCP and Side to end anastomosis in the early and medium term in the post-operative period, However, fragmentation is a problem in TCP when compared with the colon J-pouch.

The fact that evacuation dysfunction can occur as frequently after straight coloanal anastomosis as it can with a pouch shows that the reconstruction procedure is only one of several factors which cause these disorders. Damage to the internal sphincter and the autonomic nerves and interruption to the intrinsic nervous system also play a part.

6. Anastomotic leaks with a pouch and with straight coloanal anastomosis (SCA)

According to the recent the Cochrane review (15) anastomotic leaks do not occur more frequently after SCA than with the colon J-pouch and according to a recent meta-analysis which includes six randomized studies (93), there is no difference in leakage rate between the colon J-pouch and the TCP. Leakage rate in side to end anastomosis does not differ with the CLP.

7. Voiding disorders after LAR

The consequences of damage to the autonomic nerves which supply the bladder are well known from the process of lateral lymph node dissection in low advanced rectal cancer, which is sometimes performed in Japan. Extensive bilateral resection of the inferior hypogastric plexus leads to a neurogenic bladder in 78 % of patients in the third post-operative week, in 58% of patients spontaneous voluntary evacuation was not restored after 2 months (59). After unilateral resection the majority of patients can urinate spontaneously again only after 2 months. (59,99). Vesicourethral dysfunction occurs after LAR and APE in the early post-operative phase in 30 -70 % of patients if the autonomic nerves are not specifically preserved or cannot be correctly identified in an effort to preserve the nerves (1,76,77) Obstructive disorders after surgery attract more attention as they have to be treated acutely, although continence disorders are also common. A retrospective study (166) showed an increase of 19 % in imperative need to urinate post-operatively compared with 4% pre-operatively, from 9% to 26 % in pollakiuria and from 46.4% to 63% in nocturia, from

1.8% to 7.6 % in stress incontinence grade 2 and from 0.7% to 5.8 % in grade 3, complete incontinence. If they are not preexistent and if the autonomic nerves are not damaged bilaterally obstructive disorders are transient. According to a prospective study (151), 24 % of patients suffered from a voiding dysfunction which required treatment until the 14th day post-operatively, and only 8 % after two months.

7.1 Evaluating vesicourethral function

The IPSS covers 7 symptoms (75). The score allows a semi-quantitative assessment of the dysfunction. However, the IPSS should be augmented by a survey on urge incontinence and stress incontinence. The additional determination of residual urine volume is diagnostically meaningful in assessing dysfunction.

7.2 Physiology and innervation of the bladder

The external voluntary urethral sphincter is controlled by the pudendal nerve. The pudendal nerve also contains afferents which pass on bladder filling and wall tension. The smooth-muscled internal sphincter is contracted during the storage phase of the bladder. This muscle is controlled by the N. sympathicus. During the storage phase, the smooth-muscled detrusor is also inhibited by the N. sympathicus. When the bladder is emptying the external and internal sphincters relax, while the detrusor, which is subject to parasympathetic innervation, contracts. The storage phase is regulated by the spinal urine storage reflex: Contraction of the internal sphincter increases as the bladder becomes fuller. Micturition is initiated via the pontine micturation reflex: The increasing filling of the bladder activates the pontine micturation center which is responsible for inhibiting the urine storage reflex, resulting in activation of the detrusor and relaxation of the internal sphincter. The urethra-bladder reflex - during micturation the flow of urine affects detrusor contraction - serves to ensure the bladder is completely emptied.

7.3 Voiding dysfunction (VD) in preserving autonomic nerve procedure (PANP)

The fact that bladder dysfunction is caused by injury to the autonomic nerves has been established in a prospective study (70): where the autonomic nerves were completely identified during the LAR only 5.6 % of patients developed a VD compared with 38.5 % when identification was not possible. The connection between preservation of the nerves and preservation of bladder function could be demonstrated by intra-operative neuro-monitoring (77).In patients with an positive test regarding an adequate increase in bladder pressure,the IPPS items weak stream,incomplete emptying and frequency of micturition varied significantly from those with negative test result.

According to various studies, if the autonomic nerves are identified the VD rate can be expected to fall significantly to between 0 and 23 %, whereby generally rates of about 10 % and lower are given and some of the patients had a pre-existing VD (2,6,35,46,70,75,77,99,114,133). Risk factors for VD are pre-existing disorders, tumor size over 5 cm (75), deep-seated tumor and APE (155,157), blood loss (84), age > 65 years (155).

8. Sexual dysfunction

Sexual dysfunction occurs in 10 - 80 % of men after surgery for rectal cancer (8,21,22,27,36,47,60,151,157,167). When evaluating post-operative sexual function, the not infrequent pre-existing disorders and non-somatic causes must first be identified. Post-operative sexual dysfunction is predominantly caused by nerve lesions. A lesion of the hypogastric nerve or the superior hypogastric plexus (SHP) causes retrograde ejaculation. A lesion of the parasympathetic fibers (n. erigentes) causes erectile dysfunction(ED). The extent of nerve injury correlates with the degree of dysfunction. 76% of patients suffered from severe ED after ilio-pelvic lymphadenectomy (59); 48% (103) and 61 %(152) of patients experienced ED where the autonomic nerve was preserved unilaterally, and 70 % when the lesion was more extensive. The incidence is particularly high in APE because damage to the nerves is difficult to avoid in this case due to the proximity of the nerves ,which supply the corpora cavernosa. It has been recognized as a risk factor in several studies (46,47,114,155). Advanced tumors, prior surgery in the pelvis (70,147)and age > 60 years (75) have been described as further risk factors. In contrast to voiding dysfunction, sexual dysfunction is normally permanent. As with voiding dyxfunction, the rate of sexual dysfunction can be clearly reduced - to between 5 and 33 %, if the autonomic nerves are identified: (6,46,75,77,99,114,147).

8.1 Dissection techniques and outcome

During dissection it is important on the one hand to identify the autonomic nerves (AN), and on the other to avoid lesions as a result of the technique applied. Of the different procedures, such as dissection with monopolar or bipolar current, with ultrasonic instruments, the so-called bloody dissection with scissors or with a capillary high-pressure water jet (hydrojet)(Fig2), the latter two do not cause thermal lesions. According to the few studies in which the rate of identification of the AN has been examined, hydrojet dissection is the technique with which the nerves can always be represented (6,35), whereas the success rate is less successful with other techniques. Although the hypogastric nerves can almost always be identified with every technique, this is not the case with the splanchnic nerves, the IHP or the nerve fibers which emanate from them. 72 % of the AN (70) and 51 % (114) of the N. erigentes could be identified using the conventional technique. However, the success rate can be significantly improved with neuro-monitoring (23,77)

The only controlled study, a matched pair analysis also showed hydrojet dissection to be superior to the conventional technique with regard to complete loss of function (7.1% v 42.9%) as well as to the IIEF-5 (International Index of erectile function) (13.5 v 7.2),(6). However, the proportion of our own patients with ED, 26.1 % when the IIEF - 5 score was not taken into account, did not differ from the other studies (75,77,99,114,147)

8.2 Sexual dysfunction after laparoscopic surgery

The results with regard to sexual function after laparoscopic surgery for rectal cancer in men are contradictory. In the controlled studies, an advantage for the laparoscopic operation with an ED of 5 % (laparoscopic) v 29 % (open) (7) has been established, as well as a disadvantage with 41% (laparoscopic) compared with 4.5 % (open) (136). In the Classic trial (65) there was a trend to a higher rate of ED after the laparoscopic operation. After laparoscopic proctocolectomy with ileoanal pouch (85), a significantly higher rate of orgasm dysfunction was found in men compared with open surgery. In two further studies (119,148) no difference could be established between open and laparoscopic surgery. In the non-controlled studies, the rates of complete functional failure and of ED are not insignificant at 23% (144), 21.9% (92) and 31.1% (112). In the two first studies (92,144) an ED was found in 41 % and 15.9 % respectively. In a further study (68) based on extensive experience in laparoscopic colorectal surgery, only 6 % ED was reported. The different results may be due to different dissection techniques, which were not described. For instance ultrasonic instruments and dissection using monopolar or bipolar current can cause thermal lesions. These techniques are used laparoscopically.

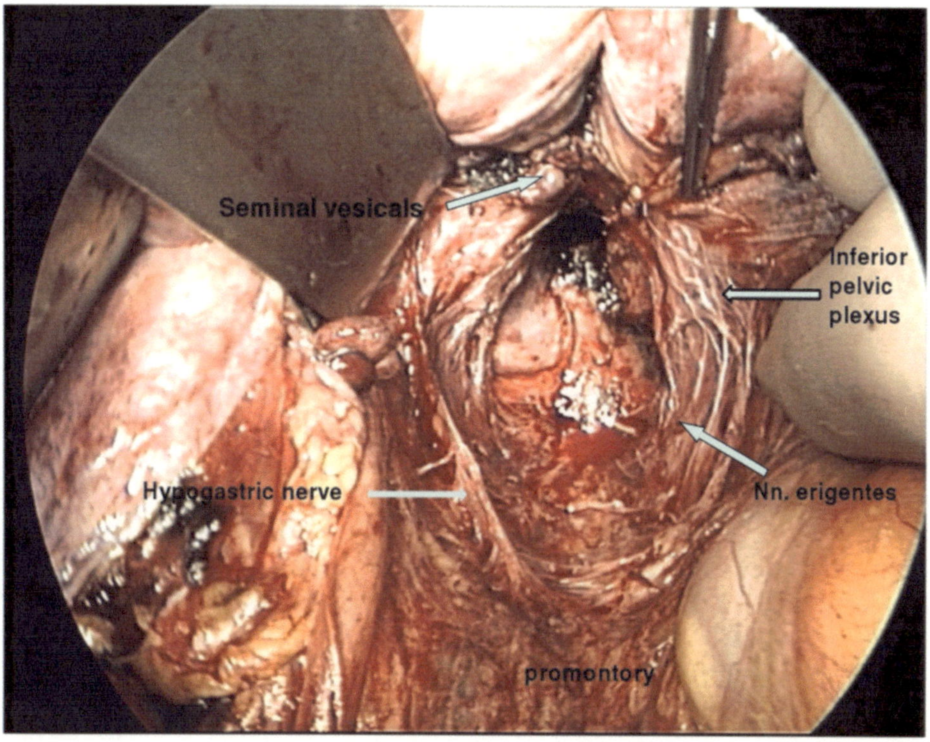

Fig. 2. Pelvic autonomic nerve identified by hydrojet dissection .View from the head of the patient. The rectum is removed.

9. Anastomotic leakage and anal continence

An anastomotic fistula always leaves scarring after healing. The extent of scarring depends on the size of the abscess, and may also cause symptomatic stenosis. As two studies have shown, these changes usually also result in decreased anal continence: patients with anastomotic leakage suffered more than patients without leakage from increased stool frequency, imperative urge to defecate and evacuation problems (44,115). A correspondingly lower compliance of the neorectum in this patient group was also measured. Not only clinically apparent leakages, but also inapparent ones can affect continence (95).

10. Adjuvant and neoadjuvant radio- and radio-chemotherapy and dysfunction

Neoadjuvant radio- and radio-chemotherapy and adjuvant radio-chemotherapy are risk factors for anal continence disorders, whereby post-operative treatment naturally presents the greater risk, because, in contrast to pre-operative therapy, a late radiation reaction can always occur in the neorectum. Several trials established significantly worse continence in patients who underwent adjuvant radiotherapy compared with patients without radiotherapy (81,97). Poorer continence manifested itself as more frequent bowel movement, more frequent urge and soiling. Both neorectal compliance and capacity were significantly diminished in patients who underwent adjuvant radio-chemotherapy. In a non-controlled study (98) 39% had poor continence after a mean follow-up time of 10 years. Several studies also found significantly worse continence after neoadjuvant radiotherapy and radio-chemotherapy compared with patients who had not been pre-treated (18,126,129,134). In two non-controlled studies (20.135) only 14 % and 25% of patients had normal continence. Radio-chemotherapy on its own can trigger anal dysfunction, regardless of surgery (94).

As with anal dysfunction, both neoadjuvant radiotherapy and radio-chemotherapy and adjuvant radio-chemotherapy are risk factors for sexual dysfunction: Male patients who underwent adjuvant radio-chemotherapy showed a significant deterioration in sexual function eight months after treatment (48). In the Norwegian cancer register a significant deterioration in sexual function was also seen 4.5 years after treatment in male patients who underwent adjuvant radio-chemotherapy or neoadjuvant radiotherapy (17) compared with patients who did not undergo such therapy. After neoadjuvant radio-chemotherapy sexual function in men was significantly worse compared with patients who did not receive neoadjuvant treatment (126,135,167). In contrast, in women sexual function is not affected to the same extent by radiation therapy (16,126,132).

Low anterior resection is the operation of choice in rectal cancer and is always possible without violating oncological principles if the sphincter is not tumor-involved. If the circumferential margin is not affected the autonomic nerves can be identified in TME using suitable dissection techniques, such as hydrojet dissection or sharp dissection, and thus preserved. The risk of thermal lesions to the nerves is always present when ultrasonic instruments are used, or in dissection with mono- or bipolar current. This is probably the reason why some higher rates of sexual dysfunction have been observed in laparoscopic LAR and TME. Damage to nerves not only causes sexual dysfunction, which is generally persistent, but also vesicourethral dysfunction, which is only permanent if the nerve lesions are extensive. Damage to the pelvic autonomic nerves and to the N. levator also contribute to disorders of anal continence. Stretching trauma to the anal sphincter is unavoidable if a peranal anastomosis is performed, particularly during inter-sphincteral resection. Stretching trauma caused by the circular stapler or by the double stapling technique can be avoided by using the inverse technique, in which the pressure plate is introduced anally and the stapler in the open limb of the colon J-pouch, or side to end anastomosis. The open limb is then closed with a linear stapler. It is not possible to use the inverse technique in coloplasty. Continence is significantly improved with the construction of a pouch. The different types of pouch, including side to end anastomosis, are all comparable in regard to continence and complication rates.

Anastomosis complications involve poor continence. It follows from this that a protective ileostomy or colostomy should be a routine in TME in order to avoid the clinical consequences of a leakage, and hence a long-term disturbance in anal function. Although the side-effects of radiotherapy have been largely reduced as a result of new techniques, the risk of anal continence dysfunction, which is not inconsiderable with adjuvant therapy, remains. Neoadjuvant therapy should always be preferred over adjuvant therapy because of the lesser risk. Radiotherapy, whether adjuvant or neoadjuvant, frequently causes sexual dysfunction in men. The general indication of neoadjuvant radio-chemotherapy in patients with infiltration of the mesorectum (T3) is probably excessive (71) if the circumferential resection margin is not affected and an exact TME is performed. Over-treatment can be avoided with an MRT-based indication for neoadjuvant radio-chemotherapy.

11. References

[1] Aagaard J, Thomas C, Gerstenberg TC, Knudsen JJT. Urodynamic investigation predicts bladder dysfunction at an early stage after abdominoperineal resection of the rectum for cancer. Surgery 1986; 90: 564-568

[2] Ameda K, Kakizaki H, Koyangi T, Hirakawa K, Kusumi T, Hosokawa M. The long-term voiding function and sexual function after pelvic nerve–sparing radical surgery for rectal cancer. Int J Urol 2005;12:256-63

[3] Amin AI, Hallböök O, Lee AJ, Sexton R, Moran BJ, Heald RJ. A 5 cm J pouch coloanal reconstruction following anterior resection for low rectal cancer results in acceptable evacuation and continence in the long term. Colorectal Dis 2003;5:33-37

[4] Andersen IS, Buntzen S, Rijkhoff NJ, Dalmose AL, Djurhuus JC, Laurberg S. Anorectal motility responses to pelvic hypogastric and pudendal nerve stimulation in the Göttingen minipig. Neurogastroenterol Motil 2006;18:153-161

[5] Araki Y, Isomoto H, Tsuzi J, Matsumoto A, Yasunaga M, Yamauchi K, Hayashi K, Kodama T. Functional results of colonic j-pouch anastomosis for rectal cancer. Surg Today 1999 ;29:597-600

[6] Arndt A. Urogenitale Dysfunktionen nach Rektumresektion mit TME unter Anwendung der Nerven schonenden Wasserstrahldissektion. Dissertation 2010 ; Universitätskrankenhaus Eppendorf Hamburg

[7] Asoglu O, Matlim T, Karanlik H, Atar M, Muslumanoglu M, Kapran Y;Igci A, ÖmenV, Kecer M, Parlak M. Impact of laparoscopic surgery on bladder and sexual function after total mesorectal excision for rectal cancer. Surg Endosc 2009;23:296-302

[8] Balsev I. , Harling H. Sexual dysfunction following operation for carcinoma of the rectum. Dis Colon Rectum 1983; 26: 785-788

[9] Barisic G, Markovic V, Popovic M, Dimitriijevic I, Gavrilovic P, Krivokapic Z. Function after intersphincteric resection for low rectal cancer and its influence on quality of life. Colorectal Dis 2011;13:638-641

[10] Barrier A, Martel P, Gallot D, Dugue L, Sezeur A, Malfosse M. Long-term functional results of colonic j pouch versus straight coloanal anastomosis. Br J Surg 1999;86:1179-1186

[11] Berger A, Tiret E, Parc R, Frileux P, Hannoun L, Nordlinger B, Ratelle R, Simon R. Excision of the rectum with colonic j pouch-anal anastomosis for adenocarcinoma of the low and midrectum. World J Surg 1992;16:470-477

[12] Bernoist S, Panis Y, Boleslawski E, Hautefeuille P, Valleur P. Functional outcome after coloanal versus low colorectal anastomosis for rectal carcinoma J Am Coll Surg 1997:185:114-119

[13] Bittdorf B, Stadelmeier U, Gohl J, Hohenberger W, Matzel KE. Functional outcome after intersphincteric resection of the rectum with coloanal anastomosis in low rectal cancer. Eur J Surg Oncol 2004 ;30:260-265

[14] Bretagnol F, Rullier E, Laurent C, Zerbib F, Gontier R, Saric J. Comparison of functional results and quality of life between intersphincteric resection and conventional coloanal anastomosis for rectal cancer. Dis Colon Rectum 2004;47: 832-838

[15] Brown CJ, Fenech D, Mc Leod RS. Reconstructive techniques after rectal resection for rectal cancer The Cochrane Library 2009 issue 4.

[16] Bruheim K, Tveit KM, Skovlund E, Balteskard L, CarlsenE, Fossa SD, Guren MG. Sexual function in females after radiotherapy for rectal cancer. Acta Oncol 2010, 49:826-832

[17] Bruheim K, Guren MG, Dahl AA,, Skovlund E, Balteskard L, CarlsenE, Fossa SD, Tveit KM. Sexual function in males after radiotherapy for rectal cance. r. Int J Radiat Oncol Biol Phys 2010 ;76:1012-1027

[18] Canda AE, Terzi C, GorkenIB, Oztop I, Sokmen S, Fuzun M. Effects of preoperative chemoradiotherapy on anal sphincter functions and quality of life in rectal cancer patients. Int J Colorectal Dis 2010;25:197-204

[19] Carlstedt A, Nordgren S, Fasth S, Appelgren L, Hulten L. Sympathetic nervous influence on the internal anal sphincter and rectum in man. Int Colorectal Dis 1988 :3:90-95

[20] Coco C, Valentini V, Manno A, Rizzo G, GambacortaMA, Mattana C, Verbo A, Picciocchi A. Functional results after radiochemotherapy and total mesorectal excisison for rectal cancer. Int J Colorectal Dis 2007;22:903-910

[21] Cunsolo A, Bragaglia RB, Manara G, Poggioli G, Gozzetti G. Urogenital dysfunction after abdominoperineal resection for carcinoma of the rectum. Dis Colon Rectum 1990; 33: 918-922

[22] Danzi M, Ferulano GP, Abate S, Califano G. Male sexual function after abdominoperineal resection for rectal cancer. Dis Colon Rectum 1983; 26: 665-668

[23] Da Silva GM, Zmora O, Börjesson L, Mizhari N, Daniel N, Khnándwala F, Efron J, Weiss EG, Nogueras JJ, Vernava AM, Wexner SD. The efficacy of a nerve stimulator(Cavermap)to enhance autonomic nerve identification and confirm nerve preservation during total mesorectal excision. Dis Colon Rectum 2005;47:2032-2038

[24] Dehni N, Schlegel D, Tiret E, Singland JD, Giguet M, Parc R. Effects of aging on the functional outcome of coloanal anastomosis with colonic j-pouch. Am J Surg 1998;175:209-212

[25] van Duijvendijk P, Slors F, Taat C, Heisterkamp SH, Obertop H, Boeckxstaens GEE. A prospective evaluation of anorectal function after total mesorectal excision in patients with a rectal carcinoma. Surgery 2003;133:56-65

[26] Eigler FW, Gross E. Kontinenzleistung nach totaler und subtotaler Rektumresektion mit peranaler Anastomosierung. In Postoperative Fogezustände S. 399, (ed). R. Häring Überreuter Verlag Wien 1988

[27] Enker WE, Stearns MW, Janov AJ. Peranal coloanal anastomosis following low anterior resection for rectal cancer. Dis Colon Rectum 1985; 28:576-581

[28] Farouk R, Duthie GS, Lee PW, Monson JR. Endosonographic evidence of injury to the internal anal sphincter after low anterior resection: long-term follow up. Dis Colon Rectum 1998;41:888-891

[29] Fazio VW, Zutshi M, Remzi F, Parc Y, Ruppert R, Fürst A, Celebrezze J, Galanduik S, Orangio G, Hyman N, Bokey L, Tiret E, Kirchdorfer B, Medich D, Tietze M, Hull T, Hammel J. A randomized multicentre trial to compare long-term functional outcome, quality of life and complications of surgical procedures for low rectal cancer. Ann Surg 2007;246:481-490

[30] Flühe v. d MO, Degen LP, Beglinger C, Hellwig AC, Rothenbühler JM, Harder FH. Ileocecal reconstruction with physiologic function after total mesorectal cancer excision. Ann Surg 1996;224:204-212

[31] Frenckner B, Ihre T. Influence of autonomic nerves on the internal anal sphincter in man. Gut 1976;17:306 - 312

[32] Fürst A, Burghofer K, Hutzel J, Jauch KW. Neorectal reservoir is not the functional principle of the colonic j-pouch: the volume of a short colonic j-pouch does not differ from a straight coloanal anastomosis. Dis Colon Rectum 2002;45:660-667

[33] Fürst A, Suttner S, Ayman A, Beham A, Jauch KW. Colonic j-pouch vs coloplasty following resection of distal rectal cancer Dis Colon Rectum 2003;46:1161-1166

[34] Garrett JR, Howard ER, Jones W. The internal sphincter in cat:a study of nervous mechanism affecting tone and reflex acitivity. J Physiol 1974;243. 153-166

[35] Geers P, Moesta KT;Yildirim C, Thon WF, Köckerling F. Urodynamic outcome of waterjet-assisted total mesorectal excisison. Br J Surg 2007;94:1543-1547

[36] Gerstenberg TC, Nielsen ML, Clausen S, Blaabjerg J, Lindenberg J. Bladder function after abdominoperineal resection of the rectum for anorectal cancer. Urodynamic investigation before and after operation in a consecutive series. Ann Surg 1980; 191: 81-86

[37] Götzinger P, Wamser P, Herbst F. Coloanale Anastomose :Verbesserung der funktionellen Frühergebnisse durch Rekonstruktion mit Colonpouch. Chirurg 2001 ;72:49-53

[38] Gosselink MP, West RL, Kuipers EJ, Hansen BE, Schouten WR. Integrity of the anal sphincters after pouch-anal anastomosis: evaluation with the three-dimensional endoanal ultrasonography. Dis Colon Rectum 2005 ;48:1728-35

[39] Gross E, Beersiek F, Eigler FW. Sphinkterfunktion nach peranalen Anastomosen. Langenbecks Arch Surg 1980;353:207-216

[40] Gross E, Amir-Kabirian H:Koloanaler Pouch nach totaler Rektumresektion. Zentralbl Chir; 1994;119:878-885

[41] Hallböök O, Pahlmann L, Krog M, Wexner St, Sjödahl R. Randomized comparison of staight and colonic j-pouch anastomosis after low anterior resection. Ann Surg 1996;224:58-65

[42] Hallböök O, Nyström P-O, Sjödahl R. Physiological characteristics of straight and colonic j-pouch anastomosis after rectal excision for cancer. Dis Colon Rectum 1997;40:332-338

[43] Hallböök O, Sjödahl R. Comparison between the colonic j -pouch-anal anastomosis and healthy rectum: clinical and physiological function. Br J Surg 1997; 84:1437-1441

[44] Hallböök O, Sjödahl R. Anastomotic leakage and functional outcome after anterior resection of the rectum Br J Surg 1996 ;83:60-62
[45] Harris GJC, Lavery IC, Fazio VW. Function of colonic pouch continues to improve with time. Br J Surg 2001;88:1623-1627
[46] Havenga K, Enker WE, McDermott K, Cohen AM, Minsky BD, Guillem J. Male and female sexual and urinary function after total mesorectal excision with autonomic nerve preservation for carcinoma of the rectum. J Am Coll Surg 1996; 182: 495-502
[47] Hendren SK, O`Connor BI, Liu M, Asano T, Cohen Z, Swallow CJ, Mc Rae HM, Gryfe R, Mc Leod R. Prevalence of male and female sexual dysfunctions high following surgery for rectal cancer. Ann Surg 2005;242:212-223
[48] Heriot A G, Tekkis PP, Fazio VW, Neary P, Lavery JC. Adjuvant radiotherapy is associated with increased sexual dysfunction in male patients undergoing resection for rectal cancer. Ann Surg 2005;242:502 -511
[49] Heriot A G, Tekkis PP, Constantinidis V, Paraskevas P, Nicholls R J, Darzi A, Fazio V. Meta-analysis of colonic reservoirs versus straight coloanal anastomosis after anterior resection. Br J Surg 2006;93:19-32
[50] Hida J, Yatsunomi M, Fujimoto K, et al. Functional outcome after low anterior resection with low anastomosis for rectal cancer using the colonic j-pouch: prospective randomized study for determination of optimum pouch size. Dis Colon Rectum 1996;39:986-981
[51] Hida J, Yasutomi M, Maruyama T, Yoshifuji T, Tokoro T, wakano T, Uchida T, Ueda K. Detection of a rectocele-like prolapse in the colonic-j pouch using pouchography:cause or effect of evacuation difficulties. Surg Today 1999;29:1237-1242
[52] Hida J, Yoshifuji T, Tokoro T, Inoue K, MatzuzakibT, Okuno K, Shiozaki H, Yasutomi M. Comparison of long-term functional results of colonic j-pouch and straight anastomosis after low anterior resection for rectal cancer. A five year follow- up, Dis Colon Rectum 2004;47:1578-1585
[53] Hirano A, Koda K, Kosugi C, Yamazaki M, Yasuda H. Dmage to the anal sphincter/levator ani muscles caused by operative procedure sphincter-preseving operation for rectal cancer. Am J surg 2011;201:508-513
[54] Ho YH, Tan M, Seow -Cheon F. Prospective randomized trial controlled study of clinical function and anorectal physiology after low anterior resection : comparison of straight and colonic j pouch anastomosis. Br J Surg 1996;83:978-980
[55] Ho YH, Tan M, Leong A, Eu, KW, Nyram D, Seow-Cheon F. Anal pressures impaired by stapler insertion during colorectal anastomosis. Dis Colon Rectum 1999;42:89-95
[56] Ho YH, Seow-Choen F, Tan M. Colonic j-pouch function at six months versus straight coloanal anastomosis at two years :randomized controlled trial. World J Surg 2001 ;26:876-81
[57] Ho YH, Tan, M, Leong AFPK, Seow-Choen F. Ambulatory manometry inpatients with colon-J pouch and straight coloanal anastomosis. Dis Colon Rectum 2000;43:793-799
[58] Ho YH, Brown S, Heah SM, Tsang C, Seow Chon. Comparison of j-pouch and coloplasty pouch for low rectal cancer : an randomized, controlled trial

investigating functional results and comparative anastomotic leak rates. Ann Surg 2002;236:49-55

[59] Hojo K, Sawada T, Morya Y. An analysis of survival and voiding, sexual function after wide iliopelvic lymphadenectomy in patients with carcinoma of the rectum compared with conventional lymphadenectomy. Dis Colon Rectum 1989;32:128-133

[60] Hojo K, Vernava AM III, Sugihara K, Katumata K. Preservation of urine voiding and sexual function after rectal cancer surgery. Dis Colon Rectum 1991; 34: 532-53

[61] Horgan PG, O`Conell PR, Shinkwin CA, Kirwan WO. Effect of anterior resection on anal sphincter function Br J Surg 1989;76:783-786

[62] Horgan AF, Molloy RG, Cpulter J, Sheehan M, Kirwan WO. Nerve regeneration across colorectal anastomoses after low anterior resection in a canine model. Int J Colorectal Dis 1993;8:167 -169

[63] Huber FT, Herter B, Siewert JR. Colonic pouch vs side -to -end anastomosis in low anterior resection. Dis Colon Rectum 1999 ;42:896-902

[64] Ikeuchi H, Kusunoki M, Shoji Y, Yamamura T, Utsonomiya J. Functional results after high coloanal anastomosis and "low" coloanal anastomosis with a colonic j-pouch for rectal carcinoma. Surg Today 1997:27:702-705

[65] Jayne DG, Brown JM, Thorpe H, Walker J. Quirke P, Guillou PJ, Bladder and sexual function following resection for rectal cancer in a randomized clinical trial of laparoscopic versus open technique. Br J Surg 2005; 92:1124-1132

[66] Jehle EC, Haehnel T, Starlinger MJ, Becker HD. Level of anastomosis does not influence functional outcome after anterior resection for rectal cancer. Am J Surg 1995;169:147-153

[67] Jiang L-K, Yang S-H, Lin J-K. Transabdominal anastomosis after low anterior resection :a prospective randomized, controlled trial comparing long term results between side- to-end anastomosis and colonic j- pouch. Dis Colon Rectum 2005;48:2100-2110

[68] Jones OM, Stevenson AR, Stitz RW, Lumley JW. Preservation of sexual and bladder function after laparoscopic rectal surgery. Colorectal Dis 2009;11:489-495

[69] Joo JS, Latulippe JF, Alabaz O Weiss EG, Nogueras JJ, Wexner SD. Long-term functional evaluation of straight coloanal anastomosis and colonic j-pouch :is functional superiority of colonic j-pouch sustained? Dis Colon Rectum 1998;41:740-741

[70] Junginger T, Kneist W, Heintz A,. influence of identification and preservation of pelvic autonomic nerves in rectal cancer surgery on bladder dysfunction after total mesorectal excision. Dis Colon Rectum 2003;46;621-628

[71] JungingerT, Hermanek P, Oberholzer K, Schmidberger H. Rectal carcinoma:Is too much neoadjuvant therapy performed? Proposals for a more selective MRI based indication. Zentralbl Chir 2006, 1311:275-231

[72] Kakodkar R, Gupta S, Nundy S. Low anterior resection with total mesorectal excision for rectal cancer : functional assessment and factors affecting outcome. Colorectal Dis 2006;8:650-656

[73] Karania ND, Schache DJ, Heald RJ. Function of the distal rectum after low anterior resection for carcinoma. Br J Surg 1992;79:114-116

[74] Kienle P, Stern J, Herfarth Ch. Restaurative Proktektomie. Vergleich direkter coloanaler und colonpouchanaler Anastomosen zur Kontinuitätswiederherstellun. Chirurg 1997;68:630-63

[75] Kim NK, Aahn TW, Park JK, Lee KY, Lee WH, Sohn SK, Min JS. Assessment of sexual and voiding function after total mesorectal excision with pelvic autonomic nerve preservation in males with rectal cancer. Dis Colon Rectum 2002; 45: 1178-1185

[76] Kinn AC, Ohman U. Bladder and sexual function after surgery for rectal cancer. Dis Colon Rectum 1986;29:43-48

[77] Kneist W, Junginger T. Male urogenital function after confirmed nerve sparing total mesorectal excision with dissection in front of Denonvillier`s fascia. World J Surg 2007;31:1321-1328

[78] Kneist W, Knauff D W, Roman K, Rahimi N, Rink AD, Heimann A, Somerlik K, Koch KP, Doerge T, Lang H. Intraoperative pelvic nerve stimulation performed under continous electromyography of the internal anal sphincter. Int J Colorectal Dis 2010;25:1325-1331

[79] Kneist W, Kuhn E, Berger S, Knabe J, Ekkert B, Junginger T. Kontinenz nach Chirurgie des Rektumkarzinoms - Bedeutung des Nervenerhaltes und Wertigkeit der intraoperativen Neurostimulation:in Deutsche Kontinenz Gesellschaft(eds). Inkontinenz –eine soziale Herausforderung. Stuttgart Thieme 2006 p71

[80] Köhler A, Athanasiadis S, Ommer A, Psarakis E. Long-term results of low anterior resection with intersphincteric anastomosis in carcinoma of the lower third of the rectum:analysis of 31 patients. Dis Colon Rectum 2000 ;43:843-850

[81] Kollmorgen CF, Meagher AP, Wolff BG, Pemberton JH, Martenson JA, Ilstrup DM. The long-term effect of adjuvant postoperative chemoradiotherapy for rectal carcinoma on bowel function. Ann Surg 1994;220:576-682

[82] Kusunoki M, Shoji Y, Yanagi H, Hatada T, Fujita S, Sakanoue T, Yamamura T, Utsunomiya J. Function after anoabdominal rectal resection and colonic J pouch–anal anastomosis. Br J Surg 1991 ;78:1434 -1438

[83] Lane RH, Parks AG. Function of the anal sphincters following colo-anal anastomosis. Br J Surg 1977; 64:596-599

[84] Lange MM, Maas CP, Marijnen CA, Wiggers T, Rutten HJ, Kranenberg EK, van der Welde CJ, Cooperative clinical investigation of the dutch total mesorectal trial. Urinary function after rectal cancer treatment is mainly caused by surgery. Br J Surg 2008;95:1020-1028

[85] Larson DW, Davies MM, Dozois EF, Cima RR, Piotrowicz K, Anderson K, Barnes SA, Harmsen WS, Young-Fadok TM, Wolff BG, PembertonJH. Sexual function, body image and quality of life after laparoscopic and open pouch –anal anastomosis Dis Colon Rectum 2008:51:392-396

[86] Lazorthes F, Fages P, Chiotasso P, et al : Resection of the rectum with construction of a colonic reservoir and coloanal anastomosis for carcinoma of the rectum. Br J Surg 1986;73:136-38

[87] Lazorthes F, Gamagami R, Chiotasso P, et al. Prospective radomized study comparing clinical results between small and large colonic j-pouch following coloanal anastomosis. Dis Colon Rectum 1997;40:1409- 1413

[88] Lazorthes F, Chiotasso P, Gamagami RA, Istvan G, Chevreau P. Late clinical outcome in a randomized prospective comparison of colonic j-pouch and straight coloanal anastomosis. Br J Surg 1997;84:1449-1451

[89] Lee SJ, Park YS. Seriel evaluation of anorectal function following low anterior resection of the rectum. Int J Colorectal Dis 1998;13:241-246

[90] Lewis WG, Holdsworth PJ, Stephenson BM, Finan PJ, Johnston D. Role of the rectum in the physiological and clinical results of coloanal and colorectal anastomosis after anterior resection for rectal carcinoma Br J Surg1992;79:1082 -1088

[91] Lewis WG, Martin IG, Williamson ME et al. Why do some patients experience poor functional results after anterior resection of the rectum for carcinoma. Dis Colon Rectum 1995;38:259-263

[92] Liang JT, Hong SL, Lee PH. Laparoscopic pelvic autonomic nerve-preserving surgery for patients with lower rectal cancer after chemoradiation therapy. Ann Surg Oncol 2007;14:1285-1287

[93] Liao C, Cao F, Cao Y, Tan A, Li X, Wu D. Meta-analysis of the colo-J pouch vs transversoplasty pouch after anterior resection for rectal cancer. Colorectal Dis 2010, 12:624-631

[94] Lim Jf, Tiandra JJ, Hiscock R, Chao MW, Gibbs P. Preoperative chemoradiation for rectal cancer causes prolonged pudendal nerve terminal motor latency. Dis Colon Rectum 2006;49:12 -19

[95] Lim M, Akhtar S, Sasapu K, Keith H, Burke d, Sagar P, Finan P. Clinical and subclinical leaks after low colorectal anastomosis:a clinical and radiological study. Dis Colon Rectum 2006;49:1611-1619

[96] Lubowski DZ, Nicholls RJ, Swash M, Jordan MJ. Neural control of internal anal sphincter function. Br J Surg 1987 ;74:668-670

[97] Lundby L, Krogh K, Jensen VJ, Gandrup P, Qvist N, Overgaard J, Laurberg S. Long-term anorectal dysfunction after postoperative radiotherapy for rectal cancer. Dis Colon Rectum 2005;48:1343-1349

[98] Lupatelli M, Mascioni F, Bellavita R, Draghini L, Tarducci R, Castagnoli P, Russo G, Aristei C. Long term anorectal function after preoperative chemoradiotherapy in high –risk rectal cancer patients. Tumori 2010; 96:34-41

[99] Maas CP, Moriya Y, Steup WH, Kiebert GM, Kranenberg WMK, van de Velde CJH. Radical and nerve-preserving surgery for rectal cancer in the Netherlands: a prospective study on morbidity and functional outcome. Br J Surg 1998; 85: 92-97.

[100] Machado M, Nygren J, Goldman S, Ljungqvist O. Similar outcome after colonic j - pouch and side-to -end anastomosis in low anterior resection for rectal cancer:a prospective randomized trial. Ann Surg 2003;238:214-220

[101] Machado M, Nygren J, GoldmannS, Ljungqvist O. Functional and physiologic assessmant of the colonic reservoir or side-to end anastomosis after low anterior resection for rectal cancer: a two year follow up. Dis Colon Rectum 2005;48:29-36

[102] Manthyh CR, Hull TL, Fazio VW. Coloplasty in low colorectal anastomosis :manometric and functional comparison with straight and colonic j pouch anastomosis. Dis Colon Rectum, 2001;44:37-42

[103] Masui H, Ike H, Yamaguchi S, Oki S, Shimada H. Male sexual function after autonomic nerve-preserving operation for rectal cancer. Dis Colon Rectum 1996; 39: 1140-1145

[104] Matsfuji H, Yokoyama J. Neural control of the internal anal sphincter motility. J Smooth Muscle Res 2003;39:11 -20

[105] Matzel KE, Stadelmeier U, Muehldorfer S, Hohenberger W. Coninence after colorectal reconstruction following resection: impact of level of anastomosis. Int J Colorectal Dis 1997;12:82-87

[106] Matzel, KE, Bittdorf B, Günther K, Stadelmaier U, Hohenberger W. Rectal resection with low anastomosis:functional outcome. Colorectal Disease 2003 ;5:458-464

[107] Mc Anena OJ, Heald RJ, Lockhart-Mummery HE. Operative and functional results of total rectal excision with ultra-low anterior resection in the management of carcinoma of the lower one third of the rectum. Surg Gyn Obstet 1990;170:517-521

[108] Mauroy B, Demondion X, Bizet B, Claret A, Mestdagh P, Hurt C. The female inferior hypogastric (pelvic)plexus: anatomical and radiological description of the plexus and its afferences - applications to pevic surgery. Surg Radiol Anat 2007;29:55-66

[109] Mauroy B, Demondion X, Drizenko A, Goullet E, Bonnal J. -l, Biserte J, Abbou C. The inferior hypogastric plexus (pelvic plexus):its importance in neural preservation techniques. Surg Radiol Anat 2003;25: 6-15

[110] Miller AS, Lewis WG, Williamson ME et al. Factors that influence functional outcome after coloanal anastomosis for carcinoma of the rectum. Br J Surg 1995;82:1327-1330

[111] Montesani C, Pronio A, Santella S, Boschetto A, Aguzzi D, Pirozzi R, D`Amato A, Vestri A. Rectal cancer surgery with sphincter preservation: functional results related to the level of anastomosis. Clinical and instrumental study. Hepatogastroenterology 2004;51:718-721

[112] Morino M, Parini U, Allaix ME,, Monasterolo G, Contul RB, Garrone C. Male sexual and urinary function after lapaoscopic total mesorectal excision. Surg Endosc 2009;23:1233-1240

[113] Mortensen NJ, Ramirez JM, Takeuchi N, Humphreys MM: Colonic j pouch -anal anastomosis after rectal excision for carcinoma: functional outcome. Br J Surg 1995;82:611-613

[114] Nesbakken, A, Nygaard K, Bull-Njaa T, Carlsen E, Eri LM. Bladder and sexual dysfunction after mesorectal excision for rectal cancer. Br J Surg 2000; 87: 206-210

[115] Nesbakken A, Nygaard K, Linde OC. Outcome and late functional results after anastomotic leakage following mesorectal excision for rectal cancer. Br J Surg 2001;88:400-404

[116] Nesbakken A, Nygard K, Lunde O. Mesorectal excision for rectal cancer :functional outcome after low anterior resection and colorectal anastomosis without reservoir. Colorectal Dis 2002 ;4:172-176

[117] Neuhuber WL, Appelt M, Pollak JM. Rectospinal neurons. Neuroscience 1993;56:367-378

[118] Nicholls RJ, Lubowski DZ, Donaldson DR. , Comparison of colonic reservoir and straight coloanal reconstruction after rectal excision. Br J Surg 1988;75:318-320

[119] Nitori N, Hasegawa H, Ishij Y, Endo T, Kitajima M, Ktagawa Y. Sexual function in men with rectal and rectosigmoid cancer after laparoscopic and open surgery. Hepatogastroenterology 2008;55:1304-1307

[120] O`Kelly T J, Davies J R, Brarding A F. Distribution of nitrioxid synthase containing neurons in the rectal myenteric plexus and anal canal. Dis Colon Rectum 1994;37 :350

[121] O`Riordan MG, Molloy RG, Gillen P, Horgan A, Kirwan WO. Rectoanal reflex following low stapled anterior resection of the rectum. Dis Colon Rectum 1992;35:874-878

[122] Ortiz H, De Miguel M, Armendariz P, Rodriguez J, Chocarro C. Coloanal anastomosis:Are functional results better with a pouch ? Dis Colon Rectum 1995;38:375-377

[123] Oya M, Komatsu J, Tkase Y, Nakamura T, Ishikawa H: Comparison of defacatory function after colonic-j pouch anastomosis and straight anastomosis for stapled low anterior resection:results of a prospective randomized trial. Surg Today 2002;32:104-110

[124] Pappalardo G, Toccaceli S, Dionisio P, Castrinis G, Ravo B. Preoperative and postoperative evaluation by manometric study of the anal sphincter after coloanal anastomosis for carcinoma. Dis Colon Rectum 1988;31:119-122

[125] Parc R, Tiret E, Frileux P, et al. Resection and coloanal anastomosis with colonic reservoir for rectal carcinoma. Br J Surg 1986;73:139-141

[126] Parc Y, Zutshi M, Zalinski S, ruppert R, Fürst A, Fazio VW. Preoperative radiotherapy is associated with worse functional results after coloanal anastomosis for rectal cancer. Dis Colon rectum2009;52:2004-2015

[127] Parks AG, Pecy JP. Rectal carcinoma ;restorative resection using a sutured colo-anal anastomosis. Int Surg 1983;68:7-11

[128] Pedersen IK, Hint K, Olsen J. Christiansen J, Jensen P, Mortensen PE. Anorectal function after low anterior resection for carcinoma. Ann Surg 1986;204:133-135

[129] Peeters KCMJ, van de welde CJH, Leer JWH, Mrtijn H, Junggeburt JMC, Klein E, Kranenberg WH, Steup WH, Wiggers T, Rutten HJ, Marijnen CAM. late bsideeffects of short course preoperative radiotherapy combined with total mesorectal excision for rectal cancer. Increased bowel dysfunction in irradiated patients. - a dutch colorectal cancer group study. J Clin Oncol 2005;23:6199-6206

[130] Pelissier EP Blum D, Bachour A, Bosset JF. Functional results of coloanal anastomosis with reservoir. Dis Colon Rectum 1992;35:843-846

[131] Pimentel JM, Duarte A, Gregorio C, Souto P, Patricio J. Transverse coloplasty pouch and colonic j-pouch for rectal cancer: a comparative study. Colorectal Dis 2003;5:465-470

[132] Platell CF, Thompson PJ, Makin GB. Sexual health in women following pelvic surgery for rectal cancer. Br J Surg 2004;91:465-468

[133] Pocard M, Zinzindohone F, Haab F, Caplin S, Parc R, Tiret E. A prospective study of sexual and urinary function after total mesorectal excision with autonomic nerves preservation for rectal cancer. Surgery 2002; 131: 368-372

[134] Pollack J, Holm T, Cedermark B, Altman D, Holmström B, Glimelius B, MellgrenA. Late adverse effect of short -course preoperative radiotherapy in rectal cancer. Br J Surg 2006;93:1519-1525
[135] Puciarelli S, Del BiancoP, Efficace F, Serpentini S, Capirci C, De Paoli A, Amato A, Cuicchi D, Nitti D. Patient - reported outcomes after neoadjuvant chemoradiotherapy for rectal cancer. A multicentre prospective observational study. Ann Surg 2011; 253:71-77
[136] Quah HM, Jayne DG, Eu KW, Seow-Choen F. Bladder and sexual dysfunction following laparoscopically assisted and conventional open mesorectal resection for cancer. Br J Surg 2002; 89: 1551-1556
[137] Rasmussen OO, Petersen IK, Christiansen J: Anorectal function following low anterior resection. Colorectal Dis 2003;5:258-261
[138] Rink AD, Haaf F, Knupper N, Vestweber KH. Prospective randomized trial comparing ileocaecal interposition anmd colon -j-pouch as rectal replacement after total mesorectal excision. Int J Colorectal Dis 2007;22:153-60
[139] Rink AD, Sgourakis G, Sotiropoulos GC, Lang H, Vestweber KH. The colon J-pouch as a cause of evacuation disorders after rectal resection:myth or fact. Langenbecks Arch Surg 2009;394:79-91
[140] Romanos J, Stebbing JF, Humphreys MM et al. Ambulatory manometric examination in patients with colonic j-pouch and in normal controls. Br J Surg1996;83:1744-1746
[141] Saigusa N, Belin BM, Choi HJ, Efron JE, Weiss EG, Nogueras JJ, Wexner SD. Recovery of the rectoanal inhibitory reflex after restorative proctocolectomy : does it correlate with nocturnal continence? Dis Colon Rectum 2003 ;46:168-172
[142] Sailer M, Debus ES, Fuchs KH, Fein M, Beyerlein J, Thiede A. Comparison of different J-pouches vs straight and side-to- end coloanal anastomoses: experimental study in pigs. Dis Colon Rectum 1999;42:590-595.
[143] Sailer M, Fuchs KH, Fein M, Thiede A. Randomized clinical trial comparing quality of life after straight and pouch coloanal reconstruction. Br J Surg 2002;89:1108-1117
[144] Sartori CA, Sartori A, Vigna S, Occhipinti R, Biaocchi GL. Urinary and sexual disorders after laparoscopic TME for rectal cancer. J Gastrointest Surg 2011;15:637-643
[145] Schiessl R, Karner -Hanusch J, Herbst F, Teleky B, Wunderlich M. Intersphincteric resection for low rectal tumors Br J Surg 1994;81:1376-1378
[146] Seow-Choen F, Goh HS. Prospectve randomized trial comparing pouch anal anastomosis and straight coloanal reconstruction. Br J Surg 1995 ;82:608- 610
[147] Shirouzu K, Ogata Y, Araki Y. Oncologic and functional results of total mesorectal excision and autonomic nerve-preserving operation for advanced lower rectal cancer. Dis Colon Rectum 2004;47:1442-1447
[148] Stamopoulos P, Theodoropoulos GE, Papailiou J, Savidis D, Golemati C, Bramis K, Panoussopoulos SCE. Prospective evaluation of sexual function after open and laparoscopic surgery for rectal cancer. Surg Endosc 2009;May 23 epub

[149] Stelzner F, Biersack H, von Mallek D. Unteres, kloakogenes Rektumviertel. Anatomie und chirurgische Bedeutung für Mastdarmvorfall, Inkontinenz, Rektozele und Radikaloperation beim Rektumkarzinom. Chirurg 2006;77:273-280

[150] Stelzner F. Die Nervenversorgung des anorektalen Kontinenzorgans In:. Chirurgie an viszeralen Abschlußsystemen. Thieme Verlag Stuttgart 1998 pp. 131

[151] Sterk P, Shekarriz B, Günter S, Nolde J, Keller R, Bruch HP, Shekarriz H. Voiding and sexual dysfunction after deep rectal resection and total messorectal excision. Int J Colorectal Dis 2005;20:223 - 227

[152] Sugihara K, Morya Y, Fujita S. Pelvic autonomic nerve preservation for patients with rectal carcinoma:oncological and functional outcome. Cancer 1996 ;78:1871-1880

[153] Sun WM, Read NW, Katsinelos P, Donelly TC, Shorthaus AJ. Anorectal function after restorative proctocolectomy and low anterior resection with coloanal anastomosis. Br J Surg 1994;81:280-284

[154] Suzuki H, Matsumoto K, Amano S, Fujioka M, Honzumi M. Anorectal pressure and rectal compliance after low anterior resection. Br J Surg 1980;67:655-657

[155] Tekkis PP, Cornish JA, ; Remzi FH, Tilney HS, Strong SA, Church JM, Lavery IC, Fazio VW. Measuring sexual and urinary outcomes in women after rectal cncer excision. Dis Colon rectum 2009;52:46 -54.

[156] Temple LK, Bacik J, Savatta SG, Gottesman L, Paty PB, Weiser MR, Guillem JG, Minsky BD, Kalman M, Thaler HT, Schrag D, Wong WD. The development of a validated instrument to evaluate bowel function after sphincter-preserving surgery for rectal cancer. Dis Colon Rectum 2005;48:1353-1365

[157] Varpe P, Huhtinen H, Rantala A, Salminen P, Rautava P, Hurme S, Grönroos J. Quality of life after surgery for rectal cancer with special reference to pelvic floor dysfunction. Colorectal Dis 2011;13. 399-405

[158] Vassilakis JS, Pechlivanides G, VrachasotakisN Chrysos E, Tzovaras G, Xynos E:Anorectal function after low anterior resection of the rectum. Int J Colorectal Dis 1993;10:101-106

[159] Wallner C, Lange MM, Bonsing BA,, Maas CP, Wallace CN, Dabohoiwla NF, RuttenHJ, Lamers WH; De Ruiter MC, van de Welde CJH. Caues of fecal and urinary incontinence after total mesorectal excision for rectal cancer based on cadaveric surgery: study from the cooperative clinical investigators of the dutch total mesorectal excision trial. J Clin Oncol 2008;26. 4466-4472

[160] Wang JW, You YT; Chen HH, Chiang JM, Yeh CY, Tang R. Stapled colonic j-pouch anal anastomosis without diverting colostomy for rectal carcinoma. Dis Colon Rectum 1997;40:30-34

[161] Williamson ME,, Lewis WG, Finan PJ, Miller AS, Holdsworth PJ, Johnston D. Recovery of physiologic and clinical function after low anterior resection of the rectum for carcinoma:myth or reatlity ? Dis Colon Rectum 1995;38:411-418

[162] Willis S, Kasperk R, Braun J, Schumpelick V. Comparison of colonic j-pouch reconstruction and straight coloanal anastomosis after intersphincteric rectal resection. Langenbecks Arch Surg 2001;386:193- 199

[163] Wunderlich M, Teleki B, Schiessel R. Sphincter function following coloanal anastomosis. Langenbecks Arch Chir 1986;367:259-269

[164] Yamamoto G, Satoni H, Ise H. Sacral spinal innervation of the rectal and vesical smooth muscles and sphincter striated muscles. Neuroscience 1978;7:41 -47
[165] Z`graggen K, Maurer CA, Birrer S, Giachino D, Kern B, Büchler MW. A new surgical concept for rectal replacement after low anterior resection :the transverse coloplasty pouch. Ann Surg 2001; 234:780-787
[166] Zugor V, Miskovic I, Matzel K, Hohenberger W, Neuhuber W, Labanaris A, Schott GE. Harnblasenentleer ungsstörungen nach Rektumoperationen. Chirurg 2010:81;56-60
[167] Zugor V, Miskovic I, Lausen B, Matzel K, Hohenberger W, Schreiber M,, Labanaris A, Neuhuber W Witt J, Schott GE. Sexual dysfunction after rectal surgery :a retrospective study of men without disease recurrence. J Sex Med 2010;7:3199-31205

Part 4

Adjuvant and Neo-Adjuvant Treatments

14

Role of Tumor Tissue Analysis in Rectal Cancer Pharmacogenetics

Emilia Balboa et al.*
[1]*Grupo Medicina Xenomica - CIBERER*
Fundación Publica Galega de Medicina Xenómica, Santiago de Compostela
Spain

1. Introduction

Cancer management has experienced an important progress in the last years due to the discovery of new treatments and an improvement in the early detection methods. These improvements have had an important repercussion in patients´ life span, having an impact in both time and quality life (Berardi et al., 2009). At the same time, knowledge of the specific characteristics of each tumor has led us, in recent times, to be aware of the need of study the unique identity of the cancer (Li & Lai, 2009).

For rectal cancer patients, 5-fluorouracil (5-FU)- based chemoradiotherapy before total mesorectal excision (TME) is the gold standard treatment for stage II and III (Sauer et al., 2004; Wheeler et al., 2004), but the overall rate of response is still about 46-74% (Wheeler et al., 2004; Chen et al.,1994) Research has focused in the discovery of more specific treatments for each cancer and, at the same time, has tried to identify the particular features of cancer cells with the purpose of design target drugs for these cells in order to avoid affect normal cells. Recently, several studies aim at adding to this regimen several different currently available chemotherapeutics in colon cancer treatment, such as the 5-FU prodrug, capecitabine (Carlomagno et al., 2009; Ugidos et al., 2009), oxaliplatin (Carlomagno et al., 2009), irinotecan (Ugidos et al., 2009), cetuximab (Bertolini et al., 2009) or bevacizumab (Willett et al., 2009).

But these treatments are not devoid of adverse effects that could put at risk patients lives due to the treatment itself, so, in these state of affairs,there is a need for identify patients that are going to experience important adverse effects or try to recognize the patients in which the drug benefits will be more than the adverse effects produced; with this purpose, pharmacogenomics and more specific pharmacogenetics studies arise, that so far, have a bright and a dark side.

---

* Goretti Duran[2], Maria Jesus Lamas[2], Antonio Gomez-Caamaño[3], Catuxa Celeiro-Muñoz[4], Rafael Lopez[5], Angel Carracedo[1,6] and Francisco Barros[1]
[1]*Grupo Medicina Xenomica - CIBERER. Fundación Publica Galega de Medicina Xenómica. Santiago de Compostela, Spain*
[2]*Servicio de Farmacia, Complejo Hospitalario de Santiago de Compostela (CHUS). Santiago de Compostela, Spain*
[3]*Servicio de Oncología Radioterápica, CHUS, Spain*
[4]*Servicio de Anatomía Patológica, CHUS, Spain*
[5]*Department of Medical Oncology, CHUS, Spain*
[6]*Grupo Medicina Xenomica - CIBERER. Universidad de Santiago de Compostela, Spain*

In the bright side, there are a few markers with consistent results across studies. Regarding oncology field, hematology has been the pharmacogenomic area with the more important improvement, being several drugs developed for the treatment of different leukemias depending on the genetic of the disease. Development of the first target drug Gleevec supposed an important advance for Chronic Myeloid Leukemia treatment (Buchdunger et al., 1996), and detection of mutations that confer drug resistance (von Bubnoff et al., 2002) allowed to switch to a most favorable treatment depending on the patients´ pharmacogenetics (Hiwase et al., 2011).
Concerning to colorectal cancer treatment and even though it is still necessary to establish a definitive pattern across populations and an extensive research is being realized in that field. From these researches, it has been establish that one of the markers more studied and whose pharmacogenetic association has been more consistently replicated, is high risk of developing severe irinotecan toxicity due to a deficiency in the detoxifying enzyme UGT1A1 (Innocenti et al., 2004; Fujiwara et al., 2010).
Another important detoxifying enzyme related to colorectal cancer treatment is dihydropyrimidine dehydrogenase (DPD). DPD deficiency, the main enzyme related to 5-fluorouracil catabolism, is associated to severe toxicity, patients with this protein deficiency experience mucositis, neutropenia and neurological symptoms under treatment (Johnson & Diasio, 2001; Van Kuilenburg, 2004).

1.1 Germline vs tumoral tissue in pharmacogenetics

But, despite the existence of solid studies supporting the relationship between germline polymorphisms and toxicity of treatment, the efforts of pharmacogenetics studies trying to get information of treatment efficiency from germline polymorphisms have not been as rewarded (Contopoulos-Ioannidis et al., 2006).
One of the genes more studied, mainly related to treatment efficiency but also toxicity is TYMS gene. Polymorphisms in this gene have been associated to different gene expression degree and this to a different protein level (Horie et al., 1995; Kawakami et al., 2001; Mandola et al., 2003, 2004). Although numerous studies have indicated association of germline low-expression alleles in this gene to an increase survival in patients undergoing treatment with 5-Fluorouracil (Mandola et al., 2003; Kawakami & Watanabe, 2003), contradictory results and even no association have been reported. (Showalter et al., 2008)
So far, the only pharmacogenetics markers label by the FDA in colorectal cancer treatments for their study, prior to drug administration, are tumoral expression of EGFR measure by immunohistochemical and KRAS mutation in codon 12 or 13 (FDA, 2011).
Germline pharmacogenetics studies of efficiency are based on the premise of non mutability of the markers in the tumor (McWhinney & McLeod, 2009), nevertheless, being cancer a disease resulting from accumulation of mutations which drives its progression, such assumption, does not appear to have any evidence based support neither from an experimental or literature point of view (Biankin & Hudson, 2011).
To date there is 70 drugs with pharmacogenomic biomarkers in drug labels approved by the FDA. Of these, 21 are oncology- hematology drugs. In Table 1 is shown the kind of information acquired from each gene and the tissue required for its study (FDA, 2011).
The table reflects the utility of the analysis performed in blood related to toxicity but it is noticeable to point out that the FDA recommendations state the necessity of analyze the tumor tissue when performing studies of effectiveness. It remarkable to highlight too, that just a few genes (EGFR, KRAS, Estrogen receptor, Her2/neu and C-kit) are used as

pharmacogenetic markers of effectivity in solid tumors, which indicates that just the association of these genes have been consistently replicated across the studies.

Drug Biomarker	FDA recommendation	Related to	Tissue analyzed
Arsenic Trioxide			
PML/RARα translocation	Positive for PML/RAR-alpha.	Effectivity	Blood
Busulfan			
Chr. Ph	Positive for Philadelphia chromosome.	Effectivity	Blood
Capecitabine			
DPD	Contraindicated in patients with known dihydropyrimidine dehydrogenase (DPD) deficiency.	Toxicity	Blood
Cetuximab			
EGFR	Colorectal cancer. Immunohistochemical evidence of EGFR tumor expression	Effectivity	Tumor
KRAS	Use of Erbitux is not recommended for the treatment of colorectal cancer with KRAS mutations in codon 12 or 13	Effectivity	Tumor
Dasatinib			
Ph+	Positive for Philadelphia chromosome.	Effectivity	Blood
Erlotinib			
EGFR	Patients with EGFR immunohistochemistry (IHC) positive tumors.	Effectivity	Tumor
Fulvestrant			
Estrogen receptor	Hormone receptor positive metastatic breast cancer.	Effectivity	Tumor
Gefitinib			
EGFR	Positive for EGFR	Effectivity	Tumor
Imatinib			
C-Kit	Adult patients with ASM without the D816V c-Kit mutation or with c-Kit mutational status unknown. Patients with Kit (CD117) positive unresectable and/or metastatic malignant GIST. Adjuvant treatment of adult patients following resection of Kit (CD117) positive GIST.	Effectivity	Tumor
Ph+	Newly diagnosed patients with Ph+ CML in CP. Patients with Ph+ CML in BC, AP, or in CP after failure of interferon-alpha therapy. Adult patients with relapsed or refractory Ph+ ALL	Effectivity	Blood

PDGFR gene re-arrangements	Adult patients with MDS/MPD disease associated with PDGFR gene re-arrangements	Effectivity	Blood
FIP1L1-PDGFRα fusion	Adult patients with HES and/or CEL who have the FIP1L1-PDGFRα fusion kinase (mutational analysis or FISH demonstration of CHIC2 allele deletion) and for patients with HES and/or CEL who are FIP1L1-PDGFRα fusion kinase negative or unknown	Effectivity	Blood
Irinotecan			
UGT1A1	A reduction in the starting dose by at least one level of CAMPTOSAR should be considered for patients known to be homozygous for the UGT1A1*28 allele	Toxicity	Blood
Lapatinib			
Her2/neu	Hormone receptor positive metastatic breast cancer that overexpresses the HER2 receptor for whom hormonal therapy is indicated.	Effectivity	Tumor
Lenalidomide			
Chr.5q	Chromosome 5q deletion	Effectivity	Blood
Mercaptopurine			
TPMT	Substantial dose reductions are generally required for homozygous-TPMT deficiency patients and for heterozygous patients when clinical evidences of severe toxicity, particularly myelosuppression, TPMT testing should be considered.	Toxicity	Blood
Nilotinib			
Ph+	Patients positive for Philadelphia chromosome	Effectivity	Blood
UGT1A1	Tasigna can increase bilirubin levels. A pharmacogenetic analysis the (TA)7/(TA)7 genotype was associated with a statistically significant increase in the risk of hyperbilirubinemia relative to the (TA)6/(TA)6 and (TA)6/(TA)7 genotypes.	Toxicity	Blood
Panitumumab			
EGFR	Detection of EGFR protein expression is necessary for selection of patients.	Effectivity	Tumor
KRAS	Use of Vectibix is not recommended for the treatment of colorectal cancer with in patients whose tumors had KRAS mutations in codon 12 or 13.	Effectivity	Tumor
Rasburicase			
G6PD	Do not administer Elitek to patients with glucose-6-phosphate dehydrogenase (G6PD) deficiency.	Toxicity	Blood

Tamoxifen			
Estrogen receptor	Available evidence indicates that patients whose tumors are estrogen receptor positive are more likely to benefit from NOLVADEX therapy.	Effectivity	Tumor
Thioguanine			
TPMT	Inherited deficiency of the enzyme thiopurine methyltransferase (TPMT) may be unusually sensitive to the myelosuppressive effects of thioguanine and prone to developing rapid bone marrow suppression following the initiation of treatment.	Toxicity	Blood
Tositumomab			
CD20 antigen	The BEXXR therapeutic regimen is indicated for the treatment of patients with CD20 antigen expressing relapsed or refractory, low grade, follicular, or transformed non-Hodgkin´s lymphoma, including patients with Rituximab-refractory non-Hodgkin´s lymphoma.	Effectivity	Blood
Trastuzumab			
Her2/neu	Detection of HER2 protein overexpression is necessary for selection of patients appropriate for Herceptin therapy.	Effectivity	Tumor
Warfarin			
CYP2C9 VKORC1	Not all factors causing warfarin dose variability are known. The maintenance dose needed to achieve a target PT/INR is influenced genetic factors (CYP2C9 and VKORC1 genotypes) patients. Dose adjustments are required.	Effectivity	Blood

Table 1. Pharmacogenomic Biomarkers in Drug Labels in Oncology-Hematology labeled by FDA

In line with the pharmacogenetic markers are the pharmacogenetic methods used to test them. A review by Beaulieu et al., make an analysis of the evaluation of the pharmacogenomic tests implemented by some organizations. The authors state: A high degree of heterogeneity between evaluations was observed even within studies evaluating the same pharmacogenomic test" (Beaulieu et al., 2010).

Interestingly, of the 44 markers analyzed by the review, only the analysis of HER-2 gene amplification and HER-2 protein overexpression related to the breast cancer treatment, Trastuzumab, and EGFR overexpression related to NSCLC treatment, Erlotinib, was assessed or referred by the four organizations mentioned, and there is only 7 and 10 markers that were evaluated by three and two of them, respectively. This reflects the lack of consensus in the genetic markers utilized for the pharmacogenetic approach of the treatments (Beaulieu et al., 2010).

The analysis, realized by the authors, highlights some issues in some of the studies, like, the poor definition of the genetic group classification used for the evaluation of the markers, as well as the management of the possible false results that were not considered in some of them. In one of the studies, the authors used inappropriate information to infer the genotype, and in another there is not a clear presentation of the drug dose administrated based on the genetic data. The authors pointed out the need of a confirmatory assay for the evaluation of the markers when a standardized screening method do not exist, confirmation, that it is not always performed. Finally, they underline the confusing assignment of the intermediate phenotype that can lead to a wrong classification of the patients into the groups (Beaulieu et al., 2010).

Regardless these polymorphisms seem to be implicated in the treatment outcome, the lack of replication of these studies together with the fact that most replicated studies are done in tumor samples, bring in relevance the importance of the study of the tumoral tissue (Contopoulos-Ioannidis, 2006; FDA, 2011).

If following the stated lines for this approach, it appears evident that the optimal situation would be the analysis of tumor samples at different times in order to provide updated information enabling a better treatment selection, as it is already done in different leukemias (Baccarani et al., 2006).

However, the difficulty of this practical approach in solid cancers point out the importance of defining the somatic footprinting of the tumor.

Since each tumor has its specific genetic pattern that could be modified because of the addition of new variables, we seek to evaluate the impact of cancer treatments in the modulation of these patterns.

With this aim, following our previous study, where pharmacogenetic markers were studied in pre-treatment tumoral samples, we studied post-treatment tumoral samples in the same cohort of patients with the purpose of try to establish the direction of the somatic mutations under the influence of cancer treatment that we expect will help us, in the future, to find out to find out the mutational mechanisms trigger in rectal cancer that have an impact in the pharmacogenetics markers (Balboa et al., 2010).

1.2 Molecular events produced in a rectal cancer

Even though the adenoma-carcinoma sequence drives the colorectal cancer development (Gloor, 1986), specific molecular events differentiate rectal versus colon cancer (Lindblom, 2001). The proximal colon tumor is more prone to microsatellite instability than rectal and distal areas, whereas distal and rectal colon tumors have been associated with chromosomal instability and microsatellite stability (Li & Lai, 2009; Fernebro et al., 2002; Gervaz et al., 2004).

Other genetic alterations, such as over-expression of *TP53* and *COX-2* genes, and the pattern of mutational frequencies or chromosomal alterations can explain the worse prognosis of patients with rectal cancer (Slattery et al., 2009), but it is noteworthy that patients with different tumors but similar genetic and molecular background seem to have similar survival (Kalady et al., 2009).

In the same way, the existence of mutually exclusive mutations in the same tumor type highlights the importance of differentiate subgroups. These observations reveal the importance of identify the tumor specific genetic pattern (Yeang et al., 2008).

1.3 Pharmacogenomics of Neoadjuvant chemoradiation in rectal cancer

5-Fluorouracil (5-FU), is an antimetabolite of the pyrimidine analogue type which inhibits the DNA and RNA synthesis. The main target for 5-FU is Thymidylate synthase (TYMS); 5-FU acts preventing methylation of the deoxyuridine monophosphate (dUMP) to deoxythymidine monophosphate (dTMP) by forming a stable complex 5-FU-TYMS, causing a thymine deficiency (Zhang, 2008). The methylation reaction requires the availability of methyl donors, in this case the 5,10-methylenetetrahydrofolate (CH_2THF), which concentration is regulated by several enzymes such as Methylenetetrahydrofolate Reductase (MTHFR) (Gaughan et al., 2000). Since 80-85% of drug catabolic degradation occurs in the liver by Dihydropyrimide dehydrogenase (DPYD) (Ho et al., 1986), deficiency of this enzyme leads to toxicity that can cause death (Johnson et al., 1999). Both the level of TYMS expression (Pullarkat et al., 2001) and the degree of activity of MTHFR (Cohen et al., 2003) have been associated with treatment effectiveness and toxicity, although the latter is mainly related to DPYD activity (Johnson & Diasio, 2001).

Radiotherapy uses ionizing radiation to induce cellular damage either directly or indirectly, through interactions with water-derived radicals causing in DNA both, single-strand breaks and double-strand breaks. Cells that are exposed to radiation start a process that ultimately activate cell cycle checkpoints allowing DNA enzyme repair activity; when DNA damage can not be repaired, cells undergoes apoptosis (Pawlik & Keyomarsi, 2004; Hoeijmakers, 2001). In accordance with the damage generated, different repair systems are working in cells (Hoeijmakers, 2001). Single strands breaks are repaired by a rapid global single-strand breaks repair process, being XRCC1 one of the most important proteins that mediate this process by acting as a molecular scaffold stabilizing and promoting different steps of the single-strand breaks repair process (Caldecotto, 2003): XRCC1 acts direct and indirect by interaction with other molecules in the end processing, gap filling and ligation. Double-strand breaks are repaired by non homologous end-joining, homologous recombination and single-strand annealing, being this kind of damaged which generally leads to a lethal event (Valerie & Povirk, 2003). ERCC1 is an endonuclease of the nucleotide excision repair system that acts not only in the single-strand annealing repair but also there are evidences that acts in the homologous repair of the double strand break (Murray & Rosenberg, 1996; Niedernhofer et al., 2004; Ahmad et al., 2008). Deficiency in this enzyme, and others implicated in the NER system, has also been associated with hypersensitivity to radiation (Parshad et al., 1993; Satoh et al., 1993). One of these enzymes, ERCC2, is implicated in the repair of numerous types of damage and although there are few data on the possible connection between this gene and radiotherapy response it has been hypothesized to participate in the repair of ionizing radiation damage (Rzeszowska-Wolny et al., 2005; Angelini et al., 2005).

Although the volume of the literature on pharmacogenetic markers involved in the response to 5-FU is quite large (Strimpakos et al., 2009; Huang & Ratain, 2009), there are still few studies examining the relationship between pharmacogenetic markers and response to chemoradiotherapy (Lamas et al., 2009), with most of them focused on p53, *Ki-67*, *p21*, and *bax/bcl-2* (Smith et al., 2006; Debucquoy et al., 2006; Kuremsky et al., 2009), cytochrome c oxidase II (COX-2) (Debucquoy et al., 2006), EGF receptor (*EGFR*) (Kikuchi et al., 2009) and TYMS (Kikuchi et al., 2009; Stoehlmacher et al., 2008). A summary of the principal genes studied in relation to rectal cancer are shown in Table 2. However, the clinical utility of these biomarkers remains controversial (Kuremsky et al., 2009), with EGFR, p21 and TYMS as the most validated markers of response until now (Kuremsky et al., 2009).

At the present germline-based pharmacogenetics is useful for predicting toxicity, but has serious limitations for the prediction of treatment response. As stated in a previous study, pharmacogenetic markers should be contrasted with the mutational pattern in each particular tumor type. The study of the tumor and, more specifically, the determination of the tumoral mutational spectrum can possible improve response prediction.

Drug	Gene	Cell function	Mutation or polymorphism	Effect	Hypothesis to test *
CRT (chemoradiation)	P53				
		Implicated in genetic stability, cell proliferation, apoptosis, and inhibition of angiogenesis.	Inactivating tumor mutations	Increased genetic instability and survival of cells with damaged DNA	Loss of p-53 dependent apoptosis and a proliferation advantage. Mutant p53 resistant to CRT
	Ki-67				
		Asses proliferation.			
	p21				
		Cyclin-dependent kinase inhibitors that inhibit cells from entering the G1 to S phase.	Tumor mutations		Wild-type p21 suppresses apoptosis in the presence of DNA damage caused by CRT
	bax/bcl-2				
		BAX is a proapoptotic counterpart of Bcl-2 which inhibits cellular apoptosis.	Bax and Bcl2 expression		Protect cells from radiation-induced apoptosis
	cytochrome c oxidase II (COX-2)				
		Catalyzes the conversion of arachidonic acid to prostaglandins. These factors are important mediators of tumor invasiveness and metastatic potential.	COX-2 over-expression		Protect tumor cells from damage by generating prostaglandins as tumor survival factors

*(Kuremsky et al., 2009; Gaya Spoverato et al., 2011; Davis et al., 2004)

Drug	Gene	Cell function	Mutation or polymorphism	Effect	Hypothesis to test
5-FU	TYMS				
		DNA synthesis	5′ 28-bp repeat (rs34743033)	More repetitions increase the efficiency of translation (Horie et al., 1995)	TS protein levels inversely associated with tumor clinical response (Kawakami et al., 2001)
				High- and low-expression haplotypes (Johnston et al., 1994; Mandola et al., 2003)	
			SNP G->C (rs2853542)	High: 2R/3G,3C/3G,3G/3G	Increased survival in low-expression groups (Mandola et al., 2003;
				Low: 2R/2R, 2R/3C, 3C/3C	

				Kawakami & Watanabe, 2003)
		TS1494del6 (rs16430)	Decreases the stability of mRNA (Mandola et al., 2004)	Protective role in adjuvant treatment (Dotor et al., 2006)
	DPYD			
	Drug catabolism	DPYD*2 (IVS14+1 G->A) (rs3918290)	Decreased activity by deletion of exon 14. (van Kuilenburg et al., 2002)	
	MTHFR			
	Implicated in the regulation of the concentration of methyl donors	SNP C677T (rs1801133)	The change Val222Ala leads to a thermolabile variant of MTHFR with reduced enzymatic activity (Frosst et al. 1995)	Increased sensitivity to 5-FU (Sohn et al., 2004; Etienne et al., 2004)
		SNP A1298C (rs1801131)	The change Glu429Ala results in decreased MTHFR activity (Weisberg et al., 1998)	

	Gene Cell function	Mutation or polymorphism	Effect	Hypothesis to test
Radiotherapy Cetuximab	**EGF receptor (EGFR)**			
	Cell proliferation, apoptosis, and differentiation	EGFR overexpression CA-SSR1 (rs11568315)	Approximately 80% inhibition in alleles with 21 CA repeats (Gebhardt et al. 1999)	Response to preoperative radiotherapy (Giralt et al., 2002)
Radiotherapy Oxaliplatin	**XRCC1**			
	Protein that acts as a molecular scaffold, stabilizing and promoting different steps of the SSB repair process, directly and indirectly by interacting with other molecules in the end processing, gap filling and ligation.	Arg399Gln (rs25487)	Changes in binding capacity in the protein with the mutated allele to proteins that interact with it (Evans et al., 1997)	Ionizing radiation hypersensitivity (Hu et al., 2001) Resistance to oxaliplatin (Stoehlmacher et al., 2001)
	ERCC1			
	Endonuclease of the nucleotide excision repair system that acts in the single-strand annealing repair, there is also evidence suggesting that ERCC1 acts in the homologous repair of double-strand breaks	Asn118Asn (rs11615)	Predicts 50% decrease in the efficiency of translation of mRNA to protein (Lunn et al., 2000)	Ionizing radiation hypersensitivity (Lamas et al., 2009) Resistance to oxaliplatin

			(Stohelmacher et al., 2004)
ERCC2 (XPD)			
Implicated in the repair of numerous types of damage. Although there are few data on the possible connection between this gene and radiotherapy response, it has been hypothesized to participate in ionizing radiation repair damage	Lys751Gln (rs13181)	The wild-type allele exhibits suboptimal radiation-induced damage repair (Lunn et al., 2000)	Possible predictor of clinical outcome (Zárate et al., 2006) Resistance to oxaliplatin (Park et al., 2001)

Table 2. Pharmacogenetic biomarkers in rectal cancer treatment.

2. Material and methods

2.1 Patients & clinical data

We studied germline and tumoral samples of 65 stage II/III rectal patients. They were staged by CT scan, colonoscopy and endorectal ultra-sonography. The tumors were assessed by biopsy. Every treatment began in the 3 weeks following diagnosis and staging. The patients received 5-FU 225 mg/m2/day continuous infusion or capecitabine 825 mg/m2 twice daily during weeks 1–5, along the fractionated radiotherapy schedule (1.89 Gy per day, 50.49 Gy over the whole treat-ment). The surgery was carried out 6–8 weeks after completion of chemoradiotherapy using the TME technique. The surgical procedure included abdominoperineal resection, anterior resection and Hartmann's operation.

Tumor regression was assessed using the tumor regression grading (TRG) system of Mandard *et al*, 1994. as follows:

TRG1: absence of residual cancer and extensive fibrosis;

TRG2: rare residual cancer cells scattered through the fibrosis;

TRG3: increased residual cancer cells but fibrosis still predominating;

TRG4: residual cancer outgrowing fibrosis;

TRG5: absence of regressive changes.

Tumors were classified as good responders (TRG1 and TRG2) or poor responders (TRG3, TRG4 and TRG5). All patients gave written informed consent.

Relevant clinical data were obtained from clinical records (gender, age, TRG and treatment). Response to treatment and overall survival were also analyzed. TRG was assessed by the pathologist in the surgical specimen.

2.2 Genotyping

Genomic DNA was extracted from paired peripheral blood samples and rectal cancer tumors. Blood was obtained before any treatment began, and the tumor used for genotyping was a sample from the initial biopsy. Germline DNA was obtained from leukocytes by peripheral blood samples using a magnetic particle-based purification kit (Chemagen, Baesweiler, Germany). Tumoral DNA was extracted from formalin-fixed, paraffin-embedded sections of the tumor samples after xylene treatment. DNA extraction was performed using the QIAamp® DNA Mini Kit Extraction Column (Qiagen®, CA, USA) in accordance with the protocol. The DNA obtained was rapidly frozen at -20°C.

2.3 Pharmacogenetic polymorphisms

We analyzed a panel of pharmacogenetics markers with previous evidence of relation or possible relation with the treatment currently used in rectal cancer. The pharmacogenetic markers analyzed were polymorphisms in *XRCC1, ERCC1, ERCC2, GSTP1, MTHFR* and *DPYD* gene, indicated in Table 2.

2.4 SNaPshot assay

Polymorphisms at *XRCC1, ERCC1, ERCC2, GSTP1, MTHFR* and *DPYD* were analyzed by the SNaPshot® (SNaPshot Multiplex System, Applied Biosystems, CA, USA) method. Multiplex PCR primers and SNaPshot probes and methods were previously described (Balboa et al., 2010).

3. Results

Genotyping analysis was performed in 65 enrolled patients of rectal cancer. Their characteristics are shown in Table 3. Median age of the patients was 64 years (range 37-85) and all were submitted to total mesorectal excision (TME). Surgery was scheduled 6-8 weeks after completion of radiochemotherapy. Median time from the end of neoadjuvant treatment and surgery range from 5 to 13 weeks using the total mesorectal excision technique. Patients were divided into two groups according to the neoadjuvant-surgery interval: <8 weeks and ≥8 weeks. Forty-six patients in this study had an interval to surgery ≥8 weeks. Of that group, 20 (43.48%) were good responders. Nineteen patients underwent surgery at an interval <8 weeks and 11 (57.9%) of them were good responders.

Gender	Female	15	(23.1%)
	Male	50	(76.9%)
Age			
	Median (years)	64	
	Range	(37-85)	
Clinical Stage			
	II	20	(30.8%)
	III	45	(69.2%)
Tumor localization			
	Rectal	65	(100%)
TRG	1	19	(29.2%)
	2	12	(18.5%)
	3	20	(30.8%)
	4	10	(15.4%)
	5	4	(6.1%)
Neoadjuvant therapy			
	FU/UFT+RDT	46	(70.8%)
	CAPECIT+RDT	19	(29.2%)

Table 3. Characteristics of the 65 patients

As reported previously (Balboa et al., 2010) no significant associations were observed between good responders in patients operated before 8 weeks compared to those operated after 8 weeks, p=0.297, OR=1.798. The surgery procedure included anterior resection in 39 patients, abdominoperineal resection in 23 patients and Hartman procedure in 3 patients. A histopathologically confirmed complete resection (R0 status) of proximal and distal resection margins was achieved in 62 cases. Tumor regression parameters became apparent by T-level downsizing (comparing pretreatment cT with ypT at surgery) in 46 patients (70.8%). T-level was decreased by one level in 21 patients (32.3%), two levels in 6 patients (9.2%), three levels in 15 patients (23.1%) and four levels in 4 patients (6.2%). UICC downstaging (comparing cUICC and ypUICC) was performed in 49 patients (75.4%).
Sixty-five patients were evaluable for pathological response. Pathological staging was as follows: ypT0N0 19 patients (29.2%), ypT1N0 4 patients (6.2%); ypT2bN0 18 patients (27.7%); ypT2N1 1 patient (1.5%) and ypT3 in 23 patients (35.4%) (N0:11, N1:10; N2:2).
Complete pathologic response TRG1 was observed in 19 (29.2%) of patients and TRG2 was observed in other 12 (18.5%) patients, so the good response rate was of 47.7% in this study. Of the remaining 52.3% of patients, 20 patients (30.8%) showed TRG3, 10 patients (15.4%) TRG4 and 4 patients (6.1%) showed TRG5.
From 65 patients initially studied we obtain tumor samples after treatment in 53 cases. Germline DNA from blood, biopsy samples DNA (T0) and surgical samples DNA (T1) from the patients were genotyped for *XRCC1, ERCC1, ERCC2, GSTP1* and *MTHFR* gene polymorphisms. Genotype distribution in blood is in agreement with that predicted by the Hardy-Weinberg equilibrium. Overall frequencies of the studied polymorphisms were found to be similar to those described in previous reports. A summary of results are in Table 4.

		Blood	**T0**	**T1**
XRCC1	A/A	3	5	1
	G/A	33	42	34
	G/G	29	16	17
ERCC1	C/C	7	3	4
	C/T	31	33	24
	T/T	27	29	23
ERCC2	A/A	23	24	17
	A/C	38	39	33
	C/C	4	1	1
GSTP1	A/A	36	30	26
	G/A	23	21	13
	G/G	6	6	5
MTHFR_C677T	C/C	30	26	19
	C/T	27	28	26
	T/T	8	11	7
MTHFR_A1298	A/A	28	23	20
	A/C	27	35	24
	C/C	10	7	9

Table 4. Genotypes in blood, biopsy (T0) and tumor after treatment (T1)

In Balboa et al. (2010) we described the differences between the genotypes when blood and biopsy are analyzed. When blood sample is used a significant association with response to treatment is given with TS gene 5'UTR, but this significance is lost in the analysis of biopsys, arising an association between better response and genotype AA of XRCC1 gene. However, many differences between the genotype determined in blood and tumor samples were found. Loss of heterozygosity but no microsatellite instability was observed in the study. Some patients, harbouring several mutations and high somatic mutational rate allow us to classify them as hipermutable. The C:G to T:A transitions was the most prevalent changes and C:G to G:C transversions more rare, these percentages, that are conditioned by the initials genotypic frequencies of each gene in the patients cohort, it is driven by the specific mutational mechanisms asociated to each gene in each tumor.

By contrast XRCC1 appeared significant due to the increase of allele A, as results of the transition C:G to T:A. The latter could not happen with the ERCC1 presumably because the allele involved is the C, and that allele is the least frequent. This loss will have little effect on the association analysis, even if such association actually exists.

Table 5 and 6 show the results, of the study of these same patients cohort, after treatment.

As we can observe the tumor after treatment genotypes are more similar to the germline (blood), related to the effectiveness of treatment, able to reverse the genotypes. However a more detailed analysis of data reveals interesting aspects. First, although the genotypes of T1 tumor are more similar to blood, this effect is more pronounced for LOH than for gain of alleles. Yet, for almost all the markers after treatmen we reveal a drop of LOH to 0% except ERCC1 (4.5%) and MTHFR C677 (4.3%). In contrast, individuals who were homozygous in blood and heterozygotes in biopsy (16.9% average, with range from 40% for XRCC1 gene to 8,6% for GSTP1) are reduced in the second tumor in 11.6% (reduction in MTHFR is more pronounced (Balboa et al., 2010).

Thus, regardless of the specific tumor marker and taking into account the possible influence of tissue analyzed (more or less rich in tumor cells) we can broadly see in that reduction of genotype differences (which can be attributed to a reduction of tumor tissue related to tumoral treatment), a clear distinction between the two underlying mechanisms: recovery of LOH and gain of alleles. So, regardless of whether the cells are actually affected by the treatment, is clear that this treatment affects more strongly the former mechanism than the latter. If we establish a connection between genomic instability and LOH versus altered sequence repair mechanisms and gain of alleles seems that a selection is occurring against the first mechanism and not so intense in the second, and the survival cells were those maintain this altered mutational mechanism.

Taking a look at individual markers, it provides valuable information about previously proposed pharmacogenetic hypothesis. So for XRCC1 gene, we have 65 blood, 62 biopsy and 52 resection genotypes. From individuals that were homozygous analyzing blood, we can observe the 11 heterozygous genotypes (AG) in the biopsy analysis and 9 AG genotypes in the second tumor sample. The A allele is described as related to a ineffective protein and consequently associated to a more effective treatment. In our patients there are 4 individuals who revert to a normal (GG) genotype, which would be consistent with the hypothesis but an individual who reverts to AA. Since there have been a reduction in the tumor regression would be expected that cells with A allele would be greatly compromised in their ability to survive. If treatment is not completely effective in GG harbouring cells, the sample should be enriched with G alleles, but not with A ones. Furthermore, 3 individuals whose initial tumor was GG appear after treatment with GA.

	XRCC1 (%)		ERCC1 (%)		ERCC2 (%)		GSTP1 (%)		MTHFR_ C677 (%)		MTHFR_ A1298 (%)		Total (%)4	
LOH[1]														
T0	3	9,1%	2	6,5%	3	8,1%	3	13,6%	6	22,2%	0	0,0%	17	30,4%
T1	0	0,0%	1	4,5%	0	0%	0	0,0%	1	4,3%	0	0,0%	2	8,3%
Gain of allele[2]														
T0	12	40,0%	4	11,8%	5	18,5%	3	8,6%	7	18,4%	8	21,1%	39	69,6%
T1	9	32,1%	3	10,3%	3	15%	1	3,1%	4	13,8%	2	6,7%	22	91,7%
Total[3]														
T0	15	23,8%	6	9,2%	8	12,5%	6	10,5%	13	20,0%	8	12,3%	56	100,0%
T1	9	20,9%	4	9,5%	3	7,1%	1	2,7%	5	11,6%	2	4,5%	24	100,0%

Table 5. Germline changes versus tumor changes (T0 and T1): loss of heterozygosity and gain of alleles in *XRCC1, ERCC1,* ERCC2, *GSTP1* and *MTHFR* genes.

	XRCC1 (%)		ERCC1 (%)		ERCC2 (%)		GSTP1 (%)		MTHFR_ C677 (%)		MTHFR_ A1298 (%)		Total (%)4	
Substitutions at C:G base pairs														
C:G>T:A[5]														
T0	14	16,1%	6	13,3%			3	9,4%	10	11,5%			33	58,9%
T1	9	11,5%	4	11,1%			0	0,0%	4	6,0%			17	70,8%
C:G >A:T[5]														
T0					6,0	13,3%					3	6,4%	9	16,1%
T1					2	5,6%					1	2,4%	3	12,5%
Substitutions at T:A base pairs														
T:A>C:G[5]														
T0	1	2,6%	0	0%			3	3,7%	3	7,0%			7	12,5%
T1	0	0,0%	0	0%			1	1,5%	1	2,7%			2	8,3%
T:A >G:C[5]														
T0					2	2,4%					5	6,0%	7	12,5%
T1					1	1,5%					1	1,5%	2	8,3%
Total[6]														
T0	15	26,8%	6	10,7%	8	14,3%	6	10,7%	13	23,2%	8	14,3%	56	100,0%
T1	9	37,5%	4	16,7%	3	12,5%	1	4,2%	5	20,8%	2	8,3%	24	100,0%

Table 6. Germline changes versus tumor changes (T0 and T1): single base substitutions in *XRCC1, ERCC1,* ERCC2, *GSTP1,* and *MTHFR* genes.

This case illustrates some of the issues involved in the pharmacogenetic studies:

- Confounding factors. The coexistence of markers related to opposite associations could mask the results (Showalter et al., 2008).
- The association to treatment efficacy may be a statistical artifact, in fact not related to the marker but to the mutational mechanism of the tumor. For example, as already described previously (Sjoblom et al., 2006; Balboa et al., 2010), in rectal cancer the C:C to T:A transitions are the most prevalent changes and consequently the new alleles arising will be mainly A (GG to GA, GA to AA genotypes) but not G (no cases of AA to GA genotypes). Thus, for this marker, the mutagenic mechanism related to the specific G to A changes, determine the appearance of this allele in the tumor and possibly the subsequent association. As we have seen this mutagenic mechanism remains in the tumor after cancer treatment.

Yeang et al. (2008) detected significant different mutational patterns between cell lines and tumor samples. The effect of a polymorphism or somatic mutation in a protein is firstly tested in a cell line. So, another confounding source in the pharmacogenetics studies is due to that data supporting their functional effect come from ¨in vitro¨ studies and the effect observed of these mutations or polymorphisms in the cell lines could not be the same ¨in vivo¨. When these markers are tested in patient samples studies a lack of replication has been observed.

Quantification of the mutations along the different stages could helps us to identify the effective mutations, since it is expected an increase in the population of the cells that carry beneficial mutations for the tumor along the cancer development, but these increase in the number of cells that carry somatic mutations in one stage, but that are not kept across the stages could be explained too by a momentary increase of the uncontrolled cell population that are going to die due to the high number of harmful mutations.

4. Discussion

The difficult of analyzing tumor samples rises from the heterogeneity found in cancer cells that are subdue to different conditions depending on its location in the tumor (Michor et al., 2010). Besides, tumor samples are a mixture of these differents tumor cells and normal cells (Biankin & Hudson, 2011). These circumstances explain the difficult of interpret the results of pharmacogenetic markers in tumor samples.

To analyze tumor samples is important to differentiate too, the genetic background of the patient from the genetic of the tumor, and differenciate these from the response of the tumors to the treatment.

Tumor have an inherent progression, even though this is going to be affected by the patient´s genetic background, there are a pattern of genetic alterations, typical of each tumor. So, when a gene, that are tested in pharmacogenetic studies, is implicated in cancer progression, even though it should be expected a similar trend between patients, different results could be obtained, that are related to the different circumstances that the cells analyzing are being subjected. An example of this is p53, a gene implicated in the adenoma-carcinoma sequence. Overexpression of this gene has been linked to rectal cancer but, analysis of the tumor has shown different expression rates measure by IHC (Kuremsky et al., 2009; Gaya Spoverato et al., 2011). Another example of this is the proliferating cell nuclear antigen (Ki-67) used to assess cell proliferation. A cancer actively growing should have high Ki-67 expression but these will be depending on the stage, the status and the localization of the cells being tested.

Another important point to take into account is that even though cancer treatments are design to act mostly over high proliferative tumor cells, this is dependent of the genetic background of cell tumor. So, although it should be expected that a tumor with high cell proliferative rates, should experience higher efficiency and have a better prognostic, different results can be obtained, depending on the genetic background of cell tumor. If we take as example the meaning of the results of Ki-67, it should be expected that cells with a high proliferative rate, have a high Ki-67 expression, and experience a high treatment efficiency with a good prognostic, but studies by IHC show contradictory results or no correlation with the prognosis, indicating that in tumor cells are being produced a set of different changes that lead to achieve a result which are not explained by the analysis of single markers.(Kuremsky et al., 2009; Gaya Spoverato et al., 2011)

So, to interpret the results from pharmacogenetics studies and to extract information from them, it is of main importance understand the circumstances to which tumor are subjected, and identify the driver mutations, that are produced on them, that will lead its developed and its response to the environment (Stratton et al., 2009)

4.1 Ecology of the cancer

All biological system is affected by the interaction of the environment that surrounds it, and it is the response to signals from that environment a major factor that determines the system behavior (Kenny et al., 2006; Crespi & Summers, 2005).

Tumors, as any other biological system, need to survive and proliferate using the resources from their environment. Thus, the environment, where the different cancers are submerged, will shape the pathways that will be chosen by the cancer for its development. And, the response to the different signals received from the different environments over the progression of the cancer will configure the adjustment of the molecular pathways. These adjustments are executed at different levels, being the genetic level the first step of regulation, mainly through somatic mutations and epigenetic. (Stratton et al., 2009)

In this sense, a plethora of mutational events are shared in cancer but the predominance of one over the others is the specific hallmark of each cancer. Identify and determine the meaning of the changes in these molecular pathways in each cancer is key for understand the mechanisms of cancer progression (Slattery et al., 2009).

With this purpose, tumors have to redirect molecular pathways highly organized and controlled by many checkpoints in order to escape from the self-defense mechanisms, apoptosis, and grow in a not favorable environment. To achieve this aim, cells undergo changes at both phenotypic and genotypic levels that allow cancer cells to overgrow normal cells.

Even within the tumor, cells are subjected to different conditions due to a differential oxygen pressure and nutrients input. These conditions determine the adjustments that cells, according to their localization, have to undergo within the tumor. As the tumor grows, cells, in the core of the tumor, experience a decrease in oxygen and nutrients contribution due to a lack of blood supply. These restricted circumstances cause the switch to an anaerobic metabolism which increase the genetic instability in the cells and induce the segregation of angiogenesis proteins (Allen & Louise Jones, 2011).

At the same time, when tumor gets to a critical mass and the conditions for its development have been exhausted, cells in the tumor periphery initiate changes for its migration to localizations where conditions are more favorable. In this transforming process, cells are subject to a stochastic number of mutations that have a different fitness for the cell. Harmful mutations will inevitably cause cell death and beneficial mutations will be more or less efficient depending on in which cells and moment these mutations happen (Bindra et al., 2005)

But not only the tumor undergoes changes, this interaction is exerted in both ways, the tumor induces a transformation of its environment for its own benefit, inducing changes in the normal cells that support it (genetic alterations in the normal stroma have also been reported) (Kurose et al., 2001; Nosho et al., 2010). Not only cells from the stroma, hypoxia also plays a role in determining the phenotype of infiltrating monocytes, which have an impact on tumor cell behavior, since the inflammatory response have an effect in tumor progression, that can be either pro-tumoral or anti-tumoral (Allen & Louise Jones, 2011).

5. Concluding remarks

As the cancer evolves, different mechanisms drive their progression. The introduction of an additional variable as it is cancer treatments should have an important impact in cancer behavior.

Cancer treatment research, try to identify specific hallmarks of cancer cells that could differentiate them from healthy cells in order to avoid the adverse effects when these treatments are given to the patients. These differential features, can be the formation of new chromosomal entities as it happens in some leukemias or can be a differential regulation of pathways at different levels that are already acting in normal cells.

The importance of study the tumoral samples, before drug administration, raises from the fact that cancer treatments are design to exert their action in cells where these changes had happen.

Introduction of cancer treatment cause a new alteration in the system, tumoral cells have to respond to a new adverse factor, so they again have to module their behavior in order to survive. Once the treatment is given to the patients, two mechanisms of selection should be acting in cancer cells, mechanisms of selection for tumor progression and mechanisms of selection to survive to cancer treatment.

Cancer treatments have a percent of ineffectiveness that can be due to both, drug inefficiency or inaccurate dose so, the number of cells that persist under the treatments and the time that these cells dispose to rearrange the survival and proliferative pathways for its adaptation to the new conditions, will increase the probabilities of emergence of resistance cells to the drug administrated. Since cancer treatments are design to act principally in high proliferative cells, cells that have acquire the mechanisms to proliferate at a higher rate will be the more affected unless this cells posses any mechanisms to avoid it.

The specific mutational pattern in each gene helps to understand their meaning and the impact of these changes in tumor´s behavior (Kim et al., 2008). Different mutational patterns in tumor progression respond to an adjustment of the tumor to the different conditions and stages, depending on the tumor´s needs, in that sense, different mutational patterns should be expected across the stages.

This approach has been used in several studies, were tumors at different stages have been analyzed. In these studies persistence of somatic mutations detected in the primary tumor through the different stages has been observed, but at different frequencies, indicating, as stated Li Ding et al, that the metastasis arises from a minority of cells in the primary tumor (Ding et al., 2010) The analysis of post-treatment tumor samples helps to analyze if the mutational mechanisms, produced during tumor development, that were analyzed in pre-treatment samples, persist under the cancer treatment, and what changes the cells have undergone to be resistant to treatment.

6. Acknowledgment

This work was supported by grants from Fundación Ramón Areces and from Fundación Barrie de la Maza (Programa DIANA). The authors appreciate access to CHUS Tumor Tissue Bank from Dr. Jerónimo Forteza.

7. References

Ahmad A, Robinson AR, Duensing A *et al.*: ERCC1-XPF endonuclease facilitates DNA double strand break repair. *Mol. Cell. Biol.* 28, 5082–5092 (2008).

Allen M, Louise Jones J. Jekyll and Hyde: the role of the microenvironment on the progression of cancer. *J Pathol.* 223(2): 162-76 (2011).

Angelini S, Kumar R, Carbone F *et al.*: Micronuclei in humans induced by exposure to low level of ionizing radiation: influence of polymorphisms in DNA repair genes. *Mutat. Res.* 570: 105–117 (2005).

Baccarani M, Saglio G, Goldman J, Hochhaus A, Simonsson B, Appelbaum F, Apperley J, Cervantes F, Cortes J, Deininger M, Gratwohl A, Guilhot F, Horowitz M, Hughes T, Kantarjian H, Larson R, Niederwieser D, Silver R, Hehlmann R; European LeukemiaNet. Evolving concepts in the management of chronic myeloid leukemia: recommendations from an expert panel on behalf of the European LeukemiaNet. *Blood.* 108(6):1809-20 (2006).

Balboa E, Duran G, Lamas MJ, Gomez-Caamaño A, Celeiro-Muñoz C, Lopez R, Carracedo A, Barros F. Pharmacogenetic analysis in neoadjuvant chemoradiation for rectal cancer: high incidence of somatic mutations and their relation with response. *Pharmacogenomics.* 11(6): 747-61 (2010)

Beaulieu M, de Denus S, Lachaine J. Systematic review of pharmacoeconomic studies of pharmacogenomic tests. *Pharmacogenomics.* 11(11): 1573-90 (2010).

Berardi R, Maccaroni E, Onofri A, Giampieri R, Bittoni A, Pistelli M, Scartozzi M, Pierantoni C, Bianconi M, Cascinu S. Multidisciplinary treatment of locally advanced rectal cancer: a literature review. Part 1. *Expert Opin Pharmacother.* 10(14):2245-58 (2009).

Bertolini F, Chiara S, Bengala C *et al.*: Neoadjuvant treatment with single-agent cetuximab followed by 5-FU, cetuximab, and pelvic radiotherapy: a Phase II study in locally advanced rectal cancer. *Int. J. Radiat. Oncol. Biol. Phys.* 73: 466–472 (2009).

Biankin AV, Hudson TJ. Somatic variation and cancer: therapies lost in the mix. *Hum Genet.* Jun 5. (2011)

Bindra RS, Schaffer PJ, Meng A, Woo J, Måseide K, Roth ME, Lizardi P, Hedley DW, Bristow RG, Glazer PM. Alterations in DNA repair gene expression under hypoxia: elucidating the mechanisms of hypoxia-induced genetic instability. *Ann N Y Acad Sci.* 1059: 184-95 (2005)

Buchdunger E, Zimmermann J, Mett H, Meyer T, Müller M, Druker BJ, Lydon NB. Inhibition of the Abl protein-tyrosine kinase in vitro and in vivo by a 2-phenylaminopyrimidine derivative. *Cancer Res.* 56(1): 100-4 (1996).

Caldecotto KW: *XRCC1* and DNA strand break repair. *DNA Repair.* 2: 955–969 (2003).

Carlomagno C, Farella A, Bucci L *et al.*: Neo-adjuvant treatment of rectal cancer with capecitabine and oxaliplatin in combination with radiotherapy: a Phase II study. *Ann. Oncol.* 20: 906–912 (2009).

Chen ET, Mohiuddin M, Brodovsky H, Fishbein G, Marks G: Downstaging of advanced rectal cancer following combined preoperative chemotherapy and high dose radiation. *Int. J. Radiat. Oncol. Biol. Phys.* 30, 169–175 (1994)

Cohen V, Panet-Raymond V, Sabbaghian N, Morin I, Batist G, Rozen R: Methylenetetrahydrofolate reductase polymorphism in advanced colorectal cancer: a novel genomic predictor of clinical response to fluoropyrimidine-based chemotherapy. *Clin. Cancer Res.* 9, 1611–1615 (2003).

Contopoulos-Ioannidis DG, Alexiou GA, Gouvias TC, Ioannidis JP: An empirical evaluation of multifarious outcomes in pharmacogenetics: b-2 adrenoceptor gene polymorphisms in asthma treatment. *Pharmacogenet. Genomics.* 16: 705–711 (2006).

Crespi B, Summers K. Evolutionary biology of cancer. *Trends Ecol Evol.* 20(10): 545-52 (2005).

Davis TW, O'Neal JM, Pagel MD, Zweifel BS, Mehta PP, Heuvelman DM, Masferrer JL. Synergy between Celecoxib and Radiotherapy Results from Inhibition of Cyclooxygenase-2-Derived Prostaglandin E2, a Survival Factor for Tumor and Associated Vasculature. *Cancer Res.* 64(1): 279-85 (2004).

Debucquoy A, Goethals L, Geboes K, Roels S, McBride WH, Haustermans K: Molecular responses of rectal cancer to preoperative chemoradiation. *Radiother. Oncol.* 80: 172–177 (2006).

Ding L, Ellis MJ, Li S, Larson DE, Chen K, Wallis JW, Harris CC, McLellan MD, Fulton RS, et al. Genome remodelling in a basal-like breast cancer metastasis and xenograft. *Nature.* 464(7291): 999-1005 (2010).

Dotor E, Cuatrecases M, Martínez-Iniesta M *et al.*: Tumor thymidylate synthase 1494del6 genotype as a prognostic factor in colorectal cancer patients receiving fluorouracil-based adjuvant treatment. *J. Clin. Oncol.* 24(10): 1603–1611 (2006).

Etienne MC, Ilc K, Formento JL *et al.*: Thymidylate synthase and methylenetetrahydrofolate reductase gene polymorphisms: relationships with 5-fluorouracil sensitivity. *Br. J. Cancer.* 90(2): 526–534 (2004).

Evans E, Moggs JG, Hwang JR, Egly JM, Wood RD: Mechanism of open complex and dual incision formation by human nucleotide excision repair factors. *EMBO J.* 16(21): 6559–6573 (1997).

FDA. *Table of pharmacogenomic biomarkers in drug lables.* 1.06.2011. Available from: http://www.fda.gov/Drugs/ScienceResearch/ResearchAreas/Pharmacogenetics/ucm083378.html

Fernebro E, Halvarsson B, Baldetorp B, Nilbert M: Predominance of CIN versus MSI in the development of rectal cancer at young age. *BMC Cancer.* 2: 25 (2002).

Frosst P, Blom HJ, Milos R *et al.*: A candidate genetic risk factor for vascular disease: a common mutation in methylenetetrahydrofolate reductase. *Nat. Genet.* 10(1): 111–113 (1995).

Fujiwara Y, Minami H. An overview of the recent progress in irinotecan pharmacogenetics. *Pharmacogenomics*. 11(3): 391-406 (2010)

Gaughan DJ, Barbaux S, Kluijtmans LA, Whitehead AS: The human and mouse methylenetetrahydrofolate reductase (*MTHFR*) genes: genomic organization, mRNA structure and linkage to the *CLCN6* gene. *Gene*. 257: 279–289 (2000).

Gaya Spolverato , Salvatore Pucciarelli , Roberta Bertorelle, Anita De Rossi and Donato Nitti. Predictive Factors of the Response of Rectal Cancer to Neoadjuvant Radiochemotherapy *Cancers*. 3: 2176-2194 (2011).

Gebhardt F, Zänker KS, Brandt B: Modulation of epidermal growth factor receptor gene transcription by a polymorphic dinucleotide repeat in intron 1. *J. Biol. Chem.* 274(19): 13176–13180 (1999)

Gervaz P, Bucher P, Morel P: Two colons-two cancers: paradigm shift and clinical implications. *J. Surg. Oncol.* 88: 261–266 (2004).

Giralt JL, Aranzazu E, Manuel D *et al.*: Prognostic significance of epidermal growth factor receptor (EGFR) in patients with rectal cancer treated with preoperative radiotherapy: a GICOR study. *Int. J. Radiat. Oncol. Biol. Physics* 54: 98–99 (2002).

Gloor FJ. The adenoma-carcinoma sequence of the colon and rectum. *Soz Praventivmed.* 31(2): 74-5 (1986).

Hiwase DK, Yeung DT, White DL. Optimizing the selection of kinase inhibitors for chronic myeloid leukemia patients. *Expert Rev Hematol.* 4(3): 285-99 (2011).

Ho DH, Townsend L, Luna M, Bodey GP: Distribution and inhibition of dihydrouracil dehydrogenase activities in human tissues using 5-fluorouracil as substrate. *Anticancer Res.* 6: 781–784 (1986).

Hoeijmakers JH: Genome maintenance mechanisms for preventing cancer. *Nature.* 411: 366–374 (2001).

Horie N, Aiba H, Oguro K, Hojo H, Takeishi K: Functional analysis and DNA polymorphism of the tandemly repeated sequences in the 5´-terminal regulatory region of the human gene for thymidylate synthase. *Cell Struct. Funct.* 20(3): 191–197 (1995).

Hu JJ, Smith TR, Miller MS, Mohrenweiser HW, Golden A, Case LD: Amino acid substitution variants of *APE1* and *XRCC1* genes associated with ionizing radiation sensitivity. *Carcinogenesis.* 22(6): 917–922 (2001).

Huang RS, Ratain MJ: Pharmacogenetics and pharmacogenomics of anticancer agents. *CA Cancer J. Clin.* 59: 42–55 (2009).

Innocenti F, Undevia SD, Iyer L et al.: Genetic variants in the UDP-glucuronosyltransferase 1A1 gene predict the risk of severe neutropenia of irinotecan. *J. Clin. Oncol.* 22(8): 1382–1388 (2004).

Johnson MR, Diasio RB: Importance of dihydropyrimidine dehydrogenase (DPD) deficiency in patients exhibiting toxicity following treatment with 5-fluorouracil. *Adv. Enzyme Regul.* 41: 151–157 (2001).

Johnson MR, Hageboutros A, Wang K, High L, Smith JB and Diasio RB: Life-threatening toxicity in a dihydropyrimidine dehydrogenase-deficient patient after treatment with topical 5-fluorouracil. *Clin. Cancer Res.* 5, 2006–2011 (1999).

Johnston PG, Fisher ER, Rockette HE *et al.*: The role of thymidylate synthase expression in prognosis and outcome of adjuvant chemotherapy in patients with rectal cancer. *J. Clin. Oncol.* 12(12): 2640–2647 (1994).

Kalady MF, Sanchez JA, Manilich E, Hammel J, Casey G, Church JM: Divergent oncogenic changes influence survival differences between colon and rectal adenocarcinomas. *Dis. Colon Rectum.* 52: 1039–1045 (2009).

Kawakami K, Salonga D, Park JM *et al.*: Different lengths of a polymorphic repeat sequence in the thymidylate synthase gene affect translational efficiency but not its gene expression. *Clin. Cancer Res.* 7(12): 4096–4101 (2001).

Kawakami K, Watanabe G: Identification and functional analysis of single nucleotide polymorphism in the tandem repeat sequence of thymidylate synthase gene. *Cancer Res.* 63(18): 6004–6007 (2003).

Kenny PA, Nelson CM, Bissell MJ. The Ecology of Tumors: By perturbing the microenvironment, wounds and infection may be key to tumor development. *Scientist.* 20(4):30 (2006)

Kikuchi M, Mikami T, Sato T *et al.*: High Ki67, Bax, and thymidylate synthase expression well correlates with response to chemoradiation therapy in locally advanced rectal cancers: proposal of a logistic model for prediction. *Br. J. Cancer* 101: 116–123 (2009).

Kim JC, Cho YK, Roh SA, Yu CS, Gong G, Jang SJ, Kim SY, Kim YS. Individual tumorigenesis pathways of sporadic colorectal adenocarcinomas are associated with the biological behavior of tumors. *Cancer Sci.* 99(7): 1348-54 (2008).

Kuremsky JG, Tepper JE, McLeod HL: Biomarkers for response to neoadjuvant chemoradiation for rectal cancer. *Int. J. Radiat. Oncol. Biol. Phys.* 74: 673–688 (2009).

Kurose K, Hoshaw-Woodard S, Adeyinka A, Lemeshow S, Watson PH, Eng C. Genetic model of multi-step breast carcinogenesis involving the epithelium and stroma: clues to tumour-microenvironment interactions. *Hum Mol Genet.* 10(18): 1907-13 (2001)

Lamas MJ, Balboa E, Duran G *et al.*: Analysis of pharmacogenetic biomarkers in rectal patients trated with chemoradiotherapy. *J. Clin. Oncol. ASCO Annual Meeting Proceedings (Post-Meeting Edition)* 27(15S): E15051 (2009)

Li FY, Lai MD: Colorectal cancer, one entity or three. *J. Zhejiang Univ. Sci. B* 10: 219–229 (2009).

Lindblom, A: Different mechanisms in the tumorigenesis of proximal and distal colon cancers. *Curr. Opin. Oncol.* 13: 63–69 (2001).

Lunn RM, Helzlsouer KJ, Parshad R *et al.*: *XPD* polymorphisms: effects on DNA repair proficiency. *Carcinogenesis.* 21(4): 551–555 (2000).

Mandard AM, Dalibard F, Mandard JC *et al.*: Pathologic assessment of tumor regression after preoperative chemoradiotherapy of esophageal carcinoma. Clinicopathologic correlations. *Cancer.* 73(11): 2680–2686 (1994)

Mandola MV, Stoehlmacher J, Muller-Weeks S *et al.*: A novel single nucleotide polymorphism within the 5′ tandem repeat polymorphism of the thymidylate synthase gene abolishes USF-1 binding and alters transcriptional activity. *Cancer Res.* 63(11): 2898–2904 (2003).

Mandola MV, Stoehlmacher J, Zhang W *et al.*: A 6 bp polymorphism in the thymidylate synthase gene causes message instability and is associated with decreased intratumoral TS mRNA levels. *Pharmacogenetics.* 14(5): 319–327 (2004).

McWhinney SR, McLeod HL. Using germline genotype in cancer pharmacogenetic studies. *Pharmacogenomics.* 10(3): 489-93 (2009).

Michor F, Polyak K. The origins and implications of intratumor heterogeneity. *Cancer Prev Res (Phila).* 3(11): 1361-4 (2010).

Murray D, Rosenberg E: The importance of the ERCC1/ ERCC4[XPF] complex for hypoxic-cell radioresistance does not appear to derive from its participation in the nucleotide excision repair pathway. *Mutat. Res.* 364: 217–226 (1996).

Niedernhofer LJ, Odijk H, Budzowska M *et al.*: The structure-specific endonuclease ERCC1-XPF is required to resolve DNA interstrand cross-link-induced double strand breaks. *Mol. Cell. Biol.* 24: 5776–5787 (2004).

Nosho K, Baba Y, Tanaka N, Shima K, Hayashi M, Meyerhardt JA, Giovannucci E, Dranoff G, Fuchs CS, Ogino S. Tumour-infiltrating T-cell subsets, molecular changes in colorectal cancer, and prognosis: cohort study and literature review. *J Pathol.* 222(4): 350-66 (2010).

Park DJ, Stoehlmacher J, Zhang W, Tsao-Wei DD, Groshen S, Lenz HJ: A xeroderma pigmentosum group D gene polymorphism predicts clinical outcome to platinum-based chemotherapy in patients with advanced colorectal cancer. *Cancer Res.* 61(24): 8654–8658 (2001).

Parshad R, Tarone RE, Price FM, Sanford KK: Cytogenetic evidence for differences in DNA incision activity in xeroderma pigmentosum group A, C and D cells after X-irradiation during G2 phase. *Mutat. Res.* 294, 149–155 (1993).

Pawlik TM, Keyomarsi K: Role of cell cycle in mediating sensitivity to radiotherapy. *Int. J. Radiat. Oncol. Biol. Phys.* 59, 928–942 (2004).

Pullarkat ST, Stoehlmacher J, Ghaderi V *et al.*: Thymidylate synthase gene polymorphism determines response and toxicity of 5-FU chemotherapy. *Pharmacogenomics J.* 1, 65–70 (2001).

Rzeszowska-Wolny J, Polanska J, Pietrowska M *et al.*: Influence of polymorphisms in DNA repair genes *XPD, XRCC1* and *MGMT* on DNA damage induced by g radiation and its repair in lymphocytes *in vitro. Radiat. Res.* 164: 132–140 (2005).

Satoh MS, Jones CJ, Wood RD, Lindahl T: DNA excision-repair defect of xeroderma pigmentosum prevents removal of a class of oxygen free radical-induced base lesions. *Proc. Natl Acad. Sci. USA* 90: 6335–6339 (1993).

Sauer R, Becker H, Hohenberger W *et al.*: Preoperative versus postoperative chemoradiotherapy for rectal cancer. *N. Engl. J. Med.* 351: 1731–1740 (2004).

Showalter SL, Showalter TN, Witkiewicz A *et al.*: Evaluating the drug-target relationship between thymidylate synthase expression and tumor response to 5-fluorouracil. Is it time to move forward? *Cancer Biol. Ther.* 7: 986–994 (2008).

Sjöblom T, Jones S, Wood LD et al.: The consensus coding sequences of human breast and colorectal cancers. *Science* 314, 268–274 (2006).

Slattery ML, Curtin K, Wolff RK *et al.:* A comparison of colon and rectal somatic DNA alterations. *Dis. Colon Rectum.* 52: 1304–1311 (2009).

Smith FM, Reynolds JV, Miller N, Stephens RB, Kennedy MJ: Pathological and molecular predictors of the response of rectal cancer to neoadjuvant radiochemotherapy. *Eur. J. Surg. Oncol.* 32: 55–64 (2006).

Sohn KJ, Croxford R, Yates Z, Lucock M, Kim YI: Effect of the methylenetetrahydrofolate reductase C677T polymorphism on chemosensitivity of colon and breast cancer cells to 5-fluorouracil and methotrexate. *J. Natl Cancer Inst.* 96(2): 134–144 (2004).

Stoehlmacher J, Ghaderi V, Iobal S *et al.*: A polymorphism of the *XRCC1* gene predicts for response to platinum based treatment in advanced colorectal cancer. *Anticancer Res.* 21(4B): 3075–3079 (2001).

Stoehlmacher J, Goekkurt E, Mogck U *et al.:* Thymidylate synthase genotypes and tumour regression in stage II/III rectal cancer patients after neoadjuvant fluorouracil-based chemoradiation. *Cancer Lett.* 272: 221–225 (2008).

Stoehlmacher J, Park DJ, Zhang W *et al.*: A multivariate analysis of genomic polymorphisms: prediction of clinical outcome to 5-FU/oxaliplatin combination chemotherapy in refractory colorectal cancer. *Br. J. Cancer.* 91: 344–354 (2004).

Stratton MR, Campbell PJ, Futreal PA. The cancer genome. *Nature.* 458(7239): 719-24 (2009).

Strimpakos AS, Syrigos KN, Saif MW: Pharmacogenetics and biomarkers in colorectal cancer. *Pharmacogenomics J.* 9: 147–160 (2009).

Ugidos L, Delgado S, Conill C *et al.:* Phase I trial of neoadjuvant chemoradiotherapy (CRT) with capecitabine and weekly irinotecan followed by laparoscopic total mesorectal excision (LTME) in rectal cancer patients. *Invest. New Drugs.* 27: 262–268 (2009).

Valerie K, Povirk LF: Regulation and mechanisms of mammalian double strand break repair. *Oncogene.* 22: 5792–5812 (2003).

Van Kuilenburg AB, Meinsma R, Zoetekouw L, Van Gennip AH: High prevalence of the *IVS14* + 1G>A mutation in the dihydropyrimidine dehydrogenase gene of patients with severe 5-fluorouracil-associated toxicity. *Pharmacogenetics.* 12(7): 555–558 (2002).

Van Kuilenburg AB: Dihydropyrimidine dehydrogenase and the efficacy and toxicity of 5-fluorouracil. *Eur. J. Cancer.* 40(7), 939–950 (2004)

von Bubnoff N, Schneller F, Peschel C, Duyster J. BCR-ABL gene mutations in relation to clinical resistance of Philadelphia-chromosome-positive leukaemia to STI571: a prospective study. *Lancet.* 359(9305): 487-91 (2002).

Weisberg I, Tran P, Christensen B, Sibani S, Rozen R: A second genetic polymorphism in methylenetetrahydrofolate reductase (*MTHFR*) associated with decreased enzyme activity. *Mol. Genet. Metab.* 64(3): 169–172 (1998).

Wheeler JM, Dodds E, Warren BF *et al.:* Preoperative chemoradiotherapy and total mesorectal excision surgery for locally advanced rectal cancer: correlation with rectal cancer regression grade. *Dis. Colon Rectum.* 47: 2025–2031 (2004).

Willett CG, Duda DG, di Tomaso E *et al.*: Efficacy, safety, and biomarkers of neoadjuvant bevacizumab, radiation therapy, and fluorouracil in rectal cancer: a multidisciplinary Phase II study. *J. Clin. Oncol.* 27: 3020–3026 (2009).

Yeang CH, McCormick F, Levine A. Combinatorial patterns of somatic gene mutations in cancer. *FASEB J.* 22(8): 2605-22 (2008).

Zárate RN, Arias F, Bandres E, Cubedo E, Malumbres R, García-Foncillas J: Xeroderma pigmentosum group D 751 polymorphism as a predictive factor in resected gastric cancer treated with chemo-radiotherapy. *World J. Gastroenterol.* 12(37): 6032–6036 (2006).

Zhang N, Yin Y, Xu SJ, Chen WS: 5-fluorouracil: mechanisms of resistance and reversal strategies. *Molecules.* 13: 1551–1569 (2008).

15

Tumor Markers of Neo-Adjuvant Chemo-Radiation Response in Rectal Cancer

Jacintha N. O'Sullivan, Mary Clare Cathcart and John V. Reynolds
Department of Surgery, Institute of Molecular Medicine, Trinity Centre for Health Science, St. James Hospital, Dublin, Ireland

1. Introduction

Radiation therapy alone or in combination with chemotherapy has lead to improved outcomes in the management of rectal cancer patients. Many studies have demonstrated that for locally advanced rectal cancer, preoperative chemoradiation (CRT) significantly improves local control, reduces toxicity profiles and the risk of disease recurrence (Habr-Gama, Perez et al. 2004), (Kapiteijn, Marijnen et al. 2001), (Frileux, Burdy et al. 2007), (Horisberger, Hofheinz et al. 2008), (Krook, Moertel et al. 1991), (Sauer, Becker et al. 2004). Highly radiosensitive cancers completely regress, leading to improved survival. A histology tumor grading system is used to determine the success of radiation prior to surgery. This is called a tumor regression grade (TRG). Originally described for oesophageal tumors, the TRG system has been adapted to rectal cancer (Mandard, Dalibard et al. 1994). Regression grading stratifies response based on the biological effect of radiation on tumors, dividing it into five different grades based on the ratio of fibrosis to tumor where TRG1: no residual cancer; TRG2: rare residual cancer cells; TRG3 fibrosis outgrowing residual cancer; TRG4: residual cancer outgrowing fibrosis and TRG 5: absence of regressive changes. This TRG scoring system is extremely valuable as it can highlight those tumors demonstrating large variation in biological response to radiation not undergoing a T stage change (Bouzourene, Bosman et al. 2002). In a paper by Ryan et al, they have revised the 5 point TRG system into a 3 point where grade 1 indicates a complete response, grade 2 a partial response and grade 3 no response (Ryan, Gibbons et al. 2005). Currently, only approximately 25% of patients who receive CRT treatment obtain a complete pathological response (Valentini, Coco et al. 2002; Sauer, Becker et al. 2004). Disease free survival in these patients is improved with a reduce rate of local recurrence However, up to 75% of patients receive a treatment that achieves little or no benefit and an increased risk of second cancers has been documented within or adjacent to the irradiated volume (Birgisson, Pahlman et al. 2005).

The broad and unpredictable response to tumor of patients with rectal cancer treated with preoperative chemoradiotherapeutic interventions shows that our understanding of the molecular events leading to radioresistance in patients affected with this malignancy is limited. This variation is thought to depend on tumor size but also on the biological properties of individual tumors. It is important to understand what factors within the tumor predict high sensitivity to the new-adjuvant regimen and what determines resistance, as this information may allow tailor-made individualization of therapy. Classification of responders and non responders may also spare poorly responding patients from undergoing treatment which would derive no benefit for them. In contrast, the ability to predict good response may alter the subsequent management of patients. Many studies have examined prognostic and predictive molecular marker expressions in rectal cancer treated with neo-adjuvant radio-chemotherapy. However, some of these studies only examined expression profiles in the tumor excised after surgery (Bertolini, Bengala et al. 2007). In this chapter, we will critically review the assessed predictors of histological response to new-adjuvant radiation for rectal cancer patients. There are many studies in the literature which have compared biomarker expression levels before and after new-adjuvant treatment and correlated expression differences with a measure of patient outcome. These studies however are not as useful in prospectively predicting which patients will respond to new-adjuvant therapy and are not discussed in this review.

Studies utilizing molecular response predictors from archival pre-treatment tumor tissues have identified several promising predictive markers including p21, thymidylate synthase expression, EFGF status, apoptosis markers and p53 gene status. Global gene expression studies have also been performed. We will discuss these and others in relation to their ability to predict response and resistance to new-adjuvant treatment for rectal cancer patients. A number of listed biomarkers above will be discussed in detail in relation to their potential to predict response. A number of these factors can interact together at different cellular levels (Figure 1).

In figure 1, p53 can induce apoptosis, growth arrest and or senescence. Activation of p53 can induce expression or activation of pro-apoptotic Bcl2 family proteins (eg: Bax, Puma and Noxa) that coverge on the mitochondria and induce cytochrome c release. In the cytosol, cytochrome c binds Apaf1 which activates caspase 9 which activates caspase 3. It is also proposed that p53 can impair mitochondrial function. The p53 mediated mitochondrial dysfunction triggers a cycle of DNA damage, p53 activation, a compromised mitochondria and increased ROS levels leading to additional DNA damage.

2. Biomarker analyses

2.1 p21

The p21 protein is transcriptionally activated by p53 in response to DNA damage (el-Deiry, Kern et al. 1992). This causes the cells to arrest in G1 through the alteration of cyclin dependent kinases. It has been studied as a response predictor as disruption of the cell cycle networks may be a causative factor of radioresistance (Waldman, Kinzler et al. 1995), (Brugarolas, Chandrasekaran et al. 1995). Loss of wild type p21 or the presence of mutated p21 can radiosensitise cancer cells (Lu, Yamagishi et al. 1998), (Waldman, Lengauer et al. 1996), (Wang, Elson et al. 1997), (Tian and Quaroni 1999). On the basis of in vitro studies, it is predicted that tumors with low or absent p21 expression would be more sensitive to radio/and chemotherapy, ultimately leading to improved patient outcome. The levels of p21 expression have been investigated in a small number of immunohistochemistry based studies, some of which demonstrated some association with response (Reerink, Karrenbeld et al. 2004), (Fu, Tominaga et al. 1998; Qiu, Sirivongs et al. 2000). Some of these studies showed that positive p21 tumors were associated with poor survival (Reerink, Karrenbeld et al. 2004; Bertolini, Bengala et al. 2007). Four year overall survival rates in biopsies with high p21 expression levels was 43% compared with 83% 4 year survival in biopsies with low p21 expression levels (Bertolini, Bengala et al. 2007). However, others have shown no correlation between p21 expression levels and pathologic response (Rau, Sturm et al. 2003). The inclusion of p21 screening is warranted, as the referenced studies in table 1 below had low case numbers and results between centers did not show good reproducibility.

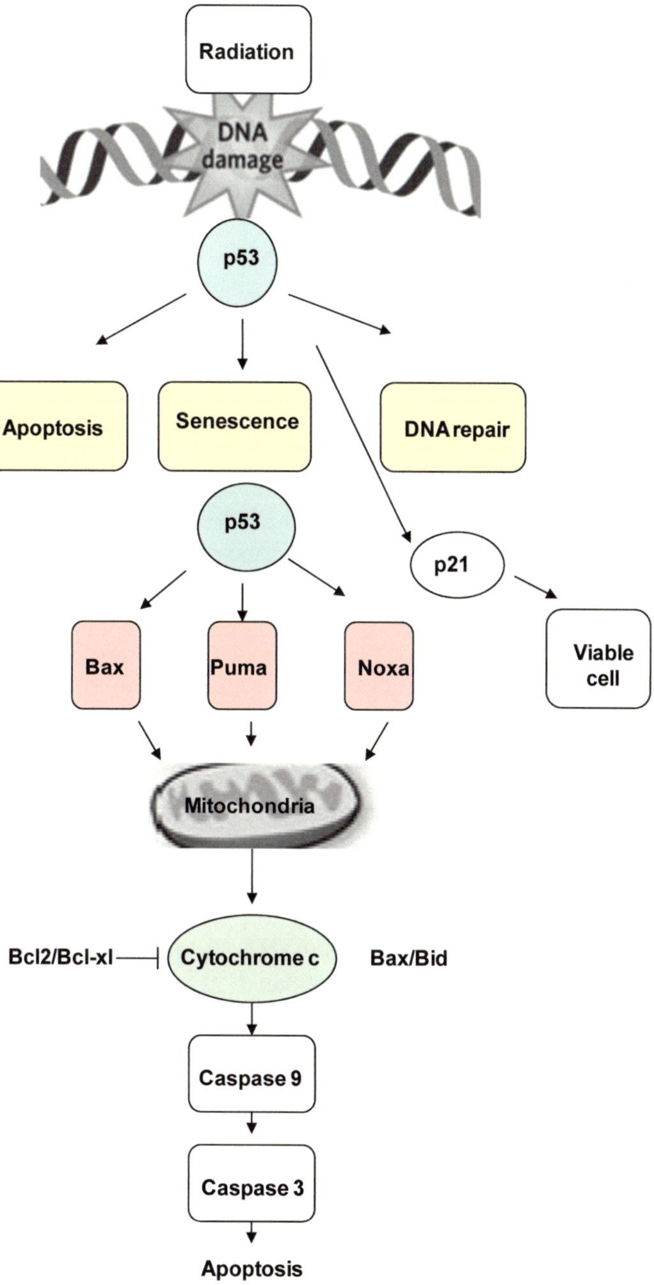

Fig. 1. p53 interaction with p21, DNA repair and mitochondrial dysfunction

Author	Technique	Study Outcome
Bertolini *et al*	IHC	Low p21 correlates with improved survival
Rau *et al*	IHC	Low p21 correlates with non responders
Charara *et al*	IHC	P21 positive tumors detected in responders
Reerink *et al*	IHC	High p21 correlates with poor survival
Kudrimoti *et al*	IHC	No correlation
Negri *et al*	IHC	No correlation
Lin *et al*	IHC	No correlation
Chang *et al*	IHC	No correlation

Table 1. Studies assessing p21 and Patient Outcome

2.2 Thymidylate synthase

Thymidylate synthase (TS) plays a crucial role in DNA synthesis. It is a primary target of 5-fluorouracil (5-FU) in the treatment of colorectal cancer. Overexpression of TS is associated with 5FU resistance and overall poor patient outcome (Salonga, Danenberg et al. 2000), (Lenz, Danenberg et al. 1998). Numerous studies assessing TS expression have found that pretreatment biopsies negative for TS were predictive of response (Saw, Morgan et al. 2003), (Diez, Ramos et al. 2003), (Jakob, Liersch et al. 2008), (Negri, Campanini et al. 2008). 3 studies revealed a better outcome with low or absent pretreatment TYMS expression, however another study demonstrated better outcome with high TYMS expression. It must be noted that the studies that did show a strong correlation between high pretreatment TYMS and outcome were performed on very small patient numbers. Therefore, the use of TYMS IHC screening is not recommended based on these small pilot studies performed. Evaluation of the TYMS allele has also been examined which determines the number of tandem repeats in the TYMS gene promoter region (Spindler, Nielsen et al. 2007), (Horie, Aiba et al. 1995), (Kawakami, Salonga et al. 2001) (44, 52,53). Villafranca et al has shown that patients homozygous for the triple repeat showed 22% downstaging compared to 60% downstaging in patients either homozygous for the double repeat (Horie, Aiba et al. 1995). TYMS DNA analyses may be valuable as a predictive biomarker, however its clinical utility needs to be evaluated in larger multi-center studies.

2.3 P53

P53 is known to play a role in apoptosis and in regulating sensitivity of tumors to radiation and chemotherapy (Bunz, Hwang et al. 1999), (Bunz, Dutriaux et al. 1998), (Kuerbitz, Plunkett et al. 1992), (Lowe, Schmitt et al. 1993), (Lowe, Ruley et al. 1993). For this reason, p53 is the most studied response predictor in rectal cancer with to date 22 different studies examining its potential to predict response to new-adjuvant treatment for rectal cancer patients. Assessment of p53 status has been performed by many different techniques including immunohistochemistry, polymorphism screening and direct gene sequencing (Reerink, Karrenbeld et al. 2004), (Rebischung, Gerard et al. 2002), (Kandioler, Zwrtek et al. 2002), (Qiu, Sirivongs et al. 2000), (Fu, Tominaga et al. 1998), (Rodel, Grabenbauer et al. 2002), (Abe, Sakaguchi et al. 2001), (Sakakura, Koide et al. 1998), (Luna-Perez, Arriola et al. 1998), (Komuro, Watanabe et al. 2003), (Spitz, Giacco et al. 1997), (Elsaleh, Robbins et al. 2000), (Saw, Morgan et al. 2003), (Scott, Hale et al. 1998), (Okonkwo, Musunuri et al. 2001), (Tannapfel, Nusslein et al. 1998), (Kim, Park et al. 2001), (Spitz, Giacco et al. 1997). The majority of work has been IHC based studies. Of these, only 18% of studies could be used to significantly predict response (Fu, Tominaga et al. 1998), (Spitz, Giacco et al. 1997; Komuro, Watanabe et al. 2003). These showed that pretreatment biopsies negative for p53 were predictive of complete tumor regression. The remaining 82% of studies did not show a positive association with levels of p53 expresison and treatment response. Some of the biggest studies were performed by Chang et al, and Bertolini et al and these revealed no correlation between mutant p53 expression and treatment outcome (Chang, Jung et al. 2005), (Bertolini, Bengala et al. 2007). Direct sequencing of the p53 gene (exons 2-10) revealed mutant p53 genotype was significantly associated with radioresistance (Rebischung, Gerard et al. 2002), (Kandioler, Zwrtek et al. 2002). These 2 studies revealed similar results however, the number of independent groups validating these results are limited. Overall, the majority of studies revealed no correlation between p53 and treatment outcome, suggesting that p53 is unlikely to serve as a predictor of response to new-adjuvant CRT.

Author	**Technique**	**Study Outcome**
Negri *et al*	IHC	High TYMS correlates with high rate of response
Saw *et al*	IHC	Lack of TYMS correlates with T stage downstaging
Bertolini *et al*	IHC	No correlation
Okonkuro *et al*	IHC	No correlation
Jakob *et al*	PCR	Low TYMS correlates with increased TRG stage
Stoehlmacher *et al*	PCR	Non significant
Spindler *et al*	PCR	TYMS2/2 levels correlate with increased TRG stage
Willafranca *et al*	PCR	TYMS2/2 levels correlate with increased TRG stage
Terrazzino *et al*	PCR	TYMS2/2 levels correlate with increased TRG stage

Table 2. Studies assessing Thymidylate Synthese and Patient Outcome

Author	Technique	Study Outcome
Jakob *et al*	IHC	No correlation
Kim *et al*	IHC	No correlation
Okonkuo *et al*	IHC	No correlation
Scott *et al*	IHC	No correlation
Kudnmoti *et al*	IHC	No correlation
Luna Perez *et al*	IHC	Positive p53 correlated with less tumor regression
Reerink *et al*	IHC	No correlation
Terzi *et al*	IHC	No correlation
Esposito *et al*	IHC	Positive p53 correlated with more tumor regression
Spitz *et al*	IHC	Positive p53 correlated with less tumor regression
Rodel *et al*	IHC	No correlation
Rau *et al*	IHC	No correlation
Lin *et al*	IHC	Negative p53 correlated with higher rate of response
Diez *et al*	IHC	No correlation
Terrazzino *et al*	IHC	No correlation
Bertolini *et al*	IHC	No correlation
Chang *et al*	IHC	No correlation

Table 3. Studies assessing p53 and Patient Outcome

2.4 Epidermal growth factor receptor (EGFR)

EGFR regulates many different cellular processes including cell proliferation, differentiation and apoptosis. It is overexpressed in 50-70% of cancers and is associated with more advanced tumor staging, poor prognosis and radiation resistance. (Akimoto, Hunter et al. 1999), (Liang, Ang et al. 2003). It has also been used as a therapeutic target with the development of new molecular targeted therapies such as Cetuximab (Eribitux) (You and Chen), (Liu, Guo et al.), (Liao, Sun et al.). There is very limited evidence on this receptor in relation to response to radiation in rectal cancer patients (Giralt, de las Heras et al. 2005), (Li, Kim et al. 2006), (Spindler, Nielsen et al. 2006), (Spindler, Nielsen et al. 2007). One study has shown an association between high EGFR levels and poor survival (Liu, Guo et al.). In tumors showing more than 50% positivity correlated with a shorter disease free survival. Multivariate analysis demonstrated low EGFR expression was a predictive factor for tumor downstaging (Liu, Guo et al.). The debate for screening EGFR levels is very weak and tenuous.

Author	Technique	Study Outcome
Spindler *et al*	IHC	No correlation
Spindler *et al*	PCR	EGFA61G SNP + EGFRSp1 with TYMS2/2 predicts Increased tumor regression
Giralt *et al*	IHC	No correlation
Bertolini *et al*	IHC	No correlation
Kim *et al*	IHC	No correlation

Table 4. Studies assessing EGFR and Patient Outcome

2.5 Ki67 and Cox2

Ki67 is required for cell cycle control (Scholzen and Gerdes 2000), (Schluter, Duchrow et al. 1993), (Linden, Ma et al. 1993). While it has been used as a prognostic factor for colorectal cancer, results have been inconclusive (Ogata, Greca et al.), (Guzinska-Ustymowicz, Pryczynicz et al. 2009), (Santagostino, Saggia et al. 2007). A small number of independent studies have examined the levels of Ki67 positivity in pretreatment biopsies from rectal cancer patients (Kudrimoti, Lee et al. 2007), (Debucquoy, Goethals et al. 2006), (Tannapfel, Nusslein et al. 1998), (Reerink, Karrenbeld et al. 2004), (Rodel, Grabenbauer et al. 2002), (Charara, Edmonston et al. 2004), Some studies have shown a positive association with Ki67 index higher in responders compared to non responders (Kim, Park et al. 2001; Jakob, Liersch et al. 2008). The remaining studies showed no correlation between Ki67 status and patient outcome. In the small number of studies that did show a positive correlation between Ki67 and response, these were conducted on a very small patient cohort. It appears unlikely that measurement of the proliferation status in pretreatment biopsies will be clinically useful.

Another molecule known to promote tumor growth is Cox 2. Cox 2 catalyses the conversion of arachidonic acid to protaglandins, especially PGE2. COX2 inhibition in conjunction with radiation can significantly enhance tumor response by blocking prostaglandin release (Kishi, Petersen et al. 2000). In laryngeal (Nix, Lind et al. 2004) and cervical cancers (Kim, Kim et al. 2004), (Kim, Kim et al. 2002), COX 2 expression in pre treatment biopsies may be indicative of treatment response to CRT. Cox2 has been evaluated in pre rectal biopsies (Watwe, Javle et al. 2005), (Kobayashi, Hashiguchi et al. 2007), (de Heer, Gosens et al. 2007), (Giralt, Navalpotro et al. 2006), (Min, Choi et al. 2008), (Smith, Reynolds et al. 2006). And its overexpression was significantly associated with poor response to treatment, suggesting that COX2 may mediate radioresponsiveness. However, study numbers are small and no multi-centre studies to validate these findings have been reported to date.

2.6 Mitochondrial proteins bcl2/bax

Bcl2 and Bax regulate caspase activation and this activation can regulate apoptosis in many disease states (Teijido and Dejean), (Thees, Hubbard et al. 2005), (Brambilla, Negoescu et al. 1996). Bcl2 and Bax are prosurvival and proapoptotic proteins respectively. Bcl2 maintains mitochondrial outer membrane integrity (Teijido and Dejean ; Luo, Budihardjo et al. 1998;

Zhang, Holzgreve et al. 2001). Bax can be activated by pro apoptotic stimuli or p53 and expression can be altered following radiation and is associated with resistance to chemotherapy (Miguel, Wajsenzon et al. 2007), (Przemeck, Duckworth et al. 2007), (Murphy, Mabruk et al. 2002), (Johnson, Xiang et al. 1998; Butt, Firth et al. 2000), (Strobel, Swanson et al. 1997), (Khanna, Wie et al. 1996). This is in contrast to overexpression of bcl2 is associated with chemotherapy resistance and protects cells from radiation induced apoptosis (Hahn, Lai et al. 2003), (Vrana, Grant et al. 1999). 12 studies have assessed these proteins, 8 for Bcl2 expression and 4 have evaluated Bax expression as predictive markers (Qiu, Sirivongs et al. 2000), (Rodel, Grabenbauer et al. 2002), (Rodel, Hoffmann et al. 2002), (Scott, Hale et al. 1998), (Okonkwo, Musunuri et al. 2001). Only one study has found that Bcl2 was an indicator of response in pre treatment biopsies, where 60% of complete responders were bcl2 positive in pretreatment biopsies compared to 16% bcl2 positive in the partial responders. One of the Bax studies showed a significant correlation between higher Bax expression in biopsies associated with treatment response. Overall, these markers do not prove useful as significant markers of response to new-adjuvant CRT.

Author	**Technique**	**Study Outcome**
Kudrimoti *et al*	IHC	Positive bcl2 expression correlates with complete response
Chang *et al*	IHC	Bax expression correlates with increases tumor regression
Scott *et al*	IHC	No correlation
Okonkwo *et al*	IHC	No correlation
Reerink *et al*	PCR	No correlation
Tannapfel *et al*	IHC	No correlation
Charara *et al*	IHC	No correlation
Rodel et al	IHC	No correlation

Table 5. Studies assessing bcl2/bax and Patient Outcome

2.7 Microsatellite instability, mis match repair and hypoxia

Evaluation of the levels of DNA repair in pretreatment biopsies may be important in predicting response or resistance to CRT. Tumors which show microsatellite instability usually have a better prognosis and have altered response to radiotherapy compared to tumors with an intact repair system (Peltomaki 2003). This effect has been evaluated in a small number of clinical trials, however screening for MSI status and presence or absence of the mis match repair proteins did not correlation with treatment response (Qiu, Sirivongs et al. 2000), (Charara, Edmonston et al. 2004), (Rau, Sturm et al. 2003) . However, assessment of

Ku70, a protein involved in double strand break repairs (Ayene, Ford et al. 2005) could predict response when combined mutant p53 status (Komuro, Watanabe et al. 2003). Markers of tumor hypoxia have also been assessed as a response predictor in rectal cancer. Qui et al have found that histological response was not correlated to VEGF expression levels in pretreatment biopsies (Qiu, Sirivongs et al. 2000). Other studies combined VEGF expression levels in serum/plasma with serial dynamic contrast-enhanced (DCE) MRI, a marker of vessel permeability. While again VEGF levels did not correlate with treatment response, higher permeability on DCE MRI significantly correlated with better response to CRT (George, Dzik-Jurasz et al. 2001).

2.8 Microarray and proteomic studies

While targeted-therapies use single marker approaches, tumor response to CRT is complex and unlikely to be attributed to one factor alone. Transcriptional profiling of tumors has shown considerable promise as a predictive approach to treatment, with commercially available microarray profiling platforms, MammaPrint and OncoTypeDX, already in place for breast cancer prognostics (van 't Veer, Dai et al. 2002; Paik, Shak et al. 2004). This has provided support for predictive genomics research in other cancer types, including rectal cancer. A number of studies carried out in recent years have aimed to identify gene and/or protein signatures predictive of response to CRT in rectal cancer. Prior to the development of genomic and proteomic screening studies, assessment of predictive markers suggested that *p53*, *Bcl2*, *Bax*, and microsatellite instability are of no predictive value as discussed above.

Ghadimi *et al.* were among the first to use gene expression profiling with the aim of predicting response to new-adjuvant CRT in rectal cancer (Ghadimi, Grade et al. 2005). A significant difference in gene expression was identified between responders and non-responders for 54 genes, while the ability of this gene profile to predict response was validated in 83% of patients (78% sensitivity, 86% specificity). While this is a promising observation, the authors noted that validation of these findings in large, independent studies would be required. Watanabe *et al.* also carried out DNA microarray analysis of gene expression profiles in response to new-adjuvant radiotherapy in rectal cancer (Watanabe, Komuro et al. 2006). They identified 33 genes with a significant difference in expression between responders and non-responders (82.4% accuracy).

While expression of pro-apoptotic genes was higher in responders, anti-apoptotic gene expression was higher in non-responders. A later study carried out gene microarray analysis on tumor tissues from 46 patients with rectal cancer, with response to CRT evaluated using Dworaks tumor regression grade. From a gene-set comprising the top-ranked 95 genes demonstrating altered expression (between partial and complete-response), response to CRT was accurately predicted in 84% of training samples and 87% of validation samples (Kim, Lim et al. 2007). Using 43 biopsy specimens from patients with locally advanced rectal adenocarcinoma, a 43-gene expression signature of response was identified by Rimkus *et al* (Rimkus, Friederichs et al. 2008). These genes mainly encoded proteins involved in nuclear processes, associated with transport function, or implicated in apoptosis regulation (caspase-1), supporting previous observations (Watanabe, Komuro et al. 2006). A subsequent small study of rectal cancer patients who underwent preoperative CRT (n=17) revealed seventeen genes with significantly altered gene expression levels. These included apoptosis, metalloproteinase, transforming growth factor beta-1, DNA repair, and cell proliferation-related genes (Nishioka, Shimada et al.). The activity of certain subsets of kinase signaling pathways has also been proposed to predict response to CRT in rectal cancer. A microarray study of 67 patients with advanced stage rectal cancer suggested that multiplex kinase activity profiling may identify biomarkers to predict tumor response to CRT, with several discriminating phosphosubstrates representing proteins derived from signaling pathways implicated in radioresistance (Folkvord, Flatmark et al.).

Using a panel of 48 cancer cell lines, a 10-gene signature of radiosensitivity was identified and used as a predictor of an intrinsic radiosensitivity index (RSI). This was applied to a rectal cancer cohort, which was treated with concurrent chemoradiation. The predicted RSI was significantly different in responders versus non-responders. This effect was also observed in head-and-neck and oesophageal cancer cohorts, a combined total of 118 patients and the first systems-based radiosensitivity model to be validated in multiple datasets (Eschrich, Pramana et al. 2009). A subsequent study used 12 colorectal cancer cell lines to examine response to CRT. The authors identified many genes involved in the MAP-kinase pathway or cell cycle genes, and suggested that both insulin and Wnt signaling pathways may have relevance for treatment response.

A recent study was carried out to examine expression profiles from pretreatment biopsies for 51 rectal cancer patients. However, the classifiers obtained from this study did not have high sensitivity/specificity, with those with highest sensitivity having poor specificity and vice versa. Validation of these classifiers with previously published data was also difficult, prompting the authors to suggest that microarray analysis is not a valuable tool for predictive studies in rectal cancer (Brettingham-Moore, Duong et al.). Alternatives approaches should therefore also be considered for future predictive studies in rectal cancer.

Author	**Technique**	**Study Outcome**
Ghadimi *et al*	DNA Microarray	54 gene panel predicts response (78% sensitivity and 86% specificity
Watanabe *et al*	DNA Microarray	33 gene panel predicts response (82% accuracy)
Kim *et al* Okonkwo *et al*	DNA Microarray	95 gene signature predicts response (87% validation)
Allal *et al*	Proteomics	Differential expression of proteins between responders and non responders. Protein targets: Tropomodulin, heat shock 42, keratin 1 and notch2

Table 6. Studies assessing array profiles and patient outcome

A small number of studies have used proteomic approaches to identify a protein signature which can predict response to CRT. The earliest of these used 2D genes and subsequent mass spectrometry to identify a small number of proteins which correlated with treatment response. These included tropomodulin, heat shock protein 42, keratin type 1 and notch-2 protein homolog. A number of these proteins are known to be associated with radioresistance (Allal, Kahne et al. 2004). The use of an integrated microarray and proteomics approach to predict response of patients on cetuximab demonstrated an enhanced predictive power, with 5 genes and 10 proteins predicting rectal cancer regression grade with 91.7% accuracy, 96.2% sensitivity and 80% specificity (Daemen, Gevaert et al. 2008). A similar approach was later taken by Debucquay *et al.*, who found that 16 genes were significantly altered following microarray analysis (Debucquoy, Haustermans et al. 2009). A decrease in proliferation gene expression was confirmed by IHC for Ki67 and further supported by an increase in TGFα in plasma samples from rectal cancer patients.

3. Concluding remarks

The relationship between biomarker expression and histological response to CRT has been investigated in a large number of studies. The vast majority of these studies have assessed single or multiple pre defined markers in small cohorts of patients. However, through these studies, a limited number of promising markers have been identified including TS expression, increased p21 and EGFR expression levels. While these markers have been assessed and have shown some promise, due to the limited number of studies assessing each marker using the same protocol, no marker to date can be considered as a clinical biomarker. The biggest problem with the studies has been the lack of statistical power. Assessment of these markers should be prospectively evaluated to elucidate their role as measures of predictive outcome, however it is unlikely that any single factor will determine response so a more global approach maybe more advantageous. The development of novel therapeutic targets for rectal cancer maybe greatly aided by the generation of global gene and protein expression profiles for responders and non-responders through microarray and proteomic studies. However, this will only be made possible by the use of large cross-institutional studies.

The discovery of specific biomarkers that could potentially predict a tumor response to treatment could prevent the above mentioned unfavorable consequence while focusing on patients that will benefit from new-adjuvant treatment. A successful biomarker(s) should predict responders versus non responders with high sensitivity and specificity levels. This biomarker should be validated prospectively in different patient cohorts from multi centre hospitals. Importantly, to conduct these prospective studies, it is vital that there is limited variation in the dose and duration of radiation, inclusion or type of chemotherapy given and pathological endpoints assessed. Another caveat is in relation to the collection and analysis. It is unknown whether the endoscopy biopsy truly reflects the biology of the tumor as a whole. Also, variability in IHC scoring systems could alter study outcomes. To date, these issues may contribute to conflicting results for the potential biomarkers as discussed in this chapter. In conclusion, the response of rectal adenocarcinoma to neo-adjuvant chemo-radiotherapy is limited to a defined group of patients. It is hoped in the future that the therapeutic course will be tailored to each patient based on analyses of initial pre treatment biopsy assessment, thus minimizing unnecessary treatment for rectal cancer patients. The next investigative step would be to conduct, initially, phase II trials prospectively to validate the predictive power of the most promising predictive markers and eventually phase III prospective trials to separate categories of patients based on the likelihood of tumor response according to expression of the different molecules.

4. References

Abe, T., Y. Sakaguchi, et al. (2001). "Apoptosis and p53 overexpression in human rectal cancer; relationship with response to hyperthermo-chemo-radiotherapy." Anticancer Res 21(3C): 2115-20.

Akimoto, T., N. R. Hunter, et al. (1999). "Inverse relationship between epidermal growth factor receptor expression and radiocurability of murine carcinomas." Clin Cancer Res 5(10): 2884-90.

Allal, A. S., T. Kahne, et al. (2004). "Radioresistance-related proteins in rectal cancer." Proteomics 4(8): 2261-9.

Ayene, I. S., L. P. Ford, et al. (2005). "Ku protein targeting by Ku70 small interfering RNA enhances human cancer cell response to topoisomerase II inhibitor and gamma radiation." Mol Cancer Ther 4(4): 529-36.

Bertolini, F., C. Bengala, et al. (2007). "Prognostic and predictive value of baseline and posttreatment molecular marker expression in locally advanced rectal cancer treated with new-adjuvant chemoradiotherapy." Int J Radiat Oncol Biol Phys 68(5): 1455-61.

Birgisson, H., L. Pahlman, et al. (2005). "Occurrence of second cancers in patients treated with radiotherapy for rectal cancer." J Clin Oncol 23(25): 6126-31.

Bouzourene, H., F. T. Bosman, et al. (2002). "Importance of tumor regression assessment in predicting the outcome in patients with locally advanced rectal carcinoma who are treated with preoperative radiotherapy." Cancer 94(4): 1121-30.

Brambilla, E., A. Negoescu, et al. (1996). "Apoptosis-related factors p53, Bcl2, and Bax in neuroendocrine lung tumors." Am J Pathol 149(6): 1941-52.

Brettingham-Moore, K. H., C. P. Duong, et al. "Pretreatment Transcriptional Profiling for Predicting Response to New-adjuvant Chemoradiotherapy in Rectal Adenocarcinoma." Clin Cancer Res 17(9): 3039-3047.

Brugarolas, J., C. Chandrasekaran, et al. (1995). "Radiation-induced cell cycle arrest compromised by p21 deficiency." Nature 377(6549): 552-7.

Bunz, F., A. Dutriaux, et al. (1998). "Requirement for p53 and p21 to sustain G2 arrest after DNA damage." Science 282(5393): 1497-501.

Bunz, F., P. M. Hwang, et al. (1999). "Disruption of p53 in human cancer cells alters the responses to therapeutic agents." J Clin Invest 104(3): 263-9.

Butt, A. J., S. M. Firth, et al. (2000). "Insulin-like growth factor-binding protein-3 modulates expression of Bax and Bcl-2 and potentiates p53-independent radiation-induced apoptosis in human breast cancer cells." J Biol Chem 275(50): 39174-81.

Chang, H. J., K. H. Jung, et al. (2005). "Bax, a predictive marker for therapeutic response to preoperative chemoradiotherapy in patients with rectal carcinoma." Hum Pathol 36(4): 364-71.

Charara, M., T. B. Edmonston, et al. (2004). "Microsatellite status and cell cycle associated markers in rectal cancer patients undergoing a combined regimen of 5-FU and CPT-11 chemotherapy and radiotherapy." Anticancer Res 24(5B): 3161-7.

Daemen, A., O. Gevaert, et al. (2008). "Integrating microarray and proteomics data to predict the response on cetuximab in patients with rectal cancer." Pac Symp Biocomput: 166-77.

de Heer, P., M. J. Gosens, et al. (2007). "Cyclooxygenase 2 expression in rectal cancer is of prognostic significance in patients receiving preoperative radiotherapy." Clin Cancer Res 13(10): 2955-60.

Debucquoy, A., L. Goethals, et al. (2006). "Molecular responses of rectal cancer to preoperative chemoradiation." Radiother Oncol 80(2): 172-7.

Debucquoy, A., K. Haustermans, et al. (2009). "Molecular response to cetuximab and efficacy of preoperative cetuximab-based chemoradiation in rectal cancer." J Clin Oncol 27(17): 2751-7.

Diez, M., P. Ramos, et al. (2003). "Preoperatively irradiated rectal carcinoma: analysis of the histopathologic response and predictive value of proliferating cell nuclear antigen immunostaining." Oncology 64(3): 213-9.

el-Deiry, W. S., S. E. Kern, et al. (1992). "Definition of a consensus binding site for p53." Nat Genet 1(1): 45-9.

Elsaleh, H., P. Robbins, et al. (2000). "Can p53 alterations be used to predict tumor response to pre-operative chemo-radiotherapy in locally advanced rectal cancer?" Radiother Oncol 56(2): 239-44.

Eschrich, S. A., J. Pramana, et al. (2009). "A gene expression model of intrinsic tumor radiosensitivity: prediction of response and prognosis after chemoradiation." Int J Radiat Oncol Biol Phys 75(2): 489-96.

Folkvord, S., K. Flatmark, et al. "Prediction of response to preoperative chemoradiotherapy in rectal cancer by multiplex kinase activity profiling." Int J Radiat Oncol Biol Phys 78(2): 555-62.

Frileux, P., G. Burdy, et al. (2007). "Surgical treatment of rectal cancer: results of a strategy for selective preoperative radiotherapy." Gastroenterol Clin Biol 31(11): 934-40.

Fu, C. G., O. Tominaga, et al. (1998). "Role of p53 and p21/WAF1 detection in patient selection for preoperative radiotherapy in rectal cancer patients." Dis Colon Rectum 41(1): 68-74.

George, M. L., A. S. Dzik-Jurasz, et al. (2001). "Non-invasive methods of assessing angiogenesis and their value in predicting response to treatment in colorectal cancer." Br J Surg 88(12): 1628-36.

Ghadimi, B. M., M. Grade, et al. (2005). "Effectiveness of gene expression profiling for response prediction of rectal adenocarcinomas to preoperative chemoradiotherapy." J Clin Oncol 23(9): 1826-38.

Giralt, J., M. de las Heras, et al. (2005). "The expression of epidermal growth factor receptor results in a worse prognosis for patients with rectal cancer treated with preoperative radiotherapy: a multicenter, retrospective analysis." Radiother Oncol 74(2): 101-8.

Giralt, J., B. Navalpotro, et al. (2006). "Prognostic significance of vascular endothelial growth factor and cyclooxygenase-2 in patients with rectal cancer treated with preoperative radiotherapy." Oncology 71(5-6): 312-9.

Guzinska-Ustymowicz, K., A. Pryczynicz, et al. (2009). "Correlation between proliferation markers: PCNA, Ki-67, MCM-2 and antiapoptotic protein Bcl-2 in colorectal cancer." Anticancer Res 29(8): 3049-52.

Habr-Gama, A., R. O. Perez, et al. (2004). "Operative versus nonoperative treatment for stage 0 distal rectal cancer following chemoradiation therapy: long-term results." Ann Surg 240(4): 711-7; discussion 717-8.

Hahn, P. J., Z. W. Lai, et al. (2003). "Bcl2-independent chromatin cleavage is a very early event during induction of apoptosis in mouse thymocytes after treatment with either dexamethasone or ionizing radiation." Radiat Res 160(5): 559-67.

Horie, N., H. Aiba, et al. (1995). "Functional analysis and DNA polymorphism of the tandemly repeated sequences in the 5'-terminal regulatory region of the human gene for thymidylate synthase." Cell Struct Funct 20(3): 191-7.

Horisberger, K., R. D. Hofheinz, et al. (2008). "Tumor response to new-adjuvant chemoradiation in rectal cancer: predictor for surgical morbidity?" Int J Colorectal Dis 23(3): 257-64.

Jakob, C., T. Liersch, et al. (2008). "Predictive value of Ki67 and p53 in locally advanced rectal cancer: correlation with thymidylate synthase and histopathological tumor regression after new-adjuvant 5-FU-based chemoradiotherapy." World J Gastroenterol 14(7): 1060-6.

Johnson, M. D., H. Xiang, et al. (1998). "Evidence for involvement of Bax and p53, but not caspases, in radiation-induced cell death of cultured postnatal hippocampal neurons." J Neurosci Res 54(6): 721-33.

Kandioler, D., R. Zwrtek, et al. (2002). "TP53 genotype but not p53 immunohistochemical result predicts response to preoperative short-term radiotherapy in rectal cancer." Ann Surg 235(4): 493-8.

Kapiteijn, E., C. A. Marijnen, et al. (2001). "Preoperative radiotherapy combined with total mesorectal excision for resectable rectal cancer." N Engl J Med 345(9): 638-46.

Kawakami, K., D. Salonga, et al. (2001). "Different lengths of a polymorphic repeat sequence in the thymidylate synthase gene affect translational efficiency but not its gene expression." Clin Cancer Res 7(12): 4096-101.

Khanna, K. K., T. Wie, et al. (1996). "Expression of p53, bcl-2, bax, bcl-x2 and c-myc in radiation-induced apoptosis in Burkitt's lymphoma cells." Cell Death Differ 3(3): 315-22.

Kim, I. J., S. B. Lim, et al. (2007). "Microarray gene expression profiling for predicting complete response to preoperative chemoradiotherapy in patients with advanced rectal cancer." Dis Colon Rectum 50(9): 1342-53.

Kim, N. K., J. K. Park, et al. (2001). "p53, BCL-2, and Ki-67 expression according to tumor response after concurrent chemoradiotherapy for advanced rectal cancer." Ann Surg Oncol 8(5): 418-24.

Kim, Y. B., G. E. Kim, et al. (2002). "Overexpression of cyclooxygenase-2 is associated with a poor prognosis in patients with squamous cell carcinoma of the uterine cervix treated with radiation and concurrent chemotherapy." Cancer 95(3): 531-9.

Kim, Y. B., G. E. Kim, et al. (2004). "Differential cyclooxygenase-2 expression in squamous cell carcinoma and adenocarcinoma of the uterine cervix." Int J Radiat Oncol Biol Phys 60(3): 822-9.

Kishi, K., S. Petersen, et al. (2000). "Preferential enhancement of tumor radioresponse by a cyclooxygenase-2 inhibitor." Cancer Res 60(5): 1326-31.

Kobayashi, H., Y. Hashiguchi, et al. (2007). "Absence of cyclooxygenase-2 protein expression is a predictor of tumor regression in rectal cancer treated with preoperative short-term chemoradiotherapy." Dis Colon Rectum 50(9): 1354-62.

Komuro, Y., T. Watanabe, et al. (2003). "Prediction of tumor radiosensitivity in rectal carcinoma based on p53 and Ku70 expression." J Exp Clin Cancer Res 22(2): 223-8.

Krook, J. E., C. G. Moertel, et al. (1991). "Effective surgical adjuvant therapy for high-risk rectal carcinoma." N Engl J Med 324(11): 709-15.

Kudrimoti, M., E. Y. Lee, et al. (2007). "Genetic markers predictive of response to induction chemoradiotherapy for locally advanced rectal cancers." J Ky Med Assoc 105(1): 18-22.

Kuerbitz, S. J., B. S. Plunkett, et al. (1992). "Wild-type p53 is a cell cycle checkpoint determinant following irradiation." Proc Natl Acad Sci U S A 89(16): 7491-5.

Lenz, H. J., K. D. Danenberg, et al. (1998). "p53 and thymidylate synthase expression in untreated stage II colon cancer: associations with recurrence, survival, and site." Clin Cancer Res 4(5): 1227-34.

Li, S., J. S. Kim, et al. (2006). "Epidermal growth factor receptor as a prognostic factor in locally advanced rectal-cancer patients treated with preoperative chemoradiation." Int J Radiat Oncol Biol Phys 65(3): 705-12.

Liang, K., K. K. Ang, et al. (2003). "The epidermal growth factor receptor mediates radioresistance." Int J Radiat Oncol Biol Phys 57(1): 246-54.

Liao, C., Q. Sun, et al. "Targeting EGFR-overexpressing tumor cells using Cetuximab-immunomicelles loaded with doxorubicin and superparamagnetic iron oxide." Eur J Radiol.

Linden, M. D., C. K. Ma, et al. (1993). "Ki-67 and proliferating cell nuclear antigen tumor proliferative indices in DNA diploid colorectal adenocarcinomas. Correlation with histopathologic characteristics and cell cycle analysis with two-color DNA flow cytometry." Am J Clin Pathol 100(3): 206-12.

Liu, X., W. J. Guo, et al. "Cetuximab enhances the activities of irinotecan on gastric cancer cell lines through downregulating the EGFR pathway upregulated by irinotecan." Cancer Chemother Pharmacol.

Lowe, S. W., H. E. Ruley, et al. (1993). "p53-dependent apoptosis modulates the cytotoxicity of anticancer agents." Cell 74(6): 957-67.

Lowe, S. W., E. M. Schmitt, et al. (1993). "p53 is required for radiation-induced apoptosis in mouse thymocytes." Nature 362(6423): 847-9.

Lu, Y., N. Yamagishi, et al. (1998). "Mutated p21(WAF1/CIP1/SDI1) lacking CDK-inhibitory activity fails to prevent apoptosis in human colorectal carcinoma cells." Oncogene 16(6): 705-12.

Luna-Perez, P., E. L. Arriola, et al. (1998). "p53 protein overexpression and response to induction chemoradiation therapy in patients with locally advanced rectal adenocarcinoma." Ann Surg Oncol 5(3): 203-8.

Luo, X., I. Budihardjo, et al. (1998). "Bid, a Bcl2 interacting protein, mediates cytochrome c release from mitochondria in response to activation of cell surface death receptors." Cell 94(4): 481-90.

Mandard, A. M., F. Dalibard, et al. (1994). "Pathologic assessment of tumor regression after preoperative chemoradiotherapy of esophageal carcinoma. Clinicopathologic correlations." Cancer 73(11): 2680-6.

Miguel, N. C., I. J. Wajsenzon, et al. (2007). "Catalase, Bax and p53 expression in the visual system of the crab Ucides cordatus following exposure to ultraviolet radiation." Cell Tissue Res 329(1): 159-68.
Min, B. S., Y. J. Choi, et al. (2008). "Cyclooxygenase-2 expression in pretreatment biopsy as a predictor of tumor responses after preoperative chemoradiation in rectal cancer." Arch Surg 143(11): 1091-7; discussion 1097.
Murphy, M., M. J. Mabruk, et al. (2002). "The expression of p53, p21, Bax and induction of apoptosis in normal volunteers in response to different doses of ultraviolet radiation." Br J Dermatol 147(1): 110-7.
Negri, F. V., N. Campanini, et al. (2008). "Biological predictive factors in rectal cancer treated with preoperative radiotherapy or radiochemotherapy." Br J Cancer 98(1): 143-7.
Nishioka, M., M. Shimada, et al. "Gene expression profile can predict pathological response to preoperative chemoradiotherapy in rectal cancer." Cancer Genomics Proteomics 8(2): 87-92.
Nix, P., M. Lind, et al. (2004). "Expression of Cox-2 protein in radioresistant laryngeal cancer." Ann Oncol 15(5): 797-801.
Ogata, D. C., F. H. Greca, et al. "[Aberrant crypt foci and cancer of the colorectal junction: the correlation between beta-catenin/Ki-67 expression and the occurrence of early microscopic secondary lesions surrounding periphery colorectal cancer]." Rev Col Bras Cir 37(2): 114-20.
Okonkwo, A., S. Musunuri, et al. (2001). "Molecular markers and prediction of response to chemoradiation in rectal cancer." Oncol Rep 8(3): 497-500.
Paik, S., S. Shak, et al. (2004). "A multigene assay to predict recurrence of tamoxifen-treated, node-negative breast cancer." N Engl J Med 351(27): 2817-26.
Peltomaki, P. (2003). "Role of DNA mismatch repair defects in the pathogenesis of human cancer." J Clin Oncol 21(6): 1174-9.
Przemeck, S. M., C. A. Duckworth, et al. (2007). "Radiation-induced gastric epithelial apoptosis occurs in the proliferative zone and is regulated by p53, bak, bax, and bcl-2." Am J Physiol Gastrointest Liver Physiol 292(2): G620-7.
Qiu, H., P. Sirivongs, et al. (2000). "Molecular prognostic factors in rectal cancer treated by radiation and surgery." Dis Colon Rectum 43(4): 451-9.
Rau, B., I. Sturm, et al. (2003). "Dynamic expression profile of p21WAF1/CIP1 and Ki-67 predicts survival in rectal carcinoma treated with preoperative radiochemotherapy." J Clin Oncol 21(18): 3391-401.
Rebischung, C., J. P. Gerard, et al. (2002). "Prognostic value of P53 mutations in rectal carcinoma." Int J Cancer 100(2): 131-5.
Reerink, O., A. Karrenbeld, et al. (2004). "Molecular prognostic factors in locally irresectable rectal cancer treated preoperatively by chemo-radiotherapy." Anticancer Res 24(2C): 1217-21.
Rimkus, C., J. Friederichs, et al. (2008). "Microarray-based prediction of tumor response to new-adjuvant radiochemotherapy of patients with locally advanced rectal cancer." Clin Gastroenterol Hepatol 6(1): 53-61.
Rodel, C., G. G. Grabenbauer, et al. (2002). "Apoptosis as a cellular predictor for histopathologic response to new-adjuvant radiochemotherapy in patients with rectal cancer." Int J Radiat Oncol Biol Phys 52(2): 294-303.

Rodel, F., J. Hoffmann, et al. (2002). "High survivin expression is associated with reduced apoptosis in rectal cancer and may predict disease-free survival after preoperative radiochemotherapy and surgical resection." Strahlenther Onkol 178(8): 426-35.

Ryan, R., D. Gibbons, et al. (2005). "Pathological response following long-course new-adjuvant chemoradiotherapy for locally advanced rectal cancer." Histopathology 47(2): 141-6.

Sakakura, C., K. Koide, et al. (1998). "Analysis of histological therapeutic effect, apoptosis rate and p53 status after combined treatment with radiation, hyperthermia and 5-fluorouracil suppositories for advanced rectal cancers." Br J Cancer 77(1): 159-66.

Salonga, D., K. D. Danenberg, et al. (2000). "Colorectal tumors responding to 5-fluorouracil have low gene expression levels of dihydropyrimidine dehydrogenase, thymidylate synthase, and thymidine phosphorylase." Clin Cancer Res 6(4): 1322-7.

Santagostino, A., C. Saggia, et al. (2007). "Prospective study on prognostic significance of DNA ploidy and Ki-67 expression in colorectal cancer." J Biol Regul Homeost Agents 21(1-2): 13-20.

Sauer, R., H. Becker, et al. (2004). "Preoperative versus postoperative chemoradiotherapy for rectal cancer." N Engl J Med 351(17): 1731-40.

Saw, R. P., M. Morgan, et al. (2003). "p53, deleted in colorectal cancer gene, and thymidylate synthase as predictors of histopathologic response and survival in low, locally advanced rectal cancer treated with preoperative adjuvant therapy." Dis Colon Rectum 46(2): 192-202.

Schluter, C., M. Duchrow, et al. (1993). "The cell proliferation-associated antigen of antibody Ki-67: a very large, ubiquitous nuclear protein with numerous repeated elements, representing a new kind of cell cycle-maintaining proteins." J Cell Biol 123(3): 513-22.

Scholzen, T. and J. Gerdes (2000). "The Ki-67 protein: from the known and the unknown." J Cell Physiol 182(3): 311-22.

Scott, N., A. Hale, et al. (1998). "A histopathological assessment of the response of rectal adenocarcinoma to combination chemo-radiotherapy: relationship to apoptotic activity, p53 and bcl-2 expression." Eur J Surg Oncol 24(3): 169-73.

Smith, F. M., J. V. Reynolds, et al. (2006). "Pathological and molecular predictors of the response of rectal cancer to new-adjuvant radiochemotherapy." Eur J Surg Oncol 32(1): 55-64.

Spindler, K. L., J. N. Nielsen, et al. (2006). "Prediction of response to chemoradiation in rectal cancer by a gene polymorphism in the epidermal growth factor receptor promoter region." Int J Radiat Oncol Biol Phys 66(2): 500-4.

Spindler, K. L., J. N. Nielsen, et al. (2007). "Germline polymorphisms may act as predictors of response to preoperative chemoradiation in locally advanced T3 rectal tumors." Dis Colon Rectum 50(9): 1363-9.

Spitz, F. R., G. G. Giacco, et al. (1997). "p53 immunohistochemical staining predicts residual disease after chemoradiation in patients with high-risk rectal cancer." Clin Cancer Res 3(10): 1685-90.

Strobel, T., L. Swanson, et al. (1997). "Radiation-induced apoptosis is not enhanced by expression of either p53 or BAX in SW626 ovarian cancer cells." Oncogene 14(23): 2753-8.

Tannapfel, A., S. Nusslein, et al. (1998). "Apoptosis, proliferation, bax, bcl-2 and p53 status prior to and after preoperative radiochemotherapy for locally advanced rectal cancer." Int J Radiat Oncol Biol Phys 41(3): 585-91.

Teijido, O. and L. Dejean "Upregulation of Bcl2 inhibits apoptosis-driven BAX insertion but favors BAX relocalization in mitochondria." FEBS Lett 584(15): 3305-10.

Thees, S., G. B. Hubbard, et al. (2005). "Specific alteration of the Bax/Bcl2 ratio and cytochrome c without execution of apoptosis in the hippocampus of aged baboons." Restor Neurol Neurosci 23(1): 1-9.

Tian, J. Q. and A. Quaroni (1999). "Involvement of p21(WAF1/Cip1) and p27(Kip1) in intestinal epithelial cell differentiation." Am J Physiol 276(6 Pt 1): C1245-58.

Valentini, V., C. Coco, et al. (2002). "Does downstaging predict improved outcome after preoperative chemoradiation for extraperitoneal locally advanced rectal cancer? A long-term analysis of 165 patients." Int J Radiat Oncol Biol Phys 53(3): 664-74.

van 't Veer, L. J., H. Dai, et al. (2002). "Gene expression profiling predicts clinical outcome of breast cancer." Nature 415(6871): 530-6.

Vrana, J. A., S. Grant, et al. (1999). "Inhibition of the MAPK pathway abrogates BCL2-mediated survival of leukemia cells after exposure to low-dose ionizing radiation." Radiat Res 151(5): 559-69.

Waldman, T., K. W. Kinzler, et al. (1995). "p21 is necessary for the p53-mediated G1 arrest in human cancer cells." Cancer Res 55(22): 5187-90.

Waldman, T., C. Lengauer, et al. (1996). "Uncoupling of S phase and mitosis induced by anticancer agents in cells lacking p21." Nature 381(6584): 713-6.

Wang, Y. A., A. Elson, et al. (1997). "Loss of p21 increases sensitivity to ionizing radiation and delays the onset of lymphoma in atm-deficient mice." Proc Natl Acad Sci U S A 94(26): 14590-5.

Watanabe, T., Y. Komuro, et al. (2006). "Prediction of sensitivity of rectal cancer cells in response to preoperative radiotherapy by DNA microarray analysis of gene expression profiles." Cancer Res 66(7): 3370-4.

Watwe, V., M. Javle, et al. (2005). "Cyclooxygenase-2 (COX-2) levels before and after chemotherapy: a study in rectal cancer." Am J Clin Oncol 28(6): 560-4.

You, B. and E. X. Chen "Anti-EGFR Monoclonal Antibodies for Treatment of Colorectal Cancers: Development of Cetuximab and Panitumumab." J Clin Pharmacol.

Zhang, H., W. Holzgreve, et al. (2001). "Bcl2-L-10, a novel anti-apoptotic member of the Bcl-2 family, blocks apoptosis in the mitochondria death pathway but not in the death receptor pathway." Hum Mol Genet 10(21): 2329-39.

16

MicroRNAs and Rectal Cancer

Miroslav Svoboda[1] and Ilona Kocakova[2]
[1]*Oncobios, Brno,*
[2]*Masaryk Memorial Cancer Institute, Brno*
Czech Republic

1. Introduction

Spontaneous rectal cancers usually arise as a consequence of somatic mutation of the APC gene followed by other mutations (K-ras mutation, DCC inactivation and p53 gene mutation), well-known today as the adenoma-to-carcinoma sequence (Kinzler & Vogelstein, 1996). This sequence covers most spontaneous rectal cancers (80%). However mutation(s) in DNA repair genes; the MSH1, MSH2, PMS1, PMS2 are also involved in certain fraction of rectal tumours, leading to microsatellite instability (Kim et al., 2006). Today about seventy different mutations, including important oncogenes and tumour suppressor genes, are known to be present in various colorectal cancers (Sjoblom, 2008). Colorectal cancers also exhibit changes in DNA methylation with hypermethylation of CpG islands and hypomethylation of oncogenes (Kang, 2007). The mutated cancer genotype is associated with changed expression in many genes, as has been demonstrated by powerful microarray analysis and Real Time PCR technology. It is now well known that mutations and changed DNA methylation pattern, as well as changes of mRNA transcription, are accompanied by changes of expression in certain microRNAs.

2. Background information

2.1 Therapy of rectal cancer

Surgical excision is the primary treatment. However locally advanced rectal cancer (LARC, T3,T4,N0, or TX, N1, N2) needs supportive pre-operative and postoperative therapy. This therapy combines pre-operative linear accelerator irradiation and chemotherapy with fluoropyrimidines, such as 5-fluorouracil or capecitabine. Postoperative therapy is based on adjuvant treatment with further doses of fluoropyrimidines combined with biological treatment where appropriate. (for details, see Lee et al., 2008). Supportive therapy is necessary for downsizing and downstaging of LARC tumours before surgery. Downsizing and downstaging during pre-operative treatment increases the frequency of operations in which the sphincter is saved (Lee et al., 2008). Moreover, this pre-operative treatment may also lower the risk of cancer dissemination during surgery. Seventy to seventy-five percent of patients react with some downstaging and downsizing of rectal tumours following chemoradiotherapy before surgery. However, only about 30% of patients exhibit substantial downstaging and downsizing tumour response and only 10-20% of them exhibit complete tumour eradication through this pre-operative procedure (Kim, 2007). The reasons for these differences in tumour response are not yet well understood. It is widely known that irradiation or anticancer drug treatment of cell lines causes extensive changes in gene expression as well as changes in certain microRNAs, and that differences in responsiveness of cell lines to irradiation and drug treatment are dependent on individual genetic background and the presence of certain mutations in certain oncogenes or tumour suppressor genes. However information is very limited concerning molecular events associated with tumour response to therapy in vivo.

2.2 MicroRNA- basic information

MicroRNAs, also known as miRNAs, are small regulatory molecules (19-25 nucleotides long) that play an important role at the post-translational level of gene regulation (Ambros, 2001). MicroRNAs are widespread molecules, present in all eukaryotic organisms studied to date, including fungi, green plants and animals. MicroRNAs were first described in Western literature in 1993 and were found to play an irreplaceable regulatory role in the spatiotemporal development of the nematode worm *Caenorhabditis elegans* (Lee, 1993). Some 1800 different microRNAs and their sequence variants have been discovered in humans to date. Mature molecules are processed from primary transcripts (pri-miRNAs) that are 1000 nucleotides or more long (Winter et al., 2009). Primary microRNA transcripts originate either at intergenic locations or from intronic sequences of certain actively transcribed genes. If located at intronic sites, microRNAs may be transcribed both as sense and antisense sequences of these actively transcribed genes. Primary transcripts are processed in the nucleus by the specific nuclease Drosha to form approx. 70-nucleotide-long double-stranded pre-miRNAs (see also Scheme 1. for details). These pre-mature microRNA molecules are transported through nuclear pores of the nuclear membrane via the exportin 5 complex to the cytoplasm. Once within the cytoplasm, pre-miRNAs are processed by nuclease Dicer to form 19-25-nucleotide long, double-stranded molecules of sense miRNA and antisense miRNA*. Single stranded microRNAs finally bind to an RNA-silencing protein complex (known as RISC) and target complementary sequences present at the 3' end of the mRNA molecules. If a complex of target mRNA-miRNA-RISC is generated, translation inhibition of mRNA occurs. In humans approximately one-third of mRNA coding genes also contain target sites for one or more of several different types of microRNA. The same target sequence for a given microRNA may be present in mRNAs transcribed from many different genes.

Thus one type of microRNA may regulate many different genes simultaneously. Moreover, since several target sites for different microRNAs may be present in one mRNA and its gene, one gene can be regulated by several microRNAs. Thus post-translational regulation of gene expression by microRNAs is a very complex process; it is not yet fully understood.

2.3 MicroRNAs as regulatory molecules

MicroRNAs were originally discovered as important regulators of spatiotemporal development in the nematode worm *Caenorhabditis elegans* (Slack and Ruvkun, 1997) and were thought to have a canalisation function (i.e. phenotype stabilizing) in the organism (Hornstein and Shomron, 2006). Other authors later found that microRNAs may also have a buffering function in the regulation of gene expression (Cui and Yu, 2007). It is accepted today that microRNAs may play both the above roles (Wu et al., 2009). MicroRNAs are integrated into many regulatory circuits influencing cell cycle progression, genome maintenance, apoptosis and differentiation (Ambros, 2004; Re et al., 2009).

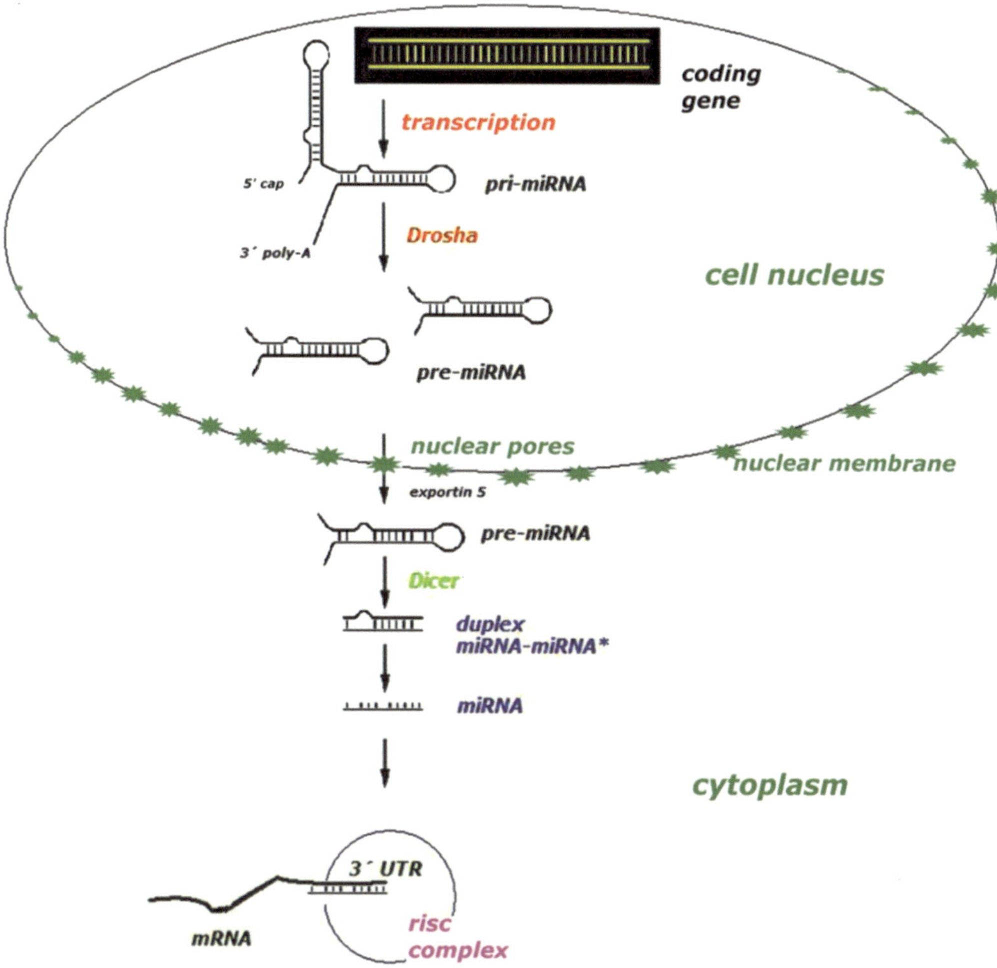

Scheme 1. MicroRNA processing.

2.4 MicroRNAs and exosomes

The term "exosome" has become somewhat ambiguous over time. It was originally applied to the extrachromosomal DNA elements mediating non-Mendelian inheritance of certain traits in the fruit fly *Drosophila melanogaster* (Fox et al., 1970). Later the term "exosome complex" came to designate the supermolecular aggregates responsible for RNA degradation in eukaryotic cells (Mitchell, 1997). Finally, since the 1980's, the term "exosome vesicles" or "exosomes" came to be consistently applied to the membrane vesicles that are exported from the cytoplasmic membrane of mammalian cells to the surrounding milieu (Trams et al., 1981). Any further mention of exosomes in this paper refers to this third meaning of the term. Exosomes may function as tools of intercellular communication (Simons et al., 2009). They may influence such an important processes as immunity responses (Lee et al., 2011). Moreover, since exosomes are exported to the bloodstream, they may transfer information to cells that are distant from the site at which the exosomes themselves are produced in the body. Thus something like "long distance calls" may occur by means of exosome extravasation by one kind of cell at one body site and exosome intravasation to other cells at a second site, and vice versa. Exosomes may transport not only proteins, but also mRNAs, DNAs and microRNAs. It has been demonstrated that the information carried can be exploited by cells that intravasate exosomes. Intravasated mRNA can be translated to a functional product, while transferred microRNA may inhibit translation of target proteins in cells to which exosome microRNAs have been admitted(Keller et al., 2011). Apart from the establishment of exosomes as a new platform for intercellular communication, exosomes can serve as a diagnostic tool, since cancer cells extravasate a different spectrum of microRNAs compared to normal cells (Keller et al., 2011). Moreover, microRNAs in exosomes secreted to the blood are relatively stable (Wittman et al., 2011). It is well proven that plasma microRNA profiles from cancer patients have different spectra of microRNAs compared to microRNA profiles from healthy people (Kosaka et al., 2011). However, multi-centre studies are required to investigate the clinical diagnostic validity of results obtained to date, since the majority of the studies have involved relatively small numbers of clinical samples, usually from fewer than a hundred patients.

2.5 MicroRNA expression profiles in cancer

It is widely accepted that microRNA expression profiles are different in all types of cancer when compared with non-tumourous tissue counterparts studied to date, including for example sarcoma, glioma, carcinoma and haematological malignancies (Volinia, 2006) MicroRNAs actively involved in carcinogenesis operate by inhibiting tumour suppressor genes or by activation of cellular proto-oncogenes. Both the suppressing role and the activating role are most frequently mediated by the inhibitory role of microRNAs in translation of target mRNAs containing complementary sequences. Thus the first mode of miRNA action (suppression) is mediated directly, while the second mode, i.e. proto-oncogene activation, must take place indirectly through negative feedback, inhibiting translation of certain proto-oncogene suppressors. However, some microRNAs may well activate target genes by an as-yet-undisclosed mechanism (Iwasaki and Tomari, 2009).

2.6 Changes of microRNA expression in rectal cancer

Several microRNAs exhibit specific differences of expression levels in rectal and colon cancer when compared with healthy or non-tumourous tissue. Colorectal cancers show decreased levels of miR-143, miR-145 and Let-7a-1 microRNAs (Michael, 2003; Akao, 2006). These microRNAs are known to function as tumour suppressors since they inhibit expression of the known cellular proto-oncogenes c-myc and K-ras (Akao, 2006). Levels of these microRNAs are also lowered in other cancers, including haematological malignancies (Akao, 2007). A further microRNA, miR-21, acts as an oncogene, since it inhibits apoptotic processes and induces cancer cell proliferation (Si, 2007). This microRNA is significantly overexpressed in higher states of colon and rectal cancers and higher miR-21 levels are associated with worse prognosis (Schetter, 2008). Recently miR-95 was found to be overexpressed in approximately 50% of CRC tumours (Huang, 2011). This microRNA promotes proliferation by direct repression of sorting nexin 1 (Huang, 2011). Nowadays, several dozen different microRNAs are known to exhibit changed expression levels in association with CRC (Volinia, 2006; Bandres, 2006).

2.7 Potential role of microRNAs in modulating anticancer drug and radiation response

Drug resistance and the comparative impact of radiation has been fairly frequently studied in cancer cells in vitro (Bandres, 2007; DiGennaro, 2009). However, our knowledge of the molecular events that take place in response to anticancer drugs and radiation in human tumours in vivo is very limited, and this is even more true of microRNA expression changes induced by these events. It has been demonstrated that several microRNA levels are significantly changed in response to 5-fluorouracil in CRC cell lines in vitro (Rossi, 2007). MicroRNAs miR-27a a miR-451 have been found to stimulate expression of multidrug resistance protein MDR1, thus increasing resistance to several anticancer drugs in vitro (Zhu, 2008). Two further important microRNAs, miR-181b and Let-7g, have been found to be involved in responses to the S-1 anticancer drug in colon cancer cells (Nakajima, 2006). Several studies have also been dedicated to the role which 5-fluorouracil therapy may play in the induction of microRNA level changes in clinical samples of cancers. It has been disclosed that 5-fluorouracil therapy induces changes in several microRNAs in gastric cancer (Takagi, 2009) and breast cancer (Salter, 2008). One of our previously-published papers addressed the induction of miR-125b and miR-137 in rectal cancer in response to pre-operative chemoradiotherapy (Svoboda et al., 2008). A German research group has recently noted that miRNAs are returned to normal levels after successful pre-operative chemoradiotherapy and subsequent surgery of locally advanced rectal cancer (Drebber et al., 2011).

2.8 MicroRNAs as prognostic and predictive markers

This subject has recently been reviewed by (Dong et al., 2011). The expression levels of several microRNAs are associated with the TNM state of rectal cancer and might be used for prognosis. MicroRNA miR-21 is upregulated in rectal cancer and higher levels are associated with node positivity, metastasis, and poor survival (Kulda 2010, Schetter 2008, Slaby 2007). High miR-21 stromal expression levels are associated with short disease-free intervals in stage II colorectal cancer patients (Nielsen et al., 2011). MicroRNAs miR-143 and miR-145 are downregulated in rectal cancer. Lower levels are related to large tumour sizes and to disease-free intervals (Slaby et al., 2007; Motoyama et al., 2009; Wang et al., 2009). MiR-31 and miR-106a are upregulated in CRC and reflect tumour states (Bandres et al., 2006; Schetter 2008). Several microRNAs have also been found to be associated with tumour response to therapy or response of cell lines to anticancer drugs. Patients who responded to fluoropyrimidine S-1 showed lower levels of miR-181b and Let-7g. However neither microRNA was associated with survival (Nakajima 2006). MiR-215 increased resistance of cancer cell lines to methotrexate and tomudex (Song 2010). We have previously noted that microRNAs miR-125b and miR-137 are upregulated in response to pre-operative chemoradiotherapy, and higher levels of expression have been associated with worse response to therapy (Svoboda 2008). Various modalities of X-irradiation may give rise to different microRNA expression in vitro (Ahmed 2009). Ragusa suggested that microRNAs let-7b, let 7e and miR-17-3p might be potential predictors of cetuximab resistance (Ragusa et al 2010). MicroRNAs are embedded in exosomes in blood plasma. Since molecules embedded in exosomes are relatively stable for a period of time (up to several days), microRNA expression may simply be monitored from patients' blood (Ng 2009).

3. Aims of the study

The aim of this study was to test the possible involvement of the miR-21, miR-125b, miR-137 and miR-145 in tumour responses to standard pre-operative capecitabine chemoradiotherapy. A further aim was to evaluate the possibility of using mentioned microRNAs as predictors of antiacancer drug response or as prognostic markers.

4. Patients and methods

4.1 Patients

Patients aged 33-76 years, median age being 59, 31 man and 12 woman, ECOG performance status of 0-2, who had histologically confirmed locally advanced rectal adenocarcinoma (LARC) without distant metastases, stages II-III (cT3 - cT4, cN0, cM0 or T2 –T4, cN+,cM0) according to IUCC (Wittekind, 2002) were included in the study. The Ethics Committee of the Masaryk Memorial Cancer Institute approved the treatment protocol. All patients gave written informed consent.

4.2 Methods

Preoperative capecitabine was administered orally, at a dose of 825 mg/m^2 twice a day, two hours prior to radiotherapy for approximately 5.5 weeks from the first to the last day of radiotherapy. Radiation therapy was given in conventional fractionation in locally curative dosage. The daily fraction dose was 1.8 Gy, applied in five days per week up to cumulative dose of 45 Gy, boosting up to 50,4 Gy, during the period of 5.5 weeks. The standard total rectal resection or amputation (Faerden, Naimy et al. 2005), leaving tumor-free resection margins including total mesorectal excision (TME) was performed within the 6th week after completion of radiotherapy. Clinical cTNM stage (preceding a therapy) was based on the endorectal ultrasonography, CT and colonoscopy. Pathological examination after surgery involved the former tumor-bearing area and its macroscopic and microscopic description. The tumor response to therapy was investigated microscopically. Our department of pathology has routinely been using tumor regression (TRG 1-5) criteria adapted to colon cancer (Bouzourene et al., 2002). Tumor biopsies (1-3 mm^3) were taken before starting therapy and again after two-week therapy. Tumor samples were immersed immediately in RNA Later solution (Quiagen GmbH, Germany). The RNAs from bioptic samples were isolated by the standard Trizol method (Chomczynski 1993). RNAs were quantified using Eppendorf spectrophotometer (Eppendorf, Germany). Quality of RNA was tested by standard denaturing electrophoresis. The microRNA levels in pre-treatment and treatment samples were determined by means of stem-loop RT-Real Time PCR and TaqMan detection (Chen, Ridzon et al. 2005). Reverse transcription of cDNA was performed using gene-specific primers, TaqMan MicroRNA Reverse Transcription Kit and 10 ng RNA according to TaqMan MicroRNA Assay Protocol. Stem-loop RT primer (50nM), 1x RT buffer, 10mM dNTP each, RNase inhibitor 0.19ul, MultiScribe reverse transcriptase 1ul, water and RNA were mixed in 15ul final reaction volume and incubated for 30 min at 16°C, 30 min at 42°C, 5 min at 85°C, cooled and kept at 4°C. Real Time PCR mix contained 10ul TaqMan Universal Master Mix No Amp Erase UNG, 1ul 20x Assay Mix from TaqMan MicroRNA Assay Kit (both from Applied Biosystems, Foster City, USA), RT product 1.33ul and water in final volume of 20ul.Real Time PCR was performed on Applied Biosystems 7000 instrument in a

96- well optical plate under following conditions: 95oC 10min initial denaturation, 40 cycles of 95oC for 15s and 60oC for 40s. RNU6B RNA was used as an reference endogenous control. The threshold cycle CT was determined using default instrument settings. Adjacent non-tumorous mucosa before treatment was used as a calibrator.

4.3 Data analysis

We used comparative C_T method approach ($2^{-\text{delta delta Ct}}$) for the calculation of relative miRNA expression (Applied Biosystems User Bulletin #2, P/N 4303859). Expression of miRNA was related to RNU6B RNA as an endogenous active reference. The data before starting therapy were designated as a control group versus a sample group representing data two weeks after starting therapy. Standard statistical analyses were calculated using MedCalc and Statistica version 7 software.

5. Results

5.1 Clinical data

Table 1 summarizes data of patients under study. Forty- three patients were recruited. Nine patients exhibited recurrent disease within follow-up period. Eight of them died. One patient died from comorbidity. All recurrent diseases occured within the three-years period after surgery.

Patients	Attribute	%	Value range
man/woman	31/12	74/26	
Age (median and range)			59 (33-76)
Patients undergoing surgery	42	98	
Number of recidives	9	21	
Median follow-up (months) Local recidives	 2	 5	49
Median disease-free period to local recidive			23 (10-36)
Distant metastases	7	17	
Median disease-free period to distant metastase recurrence			19 (10-58)
Secondary malignities	0	0	
Number of deaths	9	21	
Deaths owing to cancer recurrence	8	19	
a) local	2	5	
b) distant	6	14	
Comorbidities	1	2	
Postoperative complications	0	0	

Table 1. Basic clinical data of recruited patients.

5.2 Non-parametric distribution of statistical data

Statistical analysis of microRNA expression levels determined by standard comparative C_T method shows non-parametric distribution of data (Shapiro-Wilk and Lilliefors tests). We therefore used non-parametric testing for all data (Wilcoxon paired test and Mann-Whitney-U-test).

5.3 MicroRNA expression levels

Our results show that median levels of miR-21, miR-125b and miR-145 were upregulated two weeks after starting therapy. Expression level of miR-137 is not included since we already published its upregulation (Svoboda et al., 2008).

miR21	No.samples	Median	95% confidence interval		p Mann-Whitney U-test (two- sided)	p Wilcoxon (paired, two-sided)
before	42	9,318	0,057	26,173	0,1129	0,0464
two weeks	35	16,450	5,637	29,651		(N=35)

a) miR-21 induction

Mann-Whitney U-test (two- sided)	No.samples	Median	95% confidence í interval		p
miR125b before	42	0,463	0,045	5,618	0,03054
miR125b , two weeks	35	1,173	0,129	8,282	

b) miR-125b induction

Mann-Whitney U-test (two- sided)	No.samples	Median	95% confidence interval		p
miR145 before	42	0,145	0,078	1,279	0,000001
miR145 , two weeks	35	1,661	0,483	9,383	

c) miR-145 induction

Table 2. a,b,c. Induction of microRNA expression by the preoperative chemoradiotherapy.

MicroRNAs exhibited extensive intertumoral level variability both before treatment and in samples taken two weeks after starting therapy (see 95% confidence intervals in Tables 3.,4.). The observation of frequent upregulation after starting therapy may support our initial hypothesis that miRNA levels tend to change to normal levels after efficient tumor destruction as both miR125b and miR137 are known to be down-regulated either in CRC lines or colorectal and breast carcinomas (Iorio, Ferracin et al. 2005). Nevertheless, miR-21 is upregulated in most colorectal cancers and functions as an oncogene (Nielsen et al., 2011).

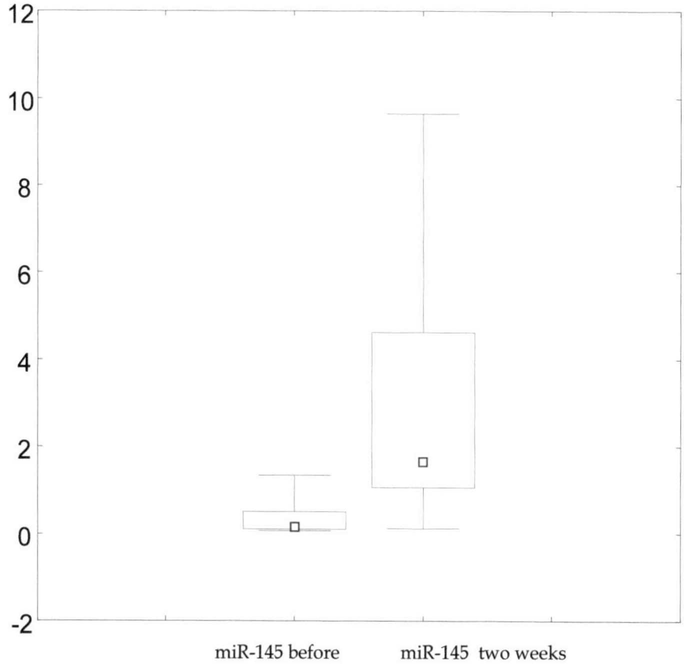

Table 3. Variability of microRNA miR-145 expression levels before and two weeks after starting preoperative chemoradiotherapy

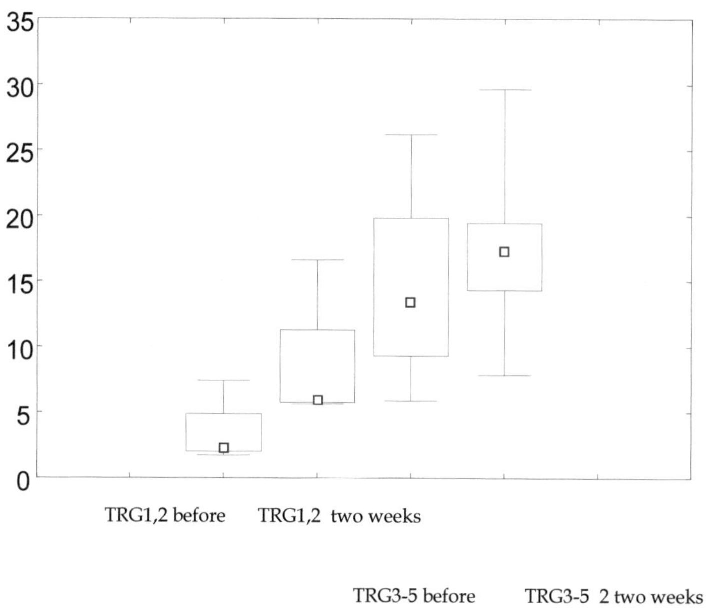

Table 4. a) Box-plot graph of the relative expression of miR-21. Role of tumour regression grade TRG.

Therefore, we investigated whether the changes of miRNA levels are reflected within immediate tumor responses and downstaging. As table 2 shows., miR-21 is upregulated in rectal cancer two weeks after starting preoperative chemoradiotherapy. Moreover, there are statistically significant differences between responsive (TRG1,2) and non-responsive group (TRG 3-5) before starting therapy and different ypT stages respectively (tables 4. and 5.).

Mann-Whitney U-test (two-sided)	Median relatve expression	95% confidence interval		p
miR21 TRG1,2 before	2,312	1,731	7,438	0,014
miR21 TRG3-5 before	13,404	5,897	26,173	
miR21 TRG1,2 two wks.	5,849	5,637	16,641	0,077
miR21 TRG3-5 two wks.	17,749	7,863	29,651	

Table 4. b) Median levels of relative miR-21 expression. Role of tumour regression grade TRG.

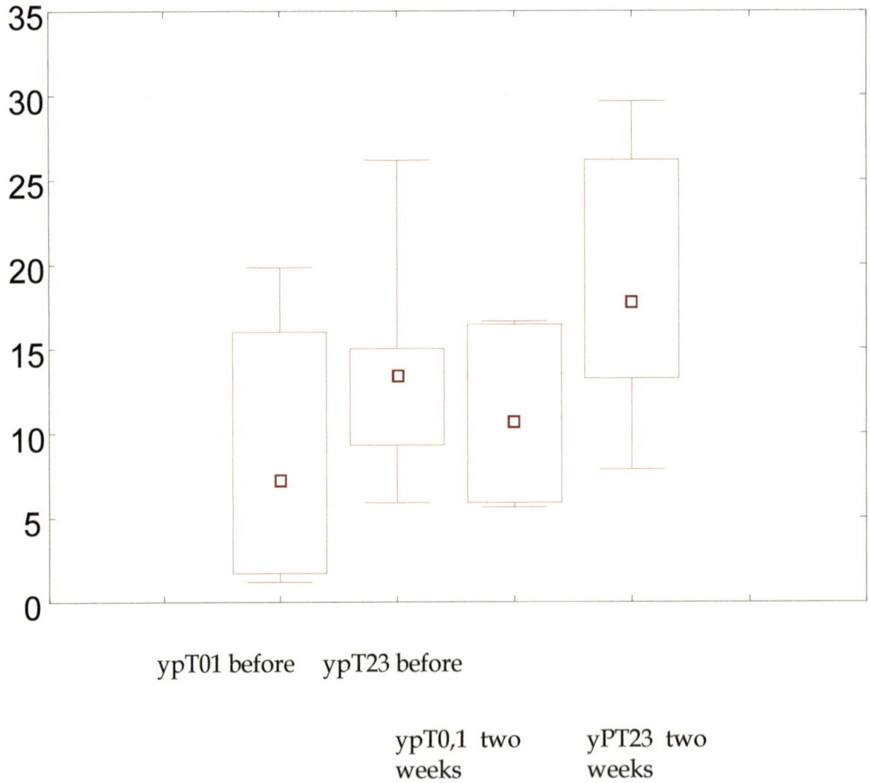

Table 5. a) The Box-plot graph of relative miR-21 expression. Role of ypT.

Mann-Whitney U-test (two-sided)	Patients ypT0,1	Patients ypT2,3	p
ypT0,1 vs. ypT2,3 before	16	26	0,1088
ypT0,1 vs. yPT2,3 two weeks	10	25	0,0185

Table 5. b) Median levels of relative miR-21 expression. Role of ypT.

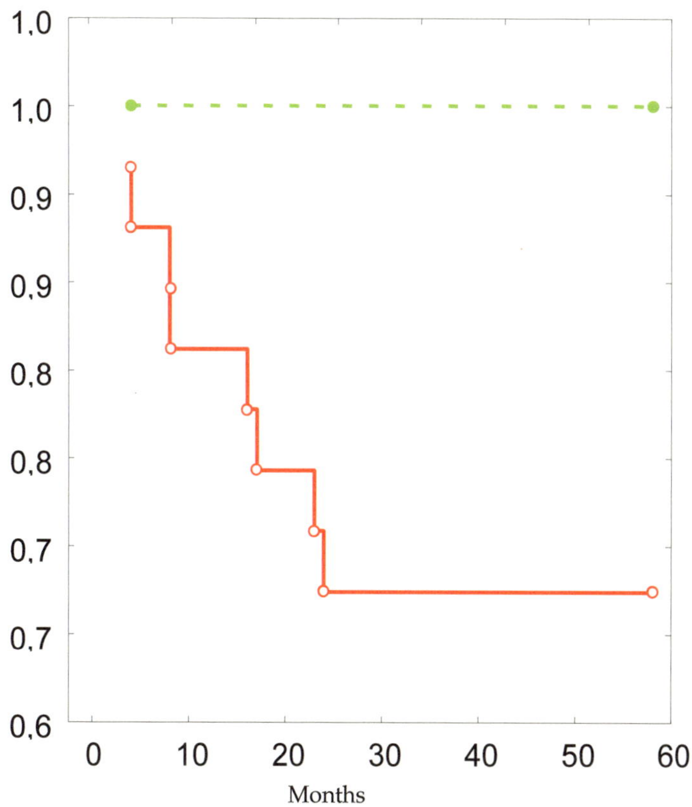

Log-Rank Test p = ,15754

Table 6. Kaplan-Meyer graph of disease-free survival. Red line: patients with high-level miR-21 tumours suffer from recurrent disease. Green line: patients with low-level miR-21 tumours. Median level of relative miR-21 expression is the cut-off value discriminating between high-level miR-21 tumours and low-level miR-21 tumours respectively.

Although 125b is upregulated in all ypT groups, the highest and the only statistically significant change is observed in the group ypT3 patients (no downstaging). It is well known that T3/4 stage or node involvement is usually associated with worse prognosis than T0-T2, N0. Therefore, higher induction of miR125 is associated with a worse prognosis.

miR-125b	Patients	Median expression	95% confidence interval		p (Wilcoxon paired)
TRG12 before	25	0,393	0,092	2,761	0,005
TRG12 two weeks	21	0,905	0,329	9,646	(N=21)
TRG3-5 before	17	0,694	0,188	1,414	0,059
TRG 3-5 two weeks	14	1,131	0,189	3,204	(N=14)

Table 7. a) Dependence of induced miR-125b levels on the tumour regression grade. Wilcoxon paired test

Mann-Whitney U- test	TRG1-2	TRG3-5	p
TRG12 vs TRG3-5 before	25	17	0,109
TRG12 vs TRG3-5 two weeks	21	14	0,391

Table 7. b) Dependence of induced miR-125b levels on the tumour regression grade. Comparison of different TRG groups.

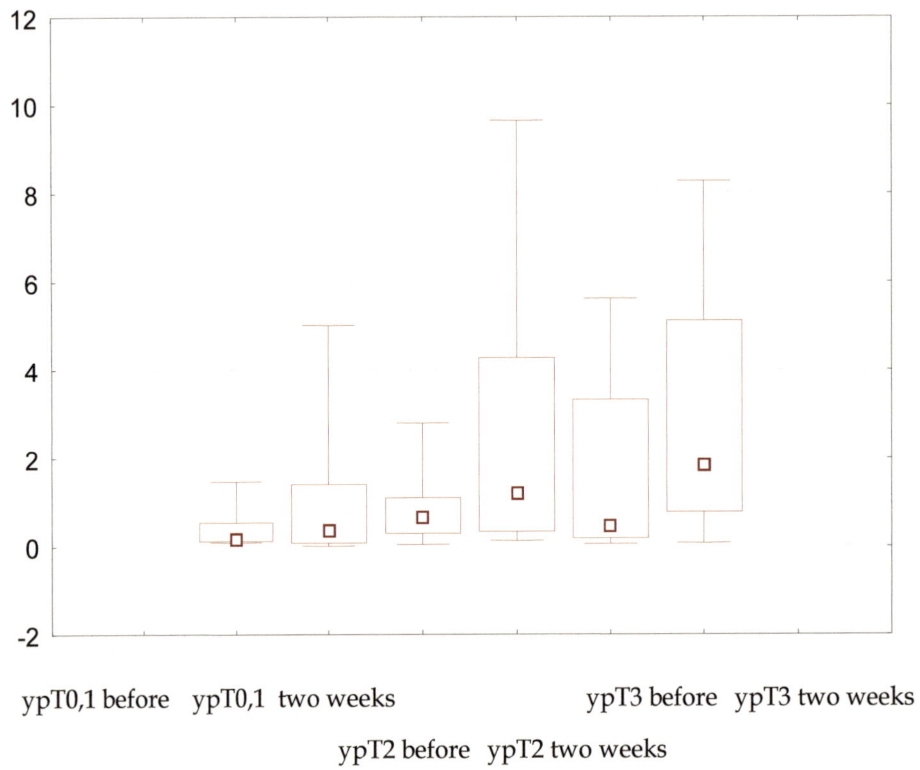

Table 8. a) Dependence of induced miR-125b levels on the tumour state ypT. Box-plot graph.

There are profound differences of miR125b levels between ypT0,1, and ypT3 patient groups after starting therapy (Table 8). Patients with low stage tumours have lower miRNA induction than patients with more advanced cancers. These results tell us that we should use carefully term oncogene or tumour suppresor in connection with certain miRNAs. MicroRNA miR125b is downregulated in several cancers and may be therefore considered a tumor suppressor from this point of view. However, in this study we show no downstaging and less regression (bad response) in the tumors with the highest upregulation of miR125b level two weeks after starting therapy. Non-responding tumors exhibited induction of miR125b level close to and above normal levels of adjacent non-tumorous mucosa.

miR-125b	Patients	Median	95% confidence interval		p Wilcoxon (paired, two-sided)
ypT0,1 before	16	0,158	0,092	1,464	0,4446
ypT0,1 two weeks	10	0,362	0,011	5,011	
ypT2 before	14	0,662	0,045	2,796	0,0843
ypT2 two weeks	13	1,186	0,129	9,646	
ypT3 before	12	0,463	0,054	5,618	0,0164
ypT3 two weeks	12	1,828	0,073	8,282	

Table 8. b) Dependence of induced miR-125b levels on the tumour state ypT. Wilcoxon paired test.

Mann-Whitney U-test (two-sided)	Patients ypT0,1	Patients ypT2 ypT3	p
ypT0,1 vs pT2 before	16	14	0,1223
ypT0,1 vs pT2 two weeks	10	13	0,1375
ypT0,1 vs pT3 before	16	12	0,1971
ypT0,1 vs pT3 two weeks	10	12	0,0295

Table 8. c) Dependence of induced miR-125b levels on the tumour state ypT. Comparison of different ypT states by Mann-Whitney two-sided test.

Our results show that miR137 is significantly upregulated in both responder groups (Table 9.a). However there is no association of miR137 induction with tumour response (Table 9.b). Interestingly, on the contrary to the above-mentioned miR125b although upregulated, miR137 in tumors never reached the original median value of normal tissue. We therefore speculate that low miR137 levels may be important to maintain tumour state.

miR-137	Patients	Median	Confidence interval		p (Wilcoxon paired)
TRG1,2 beforer	25	0,037	0,003	0,688	0,027
TRG1,2 two weeks	21	0,162	0,012	0,766	(N=21)
TRG3-5 before	17	0,035	0,006	0,646	0,006
TRG3-5 two weeks	14	0,301	0,005	0,655	(N=14)

Table 9. a) Dependence of induced miR-137 levels on the tumour regression grade. Wicoxon paired test.

Mann-Whitney U-test (two-sided)	Patients TRG1,2	Patients TRG3-5	p
TRG12 vs. 3-5 before	25	17	0,538
TRG12 vs. 3-5 two weeks	21	14	0,373

Table 9. b) Comparison of miR-137 levels between responders and non-responders. Mann-Whitney two-sided test.

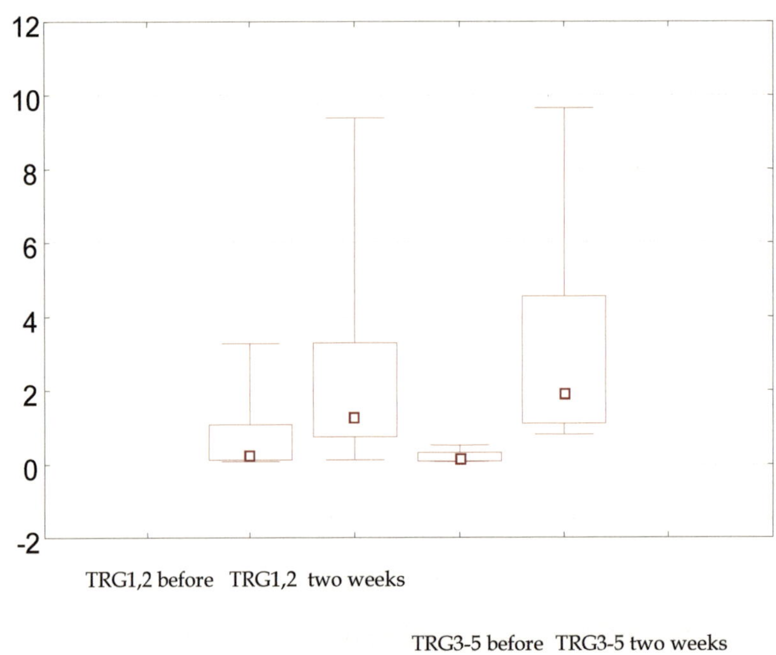

Table 10. a) Dependence of induced miR-145 levels on the tumour state ypT.

MicroRNA miR-145 is significantly upregulated both in responders and non-responders respectively (Tables 10 a,b). Moreover, miR-145 has significantly higher expression in tumors from responders before therapy (Table 10 c). Similar effect we can observe in the ypT state groups: patients with ypT0,1 tumours (better prognosis) have higher miR-145 levels. This is in accordance with known tumour-supressive role of miR-145.

miR-145	Valid N	Median expresion	95% confidence interval		p (Wilcoxon paired t.)
TRG1,2 before	25	0,226	0,078	3,279	0,0021
TRG1,2 two weeks	21	1,248	0,126	9,383	(N=21)
TRG3-5 before	17	0,115	0,075	0,518	0,0003
TRG3-5 two weeks	14	1,886	0,812	9,646	(N=14)

Table 10. b) Dependence of induced miR-145 levels on the tumour regression grade.

Mann-Whitney U-test	Patients TRG 1,2	Patients TRG 3-5	p (two sided)
TRG 1,2 vs.3-5 before	25	17	0,013
TRG1,2 vs. 3-5 two weeks	25	17	0,274

Table 10. c) Dependence of induced miR-145 levels on the tumour regression grade. Comparison of diffferent TRG groups.

miR-145	Valid N	Median	95% confidence interval		p Wilcoxon (paired, two sided test)
ypT0,1 before	16	0,226	0,111	1,338	0,0004
ypT0,1 two weeks	10	1,586	0,483	9,383	(N=10)
ypT2 before	14	0,132	0,078	3,279	0,1361
ypT2 two weeks	13	1,227	0,126	9,646	(N=13)
ypT3 before	12	0,133	0,075	0,518	0,0010
ypT3 two weeks	12	1,621	0,812	4,691	(N=12)

Table 10. d) Dependence of induced miR-145 levels on the tumour state ypT.

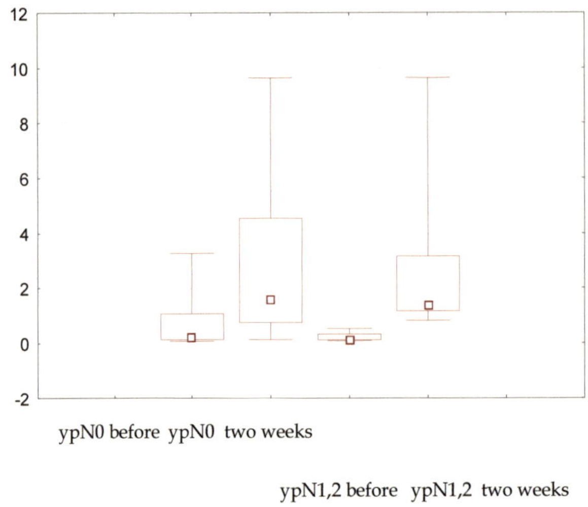

Table 11. a) Dependence of pre-therapeutic and induced miR-145 levels on the node state pN. Box-plot graph.

miR-145	Patients	Median	95% confidence interval		p Wilcoxon (paired, two sided t.)
ypN0 before	25	0,226	0,075	3,279	0,0010
ypN0 two weeks	23	1,586	0,126	9,646	(N=23)
ypN1,2 before	17	0,115	0,078	0,518	0,0003
ypN1,2 two weeks	12	1,357	0,812	9,646	(N=12)

Table 11. b) Dependence of pre-therapeutic and induced miR-145 levels on the node state pN .

Mann-Whitney U-test (two-sided)	Patients pN0	Patients pN1,2	p
ypN0 vs. ypN1,2 before	25	17	0,0283
ypN0 vs. ypN1,2 two weeks	23	12	0,8196

Table 11. c) Dependence of pre-therapeutic and induced miR-145 levels on the node state pN. Comparison of ypN0 and ypN1,2 groups.

We have also investigated the role of node involvement. Table 11 shows that miR-145 levels of ypN0 patients differ significantly from ypN1,2 before starting therapy. The upregulation of miR-125b was published previously (Svoboda, 2008).

6. Discussion

MicroRNAs play an important part in the regulation of many important cellular processes and target approximately a third of expressed genes. It is therefore reasonable to assume that microRNAs would be influenced by such a massive cell-destructive process as pre-operative chemoradiotherapy. This pre-operative treatment degrades the proliferative potential of many cancer cells and leads to extensive tumour regression in many patients (Bouzourene et al., 2002). Among the microRNAs we have been investigating, miR-21 exhibits the highest difference in expression levels considered in terms of response to therapy. While tumours that respond well contain low miR-21 levels, non-responders have high miR-21 levels (median level as cut-off value discriminating between low and high levels). It is crucial to note that these differences are already pronounced in samples taken from tumours before starting therapy (p=0.014). Therefore, miR-21 is not only a known prognostic factor, but it may also be used also as a predictor of tumour response to pre-operative chemoradiotherapy. This is not a surprising fact, since miR-21 is a known anti-apoptotic and pro-proliferative factor and is currently recognized as an oncogene (Zhang et al., 2008). We also show in our preliminary data that high miR-21 levels might be associated with short disease-free survival and recurrent disease, as may be seen on the Kaplan-Meyer graph (Table 6). Patients with high-level miR-21 tumours suffer from recurrent disease while patients with low-level miR-21 tumours are all disease-free within the five-year follow-up period. However since only a small number of patients has been monitored to date, statistical significance according to log-rank test remained only p=0.15 and more patients must be recruited in order to obtain statistically valid data. Epithelial-to-mesenchymal transition (EMT) is a primary event leading to the prometastatic behaviour of cancer cells (Gregory et al., 2008). TGF-beta-induced EMT leads to upregulation of miR-21 in a model system of human keratinocytes in vitro (Zavadil et al., 2007). Induction of miR-21 leads to pro-invasive behaviour in breast cell lines in vitro and metastasizing of tumours related to those lines in animals in vivo (Zhu et al., 2008). This effect is mediated by miR-21 inhibition of tropomyosin 1 activity (Zhu et al., 2008). Tropomyosin 1 is a tumour suppressor. MiR-21 also inhibits PDCD4 and maspin, further important regulators: (Zhu et al., 2008). Our data are in accordance with these in vitro findings, since high levels of miR-21 are associated with recurrent and refractory disease in our study. MicroRNA miR-125b is an ortholog of Lin-4 microRNA of the worm *Caenorhabditis elegans* (Ambros, 2003). High levels of this microRNA prolong the lifespan of the worm, probably by influencing the insulin metabolic pathway (Boehm, 2006). High levels of miR-125b give rise to similar effects in rectal cancer: tumours with highly-induced miR-125b survive chemoradiotherapy intervention and are refractory, while low-MiR-125b-level tumours are partially or completely destroyed. On the basis of the analogy with the nematode worm and of our findings, we suggest that miR-125b supports mechanisms necessary for cell survival that are undoubtedly initiated as an adaptation to the chemical and radiation stress induced as a consequence of preoperative chemoradiotherapy. On the other hand, miR-125b is known to suppress proto-oncogenes ERBB2 and ERBB3 expression in vitro (Scott et al., 2007). ERBB2 and ERBB3 are known pro-metastatic and pro-proliferative factors. We speculate that this opposite effect of miR-125b may co-exist in parallel with the previously-mentioned effect and may provide a base for explanation of the fact that, while only 30-40% of tumours are extensively shrinked, the frequency of metastasis and recurrent disease is lower in patients who have undergone preoperative chemoradiotherapy versus patients who did not in the past when this treatment modality was not yet established (Lee, 2008). The level of miR-137 is frequently suppressed in glioblastoma and CRC (Silber et al., 2008). This is caused by aberrant methylation of CpG islands near coding genes (Kozaki, 2008). Here, the observed induction of miR-137 is in accordance with the fact that this microRNA suppresses G_0 to G_1

transition (Silber et al., 2008). Suppression of cell growth is a general process accompanying chemoradiation treatment. Tables 9 a,b show that miR-137 levels are upregulated in all tumours despite TRG. We may therefore expect that miR-137 induction is a part of the general process of adaptation to chemical and radiation stress. However therapy-induced miR-137 levels never achieve their original levels, i.e. those present in non-cancerous tissue counterpart. We may therefore assume that miR-137 might be a tumour suppressor and that lower miR-137 expression helps to maintain the transformed phenotype. This is also supported by the finding that miR-137 directly targets carboxy-terminal binding protein I (CtBPI) to inhibit epithelial-to-mesencyhmal transition and induce apoptosis in melanoma cells (Deng et al., 2011). We therefore speculate that, although miR-137 does not contribute to an immediate effect of tumour regression, it may lower later cancer recurrence by inhibiting epithelial-to-mesenchymal transition processes. The relevance of this speculative construction is also supported by the fact that transfection of pre-miR-137 (a microRNA precursor molecule) stops proliferation and induces differentiation in glioblastoma cells in vitro (Silber et al., 2008). MicroRNA miR-145 is downregulated in many cancers, including carcinomas of the bladder, lung and stomach (Takagi et al., 2009; Cho et al., 2009; Ichimi, 2009). Levels of this microRNA are also downregulated in CRC (Wang&Zhou, 2009). It is recognised as a tumour suppressor, supported by the fact that transfected miR-145 precursors inhibit the growth of lung cancer cells in vitro and also inhibit the growth of MCF-7 breast cancer-derived cells (Cho et al., 2009). Moreover, miR-145 upregulation induces apoptosis in MCF-7 cells (Wang& Bian et al., 2009). According to our results, miR-145 is upregulated after starting pre-operative chemoradiotherapy. In the light of the tumour suppressor role, we assume that upregulated miR-145 participates in vivo (in vitro model analogy) in the inhibition of cancer cell growth. Our results show that microRNA miR-145 levels before starting therapy well reflect therapy outcome. Therefore, miR-145 may be used as a predictor of response to pre-operative chemoradiotherapy. This accords with the recent finding of German authors (Drebber et al., 2011).

7. Conclusion

MicroRNAs miR-21, miR-125b, miR-137 and miR-145 all display up-regulation of expression induced by preoperative chemoradiotherapy of locally advanced rectal cancer. Among microRNAs we have been investigating, miR-21 and miR-145 exhibit the highest differences in expression levels considered in terms of response to therapy. MiR-21 as well as miR-145 may be used as potential predictive and prognostic markers.

8. Acknowledgement

We wish to thank Tony Long and Simon Buxton for careful reading the manuscript.
Notice: both authors participated equally.

9. References

Ahmed, F. E., P. W. Vos, et al. (2009). "Differences in mRNA and microRNA microarray expression profiles in human colon adenocarcinoma HT-29 cells treated with either Intensity-modulated Radiation Therapy (IMRT), or Conventional Radiation Therapy (RT)." Cancer Genomics Proteomics 6(2): 109-27.

Akao, Y., Y. Nakagawa, et al. (2007). "Downregulation of microRNAs-143 and -145 in B-cell malignancies." Cancer Sci 98(12): 1914-20.
Akao, Y., Y. Nakagawa, et al. (2006). "let-7 microRNA functions as a potential growth suppressor in human colon cancer cells." Biol Pharm Bull 29(5): 903-6.
Ambros, V. (2001). "microRNAs: tiny regulators with great potential." Cell **107**(7): 823-6.
Ambros, V. (2003). "MicroRNA pathways in flies and worms: growth, death, fat, stress, and timing." Cell 113(6): 673-6.
Ambros, V. (2004). "The functions of animal microRNAs." Nature 431(7006): 350-5.
Bandres, E., E. Cubedo, et al. (2006). "Identification by Real-time PCR of 13 mature microRNAs differentially expressed in colorectal cancer and non-tumoral tissues." Mol Cancer 5: 29.
Bandres, E., R. Zarate, et al. (2007). "Pharmacogenomics in colorectal cancer: the first step for individualized-therapy." World J Gastroenterol 13(44): 5888-901.
Boehm, M. and F. J. Slack (2006). "MicroRNA control of lifespan and metabolism." Cell Cycle 5(8): 837-40.
Bouzourene, H., F. T. Bosman, et al. (2002). "Importance of tumor regression assessment in predicting the outcome in patients with locally advanced rectal carcinoma who are treated with preoperative radiotherapy." Cancer 94(4): 1121-30.
Cui, Q., Z. Yu, et al. (2007). "MicroRNA regulation and interspecific variation of gene expression." Trends Genet 23(8): 372-5.
Di Gennaro, E., F. Bruzzese, et al. (2009). "Modulation of thymidilate synthase and p53 expression by HDAC inhibitor vorinostat resulted in synergistic antitumor effect in combination with 5FU or raltitrexed." Cancer Biol Ther 8(9): 782-91.
Deng, Y., H. Deng, et al. "MicroRNA-137 targets carboxyl-terminal binding protein 1 in melanoma cell lines. " Int J Biol Sci 7(1): 133-7.
Dong, Y., W. K. Wu, et al. "MicroRNA dysregulation in colorectal cancer: a clinical perspective." Br J Cancer 104(6): 893-8.
Drebber, U., M. Lay, et al. "Altered levels of the onco-microRNA 21 and the tumor-supressor microRNAs 143 and 145 in advanced rectal cancer indicate successful neoadjuvant chemoradiotherapy." Int J Oncol 39(2): 409-15.
Fox, A. S., W. F. Duggleby, et al. (1970). "DNA-induced transformation in Drosophila: evidence for transmission without integration." Proc Natl Acad Sci U S A 67(4): 1834-8.
Gregory, P. A., C. P. Bracken, et al. (2008). "MicroRNAs as regulators of epithelial-mesenchymal transition." Cell Cycle 7(20): 3112-8.
Hornstein, E. and N. Shomron (2006). "Canalization of development by microRNAs." Nat Genet 38 Suppl: S20-4.
Huang, Z., S. Huang, et al. "MicroRNA-95 promotes cell proliferation and targets sorting Nexin 1 in human colorectal carcinoma." Cancer Res 71(7): 2582-9.
Chen, C., D. A. Ridzon, et al. (2005). "Real-time quantification of microRNAs by stem-loop RT-PCR." Nucleic Acids Res 33(20): e179.
Cho, W. C., A. S. Chow, et al. (2009). "Restoration of tumour suppressor hsa-miR-145 inhibits cancer cell growth in lung adenocarcinoma patients with epidermal growth factor receptor mutation." Eur J Cancer 45(12): 2197-206.
Chomczynski, P. (1993). "A reagent for the single-step simultaneous isolation of RNA, DNA and proteins from cell and tissue samples." Biotechniques 15(3): 532-4, 536-7.

Ichimi, T., H. Enokida, et al. (2009). "Identification of novel microRNA targets based on microRNA signatures in bladder cancer." Int J Cancer 125(2): 345-52.

Iorio, M. V., M. Ferracin, et al. (2005). "MicroRNA gene expression deregulation in human breast cancer." Cancer Res 65(16): 7065-70.

Iwasaki, S. and Y. Tomari (2009). "Argonaute-mediated translational repression (and activation)." Fly (Austin) 3(3): 204-6.

Kang, G. H. "Four molecular subtypes of colorectal cancer and their precursor lesions." Arch Pathol Lab Med 135(6): 698-703.

Keller, S., J. Ridinger, et al. "Body fluid derived exosomes as a novel template for clinical diagnostics." J Transl Med 9: 86.

Kim, D. Y., K. H. Jung, et al. (2007). "Comparison of 5-fluorouracil/leucovorin and capecitabine in preoperative chemoradiotherapy for locally advanced rectal cancer." Int J Radiat Oncol Biol Phys 67(2): 378-84.

Kim, Y. R., N. G. Chung, et al. "Novel somatic frameshift mutations of genes related to cell cycle and DNA damage response in gastric and colorectal cancers with microsatellite instability." Tumori 96(6): 1004-9.

Kinzler, K. W. and B. Vogelstein (1996). "Lessons from hereditary colorectal cancer." Cell 87(2): 159-70.

Kosaka, N., H. Iguchi, et al. "Circulating microRNA in body fluid: a new potential biomarker for cancer diagnosis and prognosis." Cancer Sci 101(10): 2087-92.

Kozaki, K., I. Imoto, et al. (2008). "Exploration of tumor-suppressive microRNAs silenced by DNA hypermethylation in oral cancer." Cancer Res 68(7): 2094-105.

Kulda, V., M. Pesta, et al. "Relevance of miR-21 and miR-143 expression in tissue samples of colorectal carcinoma and its liver metastases." Cancer Genet Cytogenet 200(2): 154-60.

Lee, R. C., R. L. Feinbaum, et al. (1993). "The C. elegans heterochronic gene lin-4 encodes small RNAs with antisense complementarity to lin-14." Cell 75(5): 843-54.

Lee, S. H., K. C. Lee, et al. (2008). "Chemoradiotherapy followed by surgery in rectal cancer: improved local control using a moderately high pelvic radiation dose." Jpn J Clin Oncol 38(2): 112-21.

Lee, T. H., E. D'Asti, et al. "Microvesicles as mediators of intercellular communication in cancer-the emerging science of cellular 'debris'." Semin Immunopathol.

Michael, M. Z., O. C. SM, et al. (2003). "Reduced accumulation of specific microRNAs in colorectal neoplasia." Mol Cancer Res 1(12): 882-91.

Mitchell, P., E. Petfalski, et al. (1997). "The exosome: a conserved eukaryotic RNA processing complex containing multiple 3'-->5' exoribonucleases." Cell 91(4): 457-66.

Motoyama, K., H. Inoue, et al. (2009). "Over- and under-expressed microRNAs in human colorectal cancer." Int J Oncol 34(4): 1069-75.

Nakajima, G., K. Hayashi, et al. (2006). "Non-coding MicroRNAs hsa-let-7g and hsa-miR-181b are Associated with Chemoresponse to S-1 in Colon Cancer." Cancer Genomics Proteomics 3(5): 317-324.

Ng, E. K., W. W. Chong, et al. (2009). "Differential expression of microRNAs in plasma of patients with colorectal cancer: a potential marker for colorectal cancer screening." Gut 58(10): 1375-81.

Nielsen, B. S., S. Jorgensen, et al. "High levels of microRNA-21 in the stroma of colorectal cancers predict short disease-free survival in stage II colon cancer patients." Clin Exp Metastasis 28(1): 27-38.
Ragusa, M., A. Majorana, et al. "Specific alterations of microRNA transcriptome and global network structure in colorectal carcinoma after cetuximab treatment." Mol Cancer Ther 9(12): 3396-409.
Re, A., D. Cora, et al. (2009). "Genome-wide survey of microRNA-transcription factor feed-forward regulatory circuits in human." Mol Biosyst 5(8): 854-67.
Rossi, L., E. Bonmassar, et al. (2007). "Modification of miR gene expression pattern in human colon cancer cells following exposure to 5-fluorouracil in vitro." Pharmacol Res 56(3): 248-53.
Salter, K. H., C. R. Acharya, et al. (2008). "An integrated approach to the prediction of chemotherapeutic response in patients with breast cancer." PLoS One 3(4): e1908.
Scott, G. K., A. Goga, et al. (2007). "Coordinate suppression of ERBB2 and ERBB3 by enforced expression of micro-RNA miR-125a or miR-125b." J Biol Chem 282(2): 1479-86.
Schetter, A. J., S. Y. Leung, et al. (2008). "MicroRNA expression profiles associated with prognosis and therapeutic outcome in colon adenocarcinoma." Jama 299(4): 425-36.
Si, M. L., S. Zhu, et al. (2007). "miR-21-mediated tumor growth." Oncogene 26(19): 2799-803.
Silber, J., D. A. Lim, et al. (2008). "miR-124 and miR-137 inhibit proliferation of glioblastoma multiforme cells and induce differentiation of brain tumor stem cells." BMC Med 6: 14.
Simons, M. and G. Raposo (2009). "Exosomes--vesicular carriers for intercellular communication." Curr Opin Cell Biol 21(4): 575-81.
Sjoblom, T. (2008). "Systematic analyses of the cancer genome: lessons learned from sequencing most of the annotated human protein-coding genes." Curr Opin Oncol 20(1): 66-71.
Slaby, O., M. Svoboda, et al. (2007). "Altered expression of miR-21, miR-31, miR-143 and miR-145 is related to clinicopathologic features of colorectal cancer." Oncology 72(5-6): 397-402.
Slack, F. and G. Ruvkun (1997). "Temporal pattern formation by heterochronic genes." Annu Rev Genet 31: 611-34.
Song, B., Y. Wang, et al. "Molecular mechanism of chemoresistance by miR-215 in osteosarcoma and colon cancer cells." Mol Cancer 9: 96.
Svoboda, M., L. Izakovicova Holla, et al. (2008). "Micro-RNAs miR125b and miR137 are frequently upregulated in response to capecitabine chemoradiotherapy of rectal cancer." Int J Oncol 33(3): 541-7.
Takagi, T., A. Iio, et al. (2009). "Decreased expression of microRNA-143 and -145 in human gastric cancers." Oncology 77(1): 12-21.
Trams, E. G., C. J. Lauter, et al. (1981). "Exfoliation of membrane ecto-enzymes in the form of micro-vesicles." Biochim Biophys Acta 645(1): 63-70.
Turchinovich, A., L. Weiz, et al. "Characterization of extracellular circulating microRNA." Nucleic Acids Res. 2011
Volinia, S., M. Galasso, et al. "Reprogramming of miRNA networks in cancer and leukemia." Genome Res 20(5): 589-99.

Wang, C. J., Z. G. Zhou, et al. (2009). "Clinicopathological significance of microRNA-31, -143 and -145 expression in colorectal cancer." Dis Markers 26(1): 27-34.
Wang, S., C. Bian, et al. (2009). "miR-145 inhibits breast cancer cell growth through RTKN." Int J Oncol 34(5): 1461-6.
Winter, J., S. Jung, et al. (2009). "Many roads to maturity: microRNA biogenesis pathways and their regulation." Nat Cell Biol 11(3): 228-34.
Wittekind, C., C. C. Compton, et al. (2002). "TNM residual tumor classification revisited." Cancer 94(9): 2511-6.
Wittmann, J. and H. M. Jack "Serum microRNAs as powerful cancer biomarkers." Biochim Biophys Acta 1806(2): 200-7.
Wu, C. I., Y. Shen, et al. (2009). "Evolution under canalization and the dual roles of microRNAs: a hypothesis." Genome Res 19(5): 734-43.
Zavadil, J., M. Narasimhan, et al. (2007). "Transforming growth factor-beta and microRNA:mRNA regulatory networks in epithelial plasticity." Cells Tissues Organs 185(1-3): 157-61.
Zhang, Z., Z. Li, et al. (2008). "miR-21 plays a pivotal role in gastric cancer pathogenesis and progression." Lab Invest 88(12): 1358-66.
Zhu, S., H. Wu, et al. (2008). "MicroRNA-21 targets tumor suppressor genes in invasion and metastasis." Cell Res 18(3): 350-9.

17

Nonoperative Management of Distal Rectal Cancer After Chemoradiation: Experience with the "Watch & Wait" Protocol

Angelita Habr-Gama[1], Rodrigo Oliva Perez[1,2], Patricio B. Lynn[1], Arceu Scanavini Neto[1,2] and Joaquim Gama-Rodrigues[1]
[1]Angelita & Joaquim Gama institute, São Paulo,
[2]Department of Gastroenterology - Colorectal Surgery Division, University of São Paulo, School of Medicine, São Paulo, Brazil

1. Introduction

Surgical treatment alone for locally advanced rectal cancer (T3/T4 or N1 tumors) has been associated with considerably high local recurrence rates. Even with appropriate total mesorectal excision (TME), radical surgery leads to excellent local disease control only in highly selected cases.(Simunovic et al. 2003) In this setting, the need for additional or complementary treatment strategies was highly warranted.

In the late 80's and early 90's it was observed that the addition of adjuvant radiotherapy with or without chemotherapy significantly improved disease control as well as survival rates in this group of patients.(Krook et al. 1991)

Later on, results from randomized controlled trials suggested that the neoadjuvant approach was superior for local disease control, even when appropriate surgical technique (total mesorectal excision) was performed when compared to adjuvant treatment. (Sauer et al. 2004) Apart from the theoretical advantage of exposing unscarred tissue with optimal oxygen delivery to chemoradiation (CRT), further benefits including reduced toxicity rates, significant tumor downstaging and downsizing, greater rates of sphincter preservation, and better functional results have been reported after neoadjuvant CRT. (Habr-Gama et al. 2004; Sauer et al. 2004)

Tumor downstaging in some patients may be so significant, that no residual cancer was detected during final pathological assessment. Still, radical surgery was associated with considerably immediate postoperative mortality and morbidity rates. In addition to usual postoperative complications, total mesorectal excision may lead to significant sexual and urinary dysfunctions. Also, even when abdominal perineal excision (and a permanent stoma) could be avoided, temporary loop ileostomies are mandatory in order to avoid potential septic consequences of anastomotic leaks in these patients. (Peter Matthiessen et al. 2007)

Therefore, in the setting of a complete tumor regression after neoadjuvant CRT, surgeons have searched for alternative management of patients in order to avoid the potential consequences of TME with or without abdominal perineal resection.

2. Factors associated with tumor response after CRT

Tumor response to neoadjuvant chemoradiation is not uniform and seems to be related to many factors such as specific treatment regimen, timing after CRT completion, tumor/patient characteristics and tumor biology.

2.1 Chemoradiation regimen

Fractionated long course chemoradiation followed by surgery after 6-8 weeks or pelvic short-course irradiation with 25Gy in five fractions followed by immediate surgery (short-course) have been the two most frequent regimens used in the preoperative treatment of patients with resectable T3-4 rectal cancer.

Even though the benefits in local disease control seem to be equivalent between short-course RT and long-course chemoradiation therapy,(Bujko et al. 2006) there are significant differences in terms of tumor downstaging between patients undergoing these two regimens. In patients undergoing short-course RT, the rates of pCR are significantly lower when compared with patients undergoing long-course neoadjuvant chemoradiation. Two aspects should be considered; first, the long-course regimen includes chemotherapy, second, cancer cells damaged after radiotherapy need time to undergo necrosis and usually in patients undergoing short-course RT, surgery is performed within 1 week after RT completion whereas long-course CRT is followed by radical surgery after at least 6–8 weeks.

The addition of chemotherapy to radiation in the neoadjuvant setting has resulted not only in improvements in local disease control (ie, lower recurrence rates) but also in tumor downstaging.(Jose G Guillem et al. 2008) In a randomized trial of patients undergoing RT with or without 5-FU- based chemotherapy, patients in the CRT group more frequently had a complete pathologic responses less lymph node metastases as well as vascular invasion. Additionally, patients treated by CRT had fewer overall lymph nodes recovered in the resected specimens and decreased tumor size. (Bosset 2005)

A review of phase II and III studies using different neoadjuvant CRT regimens for rectal cancer identified several predictive factors for complete pathologic response, including the dose of radiation therapy delivered, the method of 5-FU infusion, and the use of additional drugs to standard 5-FU based regimens. After reviewing 71 studies with over 4,000 patients treated with different regimens, complete pathologic response ranged from 0% to 42% and was significantly associated with the delivery of radiation doses higher than 45-Gy, 5-FU regimens with continous infusion, and the use of a second drug, most frequently oxaliplatin. (Sanghera et al. 2008)

Despite the suggestion that the use of additional drugs (other than 5-FU) could enhance tumor response to CRT, recently reported results from a prospective randomized trial showed that the addition of oxaliplatin to a 5-FU- based CRT regimen was not associated with significantly higher rates of pCR. In turn, patients treated with oxaliplatin experienced significantly more treatment-related toxicities. (Gérard et al. 2010)

Also, the observation of significant activity of targeted biological drugs, such as bevazicumab and cetuximab, led to its utilization in phase I and phase II trials in the neoadjuvant setting. However, the expected increase in pCR rates among patients undergoing this 'triple' therapy (5-FU, oxaliplatin, and cetuximab) was not observed in any of the trials. A review of these trials also suggested a subadditive interaction between capecitabine, oxaliplatin, and cetuximab as reflected by decreased rates of pCR (9 vs. 16%) and significant decrease in tumor regression grades (more than 50% of tumor regression) among surgical specimens from these patients when compared with patients undergoing treatment with capecitabine and oxaliplatin alone.(Weiss et al. 2010) It is not clear whether the inclusion of patients according to the K-ras status could have any influence in response to neoadjuvant CRT with this triple approach.(Glynne-Jones et al 2010)

Considering that 5FU is actually relevant for the development of complete tumor regression and that other drugs have been unsuccessful in improving rates without increasing toxicity, the use of additional cycles of 5FU in the neoadjuvant regimen has also been suggested. With the use of additional cycles of 5FU and leucovorin delivered during RT and during the interval period between CRT and tumor response assessment (also known previously as the "resting period"), increased rates of complete tumor regression without increased toxicity has been reported. (Habr-Gama et al. 2009)

2.2 Timing of assessment of tumor response

Assessment of response after CRT is crucial, and remains a real challenge even for the most experienced colorectal surgeon. The issues of when and how tumor response assessment should be performed are still under debate.

Since publication of the Lyon Trial in 1999, optimal surgical timing after neoadjuvant CRT has been accepted to be 6 weeks. In this study 201 patients with distal rectal cancer T2-3Nx were randomized before radiotherapy (39 Gy in 13 fractions) into two groups. The short interval group had surgery performed within 2 weeks after completion of radiation therapy compared to 6 weeks in the long interval group. After a median follow-up of 33 months, no differences in local relapse, morbidity and short-term survival between the two groups could be observed. On the other hand, improved clinical tumor responses ($p= .007$) and pathologic downstaging (10.3% v 26% $P = .005$) were observed in the long interval group.(Francois et al. 1999) These results provided the only prospective evidence to support a interval period of at least 6 weeks from CRT completion before surgery was performed in order to obtain maximal or optimal tumor downstaging.

Even though there was a suggestion from clinical practice that 8 weeks could probably improve the effects of CRT on tumor downstaging, only recent retrospective studies were able to provide further support that longer periods after CRT completion could be associated with higher rates of tumor downstaging. These studies have shown that patients managed by radical surgery 7 to 8 weeks after CRT completion had increased rates of complete pathological responses.(Moore et al. 2004; Tulchinsky et al. 2008;) In another retrospective review of patients managed by neoadjuvant CRT, a steep increase in complete pathological response rates was observed when surgery was performed 7 weeks after CRT completion. Even more interesting, these rates of complete response seem to stabilize after 12 weeks, perhaps suggesting no additional benefit in terms of tumor downstaging after this period. (Kalady et al. 2009) Recently, a study compared patients with rectal cancer undergoing neoadjuvant CRT followed by radical surgery after 8 or 12 weeks from CRT. Even though this study was not randomized and the longer interval group (12 weeks) had significantly more advanced disease at baseline, there was a higher rate of pCR rate in this latter but without statistical significance. Noteworthy, the authors showed no increase in postoperative surgical complications among the longer interval group (12 weeks). (Garcia-Aguilar et al. 2011)

On the other hand, the risk of leaving the tumor in situ for prolonged periods of time, with potential metastatic dissemination of tumor cells during this period has been used as an argument for performing surgery shortly (<8 weeks) after CRT completion. However, tumor cell death seems to be related to a process induced by ionizing radiation. It is thought that after exposure to a dose of 44 Gy, metastatic potential of these tumors might decrease significantly because of the potential decrease in the overall number of surviving tumor cells.(Withers and Haustermans 2004) In recent studies it was found that prolonged intervals (>8 weeks) from CRT to surgery may not have any associated oncologic compromise. In addition, these patients were associated to less postoperative morbidity, further supporting the safety of assessing tumor response at prolonged intervals.(Kerr, Norton, and R Glynne-Jones 2008)(Habr-Gama et al. 2008a)

2.3 Tumor features and biology

Several aspects of the primary rectal cancer have been considered to be predictors of tumor response or complete pathological response to neoadjuvant CRT such as initial disease staging, tumor height and extension. Even though very few studies have included patients with cT2N0 rectal treated by neoadjuvant CRT, so far there has been no data to support that these tumors would develop pCR more frequently. Still, as experience increases with these earlier tumors being treated with CRT, there is still a chance that baseline stage is indeed a predictor of response to CRT.

On the other hand, tumor extension has been shown in one retrospective study of over 500 patients to be a independent predictor of pCR after neoadjuvant CRT. In one study, circumferential tumor extent of <60% was a significant predictor of pCR. Even though tumor distance from the anal verge was not a predictor of pCR, tumors located in the distal 5cm of the rectum were more likely to develop greater tumor downstaging.(Das et al. 2007)

Finally, there is still hope that molecular biology will provide additional information regarding tumor response to neoadjuvant CRT. Few studies have addressed the role of gene expression in predicting response to CRT. (Ghadimi et al. 2005; I.-J. Kim et al. 2007; Rimkus et al. 2008) However, these studies did not seem to agree on what a "good response" was and while some of them considered only patients with pCR, others grouped together patients with significantly different ypTNM stage classification as long as less than 10% of tumor cells were present (based on tumor regression grading systems). The end-result is that all three studies suggested a set of genes capable of predicting a "good response" without a single gene in common between them.(Perez 2011) In this setting, perhaps further studies using more advanced technologies in gene expression analysis may provide more definitive and useful information.

3. Rationale for pursuing a non-operative approach

Radical surgery (with total mesorectal excision) is still considered fundamental in the treatment of distal rectal cancer, considered by many necessary regardless of tumor response to neoadjuvant CRT. However, it is associated with significant immediate morbidity and mortality. Anastomotic leak is probably the most important complication and is reported in up to 12% of cases.(Sauer et al. 2004; Chessin et al. 2005) Perioperative mortality may reach 3% and is significantly higher, reaching up to 13% when an anastomotic leak is present among patients who do not undergo temporary diversion.(P Matthiessen et al. 2004; Eriksen et al. 2005) Considering the fact that temporary stoma is almost always required, additional morbidity or even mortality related to stoma creation and take-down should be considered in the cumulative morbidity of rectal cancer management. (Perez et al. 2006). Also, even though nerve-preserving technique is now standard, the rates of urinary and sexual dysfunctions are quite significant. Finally, even though sphincteric function and quality of life among patients undergoing ultra-low anterior resections are acceptable, results are far from perfect (Denost et al 2011). Therefore, alternative treatment strategies to TME are warranted.

Considering that final disease stage (after CRT) is the most significant prognostic factor in patients with rectal cancer and that pCR is associated with improved oncological outcomes, these patients would be ideal candidates for alternative procedures avoiding TME. Unfortunately, confirmation of absence of residual microscopic disease is only possible after TME.

After all, is it justified to make our patients undergo a morbid and sometimes mutilating procedure when not even a single cancer cell is collected? In this setting, identification of patients with complete tumor regression determined by clinical, endoscopic and radiological assessment has been proposed in order to avoid immediate TME in a significant proportion of cases. Rather than providing a radical shift in the management of rectal cancer, this approach suggests close surveillance of a select group of patients with a high suspicion of complete tumor response without immediate radical surgery. Therefore, patients with no residual cancer may have a chance to be spared from a major surgical procedure while patients with residual disease and suspected for complete response may have surgery postponed or delayed without oncological compromise

4. Assessment of tumor response

Once an alternative approach to patients with rectal based on response to CRT is considered, the next step is to establish an efficient and accurate assessment of tumor response. Even though there is no perfect tool for such purpose, combination of different modalities may provide sufficient information for identification of appropriate candidates to non-immediate surgical resection. Patients with no evidence of residual disease by such assessment are considered as complete clinical responders (cCR's). Considering timing is crucial for tumor regression after CRT as discussed earlier, assessment of tumor response should be performed at least after 8 weeks from CRT and perhaps in some patients after 12 weeks from CRT.

4.1 Clinical assessment

Although clinical symptoms do subside in patients with complete clinical response, a significant proportion of patients also present with some degree of symptoms relief despite the presence of residual cancer. Therefore, the absence of clinical symptoms should not be considered as an absolute marker of complete response to CRT.

On the other hand, clinical assessment using digital rectal examination and (rigid or flexible) proctoscopy are the mainstay of clinical response assessment after CRT. Accuracy of clinical assessment of patients with rectal cancer after neoadjuvant CRT has been studied with disappointing results regarding sensitivity and specificity by others. Still, these studies were performed using 6-week intervals between CRT completion and response assessment and therefore could have detected residual disease in patients with ongoing tumor regression. In addition, the inclusion of different examiners could have biased results. (Hiotis et al. 2002)

4.2 Radiological studies

The use of radiological studies during assessment of tumor response in patients with rectal cancer after CRT completion is still a matter of controversy. Staging of primary tumor depth of penetration and distance from the circumferential margin seems to be adequately provided by endorectal ultrasound and magnetic resonance imaging.

However, after neoadjuvant CRT, distinguishing between residual cancer and transmural fibrosis may be significantly compromised by both imaging methods because these tools basically rely on morphologic features.(Mezzi et al. 2009; Suppiah et al. 2009)

For this reason CT, and endorectal ultrasound (ERUS) are probably best suited for the diagnosis of any residual extrarectal disease, such as a mesorectal enlarged nodes or masses. Thickening of the rectal wall, densification of the perirectal fat, or the presence of small perirectal nodes (less than 5 mm) should not precipitate any specific or immediate surgical attention, particular if other studies such as endoscopic and clinical assessment are normal. These findings are commonly seen in patients with cCR.

Previous studies addressed the value of rectal tumor volumetry on standard T2-weighted MR images for the assessment of response after CRT but showed conflicting results. One report did not find difference in tumor volume reduction rates between patients with pCR and those with residual disease.(Y.H. Kim et al. 2005) On the other hand a more recent report found a significant association with pCR for patients with a tumor volume reduction rate of more than 75%. (Kang et al. 2010)

With the introduction of diffusion-weighted (DW) MRI, significant amount of interest has been focused on this particular study. In a recent multicentric study, three trained radiologist reviewed 120 patients, comparing standard MRI with DW MRI and all them found improvement in sensitivity and specificity rates using DW MRI.(Lambregts et al. 2011) Another recent report showed that post-CRT volumetry on DW-MR images were significantly more accurate than on T2-weighted MR images to assess a CR after CRT. (Curvo-Semedo et al. 2011) Still further studies are needed before these tools are definitively incorporated into clinical practice.

The incorporation of positron emission tomography (PET/CT) imaging into the staging work-up provided significant additional information by overlaying metabolic activity data to standard radiological morphology. Also, PET imaging may provide an objective estimate of the metabolic activity of a specific area as represented by the standard uptake value measured at various phases of the study.

One study of 25 patients with rectal cancer compared the results of baseline PET-CT with a second PET-CT performed after 6 weeks from CRT completion. All patients included in the study experienced a decrease in maximum standard uptake values (SUVmax) between baseline and 6-week PET-CT scans. Also, the final SUVmax obtained at 6 weeks was significantly associated with primary tumor downstaging (patients with tumor downstaging exhibited significantly lower SUVmax). (Calvo et al. 2004) In another study including 15 patients undergoing baseline PET followed by a second PET 6 weeks after CRT completion, the visual response score was shown to provide superior prediction of tumor downstaging in addition of the extent of pathologic response to CRT compared to standard CT.(Guillem et al. 2000) This same group of patients was prospectively followed and outcome analysis showed that patients with greater percentual decrease between baseline and 6-week PET SUVmax values were associated with improved survival. A cutoff of a 62.5% decrease/difference between baseline and 6-week PET SUVmax values was a significant predictor of disease-free survival.(Guillem et al. 2004)

However, these results should be considered carefully, since they included only a small number of patients and none of them considered that increased interval periods between CRT and tumor response assessment might have influenced results.

In another study, 30 patients with locally advanced rectal cancer treated with CRT and surgery were assessed by pre and post-CRT PET-CT for tumor response after 7 weeks from CRT. PET/CT correctly identified six of eight patients (specificity 75 percent) with complete pathologic response. However, the sensitivity and accuracy of positron emission tomography/computer tomography was only 45 percent and 53 percent respectively. The positive and negative predictive values were 83 and 33 percent, respectively. Authors concluded that PET/CT performed was not able to predict the pathological response in locally advanced rectal cancer. (Kristiansen et al. 2008)

A prospective study with the use of PET/CT for the assessment of tumor response to CRT is currently underway in our Institution analyzing nearly 100 patients with cT2-3NxM0 after neoadjuvant CRT. The results of this study may provide significant additional information to the role of PET/CT in the assessment of tumor response.

4.3 Endoscopic biopsies after CRT

Surgeons and endoscopists are frequently faced with the issue of performing post-CRT biopsies in residual lesions within the rectal wall after neoadjuvant CRT. Even though it may sound obvious that a positive biopsy may accurately identify incomplete responses, it could also be suggested that negative biopsies could possibly help in identifying complete pathological responses despite the presence of clinically detectable disease. In fact, there is not much evidence regarding the utility of forceps' biopsies for tumor response assessment. In one retrospective review of patients undergoing post-CRT biopsies, the negative predictive value was as low as 36%.(Meterissian et al. 1994) However, it must be noted that these were unselected patients being assessed significantly earlier than 8 weeks from CRT completion.

In a retrospective review of patients undergoing neoadjuvant CRT restricted to patients with significant tumor downsizing, and therefore who were most likely to have developed pCR, post-CRT biopsies resulted in a negative predictive value of 21%.(Perez et al. 2011) In this setting, a negative biopsy of a clinically detectable lesion, even after significant tumor downsizing is not capable of ruling out residual disease and should not prevent surgeons from performing radical surgery. Alternatively, select cases may be appropriate for a excisional biopsy (through a full-thickness local excision) either as a diagnostic or therapeutic procedure.

4.4 Is there a role for CEA?

In addition to clinical, radiological and endoscopic assessment of tumor response, determination of CEA levels before and after CRT may also be useful. In a study with more than 500 patients with rectal cancer managed by neoadjuvant CRT, low CEA before treatment was a predictor of ypCR after radical surgery in univariate analysis. (Das et. al.

2007) Similar findings have been reported in a retrospective analysis of patients undergoing variable neoadjuvant CRT regimens for very low (<2.5 ng/dL) pretreatment CEA levels. (Moreno García et al. 2009)
An increase in CEA levels or persistence of at least 70% from baseline levels has also been suggested as a significant predictor of worse outcome patients with CEA levels >6 ng/ml at baseline.(C.W. Kim et al. 2011) Also, different cutoff values have been considered for patients undergoing CRT when compared to standard colorectal cancer patients. A retrospective analysis of 109 patients undergoing neoadjuvant therapy, identified a cutoff value for CEA<2.7ng/ml at 4 weeks from RT completion to be a statistically significant marker of tumor regression. (Jang et al. 2011)
The author's own experience with pre and post-CRT CEA levels suggests that only post-CRT CEA after at least 8 weeks from CRT completion was associated with the development of complete clinical response and improved disease-free survival. Both pre-treatment CEA and variation between pre and post treatment CEA levels were unpredictable of response and oncological outcomes. (Perez et al. 2009)

5. A Main concern: Lymph node assessment

In patients undergoing neoadjuvant CRT for rectal cancer, there seems to be tumor regression within the primary and perirectal nodes. This observation has been suggested by the decreased risk for the presence of lymph node metastases among patients undergoing neoadjuvant CRT when compared to patients managed by immediate radical surgery.
The presence of viable lymph node metastases within the mesorectum despite complete primary tumor regression is probably one of the most significant concerns regarding the safety of a non-immediate operative approach. The risk of residual nodal disease (N1) in patients with complete primary tumor regression (ypT0) may vary between 0% and 7%.(Stipa et al. 2004; Zmora et al. 2004; Perez et al. 2005; Pucciarelli et al. 2005) Again, these rates might reflect differences in doses of radiation therapy and timing of surgery after RT completion. Noteworthy, the higher rates of ypT0N1 are associated with patients undergoing surgery no longer than 6 weeks after CRT completion and could represent lymph node metastases that were still in the process of developing radiation-induced cell death. Additionally, the clinical relevance of microscopic residual lymph node metastases is still poorly understood. In a parallel to colorectal cancer, the presence of lymph node micrometastases has not been completely accepted as a clinically relevant finding.(Fleming et al. 2007) Even in the worst-case scenario, the risk of residual microscopic lymph node metastases after ypT0 is still less than the risk of residual microscopic lymph node metastases in patients with pT1 rectal cancer, which is around 12-13%. (Nascimbeni et al. 2002)
Still, the concept of nodal sterilization secondary to neoadjuvant CRT remains highly controversial. The finding of mucin deposits within lymph nodes that have no residual cancer cells in patients with rectal cancer who have received neoadjuvant CRT provides indirect evidence of such sterilization.(Perez et al. 2008) Recent data suggests that the presence of acellullar mucin is present in up to 27% of specimens with ypCR and 19% of them also showed acellular mucin within the nodes recovered after radical resection. Surprisingly, this finding had no negative influence on the outcomes of these patients, possibly representing evidence of tumor sterilization both within the rectum and the lymph nodes.(Smith et al. 2010)
Interestingly, the effects of RT or CRT may also be observed in the number of recovered nodes after radical surgery. Data obtained from the Surveillance, Epidemiology and End Results

(SEER) database indicates that patients undergoing neoadjuvant radiation therapy had significantly fewer retrieved nodes from the surgical specimen compared to patients undergoing surgery alone after a multivariate analysis. The number of retrieved lymph nodes was significantly higher in patients with N1 disease. (Baxter et al. 2005) This observation of an overall reduction in the number of lymph nodes among patients undergoing neoadjuvant therapy seems to be influenced by the time elapsed between radiation completion and surgical resection. One study showed that the number of recovered lymph nodes was significantly affected by the interval between CRT completion and surgery, but not by total radiation doses delivered. Exposure to longer interval periods led to recovery of fewer lymph nodes in surgical specimens. Two implications could be deduced from this: first, the critical number of lymph nodes required for proper staging of rectal cancer may not be the same for patients undergoing neoadjuvant CRT as for patients who go straight to surgery; second, the effects of radiation on lymph nodes seem to be time dependent, similarly to what has been observed for primary tumor regression. (Sermier et al. 2006)

Lymph node recovery may be further influenced by technical issues, including the use of fat-clearing solutions. In this setting, even though fat cleansing solutions were once considered too labor-intensive and potentially toxic, this technique may ultimately result in improvement in rectal cancer staging in patients undergoing neoadjuvant CRT. (Wang et al. 2009)

In a retrospective review of patients with incomplete clinical response after neoadjuvant CRT managed by radical surgery, outcomes of patients with no recovered nodes in the radical surgery specimen were slightly better than those of patients with node-negative disease, and significantly better than patients with node-positive disease. These findings suggest that patients with the absence of nodes in the resected specimen may represent a subset of patients with particularly increased sensitivity to CRT. (Habr-Gama et al. 2008b)

6. What is a complete clinical response?

One of the main limitations for the widespread use of this alternative approach without immediate surgery is the lack of a definitive or standardized definition of a complete clinical response. In this setting, clinical and endoscopic findings have been suggested as clinically useful in defining what is a complete clinical response. (Habr-Gama et al. 2010)

6.1 Clinical and endoscopic findings in cCR

Considering endoscopic assessment is performed after 8 weeks from CRT completion, a few considerations may be relevant to the decision between a complete and incomplete response:

1. Whitening of the mucosa in an area of the rectal wall may be frequently observed in patients with cCR. (Fig. 1)
2. Teleangiectasia (small derogative blood vessels seen on the rectal mucosa at the area previously harboring the primary cancer) is also frequently observed in complete clinical responders, even in long-term follow-up.
3. A subtle loss of pliability of the rectal wall harboring the scar; usually observed during manual insufflations at proctoscopy with light stiffness of the wall. In the context of no additional positive findings of residual cancer, this may also be considered as a feature of cCR
4. Whenever a tumor cannot be felt or seen, patients should be considered as complete clinical responders

6.2 Clinical and endoscopic findings of incomplete response

Some endoscopic findings should be considered to be at great risk for the presence of residual cancer. In any of these situations, a surgical action is probably warranted, at least for diagnostic purposes. In this setting, a non-surgical approach may be quite worrisome:

1. Any residual deep ulceration with or without a necrotic center.
2. Any superficial ulcer, irregularity, even in the presence of only mucosal ulceration. (Fig. 2)
3. Any palpable nodule, easily defined by digital rectal examination, even in the presence of mucosal complete integrity.

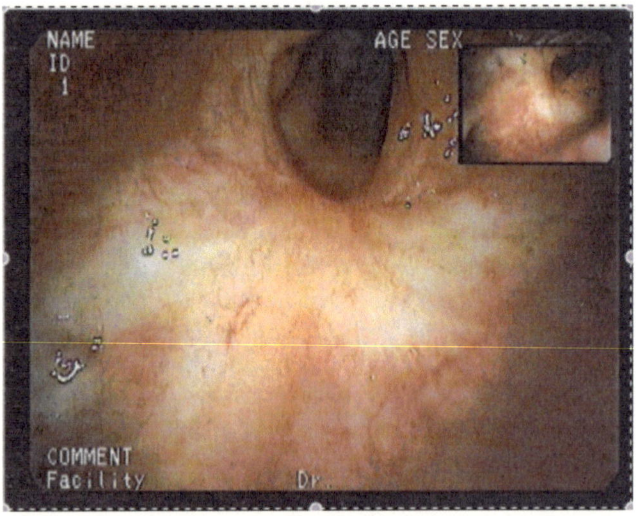

Fig. 1. Endoscopic finding in a patient with Complete Clinical response.

7. The watch-and-wait protocol algorithm

Patients with complete clinical response, either after clinical assessment or after transanal local excision (ypT0), are enrolled in a strict follow-up program (Fig. 3). Adherence to the program is critical because distinguishing between complete and near-complete responses may sometimes be difficult and final decision may only be possible after a few follow-up visits. This is why an empirical 12 month probation period has been suggested where only patients that sustain a complete clinical response are considered as cCR's (Habr-Gama et al. 1998) (Habr-Gama Ann Surg 2004).

This algorithm includes monthly follow-up visits with digital rectal examination and rigid proctoscopy in every visit for the first 3 months and every two to three months during the rest of the first year. CEA levels are determined every 2 months. As discussed previously, PET-CT is currently being investigated for its usefulness in tumor response assessment in a prospective study. Other radiological studies, including pelvic CT scans or magnetic resonance imaging, are performed at the time of initial tumor response assessment, and then every 6 months if there are no signs of tumor recurrence. Again, the main objective of these radiological studies is to rule out any sign of residual extrarectal disease, such as residual nodal disease that would require further investigation or even radical resection.

Patients are fully informed that complete clinical regression of their primary tumor may be temporary and disease recurrence or tumor regrowth may occur at any time during follow-up. In the case of obvious recurrence or tumor regrowth, radical surgery is strongly recommended. Small nodules or scars may develop over time and can be managed by full-thickness transanal excision (either standard or Transanal Endoscopic Microsurgery), primarily as a diagnostic approach.

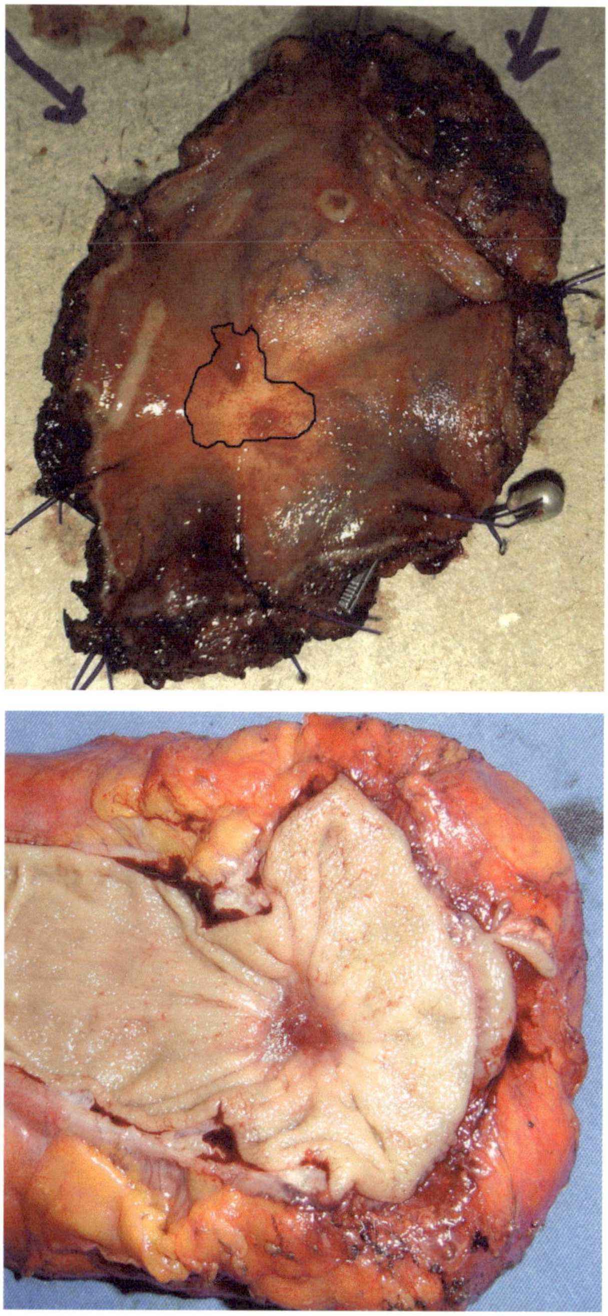

Fig. 2. Surgical specimens of rectal adenocarcinoma patients with incomplete responses to neoadjuvant chemoradiation therapy.

After 1 year of sustained, complete clinical response, patients are recommended for follow-up visits every 3 months, using the same clinical assessment tools used at initial patient assessment.

This treatment strategy evolved since the beginning of our experience in 1991. Our accuracy in clinical assessment of tumor response has probably improved significantly with growing experience. At the begining, patients were more frequently followed without immediate surgery when a near-complete clinical response was considered with the hope that time would lead to a complete clinical response. More recently, these patients have been more readily assessed using full-thickness local excision as a diagnostic procedure, and according to the pathologic report they are then either managed by strict observation or referred to immediate radical surgery. Availability of surgical techniques such as Transanal Endoscopic Microsurgery has also lowered the trigger for a excisional biopsy (Full Thickness Transanal Local Excision) in the presence of questionable residual lesions.

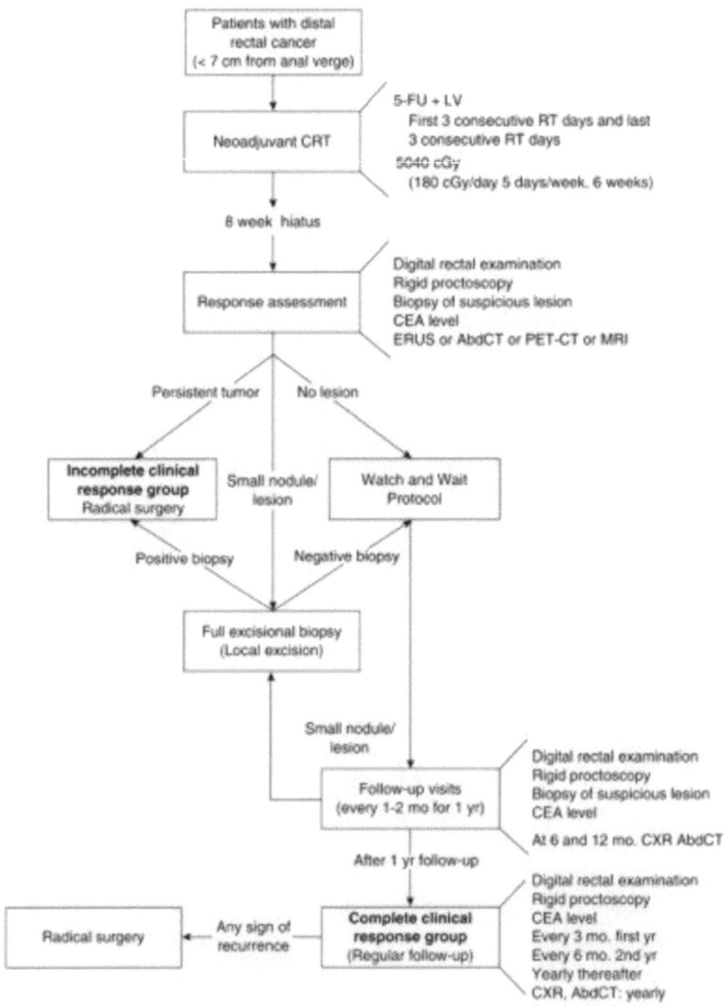

Fig. 3. Watch & Wait Algorithm

8. The extended chemoradiotherapy regimen

An interesting strategy to increase the rates of tumor response is the delivery of chemotherapy during the waiting or resting period between radiation completion and tumor response assessment. Since February 2005, this approach has been adopted at our Institution.

Radiation therapy consists of 45 Gy of radiation delivered by a three-field approach with daily doses of 1.8 Gy on weekdays to the pelvis, followed by a 9-Gy boost to the primary tumor and perirectal tissue (54 Gy total). Concomitantly, patients receive three cycles of bolus 5FU (450 mg/m2) and a fixed dose of 50 mg of leucovorin for three consecutive days every three weeks. After completion of radiation, patients received three additional identical cycles of chemotherapy every three weeks (21 days) during nine weeks. Tumor response assessment is performed immediately at 10 weeks from radiation completion. (Fig 4)

In a preliminar report of our series including T2/T3 distal rectal cancers, the sustained complete clinical response rate (>12 months) was 65% with no significant increase in chemotherapy-related toxicity rates. After a recent update of this same cohort of patients, complete clinical response rate seems to be sustained after a median follow-up of more than 36 months at 65%.(Habr-Gama et al. 2009)

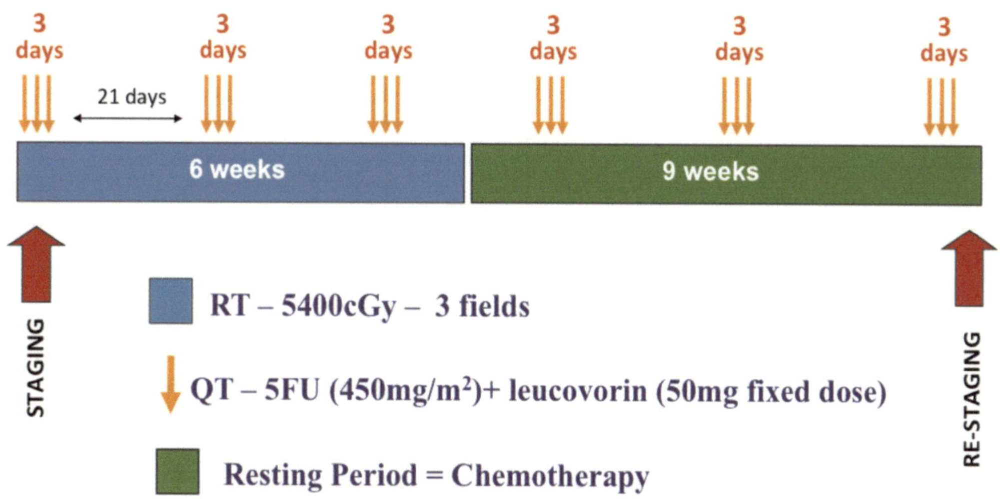

Fig. 4. The extended Chemoradiation regimen

9. Long-term results

At the beginning of our experience several patients were managed by radical surgery since residual cancer could not be confirmed or ruled out. This included patients with residual scars that were not candidates for local excision and those with partial narrowing of the rectum. In this context, many patients were operated and found to have ypT0 (absence of residual tumor). More recently, incorporation of TEM (Transanal Endoscopic Microsurgery) for diagnostic or staging purposes may lead to a significant decrease in the rates of pCR after radical TME.

In an attempt to understand the potential benefits of oncological surgery in terms of survival and local disease control, we performed a retrospective study where patients with complete pathological response (pCR) were compared to patients with cCR managed non-operatively.(Habr-Gama et al. 2004)

Patients managed by observation alone had similar outcomes to those managed by radical surgery in terms of long term survival. On the other hand, local recurrences were higher on the observation group, but noteworthy, all recurrences were within the rectal wall and amenable to surgical salvage. No pelvic relapses without endorectal component was observed.

Five-year overall and disease-free survival rates were associated to disease stage (clinical or pathological) and were 88% and 83%, respectively, in pCR group and 100% and 92% in cCR group respectively. These excellent survival rates in patients stage pCR and cCR were significantly better than those observed in patients ypII and ypIII. Curiously patients with stage ypI had intermediate results (Habr-Gama A, Perez RO, Nadalin W, et al. Long-term results of preoperative chemoradiation for distal rectal cancer correlation between final stage and survival. J Gastrointest Surg 2005;9:90-9; discussion 9-101.).

10. Survival and recurrences

Final TNM classification after neoadjuvant CRT remains the best predictor of survival in patients with rectal cancer. In a study of patients with similar baseline stages, final pathological classification distinguished those with worse and better outcomes.

Still, there is no prospective evidence favoring neoadjuvant RT over adjuvant CRT in terms of survival benefits. One explanation for this observation could be the detrimental effect of neoadjuvant CRT on host immunologic response against rectal cancer such as the potential blockade of peritumoral inflammatory as immunologic response.(Perez et al. 2007)

It has been suggested that adjuvant chemotherapy can improve survival only in highly selected patients with substantial tumor downstaging (ypT0-2).(Collette et al. 2007) These results may lead to a dramatical change in management of these patients who used to be considered for adjuvant treatment according to pretreatment staging.

An interesting observation is that in our series, systemic recurrences in cCR patients occurred considerably earlier than local recurrences. Besides intrinsic tumor behavior, this could be partly explained by the staging inaccuracy of the different available imaging modalities, which were probably not capable of detecting microscopic foci or metastasic disease at initial presentation. Also, local recurrences were observed in 10% of patients managed nonoperatively after a cCR. Interestingly, there were no extrarectal pelvic recurrences. Even though some recurrences may develop from the outer layers of the rectal wall, in all cases there was some luminal evidence of recurrence that could be detected by digital and rectoscopic examination.

Again, local recurrences developed considerably later during follow-up. This has also been observed in other series, where more than one third of patients who develop local recurrences after neoadjuvant CRT and radical surgery did so after 5 years of follow-up. In contrast, 75% of patients who develop local recurrences after radical surgery alone do so within 2 years of follow-up. This information may have implications when considering follow-up and surveillance strategies.(Habr-Gama et al. 2008a)

11. Salvage therapy

It has to be highlighted that up to now, all local recurrences in patients with cCR after neoadjuvant CRT were amenable to salvage therapy. These recurrences and their salvage procedures were performed at considerably long intervals after CRT completion (mean >50 months). In almost half of the cases an abdominoperineal resection (APR) was performed. Also, almost one third of these patients presented with low and superficial recurrences, amenable to full thickness transanal excision.(Habr-Gama et al. 2006)

A significant subgroup of patients, presented early tumor regrowth (within 12 months from CRT completion). These patients were most commonly misdiagnosed as cCR and had their definitive surgical treatment postponed for a variable period of time. This raised the issue whether these patients could have been harmed from an oncologic standpoint, by delaying definitive surgical resection. However, long-term data revealed that they fared no worse than patients with incomplete clinical response and managed by radical surgery after 8 weeks from CRT completion. Noteworthy, final pathology in this group revealed significant tumor downstaging and even lower rates of lymph node metastases, further supporting the idea that downstaging is a time-dependent phenomenon. The fact that these patients were more frequently managed by APR, could reflect the motivation (by the surgeon and the patient) to delay final decision on radical resection, knowing that tumor regression could be still going on.(Habr-Gama et al. 2008a)

12. Perspectives

Several aspects in the management of complete clinical response after neoadjuvant CRT remain unresolved and should be a focus of future clinical and basic science research.

Novel radiation therapy regimens including alternative radiation doses, delivery methods, and technical variants to maximize radiation-related tumor cell death and minimize side effects is an area of special interest. In addition, improved chemotherapy regimens might lead to an increase in the rate of complete clinical response and, possibly, improve survival rates. Some investigators have suggested the use of aggressive induction chemotherapy before the delivery of radiation to provide immediate treatment of undetected microscopic foci of metastatic tumor cells in addition to the primary tumor. These regimens are currently under investigation in controlled trials to provide data on safety and long-term benefits.(Chua et al. 2010)

Another interesting and relevant topic in rectal cancer management is the optimal interval between CRT completion and assessment of tumor response, as already said. Ongoing prospective randomized trials comparing different intervals may provide additional information regarding this particular issue in rectal cancer management. Also, perhaps data from PET/CT imaging at different intervals from CRT completion may also indicate kinetics of tumor metabolism as function of time in these patients.

Finally, development of next generation sequencing technology may allow further understanding of molecular genetic events relevant to sensitivity or resistance to neoadjuvant CRT. Perhaps identification of gene signatures will allow improvement of patient selection leading to true individualized management decisions. There is hope that studies using RNAseq technology may provide more definitive information in the near future.

13. References

Baxter NN, Morris AM, Rothenberger DA, et al. Impact of preoperative radiation for rectal cancer on subsequent lymph node evaluation: a population-based analysis. Int J Radiat Oncol Biol Phys 2005;61(2):426–31.

Bujko K, Nowacki MP, Nasierowska-Guttmejer A, Michalski W, Bebenek M, Kryj M. 2006. Long-term results of a randomized trial comparing preoperative short-course radiotherapy with preoperative conventionally fractionated chemoradiation for rectal cancer. Br J Surg 93:1215–1223.

Calvo FA, Domper M, Matute R, Martínez-Lázaro R, Arranz JA, Desco M, Alvarez E, Carreras JL. 2004. 18F-FDG positron emission tomography staging and restaging in rectal cancer treated with preoperative chemoradiation. Int. J. Radiat. Oncol. Biol. Phys. 58:528–535.

Chessin DB, Enker W, Cohen AM, Paty PB, Weiser MR, Saltz L, Minsky BD, Wong WD, Guillem JG. 2005. Complications after preoperative combined modality therapy and radical resection of locally advanced rectal cancer: a 14-year experience from a specialty service. J. Am. Coll. Surg. 200:876–82; discussion 882–4.

Chua YJ, Barbachano Y, Cunningham D, Oates JR, Brown G, Wotherspoon A, Tait D, Massey A, Tebbutt NC, Chau I. 2010. Neoadjuvant capecitabine and oxaliplatin before chemoradiotherapy and total mesorectal excision in MRI-defined poor-risk rectal cancer: a phase 2 trial. Lancet Oncol 11:241–248.

Collette L, Bosset J-F, Dulk den M, Nguyen F, Mineur L, Maingon P, Radosevic-Jelic L, Piérart M, Calais G, European Organisation for Research and Treatment of Cancer Radiation Oncology Group. 2007. Patients with curative resection of cT3-4 rectal cancer after preoperative radiotherapy or radiochemotherapy: does anybody benefit from adjuvant fluorouracil-based chemotherapy? A trial of the European Organisation for Research and Treatment of Cancer Radiation Oncology Group. J. Clin. Oncol. 25:4379–4386.

Curvo-Semedo L, Lambregts DMJ, Maas M, Thywissen T, Mehsen RT, Lammering G, Beets GL, Caseiro-Alves F, Beets-Tan RGH. 2011. Rectal Cancer: Assessment of Complete Response to Preoperative Combined Radiation Therapy with Chemotherapy--Conventional MR Volumetry versus Diffusion-weighted MR Imaging. Radiology.

Denost Q, Laurent C, Capdepont M, Zerbib F, Rullier E. Risk factors for fecal incontinence after intersphincteric resection for rectal cancer. Dis Colon Rectum. 2011 Aug;54(8):963-8

Das P, Skibber JM, Rodriguez-Bigas MA, Feig BW, Chang GJ, Wolff RA, Eng C, Krishnan S, Janjan NA, Crane CH. 2007. Predictors of tumor response and downstaging in patients who receive preoperative chemoradiation for rectal cancer. Cancer 109:1750–1755.

Eriksen MT, Wibe A, Norstein J, Haffner J, Wiig JN, Norwegian Rectal Cancer Group. 2005. Anastomotic leakage following routine mesorectal excision for rectal cancer in a national cohort of patients. Colorectal Dis 7:51–57.

Fleming FJ, Hayanga AJ, Glynn F, Thakore H, Kay E, Gillen P. 2007. Incidence and prognostic influence of lymph node micrometastases in rectal cancer. Eur J Surg Oncol 33:998–1002.

Francois Y, Nemoz CJ, Baulieux J, Vignal J, Grandjean JP, Partensky C, Souquet JC, Adeleine P, Gerard JP. 1999. Influence of the interval between preoperative radiation therapy and surgery on downstaging and on the rate of sphincter-sparing surgery for rectal cancer: the Lyon R90-01 randomized trial. J. Clin. Oncol. 17:2396.

Garcia-Aguilar J, Shi Q, Thomas CR, Chan E, Cataldo P, Marcet J, Medich D, Pigazzi A, Oommen S, Posner MC. 2011. A Phase II Trial of Neoadjuvant Chemoradiation and Local Excision for T2N0 Rectal Cancer: Preliminary Results of the ACOSOG Z6041 Trial. Ann. Surg. Oncol.

Gérard J-P, Azria D, Gourgou-Bourgade S, Martel-Laffay I, Hennequin C, Etienne P-L, Vendrely V, François E, La Roche de G, Bouché O, et al 2010. Comparison of two neoadjuvant chemoradiotherapy regimens for locally advanced rectal cancer: results of the phase III trial ACCORD 12/0405-Prodige 2. J. Clin. Oncol. 28:1638–1644.

Ghadimi BM, Grade M, Difilippantonio MJ, Varma S, Simon R, Montagna C, Füzesi L, Langer C, Becker H, Liersch T, et al 2005. Effectiveness of gene expression profiling for response prediction of rectal adenocarcinomas to preoperative chemoradiotherapy. J. Clin. Oncol. 23:1826–1838.

Glynne-Jones Rob, Mawdsley S, Harrison M. 2010. Cetuximab and chemoradiation for rectal cancer--is the water getting muddy? Acta Oncol 49:278–286.

Guillem J G, Puig-La Calle J, Akhurst T, Tickoo S, Ruo L, Minsky BD, Gollub MJ, Klimstra DS, Mazumdar M, Paty PB, et al 2000. Prospective assessment of primary rectal cancer response to preoperative radiation and chemotherapy using 18-fluorodeoxyglucose positron emission tomography. Dis. Colon Rectum 43:18–24.

Guillem Jose G, Moore HG, Akhurst T, Klimstra DS, Ruo L, Mazumdar M, Minsky BD, Saltz L, Wong WD, Larson S. 2004. Sequential preoperative fluorodeoxyglucose-positron emission tomography assessment of response to preoperative chemoradiation: a means for determining longterm outcomes of rectal cancer. J. Am. Coll. Surg. 199:1–7.

Guillem Jose G, Díaz-González JA, Minsky BD, Valentini V, Jeong S-Y, Rodriguez-Bigas MA, Coco C, Leon R, Hernandez-Lizoain JL, Aristu JJ, et al 2008. cT3N0 rectal cancer: potential overtreatment with preoperative chemoradiotherapy is warranted. J. Clin. Oncol. 26:368–373.

Habr-Gama A, de Souza PM, Ribeiro U, Nadalin W, Gansl R, Sousa AH, Campos FG, Gama-Rodrigues J. 1998. Low rectal cancer: impact of radiation and chemotherapy on surgical treatment. Dis. Colon Rectum 41:1087–1096.

Habr-Gama A, Perez RO, Nadalin W, Sabbaga J, Ribeiro U, Silva e Sousa AH, Campos FG, Kiss DR, Gama-Rodrigues J. 2004. Operative versus nonoperative treatment for stage 0 distal rectal cancer following chemoradiation therapy: long-term results. Ann. Surg. 240:711–7; discussion 717–8.

Habr-Gama A, Perez RO, Nadalin W, et al. Long-term results of preoperative chemoradiation for distal rectal cancer correlation between final stage and survival. J Gastrointest Surg 2005;9:90-9; discussion 9-101.

Habr-Gama A, Perez RO, Proscurshim I, Campos FG, Nadalin W, Kiss D, Gama-Rodrigues J. 2006. Patterns of failure and survival for nonoperative treatment of stage c0 distal rectal cancer following neoadjuvant chemoradiation therapy. J. Gastrointest. Surg. 10:1319–28; discussion 1328–9.

Habr-Gama A, Perez Rodrigo Oliva, Proscurshim I, Nunes Dos Santos RM, Kiss D, Gama-Rodrigues J, Cecconello I. 2008a. Interval between surgery and neoadjuvant chemoradiation therapy for distal rectal cancer: does delayed surgery have an impact on outcome? Int. J. Radiat. Oncol. Biol. Phys. 71:1181–1188.

Habr-Gama A, Perez Rodrigo O, Proscurshim I, Rawet V, Pereira DD, Sousa AHS, Kiss D, Cecconello I. 2008b. Absence of lymph nodes in the resected specimen after radical surgery for distal rectal cancer and neoadjuvant chemoradiation therapy: what does it mean? Dis. Colon Rectum 51:277–283.

Habr-Gama A, Perez RO, Sabbaga J, Nadalin W, São Julião GP, Gama-Rodrigues J. 2009. Increasing the rates of complete response to neoadjuvant chemoradiotherapy for distal rectal cancer: results of a prospective study using additional chemotherapy during the resting period. Dis. Colon Rectum 52:1927–1934.

Habr-Gama A, Perez RO, Wynn G, Marks J, Kessler H, Gama-Rodrigues J. 2010. Complete clinical response after neoadjuvant chemoradiation therapy for distal rectal cancer: characterization of clinical and endoscopic findings for standardization. Dis. Colon Rectum 53:1692–1698.

Hiotis SP, Weber SM, Cohen AM, Minsky BD, Paty PB, Guillem JG, Wagman R, Saltz LB, Wong WD. 2002. Assessing the predictive value of clinical complete response to neoadjuvant therapy for rectal cancer: an analysis of 488 patients. J. Am. Coll. Surg. 194:131–5; discussion 135–6.

Jang NY, Kang S-B, Kim D-W, Kim JH, Lee K-W, Kim IA, Kim J-S. 2011. The role of carcinoembryonic antigen after neoadjuvant chemoradiotherapy in patients with rectal cancer. Dis. Colon Rectum 54:245–252.

Kalady MF, de Campos-Lobato LF, Stocchi L, Geisler DP, Dietz D, Lavery IC, Fazio VW. 2009. Predictive factors of pathologic complete response after neoadjuvant chemoradiation for rectal cancer. Ann. Surg. 250:582–589.

Kang JH, Kim YC, Kim H, Kim YW, Hur H, Kim JS, Min BS, Kim H, Lim JS, Seong J, et al 2010. Tumor volume changes assessed by three-dimensional magnetic resonance volumetry in rectal cancer patients after preoperative chemoradiation: the impact of the volume reduction ratio on the prediction of pathologic complete response. Int. J. Radiat. Oncol. Biol. Phys. 76:1018–1025.

Kerr SF, Norton S, Glynne-Jones R. 2008. Delaying surgery after neoadjuvant chemoradiotherapy for rectal cancer may reduce postoperative morbidity without compromising prognosis. Br J Surg 95:1534–1540.

Kim CW, Yu CS, Yang S-S, Kim KH, Yoon YS, Yoon SN, Lim S-B, Kim JC. 2011. Clinical Significance of Pre- to Post-Chemoradiotherapy s-CEA Reduction Ratio in Rectal Cancer Patients Treated with Preoperative Chemoradiotherapy and Curative Resection. Ann. Surg. Oncol.

Kim I-J, Lim S-B, Kang HC, Chang HJ, Ahn S-A, Park H-W, Jang S-G, Park J-H, Kim DY, Jung KH, et al 2007. Microarray gene expression profiling for predicting complete response to preoperative chemoradiotherapy in patients with advanced rectal cancer. Dis. Colon Rectum 50:1342–1353.

Kim YH, Kim DY, Kim TH, Jung KH, Chang HJ, Jeong S-Y, Sohn DK, Choi HS, Ahn JB, Kim DH, et al 2005. Usefulness of magnetic resonance volumetric evaluation in predicting response to preoperative concurrent chemoradiotherapy in patients with resectable rectal cancer. Int. J. Radiat. Oncol. Biol. Phys. 62:761–768.

Kristiansen C, Loft A, Berthelsen AK, Graff J, Lindebjerg J, Bisgaard C, Jakobsen A. 2008. PET/CT and histopathologic response to preoperative chemoradiation therapy in locally advanced rectal cancer. Dis. Colon Rectum 51:21–25.

Krook JE, Moertel CG, Gunderson LL, Wieand HS, Collins RT, Beart RW, Kubista TP, Poon MA, Meyers WC, Mailliard JA. 1991. Effective surgical adjuvant therapy for high-risk rectal carcinoma. N. Engl. J. Med. 324:709–715.

Lambregts DMJ, Vandecaveye V, Barbaro B, Bakers FCH, Lambrecht M, Maas M, Haustermans K, Valentini V, Beets GL, Beets-Tan RGH. 2011. Diffusion-weighted MRI for selection of complete responders after chemoradiation for locally advanced rectal cancer: a multicenter study. Ann. Surg. Oncol. 18:2224–2231.

Matthiessen P, Hallböök O, Andersson M, Rutegård J, Sjödahl R. 2004. Risk factors for anastomotic leakage after anterior resection of the rectum. Colorectal Dis 6:462–469.

Matthiessen Peter, Hallböök O, Rutegård J, Simert G, Sjödahl R. 2007. Defunctioning stoma reduces symptomatic anastomotic leakage after low anterior resection of the rectum for cancer: a randomized multicenter trial. Ann. Surg. 246:207-214.

Meterissian S, Skibber J, Rich T, Roubein L, Ajani J, Cleary K, Ota DM. 1994. Patterns of residual disease after preoperative chemoradiation in ultrasound T3 rectal carcinoma. Ann. Surg. Oncol. 1:111-116.

Mezzi G, Arcidiacono PG, Carrara S, Perri F, Petrone MC, De Cobelli F, Gusmini S, Staudacher C, Del Maschio A, Testoni PA. 2009. Endoscopic ultrasound and magnetic resonance imaging for re-staging rectal cancer after radiotherapy. World J. Gastroenterol. 15:5563-5567.

Moore HG, Gittleman AE, Minsky BD, Wong D, Paty PB, Weiser M, Temple L, Saltz L, Shia J, Guillem JG. 2004. Rate of pathologic complete response with increased interval between preoperative combined modality therapy and rectal cancer resection. Dis. Colon Rectum 47:279-286.

Moreno García V, Cejas P, Blanco Codesido M, Feliu Batlle J, de Castro Carpeño J, Belda-Iniesta C, Barriuso J, Sánchez JJ, Larrauri J, González-Barón M, et al 2009. Prognostic value of carcinoembryonic antigen level in rectal cancer treated with neoadjuvant chemoradiotherapy. Int J Colorectal Dis 24:741-748.

Nascimbeni R, Burgart LJ, Nivatvongs S, Larson DR. 2002. Risk of lymph node metastasis in T1 carcinoma of the colon and rectum. Dis. Colon Rectum 45:200-206.

Perez OR, Habr-Gama A, Nishida Arazawa ST, Rawet V, Coelho Siqueira SA, Kiss DR, Gama-Rodrigues JJ. 2005. Lymph node micrometastasis in stage II distal rectal cancer following neoadjuvant chemoradiation therapy. Int J Colorectal Dis 20:434-439.

Perez OR, Habr-Gama A, Seid V. Proscurshim I, Sousa Jr. AH, Kiss DR, Linhares M., Sapucahy M, Gama-Rodrigues J. 2006. Loop Ileostomy Morbidity: Timing of Closure Matters. Dis. Colon Rectum. 2006; 49: 1539-1545

Perez OR, Habr-Gama A, Santos dos RMN, Proscurshim I, Campos FG, Rawet V, Kiss D, Cecconello I. 2007. Peritumoral inflammatory infiltrate is not a prognostic factor in distal rectal cancer following neoadjuvant chemoradiation therapy. J. Gastrointest. Surg. 11:1534-1540.

Perez OR, Bresciani BH, Bresciani C, Proscurshim I, Kiss D, Gama-Rodrigues J, Pereira DD, Rawet V, Cecconnello I, Habr-Gama A. 2008. Mucinous colorectal adenocarcinoma: influence of mucin expression (Muc1, 2 and 5) on clinico-pathological features and prognosis. Int J Colorectal Dis 23:757-765.

Perez OR, São Julião GP, Habr-Gama A, Kiss D, Proscurshim I, Campos FG, Gama-Rodrigues JJ, Cecconello I. 2009. The role of carcinoembriogenic antigen in predicting response and survival to neoadjuvant chemoradiotherapy for distal rectal cancer. Dis. Colon Rectum 52:1137-1143.

Perez OR 2011. Predicting response to neoadjuvant treatment for rectal cancer: a step toward individualized medicine. Dis. Colon Rectum 54:1057-1058.

Perez OR, Habr-Gama A, Vallejos Pereyra G, Lynn PB, Praskurshim I, Arruda Alves P, Viviane R, Joaquim José G-R. The Role for Biopsies in Residual Rectal Cancer following Neoadjuvant Chemoradiation after significant downsizing - Are they reliable to rule out residual cancer? Colorectal Disease. 2011 (in press).

Petersen S, Hellmich G, Mildenstein von K, Porse G, Ludwig K. 2006. Is surgery-only the adequate treatment approach for T2N0 rectal cancer? J Surg Oncol 93:350-354.

Pucciarelli S, Capirci C, Emanuele U, Toppan P, Friso ML, Pennelli GM, Crepaldi G, Pasetto L, Nitti D, Lise M. 2005. Relationship between pathologic T stage and nodal metastasis after preoperative chemoradiotherapy for locally advanced rectal cancer. Ann. Surg. Oncol. 12:111–116.

Rimkus C, Friederichs J, Boulesteix A-L, Theisen J, Mages J, Becker K, Nekarda H, Rosenberg R, Janssen K-P, Siewert JR. 2008. Microarray-based prediction of tumor response to neoadjuvant radiochemotherapy of patients with locally advanced rectal cancer. Clin. Gastroenterol. Hepatol. 6:53–61.

Sanghera P, Wong DWY, McConkey CC, Geh JI, Hartley A. 2008. Chemoradiotherapy for rectal cancer: an updated analysis of factors affecting pathological response. Clin Oncol (R Coll Radiol) 20:176–183.

Sauer R, Becker H, Hohenberger W, Rödel C, Wittekind C, Fietkau R, Martus P, Tschmelitsch J, Hager E, Hess CF, et al 2004. Preoperative versus postoperative chemoradiotherapy for rectal cancer. N. Engl. J. Med. 351:1731–1740.

Sermier A, Gervaz P, Egger JF, Dao M, Allal AS, Bonet M, Morel P. 2006. Lymph node retrieval in abdominoperineal surgical specimen is radiation time-dependent. World J Surg Oncol 4:29.

Simunovic M, Sexton R, Rempel E, Moran BJ, Heald RJ. 2003. Optimal preoperative assessment and surgery for rectal cancer may greatly limit the need for radiotherapy. Br J Surg 90:999–1003.

Smith KD, Tan D, Das P, Chang GJ, Kattepogu K, Feig BW, Skibber JM, Rodriguez-Bigas MA. 2010. Clinical significance of acellular mucin in rectal adenocarcinoma patients with a pathologic complete response to preoperative chemoradiation. Ann. Surg. 251:261–264.

Stipa F, Zernecke A, Moore HG, Minsky BD, Wong WD, Weiser M, Paty PB, Shia J, Guillem JG. 2004. Residual mesorectal lymph node involvement following neoadjuvant combined-modality therapy: rationale for radical resection? Ann. Surg. Oncol. 11:187–191.

Suppiah A, Hunter IA, Cowley J, Garimella V, Cast J, Hartley JE, Monson JRT. 2009. Magnetic resonance imaging accuracy in assessing tumour down-staging following chemoradiation in rectal cancer. Colorectal Dis 11:249–253.

Tulchinsky H, Shmueli E, Figer A, Klausner JM, Rabau M. 2008. An interval >7 weeks between neoadjuvant therapy and surgery improves pathologic complete response and disease-free survival in patients with locally advanced rectal cancer. Ann. Surg. Oncol. 15:2661–2667.

Wang H, Safar B, Wexner SD, Denoya P, Berho M. 2009. The clinical significance of fat clearance lymph node harvest for invasive rectal adenocarcinoma following neoadjuvant therapy. Dis. Colon Rectum 52:1767–1773.

Weiss C, Arnold D, Dellas K, Liersch T, Hipp M, Fietkau R, Sauer R, Hinke A, Rödel C. 2010. Preoperative radiotherapy of advanced rectal cancer with capecitabine and oxaliplatin with or without cetuximab: A pooled analysis of three prospective phase I-II trials. Int. J. Radiat. Oncol. Biol. Phys. 78:472–478.

Withers HR, Haustermans K. 2004. Where next with preoperative radiation therapy for rectal cancer? Int. J. Radiat. Oncol. Biol. Phys. 58:597–602.

Zmora O, Dasilva GM, Gurland B, Pfeffer R, Koller M, Nogueras JJ, Wexner SD. 2004. Does rectal wall tumor eradication with preoperative chemoradiation permit a change in the operative strategy? Dis. Colon Rectum 47:1607–1612.

18

Systemic Treatment in Recurrent and Metastatic Unresectable Rectal Cancer

François-Xavier Otte, Mustapha Tehfe,
Jean-Pierre Ayoub and Francine Aubin
Université de Montréal
Canada

1. Introduction

Most patients with recurrent and metastatic rectal cancer cannot be cured. Selected patients with local recurrence or liver and/or lung-limited metastatic disease are sometimes curable with radiation therapy (RT) or surgery. However, for the majority of patients, treatment is palliative and systemic therapy remains the mainstay treatment. Over the last ten years, survival of patients with unresectable metastatic or recurrent rectal cancer has considerably improved. The median survival is about two years due to availability of new chemotherapy regimens and targeted therapies. For decades, 5-fluorouracil (5-FU) was the only active and available agent. Since the year 2000, irinotecan and oxaliplatin were approved. Access to all these three active agents strongly correlates with improved survival. More progress was achieved recently with the development of targeted therapies. Bevacizumab is a monoclonal antibody targeting the vascular endothelial growth factor (VEGF). Cetuximab and panitumumab are two monoclonal antibodies targeting the epidermal growth factor receptor (EGFR). Combinations of these different drugs are now commonly used.

In non-curable patients, goals are improvement of survival and quality of life. The purpose of this chapter is to review data from clinical trials evaluating systemic therapy in unresectable recurrent or metastatic rectal cancer. Commonly used chemotherapy regimens and biologic agents will be described as well as their side effects. General principles of treatment and specific treatment recommendations will also be discussed.

2. Chemotherapy

2.1 Fluoropyrimidines

Fluoropyrimidines have been used for the treatment of metastatic colorectal cancer (mCRC) for many years. 5-FU is a fluoropyrimidine that causes inhibition of thymidylate synthase and leads to impaired DNA synthesis. Adding folinic acid (leucovorin) intensifies the cytotoxic power of 5-FU stabilizing its bind to the enzyme. Different schedules of administration have shown clinical activity in different trials. Short-term infusional schedules have gained acceptance. A French study, compared a regimen of bolus 5-FU/LV day 1 to 5 every four weeks to bimonthly 5-FU/LV bolus over two hours followed by a 22 hours 5-FU infusion for two consecutive days. The infusional regimen showed better response rate (RR) and progression free survival (PFS). It was also associated with less

hematological and gastrointestinal (GI) toxicity. This "de Gramont regimen" is now a standard (de Gramont et al. 1997).
The widely used oral form of fluoropyrimidine is capecitabine. It is a prodrug that needs to be metabolized to 5-FU by multiple sequential enzymatic reactions. In 2001, a phase 3 randomized trial showed that use of oral capecitabine in first-line mCRC patients was more active than 5-FU/LV in the induction of objective tumor responses. Time to disease progression and survival were at least equivalent for capecitabine compared with the 5-FU/LV arm. Capecitabine also demonstrated clinically meaningful benefits over bolus 5-FU/LV in terms of tolerability although hand-foot syndrome was more common (Hoff et al. 2001). Similar results were observed in another identically designed randomized study (Van Cutsem et al. 2001).
Dihydropyrimidine dehydrogenase (DPD) is an important enzyme in the metabolism of fluoropyrimidines. It is the rate limiting enzyme in 5-FU catabolism. Patients who are deficient in DPD activity may have severe, even fatal toxicities such as severe diarrhea, mucositis and pancytopenia. For these patients, an alternative to 5-FU is raltitrexed which is a pure thymidylate synthase inhibitor. In a 2002 randomized study, raltitrexed showed similar RR and overall survival (OS) to the de Gramont regimen and was easier to administer, but resulted in greater toxicity (GI and hematological) and inferior quality of life (Maughan et al. 2002).
Fluoropyrimidines alone had been the standard first-line treatment of mCRC until the development of combination regimens with irinotecan or oxaliplatin. Fluoropyrimidine monotherapy remains a valid option for patients with contraindications to combined therapies. The infusional regimen (de Gramont) is the preferred fluoropyrimidine monotherapy. Capecitabine is a safe oral alternative to 5-FU.

2.2 Irinotecan (table 1)

Irinotecan is a topoisomerase I inhibitor and has demonstrated efficacy in mCRC as a single agent or in association with a fluoropyrimidine. Irinotecan in monotherapy showed superiority to best supportive care alone after 5-FU failure. A randomized trial showed that the OS was significantly better in the irinotecan group (p=0.0001), with 36.2% 1-year survival in the irinotecan group versus 13.8% in the supportive-care group. Quality of life was also better with less tumor related symptoms. In this trial, irinotecan was given every three weeks (Cunningham et al. 1998).
A randomized trial showed an advantage in RR, time to progression (TTP) and median survival for combined treatment with irinotecan/5-FU/LV over 5-FU/LV alone in first-line mCRC. An infusional regimen was used (the Douillard regimen). Treatment was given weekly or every two weeks. There were more toxicities in the irinotecan arm (diarrhea and neutropenia) but they were manageable (Douillard et al. 2000). Results of the BICC-C study suggest that the infusional regimen (FOLFIRI) is associated with better PFS and less toxicities compared to the bolus regimen (IFL).
The use of oral capecitabine associated with irinotecan (CapeIRI) was also assessed in the BICC-C study. It was compared to FOLFIRI and IFL. It was associated with more toxicities and less efficacy (Fuchs et al. 2007).
Late diarrhea and neutropenia are the main dose-limiting toxicities from irinotecan. UGT1A1 polymorphism predicts irinotecan toxicity. Irinotecan can also cause early-onset symptoms of cholinergic excess including diarrhea, abdominal cramping, lacrimation, rhinitis and salivation.

Regimen	Irinotecan	Leucovorin	5-FU*/capecitabine	Schedule
FOLFIRI *Fuchs et al. 2007*	180 mg/m^2 IV over 90 min day 1	400 mg/m^2 IV over 2 h day 1	*400 mg/m^2 IV bolus day 1; 2400 mg/m2 IV continuous infusion over 46 h	Every two weeks
IFL *Saltz et al.2000*	125 mg/m^2 IV bolus	20 mg/m^2 IV bolus	*500 mg/m^2 IV bolus	Weekly for four weeks every six weeks
mIFL *Fuchs et al. 2007*	125 mg/m^2 IV over 90 min on days 1 and 8	20 mg/m^2 IV bolus on days 1 and 8	*500 mg/m^2 IV bolus on days 1 and 8	Every three weeks
CapeIRI *Fuchs et al. 2007*	250 mg/m^2 IV over 90 minutes day 1		Capecitabine by mouth 1000mg/m^2 twice a day on days 1 to 14	Every three weeks

Table 1. Irinotecan Regimens

2.3 Oxaliplatin (table2)

In 1998, the platinum derivative, oxaliplatin when given together with 5-FU was shown to have significant activity in mCRC (deBraud et al. 1998). The activity of oxaliplatin alone in mCRC is low (Rothenberg et al. 2003). In 2000, a study showed better PFS and RR with the addition of oxaliplatin to 5-FU/LV compared to 5-FU/LV infusional regimen alone as first-line treatment in advanced colorectal cancer (de Gramont et al. 2000).

The combination of oxaliplatin and oral capecitabine (XELOX or CAPOX) has also been studied and compared to other fluoropyrimidine/oxaliplatin combinations in multiple randomized studies. A pooled analysis of randomized trials comparing first-line CAPOX to oxaliplatin in combination to infusional 5-FU/LV showed that CAPOX resulted in lower RR, but this did not affect PFS and OS. The toxicity analysis showed thrombocytopenia and hand-foot syndrome were consistently more prominent with the CAPOX regimens (Arkenau et al. 2008). CAPOX may be considered in patients where ambulatory infusion is not possible or refused.

In 2004, Tournigand and colleagues randomly assigned previously untreated patients to FOLFOX 6 or FOLFIRI. At progression, irinotecan was replaced by oxaliplatin or oxaliplatin by irinotecan. Both strategies showed equivalent RR (about 55%) and median survival (20.6 and 21.5 months). Nausea, mucositis and alopecia were more common with FOLFIRI while neutropenia and paresthesias were more common with FOLFOX (Tournigand et al. 2004). An Italian study showed similar findings (Colucci et al. 2005).

Thus, using FOLFOX or FOLFIRI in first-line treatment and then switching to the alternate regimen at progression or treatment intolerance is widely accepted. The decision of choosing one regimen over the other will be influenced by toxicity profile and patient preference.

One of the main concerns with the use of oxaliplatin is neurotoxicity. Acute neurotoxicity and cumulative sensory neuropathy are described. The acute neurotoxicity typical symptoms are dysesthesias of hands, feet and perioral region. More rarely, pharyngeal dysesthesias can be observed. These symptoms are generally triggered by cold, are associated with higher doses of oxaliplatin and are infusion-rate dependant. In 2008, Petrioli and colleagues suggested a prolonged infusion time to reduce the acute toxicity (Petrioli et al. 2008). This acute toxicity seems to be related to hyperexcitability of the peripheral nerves which has been attributed to disruption in cell membrane ion channels (Wilson et al. 2002; Park et al. 2009). In contrast, the cumulative neuropathy is generally sensory, symmetrical and without motor involvement. Oxaliplatin-induced cumulative sensory neuropathy occurs after several cycles of therapy (Cassidy et al. 2002). In about three fourths of patients, neurotoxicity is reversible with a median time to recovery of 13 weeks after treatment discontinuation. Strategies have been developed to prevent oxaliplatin-induced cumulative neurotoxicity. First, new schedules of administration were investigated. The Optimox-1 study randomly assigned patients to FOLFOX 4 (oxaliplatin 85 mg/m2) until progression or to six cycles of FOLFOX 7 (oxaliplatin 130mg/m2) followed by maintenance 5FU-LV for 12 cycles. FOLFOX 7 was then reintroduced for non progressive patients. RR, PFS and survival were similar in both arms. Grade 3 and 4 neuropathy was reduced in FOLFOX 7 arm after the sixth cycle even though it occurred earlier. The conclusion was that oxaliplatin can be safely stopped after six cycles in a FOLFOX 7 regimen (Tournigand et al. 2006). The Optimox-2 study compared a chemotherapy-free interval with maintenance 5-FU/LV after six cycles of modified FOLFOX 7 (mFOLFOX7) chemotherapy in the first-line treatment of mCRC. mFOLFOX 7 was reintroduced for patients with progressive disease in both arms. Duration of disease control (DDC) and PFS were better in the maintenance arm (Chibaudel et al. 2009). Thus oxaliplatin-free intervals are feasible but complete discontinuation of chemotherapy may be associated with inferior outcomes. Secondly, the benefit of use of IV calcium (Ca) and magnesium (Mg) in order to diminish neuropathy symptoms was suggested in randomized trials. In 2011, Grothey and colleagues showed that IV Ca/Mg is an effective neuroprotectant against oxaliplatin-induced cumulative neuropathy in adjuvant colon cancer. The incidence of grade 2 or greater cumulative sensory neurotoxicity was significantly reduced. The onset of grade 2 or greater sensory neurotoxicity was also delayed in patients receiving Ca/Mg (Grothey et al. 2011). This study had a low statistical power due to early closure of the trial because preliminary reports from another trial (CONcePT trial) that initially suggested decreased response rates for patients getting Ca/Mg (Hochster et al. 2007). This was later proven untrue by an independent radiologic review.

2.4 Other chemotherapy combinations (table 2)

The combination of oxaliplatin and irinotecan (IROX) has been assessed in first and second line setting. In the first-line setting, IROX was shown to be inferior and more toxic in elderly patients compared to FOLFOX (Sanoff et al. 2008) and equivalent to FOLFIRI (Fischer von Weikersthal et al.2011). In the second-line setting, IROX was compared to a triple regimen of 5FU/LV with alternating irinotecan and oxaliplatin. RR (23 versus 6 percent) and median survival (12.3 versus 9.8 months) were better with IROX but the doses of irinotecan and oxaliplatin were smaller in the triple therapy arm (Bécouarn et al. 2001). The efficacy of FOLFOXIRI regimen has been evaluated in two randomized studies. An Italian study showed better RR (41 versus 66 percent), PFS (9.8 versus 6.9 months) and OS (22.6 versus 16.7 months) for FOLFOXIRI compared to FOLFIRI in the first-line setting. This was in a selected population of patients in good general condition and with favorable features. More toxicities were reported in the FOLFOXIRI arm especially in terms of neutropenia and neurotoxicity (Falcone et al.2007). This benefit and its cost in terms of toxicities were confirmed in a systematic review (Montagnani et al. 2010). In contrast, a Greek phase 3 randomized failed to show benefits to FOLFOXIRI when compared to FOLFIRI (Souglakos et al. 2006). However, compared to the Italian trial, lower doses of oxaliplatin, irinotecan and 5-FU were used.

Regimen	**Oxaliplatin**	**Irinotecan**	**Leucovorin**	**5-FU/cape**	**Schedule**
CAPOX *Hochster et al. 2008*	130mg/m^2 IV on day 1			capecitabine 1,000 mg/m^2 orally twice daily on days 1 to 15	Every three weeks
IROX *Goldberg et al. 2004*	85mg/m^2	200 mg/m^2			Every three weeks
FOLFOX 4 *Goldberg et al. 2004*	85 mg/m^2 on day 1		200 mg/m^2 day 1	bolus FU 400 mg/m^2 followed by FU 600 mg/m^2 in 22-hour infusions on days 1 and 2	Every two weeks
FOLFOX 6 *Tournigand et al. 2004*	100 mg/m^2 day 1		400 mg/m^2 day 1	bolus FU 400mg/m^2 followed by infusion 2400-3000 mg/m^2 over 46 hours	Every two weeks
FOLFOX 6 modified *Hochster et al. 2008*	85 mg/m^2 day 1		400 mg/m^2 day 1	bolus FU 400mg/m^2 followed by infusion 2400 mg/m^2 over 46 hours	Every two weeks
bFOL *Hochster et al. 2008*	85 mg/m^2 on days 1 and 15		20 mg/m^2 days 1, 8 and 15	500 mg/m^2 push days 1,8 and 15	Every four weeks
FOLFOX 7 *Tournigand et al. 2006*	130 mg/m^2 day 1		400 mg/m^2 day 1	infusion 2400 mg/m^2 over 46 hours	Every two weeks
FOLFOX 7 modified *Chibaudel et al. 2009*	100 mg/m^2 day 1		400 mg/m^2 day 1	infusion 3000 mg/m^2 over 46 hours	Every two weeks
FOLFOXIRI *Falcone et al. 2007*	85 mg/m^2 day 1	165 mg/m^2 day 1	200 mg/m^2 day 1	Infusion 3200 mg/m^2 over 48h	Every two weeks

Table 2. Oxaliplatin Regimens

3. Targeted therapies

Targeted cancer therapies are drugs that block the growth and spread of cancer by interfering with specific molecules involved in tumor growth and progression. Bevacizumab, cetuximab and panitumumab are three monoclonal antibodies which have known efficacy in mCRC.

3.1 Angiogenesis inhibitors

3.1.1 Bevacizumab

Bevacizumab is a monoclonal humanized antibody targeting the VEGF. It is assumed that bevacizumab normalizes the vascular environment and improves the chemotherapy delivery to the tumor.

Bolus IFL (irinotecan/5-FU/LV) plus bevacizumab (5mg/kg) was compared to IFL plus placebo in previously untreated patients with mCRC. They observed statistically better RR, PFS and OS (20.3 versus 15.6 months). This was the pivotal study which led to the approval of bevacizumab in the treatment of mCRC. Grade 3-4 high blood pressure (HBP) was significantly increased in the bevacizumab arm (Hurwitz et al. 2004). FOLFIRI regimen has however gained acceptance over the bolus IFL regimen due to a more favorable toxicity profile. The BICC-C trial showed a significant advantage in terms of median survival with FOLFIRI plus bevacizumab compared to mIFL plus bevacizumab (28 versus 19 months, p=0.037) (Fuchs et al. 2007). Several trials have also addressed the benefit of adding bevacizumab to an oxaliplatin-based regimen. In a phase 2 cohort study (TREE-2), three oxaliplatin-containing regimens (FOLFOX, bolus 5FU and oxaliplatin-bFOL, CAPOX) were investigated in association with bevacizumab. Median survivals were respectively 26.1, 20.4 and 24.6 months (Hochster et al. 2008). Median OS was 23.7 months for the combined group treated with bevacizumab compared to 18.2 months for patients who did not received bevacizumab.The benefit of adding bevacizumab to oxaliplatin-containing chemotherapy appeared however to be more modest in the NO16966 trial. The addition of bevacizumab to FOLFOX4 or XELOX resulted in an increase of PFS of 1.4 months but the superiority of bevacizumab was statistically evident only in the XELOX subgroup (p=0.0026). Additionally, the OS significance did not reach statistical difference (21.3 months vs. 19.9 months) and the RR was similar in both groups (47% vs. 49%) (Saltz et al. 2008). The use of bevacizumab in first line is nevertheless widely accepted with either FOLFOX or FOLFIRI. In a phase 2 randomized study 5-FU/LV plus placebo was compared to 5-FU/LV plus bevacizumab. The bevacizumab-based treatment showed significant better PFS and non significant better OS (Kabbinavar et al. 2005). Thus, 5-FU/LV plus bevacizumab remains an option for patients with contraindications to other regimens.

The addition of bevacizumab in second-line treatment was assessed in the ECOG 3200 trial. Patients previously treated with a fluoropyrimidine and irinotecan were randomly assigned to receive FOLFOX4 in combination with bevacizumab (at 10 mg/kg), FOLFOX4 or bevacizumab alone. This study showed better PFS and OS in the FOLFOX4 plus bevacizumab arm. No activity was shown with bevacizumab alone (Giantonio et al. 2007). In contrast, there is no strong enough evidence to continue bevacizumab beyond progression in first-line treatment although favorable data is suggested by the BRITE study. This cohort study showed encouraging survival rates in patients who received post-progression chemotherapy with continued bevacizumab (Grothey et al. 2008).

Bevacizumab is associated with several toxicities such as proteinuria, bleeding, HBP, arterial thromboembolic events (ATE) and gastrointestinal perforations (Kabbinavar et al. 2005). Thus high risk patients with comorbidities such as elderly patients and patients with historic of ATE or bleeding should be identified and carefully monitored if bevacizumab is administered. Also, because VEGF is involved in wound healing, bevacizumab should be stopped at least five weeks before any surgery.

3.2 Anti-EGFR monoclonal antibodies

Cetuximab and panitumumab are monoclonal antibodies targeting the extracellular domain of the EGFR (epidermal growth factor receptor). *KRAS* mutations cause permanent activation of the downstream cascade and result in failure to respond to anti-EGFR monoclonal antibodies (Bardelli et al. 2010) (figure 1). *KRAS* mutations are detected in approximately 40% of mCRC. These mutations are mainly found in codons 12 and 13. Recent studies suggest however that not all mutations confer the same resistance to anti-EGFR therapy. Nevertheless, *KRAS* mutation is a predictive biomarker for anti-EGFR therapy and tumor *KRAS* status should be determined whenever anti-EGFR therapy is considered in the treatment of mCRC. According to ASCO's provisional clinical opinion, all patients with metastatic colorectal carcinoma who are candidates for anti-EGFR antibody therapy should have their tumor tested for *KRAS* mutations in an accredited laboratory. If *KRAS* mutation in codon 12 or 13 is detected, then patients with metastatic colorectal carcinoma should not receive anti-EGFR antibody therapy as part of their treatment (Allegra et al. 2009).

Other mutations probably confer resistance to anti-EGFR therapy. *BRAF* mutation is found in 5 to 10 % of colorectal cancer tumors. *KRAS* and *BRAF* mutations are mutually exclusive. The *BRAF* mutation has been recognized as a negative prognostic marker but recent data does not confirm it as a negative predictive marker for anti-EGFR therapy. *PIK3CA* mutations/*PTEN* expression, amphiregulin and epiregulin are other potential predictive biomarkers but further supportive, preferably prospective, studies confirming their role as predictive biomarkers for anti-EGFR therapy would be necessary before considering their use in routine clinical practice in this regard.

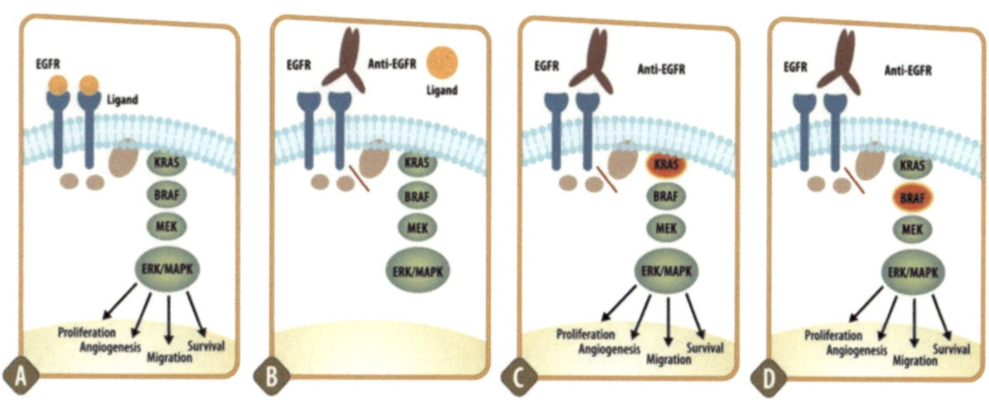

Fig. 1. EGFR Signal Transduction

Cetuximab is associated with severe infusion reaction in three percent of patients. Ninety percent occur during the first infusion and generally in the three first hours. Premedication with anti H1 antagonist and/or glucocorticoid is recommended (Wilke et al. 2008). Panitumumab is generally associated with less infusion reaction because of its 100% human origin. Cetuximab and panitumumab may be also associated with a magnesium-wasting syndrome. Serum levels of this electrolyte should be carefully monitored during treatment. Acneiform eruption occurs in two third of patients treated anti-EGFR molecules. Some studies suggest benefit from using prophylactic antibiotics such as minocyline or doxycycline and topical application of hydrocortisone-based cream (Scope et al. 2007; Lacouture et al. 2010).

3.2.1 Cetuximab (table 3)

Cetuximab is a chimeric (mouse/human) monoclonal antibody against the EGFR. In mCRC, cetuximab has shown efficacy in monotherapy as well as in combination with chemotherapy. It can be used in previously mCRC treated patients or in first-line therapy.
In 2007, cetuximab alone was compared to best supportive care (BSC) in the CO-17 trial. Patients had immunohistochemically detectable EGFR, previously been treated with fluoropyrymidines, irinotecan and oxaliplatin or had contraindications to treatment with these drugs. Survival was significantly better in the cetuximab arm (6.1 vs. 4.6 months). Quality of life was better preserved in the cetuximab group. Cetuximab was associated with a skin rash; grade 2 or higher grade rashes were strongly associated with improved survival (Jonker et al. 2007). In a subsequent analysis, in patients with mutated *KRAS* tumors, there was no significant difference between those who were treated with cetuximab and those who were treated with best supportive care. For wild-type (wt) *KRAS* patients, PFS (3.7 versus 1.9 months) and median OS (9.5 versus 4.8 months) were significantly improved by treatment with cetuximab as compared with best supportive care alone (Karapetis et al. 2008).
In the BOND study, a randomized phase 2 trial, irinotecan plus cetuximab was compared to cetuximab alone for patients refractory to irinotecan. RR and TTP were significantly better in the irinotecan plus cetuximab arm (22.9% vs. 10.8% and 4.1 vs. 1.5 months). There was a trend for better survival also in this arm as well (Cunningham et al. 2004).
In the EPIC trial, adding cetuximab to irinotecan after first-line fluoropyrimidine and oxaliplatin treatment failure, improved RR (16.4 percent versus 4.2 percent), PFS (4.0 versus 2.6 months) and quality of life compared with irinotecan alone (Sobrero et al. 2008; table 3).
Trials have also evaluated the efficacy of cetuximab in combination with chemotherapy in first-line treatment of mCRC. In the phase III CRYSTAL trial, the efficacy of cetuximab plus irinotecan, fluorouracil, and leucovorin (FOLFIRI) was investigated as first-line treatment for metastatic colorectal cancer. There was a significant advantage in RR, PFS and OS for the cetuximab group, but this benefit was limited to *KRAS*-wt patients (Van Cutsem et al. 2010).
In the randomized phase II multicenter OPUS trial, the addition of cetuximab to FOLFOX4 was associated with improved outcomes compared to FOLFOX4 alone in first-line treatment. A statistically significant better chance of response and PFS was shown in patients with *KRAS* wild-type tumors (Bokemeyer et al. 2009; table 3). Patients with mutant

KRAS tumors did not benefit, and may actually have been harmed, with the addition of cetuximab (RR of 33% vs. 49% in the FOLFOX4 alone group (p=0.106)). The phase III COIN trial is another important study which has evaluated the effect of addition of cetuximab to first-line oxaliplatin-based regimens treatment for advanced colorectal cancer. The choice of fluoropyrimidine (either 5-FU or capecitabine) was decided by the treating physician prior randomization (66% of the patients received oxaliplatin plus capecitabine). In patients with wt-*KRAS* tumor, the addition of cetuximab to oxaliplatin- based chemotherapy was associated with a small increase in best overall response (64% vs. 57%, P=0.049). In contrast to CRYSTAL and OPUS studies, however, the addition of cetuximab was not associated with any significant improvement in OS or PFS. (Maughan et al. 2011). Discrepancy between these studies remains difficult to explain.

3.2.2 Panitumumab (table 3)

Panitumumab is a fully human monoclonal antibody targeting the extracellular domain of EGFR. Similarly to cetuximab, panitumumab has shown efficacy in previously mCRC treated patients as well as in first-line therapy.

In patients refractory to 5-FU, irinotecan and oxaliplatin, panitumumab monotherapy showed significantly improved PFS from 7.3 to 8 weeks ($p<0.001$) and RR (10 percent versus 0 percent) compared to BSC alone. There was no OS benefit, likely due to panitumumab use after crossover in the BSC alone. Skin toxicities, hypomagnesaemia, and diarrhea were the most common toxicities observed (Van Cutsem et al. 2007). In this study, the effect on PFS in the wt-*KRAS* group was significantly higher than in the mutant group. Median PFS in the wt-*KRAS* group was 12.3 for panitumumab versus 7.3 weeks for BSC. RR was 17 percent for wt-*KRAS* versus 0 percent for patients with mutant *KRAS* tumors. This showed that panitumumab monotherapy efficacy is confined to wt-*KRAS* tumors and that this status should be considered in selecting patients for panitumumab monotherapy (Amado et al. 2008). In 2010, the FOLFIRI/panitumumab combination was compared to FOLFIRI alone in second-line treatment. In the *KRAS*-wt patients, when panitumumab was added to FOLFIRI median PFS was 5.9 months versus 3.9 months for FOLFIRI alone (p=0.004)(Peeters et al. 2009).

Panitumumab, in conjunction with chemotherapy regimen, has also been evaluated in first-line therapy for mCRC. In 2010, Douillard and colleagues compared FOLFOX 4 and panitumumab versus FOLFOX 4 alone as first-line chemotherapy for previously untreated mCRC (PRIME study). In the *KRAS*-wt patients, panitumumab-FOLFOX4 combination significantly improved PFS compared with FOLFOX4 (median PFS, 9.6 v 8.0 months, respectively; p=0.02). In the *KRAS*-mutant patients, outcome was significantly worse with panitumumab underscoring the importance of *KRAS* screening (Douillard et al. 2010).

Several studies have assessed the use of a dual antibody modality. The PACCE study evaluated the addition of panitumumab to bevacizumab and chemotherapy (oxaliplatin- and irinotecan-based) as first-line treatment for mCRC (Hecht et al. 2009). This study was stopped due to an interim analysis showing inferior PFS and more toxicities in the panitumumab arm. The CAIRO 2 study assigned untreated metastatic colorectal cancer to capecitabine, oxaliplatin, and bevacizumab or the same regimen plus weekly cetuximab. PFS was worse in dual antibody therapy (Tol et al. 2009).These results suggest that dual antibody therapy should not be considered outside further clinical trials.

Trial	Agent	Line	Chemotherapy	Results (**KRAS*-wt patients)
CRYSTAL *Van Cutsem et al. 2011*	Cetuximab	First	FOLFIRI	Median PFS*: 9.9 vs. 8.4 months HR 0.696 (p=0.0012) Median OS*: 23.5 vs. 20.0 months HR 0.796 (p=0.0093)
OPUS *Bokemeyer et al. 2009*	Cetuximab	First	FOLFOX 4	Overall RR*: 61% vs. 37% (p=0.011) Median PFS*: 7.7 vs. 7.2 months (p=0.0163)
COIN *Maughan et al. 2011*	Cetuximab	First	Oxaliplatin with 5FU or capecitabine	ORR*: 64% vs. 57% (p=0.049) No significant improvement in OS or PFS with the addition of cetuximab
PRIME *Douillard et al. 2010*	Panitumumab	First	FOLFOX 4	Median PFS*: 9.6 vs. 8 months (p=0.02)
EPIC *Sobrero et al.2008*	Cetuximab	Second	Irinotecan	PFS: 4 vs. 2.6 months (p<0.0001) RR: 16.4% vs. 4.2% (p<0.0001) OS: 10.7 vs. 10.0 months (p=0.71) but 46.9% of the patients in the irinotecan group received cetuximab after trial. (*KRAS* unselected)
STUDY 181 *Peeters et al.* 2010	Panitumumab	Second	FOLFIRI	Median PFS*: 5.9 vs. 3.9 months (p=0.004)

Table 3. Randomized Trials of Anti-EGFR-chemotherapy Association

4. Local recurrence

The treatment of locally recurrent disease largely depends on prior treatments. Whether the patient had prior surgery and/or radiation will determine the therapeutic approach. Surgery alone may be an option if negative surgical margins can be achieved. Extensive surgery is generally required. Combined therapies including chemotherapy and radiation (if prior radiation was not administered) are favored. In this setting the addition of chemotherapy to radiation before surgery improved local control, time to treatment failure, and cancer-specific survival compared with RT alone in a Norwegian phase 3 randomized study (Braendengen et al. 2008). Still this data has to be considered carefully because the patients in this study had primary unresectable tumors as well as local recurrences and that prior radiation was not allowed. Patients with local recurrence were more likely to be unresectable after preoperative treatment. Trends to improved local control were seen in a retrospective study from the Mayo clinic with the addition of 5-FU to external beam radiotherapy, intraoperative electron beam and surgery (Gunderson et al. 1996).

5. Summary and recommendations

Striking advances have been made in the treatment of metastatic colorectal cancer in the past fifteen years. In 2004, Grothey and colleagues reviewed seven published phase III trials in advanced CRC. Their conclusion was that the three active drugs in mCRC (5-FU/LV, irinotecan and oxaliplatin) should be available to all patients in order to maximize the OS (Grothey et al. 2004). For patients with good performance status, combination therapy (FOLFOX or FOLFIRI) should be preferred as first-line chemotherapy. The choice of regimen should be based on the different toxicity profile of these two regimens. Fragile patients are not candidates for combination therapy but can benefit from treatment with fluoropyrimidine monotherapy. Infusion regimens are associated with less toxicity and should be used in any regimen. The use of oral capecitabine in regimens such as CAPOX is also a valid option for patients for whom infusion is not possible or refused. Different strategies can be used in an attempt to prevent oxaliplatin-induced neuropathy. It remains unclear if a combination regimen such as FOLFOXIRI is superior to FOLFOX or FOLFIRI combined with bevacizumab or an anti-EGFR monoclonal antibody. FOLFOXIRI is associated with significant toxicity and its use is not yet standard in first-line treatment of mCRC. The addition of bevacizumab, a monoclonal antibody targeting the VEGF, is now widely recommended with FOLFIRI, FOLFOX or fluoropyrimidine monotherapy in first-line therapy of mCRC for patients without contraindications to this agent. The use of bevacizumab in second-line setting is also recommended in patients who did not receive this agent in first-line treatment. The benefit of its use beyond progression remains controversial and is not presently recommended. Bevacizumab is associated with potentially serious toxicities so careful attention and monitoring of expected side effects is mandatory. Anti-EGFR monoclonal antibodies, cetuximab and panitumumab, are associated with improved outcomes when used as single agents as salvage therapy in patients with chemotherapy-refractory mCRC and when used for first-line and second-line therapy of mCRC in conjunction with chemotherapy regimens. However, their benefit is restrained to patients whose tumor does not harbour *KRAS* mutation. It is unknown whether adding EGFR inhibitors to initial therapy or using it in a sequential approach as a component of second or third -line therapy gives better results. Also, for now, it is not clear whether bevacizumab or anti-EGFR inhibitor should be preferentially added to first-line therapy. Indeed, chemotherapy plus bevacizumab currently represents the most widely accepted standard for first-line treatment of mCRC. Results from the current North American CALGB/SWOG cooperative group trial of best chemotherapy plus either bevacizumab or cetuximab in untreated *KRAS*-wt metastatic colorectal patients will help in guiding this decision. Although there are no trials directly comparing panitumumab to cetuximab, these agents appear to have comparable efficacy and they are probably interchangeable. Treatment must be individualized as always, taking into account goals of therapy, *KRAS* mutation status, and the toxicity profiles of each agent. Inclusion of patients in clinical trials should always be encouraged if possible.

6. References

Allegra CJ, Jessup JM, Somerfield MR, et al. American Society of Clinical Oncology provisional clinical opinion: testing for KRAS gene mutations in patients with metastatic colorectal carcinoma to predict response to anti-epidermal growth factor receptor monoclonal antibody therapy. *J Clin Oncol.* Apr 20 2009;27(12):2091-2096.

Amado RG, Wolf M, Peeters M, et al. Wild-type KRAS is required for panitumumab efficacy in patients with metastatic colorectal cancer. *J Clin Oncol.* Apr 1 2008;26(10):1626-1634.

Arkenau HT, Arnold D, Cassidy J, et al. Efficacy of oxaliplatin plus capecitabine or infusional fluorouracil/leucovorin in patients with metastatic colorectal cancer: a pooled analysis of randomized trials. *J Clin Oncol.* Dec 20 2008;26(36):5910-5917.

Bardelli A, Siena S. Molecular mechanisms of resistance to cetuximab and panitumumab in colorectal cancer. *J Clin Oncol.* Mar 1 2010;28(7):1254-1261.

Becouarn Y, Gamelin E, Coudert B, et al. Randomized multicenter phase II study comparing a combination of fluorouracil and folinic acid and alternating irinotecan and oxaliplatin with oxaliplatin and irinotecan in fluorouracil-pretreated metastatic colorectal cancer patients. *J Clin Oncol.* Nov 15 2001;19(22):4195-4201.

Bokemeyer C, Bondarenko I, Makhson A, et al. Fluorouracil, leucovorin, and oxaliplatin with and without cetuximab in the first-line treatment of metastatic colorectal cancer. *J Clin Oncol.* Feb 10 2009;27(5):663-671.

Braendengen M, Tveit KM, Berglund A, et al. Randomized phase III study comparing preoperative radiotherapy with chemoradiotherapy in nonresectable rectal cancer. *J Clin Oncol.* Aug 1 2008;26(22):3687-3694.

Cassidy J, Misset JL. Oxaliplatin-related side effects: characteristics and management. *Semin Oncol.* Oct 2002;29(5 Suppl 15):11-20.

Chibaudel B, Maindrault-Goebel F, Lledo G, et al. Can chemotherapy be discontinued in unresectable metastatic colorectal cancer? The GERCOR OPTIMOX2 Study. *J Clin Oncol.* Dec 1 2009;27(34):5727-5733.

Colucci G, Gebbia V, Paoletti G, et al. Phase III randomized trial of FOLFIRI versus FOLFOX4 in the treatment of advanced colorectal cancer: a multicenter study of the Gruppo Oncologico Dell'Italia Meridionale. *J Clin Oncol.* Aug 1 2005;23(22):4866-4875.

Cunningham D, Humblet Y, Siena S, et al. Cetuximab monotherapy and cetuximab plus irinotecan in irinotecan-refractory metastatic colorectal cancer. *N Engl J Med.* Jul 22 2004;351(4):337-345.

Cunningham D, Pyrhonen S, James RD, et al. Randomised trial of irinotecan plus supportive care versus supportive care alone after fluorouracil failure for patients with metastatic colorectal cancer. *Lancet.* Oct 31 1998;352(9138):1413-1418.

de Gramont A, Bosset JF, Milan C, et al. Randomized trial comparing monthly low-dose leucovorin and fluorouracil bolus with bimonthly high-dose leucovorin and fluorouracil bolus plus continuous infusion for advanced colorectal cancer: a French intergroup study. *J Clin Oncol.* Feb 1997;15(2):808-815.

de Gramont A, Figer A, Seymour M, et al. Leucovorin and fluorouracil with or without oxaliplatin as first-line treatment in advanced colorectal cancer. *J Clin Oncol.* Aug 2000;18(16):2938-2947.

deBraud F, Munzone E, Nole F, et al. Synergistic activity of oxaliplatin and 5-fluorouracil in patients with metastatic colorectal cancer with progressive disease while on or after 5-fluorouracil. *Am J Clin Oncol.* Jun 1998;21(3):279-283.

Douillard JY, Cunningham D, Roth AD, et al. Irinotecan combined with fluorouracil compared with fluorouracil alone as first-line treatment for metastatic colorectal cancer: a multicentre randomised trial. *Lancet.* Mar 25 2000;355(9209):1041-1047.

Douillard JY, Siena S, Cassidy J, et al. Randomized, phase III trial of panitumumab with infusional fluorouracil, leucovorin, and oxaliplatin (FOLFOX4) versus FOLFOX4 alone as first-line treatment in patients with previously untreated metastatic colorectal cancer: the PRIME study. *J Clin Oncol.* Nov 1 2010;28(31):4697-4705.

Falcone A, Ricci S, Brunetti I, et al. Phase III trial of infusional fluorouracil, leucovorin, oxaliplatin, and irinotecan (FOLFOXIRI) compared with infusional fluorouracil, leucovorin, and irinotecan (FOLFIRI) as first-line treatment for metastatic colorectal cancer: the Gruppo Oncologico Nord Ovest. *J Clin Oncol.* May 1 2007;25(13):1670-1676.

Fischer von Weikersthal L, Schalhorn A, Stauch M, et al. Phase III trial of irinotecan plus infusional 5-fluorouracil/folinic acid versus irinotecan plus oxaliplatin as first-line treatment of advanced colorectal cancer. *Eur J Cancer.* Jan 2011;47(2):206-214.

Fuchs CS, Marshall J, Mitchell E, et al. Randomized, controlled trial of irinotecan plus infusional, bolus, or oral fluoropyrimidines in first-line treatment of metastatic colorectal cancer: results from the BICC-C Study. *J Clin Oncol.* Oct 20 2007;25(30):4779-4786.

Giantonio BJ, Catalano PJ, Meropol NJ, et al. Bevacizumab in combination with oxaliplatin, fluorouracil, and leucovorin (FOLFOX4) for previously treated metastatic colorectal cancer: results from the Eastern Cooperative Oncology Group Study E3200. *J Clin Oncol.* Apr 20 2007;25(12):1539-1544.

Grothey A, Nikcevich DA, Sloan JA, et al. Intravenous calcium and magnesium for oxaliplatin-induced sensory neurotoxicity in adjuvant colon cancer: NCCTG N04C7. *J Clin Oncol.* Feb 1 2011;29(4):421-427.

Grothey A, Sargent D, Goldberg RM, Schmoll HJ. Survival of patients with advanced colorectal cancer improves with the availability of fluorouracil-leucovorin, irinotecan, and oxaliplatin in the course of treatment. *J Clin Oncol.* Apr 1 2004;22(7):1209-1214.

Grothey A, Sugrue MM, Purdie DM, et al. Bevacizumab beyond first progression is associated with prolonged overall survival in metastatic colorectal cancer: results from a large observational cohort study (BRiTE). *J Clin Oncol.* Nov 20 2008;26(33):5326-5334.

Gunderson LL, Nelson H, Martenson JA, et al. Intraoperative electron and external beam irradiation with or without 5-fluorouracil and maximum surgical resection for previously unirradiated, locally recurrent colorectal cancer. *Dis Colon Rectum.* Dec 1996;39(12):1379-1395.

Hecht JR, Mitchell E, Chidiac T, et al. A randomized phase IIIB trial of chemotherapy, bevacizumab, and panitumumab compared with chemotherapy and bevacizumab alone for metastatic colorectal cancer. *J Clin Oncol.* Feb 10 2009;27(5):672-680.

Hochster HS, Grothey A, Childs BH. Use of calcium and magnesium salts to reduce oxaliplatin-related neurotoxicity. *J Clin Oncol.* Sep 1 2007;25(25):4028-4029.

Hochster HS, Hart LL, Ramanathan RK, et al. Safety and efficacy of oxaliplatin and fluoropyrimidine regimens with or without bevacizumab as first-line treatment of metastatic colorectal cancer: results of the TREE Study. *J Clin Oncol.* Jul 20 2008;26(21):3523-3529.

Hoff PM, Ansari R, Batist G, et al. Comparison of oral capecitabine versus intravenous fluorouracil plus leucovorin as first-line treatment in 605 patients with metastatic colorectal cancer: results of a randomized phase III study. *J Clin Oncol.* Apr 15 2001;19(8):2282-2292.

Hurwitz H, Fehrenbacher L, Novotny W, et al. Bevacizumab plus irinotecan, fluorouracil, and leucovorin for metastatic colorectal cancer. *N Engl J Med.* Jun 3 2004;350(23):2335-2342.

Jain RK. Normalization of tumor vasculature: an emerging concept in antiangiogenic therapy. *Science.* Jan 7 2005;307(5706):58-62.

Jonker DJ, O'Callaghan CJ, Karapetis CS, et al. Cetuximab for the treatment of colorectal cancer. *N Engl J Med.* Nov 15 2007;357(20):2040-2048.

Kabbinavar FF, Schulz J, McCleod M, et al. Addition of bevacizumab to bolus fluorouracil and leucovorin in first-line metastatic colorectal cancer: results of a randomized phase II trial. *J Clin Oncol.* Jun 1 2005;23(16):3697-3705.

Karapetis CS, Khambata-Ford S, Jonker DJ, et al. K-ras mutations and benefit from cetuximab in advanced colorectal cancer. *N Engl J Med.* Oct 23 2008;359(17):1757-1765.

Lacouture ME, Mitchell EP, Piperdi B, et al. Skin toxicity evaluation protocol with panitumumab (STEPP), a phase II, open-label, randomized trial evaluating the impact of a pre-Emptive Skin treatment regimen on skin toxicities and quality of life in patients with metastatic colorectal cancer. *J Clin Oncol.* Mar 10 2010;28(8):1351-1357.

Maughan TS, Adams RA, Smith CG, et al. Addition of cetuximab to oxaliplatin-based first-line combination chemotherapy for treatment of advanced colorectal cancer: results of the randomised phase 3 MRC COIN trial. *Lancet.* Jun 18 2011;377(9783):2103-2114.

Maughan TS, James RD, Kerr DJ, et al. Comparison of survival, palliation, and quality of life with three chemotherapy regimens in metastatic colorectal cancer: a multicentre randomised trial. *Lancet.* May 4 2002;359(9317):1555-1563.

Montagnani F, Chiriatti A, Turrisi G, Francini G, Fiorentini G. A systematic review of FOLFOXIRI chemotherapy for the first-line treatment of metastatic colorectal cancer: improved efficacy at the cost of increased toxicity. *Colorectal Dis.* Jan 12 2010.

Park SB, Goldstein D, Lin CS, Krishnan AV, Friedlander ML, Kiernan MC. Acute abnormalities of sensory nerve function associated with oxaliplatin-induced neurotoxicity. *J Clin Oncol.* Mar 10 2009;27(8):1243-1249.

Peeters M, Siena S, Van Cutsem E, et al. Association of progression-free survival, overall survival, and patient-reported outcomes by skin toxicity and KRAS status in patients receiving panitumumab monotherapy. *Cancer.* Apr 1 2009;115(7):1544-1554.

Petrioli R, Pascucci A, Francini E, et al. Neurotoxicity of FOLFOX-4 as adjuvant treatment for patients with colon and gastric cancer: a randomized study of two different schedules of oxaliplatin. *Cancer Chemother Pharmacol.* Jan 2008;61(1):105-111.

Rothenberg ML, Oza AM, Bigelow RH, et al. Superiority of oxaliplatin and fluorouracil-leucovorin compared with either therapy alone in patients with progressive colorectal cancer after irinotecan and fluorouracil-leucovorin: interim results of a phase III trial. *J Clin Oncol.* Jun 1 2003;21(11):2059-2069.

Saltz LB, Clarke S, Diaz-Rubio E, et al. Bevacizumab in combination with oxaliplatin-based chemotherapy as first-line therapy in metastatic colorectal cancer: a randomized phase III study. *J Clin Oncol.* Apr 20 2008;26(12):2013-2019.

Sanoff HK, Sargent DJ, Campbell ME, et al. Five-year data and prognostic factor analysis of oxaliplatin and irinotecan combinations for advanced colorectal cancer: N9741. *J Clin Oncol.* Dec 10 2008;26(35):5721-5727.

Scope A, Agero AL, Dusza SW, et al. Randomized double-blind trial of prophylactic oral minocycline and topical tazarotene for cetuximab-associated acne-like eruption. *J Clin Oncol.* Dec 1 2007;25(34):5390-5396.

Sobrero AF, Maurel J, Fehrenbacher L, et al. EPIC: phase III trial of cetuximab plus irinotecan after fluoropyrimidine and oxaliplatin failure in patients with metastatic colorectal cancer. *J Clin Oncol.* May 10 2008;26(14):2311-2319.

Souglakos J, Androulakis N, Syrigos K, et al. FOLFOXIRI (folinic acid, 5-fluorouracil, oxaliplatin and irinotecan) vs FOLFIRI (folinic acid, 5-fluorouracil and irinotecan) as first-line treatment in metastatic colorectal cancer (MCC): a multicentre randomised phase III trial from the Hellenic Oncology Research Group (HORG). *Br J Cancer.* Mar 27 2006;94(6):798-805.

Tol J, Koopman M, Cats A, et al. Chemotherapy, bevacizumab, and cetuximab in metastatic colorectal cancer. *N Engl J Med.* Feb 5 2009;360(6):563-572.

Tournigand C, Andre T, Achille E, et al. FOLFIRI followed by FOLFOX6 or the reverse sequence in advanced colorectal cancer: a randomized GERCOR study. *J Clin Oncol.* Jan 15 2004;22(2):229-237.

Tournigand C, Cervantes A, Figer A, et al. OPTIMOX1: a randomized study of FOLFOX4 or FOLFOX7 with oxaliplatin in a stop-and-Go fashion in advanced colorectal cancer--a GERCOR study. *J Clin Oncol.* Jan 20 2006;24(3):394-400.

Van Cutsem E, Peeters M, Siena S, et al. Open-label phase III trial of panitumumab plus best supportive care compared with best supportive care alone in patients with chemotherapy-refractory metastatic colorectal cancer. *J Clin Oncol.* May 1 2007;25(13):1658-1664.

Van Cutsem E, Twelves C, Cassidy J, et al. Oral capecitabine compared with intravenous fluorouracil plus leucovorin in patients with metastatic colorectal cancer: results of a large phase III study. *J Clin Oncol.* Nov 1 2001;19(21):4097-4106.

Van Cutsem E, Kohne C-H, Lang I, et al. Cetuximab plus irinotecan, fluorouracil, and leucovorin as first-line treatment for metastatic colorectal cancer: updated analysis of overall survival according to tumor KRAS and BRAF mutation status. *J Clin Oncol.* May 20 2011; 29 (15): 2011-2019..

Wilke H, Glynne-Jones R, Thaler J, et al. Cetuximab plus irinotecan in heavily pretreated metastatic colorectal cancer progressing on irinotecan: MABEL Study. *J Clin Oncol.* Nov 20 2008;26(33):5335-5343.

Wilson RH, Lehky T, Thomas RR, Quinn MG, Floeter MK, Grem JL. Acute oxaliplatin-induced peripheral nerve hyperexcitability. *J Clin Oncol.* Apr 1 2002;20(7):1767-1774.

19

Side Effects of Neoadjuvant Treatment in Locally Advanced Rectal Cancer

Karoline Horisberger[1] and Pablo Palma[2]
[1]*Department of Surgery, University Hospital Mannheim*
[2]*Division of Colon & Rectal Surgery, University Hospital HUVN Granada*
[1]*Germany*
[2]*Spain*

1. Introduction

Neoadjuvant treatment of locally advanced rectal cancer patients provides undisputable advantages regarding local control (1; 2), and it seems to afford the benefit of survival in patients with preoperative complete regression (3; 4). Furthermore, local control is an important feature in life quality of rectal cancer patients. However, due to the perspicuous interests in oncological effects, the acute and moreover late side effects tend to be neglected. The consequence is that especially late side effects have probably been underestimated until now.

Many patients would perceive a permanent stoma and loss of the anal sphincter as a stigma that lowers their self-esteem (5). Hence, sphincter preservation is a major request of the patients and developed to an important surgical concern. In fact, patients are willing to trade a considerable amount of survival to avoid a colostomy (6). And more than this, they are also disposed to trade survival in order to avoid chemotherapy (6).

Though, with regard to oncological and surgical outcome control late results are important. For all patients quality of life matters are fundamental. This particularly counts for those patients who show an incomplete regression or none and therefore do have only limited benefit from the treatment.

2. Acute side effects

The TME trial was the first large study that compared additional preoperative radiation therapy to TME (Total Mesorectal Excision) surgery alone (1). To register the acute side effects the RTOG (Radiation Therapy Oncology Group) classification 0-5 was used. In general, RTOG 0 represents no complaints and RTOG 5 is a toxicity leading to death. Mild toxic effects are grade 1 and 2; ≥ grade 3 counts as severe toxic effect. The trial showed acute side effects in 26% of the patients within three months of the start of short course radiation therapy (7). It is noticeable in the precise description of the side effects that the most frequent complications were gastrointestinal followed by neurological. 13% of the patients showed gastrointestinal symptoms, most of them grade I or II; only one patient suffered from grade III and none of grade IV (7). It is interesting to know that the scoring system for neurological symptoms was additionally implemented one year after the beginning of the

trial because observations of acute plexopathy in the antecedent Swedish Rectal Cancer Trial were published in 1996 (8). During the first full year of the 4-year trial, no neurological symptoms were recorded in any of the patients (7). In fact, the Swedish Rectal Cancer Trial also compared neoadjuvant short-course radiation with surgery alone; however, this trial was conducted in the era before TME. It has to be noticed that during the recruitment phase of the Swedish Rectal Cancer Trial, the radiation technique changed from three-beam to four-beam (8). The authors explicitly report that no plexopathy was observed after conventional fractionation of the radiotherapy (2Gy/d) but only after short-course hypofractionated 5x5Gy radiation (8).
Neoadjuvant chemoradiation correlates more closely with higher acute toxicity than short-course radiation (9); in fact, it seems to be less harmful than postoperative chemoradiation with regard to acute toxicity (2). Comparing preoperative chemoradiation and long-course radiation with 45 Gy it seems to be obvious that radiation is more tolerable in the acute phase (10; 11). Actually, in most studies only grade 3 and grade 4 toxicities are listed, though the higher rates of grade 1 and 2 toxicities are not mentioned.

Reference	No. of patients	Therapy strategy	Toxicity grade III-IV (%)	P value
Marijnen 2002	695 vs. 719	5x5 Gy versus TME	2.4 vs. 0	n.s.
Bujko 2004	155 vs. 157	5x5 Gy versus preoperative chemoradiation (5-FU)	3 vs. 18	0.001
Bosset 2004	398 vs. 400	45 Gy versus preoperative chemoradiation (5-FU)	37.7 vs. 54 *	<0.005
Gérard 2006	367 vs. 375	45 Gy versus preoperative chemoradiation (5-FU)	2.7 vs. 14.6	<0.005
Sauer 2004	404 vs. 394	Pre- versus postoperative chemoradiation (5-FU)	27 vs. 40	0.001
Gérard 2010	293 vs. 291	Cap vs. CapOx preoperative chemoradiation	10.9 vs. 25.4	<0.001

Cap: capecitabine; CapOx: capecitabine and oxaliplatin

Table 1. Acute toxicity ≥ grade III (*toxicities ≥ grade II) in randomised trials.

An impression of the difference is given in the publication of the EORTC 22921 study that listed all toxicities ≥ grade 2 and which thereby obtained a toxicity rate of 37.7 resp. 54% comparing 45 Gy with chemoradiation (11). The exclusive subsumption of grade 3 and 4 toxicities of neoadjuvant treatment obtains a toxicity rate below 20% (Table 1). It should be noted that in a direct comparison of 5-FU versus capecitabine in a phase III trial, capecitabine showed to constitute significantly more hand-footsyndrome (31 vs. 2%) but less leukopenia (25 vs. 35%) (12). Gastrointestinal and skin complications were no different between the arms.

The addition of oxaliplatin to neoadjuvant treatment, either with 5-FU treatment or capecitabine, significantly increased the acute toxicity (particularly diarrhoea) three-fold and 2.5-fold, respectively (13; 14). However, toxicity could be interpreted as feasible as particular grade III toxicities were recorded in not more than 15% of the patients. It was disappointing, however, that the rates of complete response did not change in both trials (13; 14). Unfortunately, there are no other randomised phase III trials that have compared different CRT regimens.

A pooled analysis of three phase I/II trials of patients treated with or without additional cetuximab saw no difference in question of acute toxicity (15).

3. Postoperative complications

Looking at the postoperative complications one can notice that reporting of them is performed on an irregular basis concerning the definition of some complications as well as whether they are reported at all. Few randomised studies (2; 7; 14) report in detail on perioperative complications while others outline the overall rate of complications (Tables 2/3). However, the interpretation of surgical and other complications is complex, even in the case of detailed reports. By way of example, the TME trial meticulously reports a significantly higher rate of postoperative complications in irradiated patients (7). Nevertheless, the rate of all surgical complications is the same for irradiated and non-irradiated patients, although it differs for those with abdominoperineal resection. This is caused by the rate of perineal wound dehiscence that is increased following neoadjuvant radiation, while the rate of anastomotic leakages is no different between the groups. In addition, cardiac and psychological complications that are significantly more frequent in irradiated patients aggravate the higher postoperative complication rate (7).

With regard to the risk of perineal wound dehiscence, the results of the different studies are inconsistent. While it is significantly increased for short-course radiation and chemoradiation in some trials (7; 16), others rule out an influence (2).

The early anastomotic leakage rate has been reported as 8-18% after neoadjuvant treatment and is thereby no different from rates in non-irradiated patients (Table 3) (2; 7; 10; 17; 18). A correlation between neoadjuvant treatment and anastomotic leakage rate cannot be seen in a single study (2; 7; 9; 10; 17). However, in a population-based study from Sweden, the multivariate analysis of 432 out of 6833 patients revealed preoperative radiation to be an independent risk factor for anastomotic leakage (19). The restriction of this publication, however, is the fact that the large majority of these operations were performed without TME. Though, the influence of this fact is in this regard not known.

Besides this, two single-centre studies report a positive correlation between the preoperative regression grade and the risk of anastomotic leakage (Fig. 1) (20; 21).

One main problem of anastomotic leakage reporting is the fact that there is no definition of leakage that has to be reported (Fig. 2/3). While some studies report all clinical apparent leakages as well as the abscess around the anastomosis as leakage (7; 21), others do differ between clinical and radiological leakage (20). Some do not define what they count as leakage (2), others just allude to those complications that require reintervention (9).

Until now, the influence of intensified chemoradiation using oxaliplatin is described by only one phase III trial (14). In this single trial, the rate of anastomotic leakage is no different between patients who received capecitabine and those with additional oxaliplatin (14).

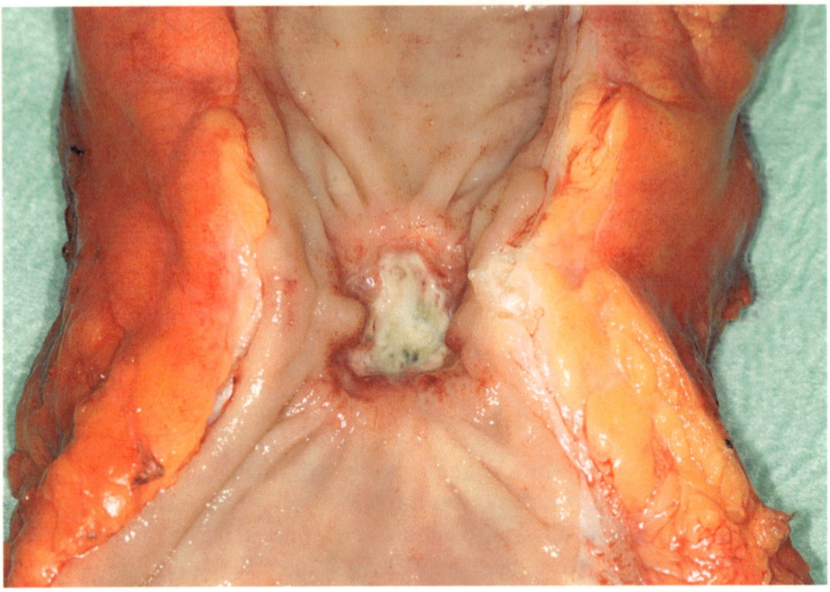

Fig. 1. Rectal cancer after neoadjuvant chemoradiation. Downstaging was histopathologically proven; a distinct fibrosis can be seen macroscopically.

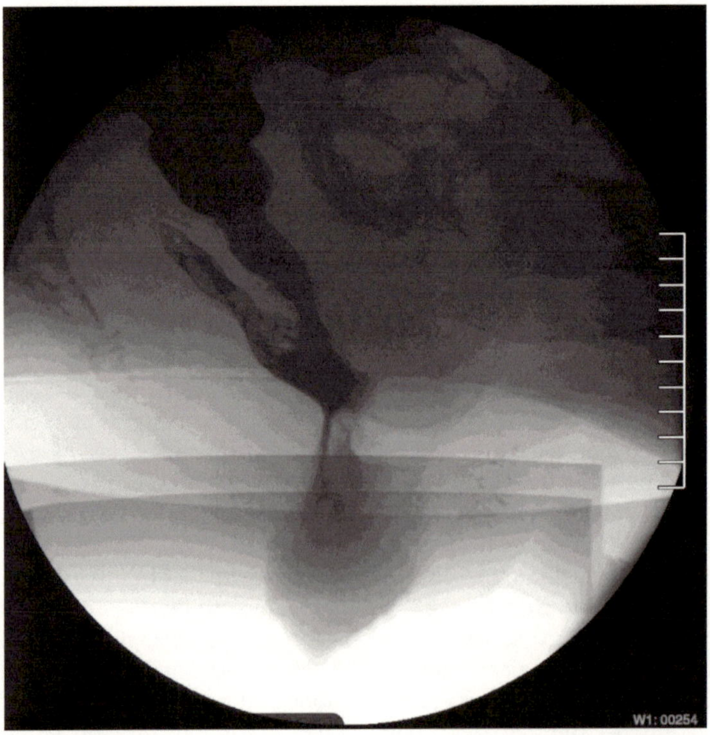

Fig. 2. Radiographically proven old anastomotic leakage that presented years later with outlet obstruction.

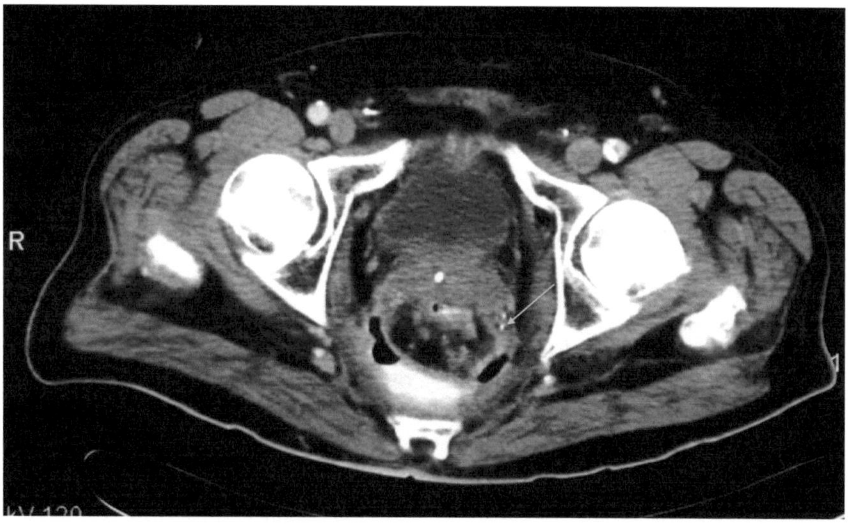

Fig. 3. Radiographically proven anastomotic leakage with extraluminal contrast agent (arrow).

Reference	No. of patients	Therapy strategy	Overall rate of postoperative complications (%)	P value
Marijnen 2002	695 vs. 719	5x5 Gy versus TME	48 vs. 41	0.008
Bujko 2004	155 vs. 157	5x5 Gy versus preoperative chemoradiation (5-FU)	23 vs. 15*	0.12
Bosset 2004	398 vs. 400	45 Gy versus preoperative chemoradiation (5-FU)	22.2 vs. 22.8*	n.s.
Gérard 2006	367 vs. 375	45 Gy versus preoperative chemoradiation (5-FU)	26.9 vs. 20.9	n.s.
Sauer 2004	404 vs. 394	Pre- versus postoperative chemoradiation (5-FU)	36 vs. 34	0.68
Gérard 2010	293 vs. 291	Cap vs. CapOx preoperative chemoradiation	33.8 vs. 30.6	n.s.

* Complication criteria not defined

Table 2. Postoperative complications in randomised trials.

Reference	Anastomotic leakage rate (%)	P value	Surgical reintervention rate (%)	P value
Marijnen 2002	11 vs. 12	n.s.	14.8 vs. 13.6	n.s.
Bujko 2004	Not reported		12 vs.9	0.38
Bosset 2004	Not reported		Not reported	
Gérard 2006	7.6 vs. 7.4	n.s.	Not reported	
Sauer 2004	11 vs. 12	0.77	Not reported	
Gérard 2010	18.9 vs. 16.7 *	n.s.	12.9 vs. 12.5	0.9

*Rate of surgically treated anastomotic fistula; Additional conservatively treated fistula: 8.5% vs. 7.7%; n.s.

Table 3. Anastomotic leakage rate and surgical reintervention rate in randomised trials.

The rate of diverting stoma creation is not mentioned in some large trials (2; 10; 11; 22). Others merely report the late rate of permanent stoma (23). In fact, only some studies have reported the rate of defunctioning stomas and identified in addition the different rates between stoma created initially and those created subsequently as a result of another complication (7; 17); altogether, the rates are hardly comparable.
Mortality rate is the same in patients with or without neoadjuvant treatment (1; 2; 9 - 11; 18; 24). It is to be noted that the intensified neoadjuvant chemoradiation with oxaliplatin does not influence the mortality rate (13; 14).

4. Late side effects

Improving the oncological results of rectal cancer patients also directed the scientific focus on late side effects, late functional results and long-term quality of life.
However, results of the late functional investigations of 597 patients of the Dutch TME trial were disappointing (Tab.4) (25). Patients with a local recurrence were excluded from this follow-up, so that the functional results were not disease-related. 5 years after the primary treatment, 68% of irradiated patients suffered from incontinence during the day and 32% from incontinence at night. These were 24% resp. 15% more than in non-irradiated patients. There were statistically significant differences in terms of bowel frequency, blood loss and mucus loss (25). Pad use as evidence of incontinence was evaluated in 56% of the irradiated patients while 33% of the directly operated patients had the same need ($p<0.001$) (25). Fractionated defecation with the sensation of incomplete evacuation is elicited in 35-58% of irradiated patients (26–28). Irradiated patients were significantly impaired in their daily activities and social function (29).
It is understandable from the information above that irradiated patients without a stoma were significantly less satisfied than non-irradiated patients. If patients had a stoma, the rate of satisfaction did not differ between those that were radiated and those that were non-irradiated (25). It is to be noted that impairment of the sphincter function may have been so

severe that significantly more patients would have been satisfied if they had had a stoma than if they had not (25). This result is interesting due to the fact that sphincter-preservation is seen to be one of the main objectives of neoadjuvant and surgical therapy (2). It is often suggested that patients with a stoma generally have lower quality of life and as a consequence, sphincter-sparing surgery has been forced (5). Already when low anastomosis started coming up, the problem of reduced social functioning of both colostomy and impaired anal sphincter was seen and could not be clearly weighed up (30). It is meaningful that the surgical and oncological aims seem not to correspond completely with the demand of the patients (31). In a survey of healthy individuals it turned out that the majority would prefer a treatment with better functional outcome even when they would have to accept a higher risk of local recurrence (31). In another study was revealed that patients and even oncologist and surgeons would trade survival for quality of life. 52% of the questioned patients - and 88 and 90% resp. of the surgeons and oncologist - would trade life to avoid colostomy (6).

A Norwegian study that evaluated the functional outcome of 199 patients 4.8 years after initial treatment found a significant correlation between incontinence of liquid stool and overall quality of life (29). In the really long-term results, 15 years after radiation, 69% of the irradiated versus 43% of the non-irradiated patients had incontinence complications (32). More than twice as many patients suffered from fecal incontinence after irradiation. However, this data was generated from the Swedish Rectal Cancer Trial, which means that the patients were operated on without using the TME procedure. Although there is no randomised trial that would compare conventional rectal cancer surgery and TME procedure - and due to the definitely favourable results of the TME procedure there will never be one - several smaller in-hospital series compare functional results of the two procedures. In those studies the postoperative impairment of urination and genital function rather improved when TME was introduced (33;34).

The poor functional results seem to be the same or even worse following chemoradiation (Tab. 4) (35; 36). Good anal function was stated in one study that compared chemoradiation with radiation in 11% versus 30%, resp. of the patients seen (p=0.04) (36).

The results concerning urinary incontinence after radiation are inconsistent. While the late results of the Dutch TME study do not find a correlation to preoperative radiation, this correlation is to be found in a Norwegian study of 199 irradiated patients (25; 29; 37).

From the Dutch TME trial, we know that former sexually active male and female patients are significantly impaired in their sexual activity in an evaluation two years after surgery (38). Two other studies that described a significant lack of lubrication or more vaginal dryness, dyspareunia and reduced vaginal dimension in irradiated patients confirmed this data. However, women were not concerned about their sexual life (36; 39). It is to be noted that one study did not discriminate between pre- and postoperative irradiation (39) and the other one was performed with initially nonresectable rectal cancer (36).

In male patients, both erection and ejaculation functions were impaired after 5x5Gy radiation therapy (38). As the impaired sexual functions differ significantly in direct comparison to only operated patients, there must be a direct influence from radiation in addition to the possible surgical damage to the pelvic autonomic nerves. Whether or not this influence consists of radiation damage to the nerves itself, a postirradiated reduced tolerance to surgery-caused ischemia or to technically hindered surgery after radiation cannot be clarified (40).

Reference	No. of patients	Therapy strategy	Follow-up (yrs; median)	Fecal incontinence (%)	P value
Peeters 2005	177 vs. 185	5x5 Gy versus TME	5.1	62 vs. 38*	<0.001
Pollack 2006	21 vs. 43	5x5 Gy versus conventional surgery	14	57 vs. 26	0.013
Brændengen 2006	18 vs. 19	Preop. RTX versus RCTX	4-12	58 vs. 38° 75 vs. 56 Δ	
Coco 2007	100	50.4Gy	12	46 Δ 14 ¥	
Urso † 2006	12	Pre- and postoperative	19 mths	75 ¥	
Bruheim † 2010	69 vs. 240	Pre- and postoperative versus TME	4.8	71 vs. 58Δ 52 vs. 13 ¥	0.01 <0.001

* Incontinence by day; Incontinence at night: 32 vs. 17%(P=0.001); ° Incontinence to stool; Δ Incontinence to gas; ¥ Defined as: requirement of pad use
†Urso (2006): Preoperative chemoradiation (50.4Gy) with 5-FU and oxaliplatin, postoperative 5-FU-based chemotherapy. Bruheim (2010): Pre- or postoperative radiation (50Gy) with chemotherapy (in 40% of neoadjuvant radiation; in 75% of adjuvant radiation).

Table 4. Late functional results; RTX: radiation therapy; RCTX: radiochemotherapy

Hip fracture is a rarely mentioned late complication but seems to be significantly increased in irradiated patients (29; 41). In the Norwegian study by Bruheim, et al. the incidence of pelvic fracture was five times higher in the irradiated patients (5% versus 1%) (29). Furthermore, in the group of irradiated patients female sex seems to be the only independent predictor for fracture (42). However, in the late follow-up of the Dutch TME trial hip fracture rate did not differ between irradiated and non-irradiated patients (25).
Reports concerning second malignancies following radiation of the Swedish Rectal Cancer Trial (43) are refuted by a large population-based analysis of 20,910 patients that showed that the rare event of second primary malignancies is not more frequent in irradiated patients (44). The occurrence of a second malignancy in an adjacent organ of the irradiated volume seems to be weighted between the radiation-induced malignancies and those spontaneous malignancies accidentally avoided by radiation (44).
Anal stricture or late anastomotic stricture is reported in some publications (35; 45). However, a difference between irradiated and non-irradiated patients is not seen in the long-term follow-up of the Dutch TME trial (25) and a difference between patients with preoperative and postoperative chemoradiation cannot be seen either (45).

5. Discussion

Besides the side effects reported above there are few further thoughts regarding neoadjuvant treatment as a source of possible harm. With the current staging methods an overtreatment is performed in probably 18% of the patients, most of them wrongly staged as cT3N0 (2). However, this overtreatment is intentional as 22% of the pT3 tumours had a previously undetected involvement of mesorectal lymph nodes and would have poorer local control with postoperative treatment (46). This means that at present the incidence of side effects in overtreated patients who would require nothing other than surgery unfortunately has to be accepted to include most of the patients to neoadjuvant treatment who really need it.

Another cause of medical discomfiture is the group of patients without any signs of regression. Those non-responders do have the correct indication for the treatment but instead of benefit they only see the side effects of the treatment. To date, there is no predictive resistance marker that could exclude those patients from neoadjuvant treatment.

For short-course radiotherapy where there is a short amount of time until the operation it must be taken into account that there is no downstaging. Patients in whom an involvement of the circumferential margin is suspected should maybe treated with chemoradiation as a preference. In case of showing an involved circumferential resection margin after neoadjuvant treatment the long-term is even worse than having an involved margin after direct surgical resection (47;48). Chemoradiation alone can provide preoperative downstaging, however, the long-term functional results are even worse than those following radiation.

Another critical point is that the improved local control of neoadjuvant short-course radiation has to be put into a certain sense of perspective by the fact that the oncological benefit may be only valid for mid-rectal cancers from 5 to 10 cm from the anal verge (47). Conversely, the low rectal cancer patients and those with tumours in the upper third seem not to profit from the benefit that short-course radiation might offer.

6. Conclusion

In addition to acute side effects that seem to be feasible, it is assumed that there are surgical and other perioperative complications that are not reported as a matter of routine. It is evident, that a regular report system of acute and late side effects concerning medical and surgical problems is not implemented yet.

In particular the late complications appear to limit the patient in their functional abilities and quality of life. Moreover, the late side effects are probably still underestimated. To date, the impairment of social life by poor anorectal function and the psychological consequences of sexual dysfunction have barely been evaluated. It has to be assumed by a lack of studies evaluating late side effects, that the unreported number of cases exceeds the published ones. A certain number of unreported cases should however also be assumed as many patients do not answer honestly due to a sense of shame. Unfortunately, the evidenced poor functional results after rectal cancer surgery seem to be worsened by neoadjuvant treatment. It is easier said than done, but the patients have to be individually balanced in terms of their potential oncological benefit against the probable functional deficiency that is likely to compound over the years.

7. References

[1] Kapiteijn E., Marijnen C.A.M., Nagtegaal I.D., Putter H., Steup W.H., Wiggers T., Rutten H.J.T., Pahlman L., Glimelius B., Van Krieken J.H.J.M., Leer J.W.H. & van de Velde C.J.H., for the Dutch Colorectal Cancer Group. (2001) Preoperative radiotherapy

combined with total mesorectal excision for resectable rectal cancer. *N Engl J Med;* 345: 638-46.

[2] Sauer R., Becker H., Hohenberger W., Rödel C., Wittekind C., Fietkau R., Martus P., Tschmelitsch J., Hager E., Hess C.F., Karstens J.H., Liersch T., Schmidberger H. & Raab R., for the German Rectal Cancer Study Group. (2004) Preoperative versus postoperative chemoradiotherapy for rectal cancer. *N Engl J Med;* 351:1731-40.

[3] Rodel C., Martus P., Papdoupolos T., Füzesi L., Klimpfinger M., Fietkau R., Liersch T., Hohenberger W., Raab R., Sauer R. & Witteking C. (2005) Prognostic significance of tumor regression after preoperative chemoradiotherapy for rectal cancer. *J Clin Oncol;* 23:8688-8698.

[4] Capirci C., Valentini V., Cionini L., De Paoli A., Rodel C., Glynne-Jones R., Coco C., Romano M., Mantello G., Palazzi S., Osti M.F., Friso M.L., Genovesi D., Vidali C., Gambacorta M.A., Buffoli A., Lupattelli M., Favretto M.S. & LaTorre G. (2008) Prognostic value of pathologic complete response after neoadjuvant therapy in locally advanced rectal cancer: Long-term analysis of 566 ypCR patients. *Int J Radiat Biol Phys;* 72:99-107.

[5] MacDonald L.D. & Anderson H.R. (1984) Stigma in patients with rectal cancer: a community study. *J Epidemiol Community Health;* 38(4): 284-90.

[6] Solomon M.J., Pager, C.K., Keshava, A., Findlay, M., Butow, P., Salkeld, G. P. & Roberts, R. (2003) What do patients want? Patients preferences and surrogate decision making in the treatment of colorectal cancer. *Dis Colon Rectum;* 46(10): 1351-1357.

[7] Marijnen C.A.M., Kapiteijn E., van de Velde C.J.H., Martijn H., Steup W.H., Wiggers T., Klein Kranenbarg E., Leer J.W.H & the Cooperative Investigators of the Dutch Colorectal Cancer Group. (2002) Acute side effects and complications after short-term preoperative radiotherapy combined with total mesorectal excision in primary rectal cancer: report of a multicenter randomized trial. *J Clin Oncol;* 20:817-25.

[8] Frykholm G.J., Sintorn K., Montelius A., Jung B., Pahlman L. & Glimelius B. (1996) Acute lumbosacral plexopathy during and after preoperative radiotherapy of rectal adenocarcinoma. *Radiother Oncol;* 38: 121-130.

[9] Bujko K., Nowacki M.P., Nasierowska-Guttmejer A., Michalski W., Bebenek M., Pudełko M., Kryj M., Oledzki J., Szmeja J., Słuszniak J., Serkies K., Kładny J., Pamucka M. & Kukołowicz M. (2004) Sphincter preservation following preoperative radiotherapy for rectal cancer: report of a randomised trial comparing short-term radiotherapy vs. conventionally fractionated radiochemotherapy. *Radiother Oncol;* 72: 15-24.

[10] Gérard J.-P., Conroy T., Bonnetain F., Bouché O., Chapet O., Closon-Dejardin M.-T., Untereiner M., Leduc B., Francois E., Maurel J., Seitz J.-F., Buecher B., Mackiewicz R., Ducreux M. & Bedenne L. (2006) Preoperative radiotherapy with or without concurrent fluorouracil and leucovorin in T3-4 rectal cancer: results of FFCD 9203. *J Clin Oncol;* 24: 4620-25.

[11] Bosset J.F., Calais G., Daban A., Berger C., Radosevic-Jelic L., Maingon P., Bardet E., Pierart M. & Briffaux A., for the EORTC Radiotherapy Group. (2004) Preoperative chemoradiotherapy versus preoperative radiotherapy in rectal cancer patients: assessment of acute toxicity and treatment compliance. Report of the 22921 randomised trial conducted by the EORTC Radiotherapy Group. *Eur J Cancer;* 40: 219-24.

[12] Hofheinz R.D., Wenz F., Post S., Matzdorff A., Laechelt S., Mueller L., Link H., Moehler M., Burkholder I. & Hochhaus A. (2009) Caecitabine (Cape) versus 5-fluorouracil (5-FU)-based (neo-) adjuvant chemoradiotherapy (CRT) for locally advanced rectal cancer (LARC): Safety results of a randomized , phase III trial. *J Clin Oncol;* 27suppl(15S): abstract4014.

[13] Aschele C., Pinto C., Cordio S., Rosati G., Tagliagambe A., Artale S., Rosetti P., Lonardi S., Boni L. & Cionini L., on behalf of STAR Network Investigator. (2009) Preoperative fluorouracil (FU)-based chemoradiation with and without weekly oxaliplatin in locally advanced rectal cancer: Pathologic response analysis of the Studio Terapia Adiuvante Retto (STAR)-01 randomized phase III trial. *J Clin Oncol;* 27suppl(18s): abstract 4008.

[14] Gérard J.-P., Azria D., Gourgou-Bourgade S., Martel-Laffay I., Hennequin C., Etienne P.-L., Vendrely V., Francois E., de La Roche G., Bouché O., Mirabel X., Denis B., Mineur L., Berdah J.-F., Mahé M.A., Bécouarn Y., Dupuis O., Lledo G., Montoto-Grillot C. & Conroy T. (2010) Comparison of two neoadjuvant chemoradiotherapy regimens for locally advanced rectal cancer: results of the phase III trial ACCORD 12/0405-Prodige 2. *J Clin Oncol;* 28: 1638-44.

[15] Weiss C., Arnold D., Dellas K., Liersch T., Hipp M., Fietkau R., Sauer R., Hinke A. & Rödel C. (2009) Preoperatove radiotherapy of advanced rectal cancer with capecitabine and oxaliplatin with or without cetuximab: a pooled analysis of three prospective phase I-II trials. *Int J Radiat Biol Phys;* 78: 472-478.

[16] Buie W.D., MacLean A.R., Attard J.P., Brasher P.M.A. & Chan A.K. (2005) Neoadjuvant chemoradiation increases the risk of pelvic sepsis after radical excision of rectal cancer. *Dis Col Rectum;* 48:1868-74.

[17] Francois Y., Nemoz C.J., Baulieux J., Vignal J., Grandjean J.-P., Partensky C., Souquet J.C., Adeleine P. & Gerard J.-P. (1999) Influnence of the interval between preoeprative radiation therapy and surgery on downstaging and on the rate of sphincter-sparing surgery for rectal cancer: the Lyon R90-01 randomized trial. *J Clin Oncol;* 17:2396-2402.

[18] Sebag-Montefiore D., Stephens R.J., Steele R., Monson J., Grieve R., Khanna S., Quirke P., Couture J., de Metz C., Sun Myint A., Bessell E., Griffiths G., Thompson L.C. & Parmar M. (2009) Preoperative radiotherapy versus selective postoperative chemoradiotherapy in patients with rectal cancer (MRC CR07 and NCIC-CTG C016): a multicentre, randomised trial. *Lancet;* 373: 811-20.

[19] Mathiessen P., Hallböök O., Andersson M., Rutegard J. & Sjödahl R. (2004) Risk factors for anastomotic leakage after anterior resection of the rectum. *Colorect Dis;* 6: 462-69.

[20] Lyall A., McAdam T.K., Townend J. & Loudon M.A. (2006) Factors affecting anastomotic complications following anterior resection in rectal cancer. *Colorect Dis;* 9: 801-807.

[21] Horisberger K., Hofheinz R.D., Palma P., Volkert A.-K., Rothenhoefer S., Wenz F., Hochhaus A., Post S. & Willeke F. (2008) Tumor response to neoadjuvant chemoradiation in rectal cancer: predictor for surgical morbidity? *Int J Colorectal Dis;* 23:257-64.

[22] Bosset J.F., Collette L., Calais G., Mineur L., Maingon P., Radosevic-Jelic L., Daban A., Bardet E., Beny A. & Ollier J.C., for the EORTC Radiotherapy Group Trial 22921.

(2006) Chemotherapy with preoperative radiotherapy in rectal cancer. *N Engl J Med;* 355:1114-23.

[23] Bujko K., Nowacki M.P., Nasierowska-Guttmejer A., Michalski W., Bebenek M. & Kryj M. for the Polish Colorectal Study Group. (2006) Long-term results of a randomized trial comparing preoperative short-course radiotherapy with preoperative conventionally fractionated chemoradiation for rectal cancer. *Br J Surg;* 93: 1215-1223.

[24] Ulrich A., Weitz J., Slodczyk M., Koch M., Jaeger D., Münter M. & Büchler M.W. (2009) Neoadjuvant treatment does not influence perioperative outcome in rectal cancer surgery. *Int J Radiat Biol Phys;* 75: 129-36.

[25] Peeters K.C.M.J., van de Velde C.J.H., Leer J.W.H., Martijn H., Junggeburt J.M.C., Klein Kranenbarg E., Steup W.H., Wiggers T., Rutten H.J. & Marijnen C.A.M. (2005) Late side effects of short-course preoperative raidiotherapy combined with total mesorectal excision for rectal cancer: Increased bowel dysfunction in irradiated patients - A Dutch Colorectal Cancer Grouo Study. *J Clin Oncol;* 23:6199-6206.

[26] Bujko K., Nowacki M.P., OleÎdzki J., Sopylo R., Skoczylas J. & Chwalinski M. (2001) Sphincter preservation after short-term preoperative radiotherapy for low rectal cancer. *Acta Oncol;* 40:593-601.

[27] Temple L.K., Wong W.D. & Minsky B. (2003) The impact of radiation on functional outcomes in patients with rectal cancer and sphincter preservation. *Sem Radiat Oncol;* 13:469-477.

[28] Coco C., Valentini V., Manno A., Rizzo G., Gambacorta M.A., Mattana A., Verbo A. & Picciocchi A. (2007) Functional results after radiochemotherapy and total mesorectal excision for rectal cancer. *Int J Colorectal Dis;* 22: 903-10.

[29] Bruheim K., Guren M.G., Skovlund E., Hjermstad M.J., Dahl O., Frykholm G., Carlsen E. & Tveit K.M. (2010a) Late side effects and quality of life after radiotherapy for rectal cancer. *Int J Radiat Biol Phys;* 76: 1005-11.

[30] Sprangers M.A.G, Taal B.G., Aaronson N.K. & te Velde A. (1995) Quality of life in colorectal cancer: Stoma vs. nonstoma patients. *Dis Colon Rectum;* 38(4): 361-369.

[31] Kennedy E.D., Schmocker S., Victor C., Baxter N.N., Kim J., Brierly J. & McLeod R.S. (2011) Do patients consider preoperative chemoradiation for primary rectal cancer worthwile? *Cancer;* 117: 2853-62.; Epub ahead of print. PMID: 21225852

[32] Pollack J., Holm T., Cedermark B., Altman D., Holmström B., Glimelius B. & Mellgren A. (2006) Late daverse effects of short-course preoperative radiotherapy in rectal cancer. *Br J Surg;* 93: 1519-25.

[33] Havenga K., Enker W.E., McDermott K., Cohen A.M., Minsky B.D., Guillem J. (1996) Male and female sexual and urinary function after total mesorectal excision with autonomic nerve preservation for carcinoma of the recum. *J Am Coll Surg;* 182: 495-502.

[34] Maurer C.A., Z'graggen K., Renzulli P., Schilling M.k., Netzer P., Büchler M.W. (2001) Total mesorectal excision preserves male genital function compared with conventional rectal cancer surgery. *Br J Surg;* 88: 1501-05.

[35] Urso E., Serpentini S., Pucciarelli S., DeSalvo G.L., Friso M.L., Fabris G., Lonardi S., Ferraro B., Bruttocao A., Aschele C. & Nitti D. (2006) Complications, functional

outcome and quality of life after intensive preoperative chemoradiotherapy in rectal cancer. *Eur J Surg Oncol;* 32: 1201-8.

[36] Brændengen M., Tveit K.M., Bruheim K., Cvancarova M., Berglund A. & Glimelius B. (2010) Late patient-reported toxicity after preoperative radiotherapy or chemoradiotherapy in nonresectable rectal cancer: resulty from a randomized phase III study. *Int J Radiat Biol Phys;* Epub ahead of print. PMID: 20932687

[37] Langc M.M., Marijnen C.A.M., Maas C.P., Putter H., Rutten H.J., Stiggelbout A.M., Meershoek-Klein Kranenbarg E., van de Velde C.J.H. & cooperative clinical investigators of the Dutch Total Mesorectal Excision trial. (2009) Risk factors for sexual dysfunction after rectal cancer treatment. *Eur J Cancer;* 45:1578-88.

[38] Marijnen C.A.M., van de Velde C.J.H., Putter H., van den Brink M., Maas C.P., Martijn H., Rutten H.J., Wiggers T., Klein Kranenbarg E., Leer J.W.H. & Stiggelbout A.M. (2005) Impact of short-term preoperative radiotherapy on health-related quality of life and sexual functioning in primary rectal cancer: report of a multicenter randomized trial. *J Clin Oncol;* 23: 1847-58.

[39] Bruheim K., Tveit K.M., Skovlund E., Balteskard L., Carlsen E., Fossa S.D. & Guren M.G. (2010b) Sexual function in females after radiotherapy for rectal cancer. *Acta Oncol;* 49: 826-32.

[40] Lange M.M., Maas C.P., Marijnen C.A.M., Wiggers T., Rutten H.J., Klein Kranenbarg E., van de Velde C.J.H. & cooperative clinical investigators of the Dutch Total Mesorectal Excision trial. (2008) Urinary dysfunction after rectal cancer treatment is mainly caused by surgery. *Br J Surg;* 95: 1020-28.

[41] Baxter N.N., Habermann E.B., Tepper J.E., Durham S.B. & Virnig B.A. (2005) Risk of pelvic fractures in older women following pelvic irradiation. *JAMA;* 294; 2587-93.

[42] Herman M.P., Kopetz S., Bhosale P.R., Eng C., Skibber J.M., Rodriguez-Bigas A., Feig B.W., Chang G.J., Delclos M.E., Krishnan S., Crane C.H. & Das P. (2009) Sacral insufficiency fractures after preoperative chemoradiation for rectal cancer: incidence, risk factors, and clinical course. *Int J Radiat Biol Phys;* 74: 818-23.

[43] Birgisson H., Pahlman L., Gunnarsson U. & Glimelius B. (2005) Occurrence of second cancers in patients treated with radiotherapy for rectal cancer. *J Clin Oncol;* 23:6126-31.

[44] Kendal W.S. & Nicholas G. (2007) A population-based analysis of second primary cancers after irradiation for rectal cancer. *Am J Clin Oncol;* 30: 333-339.

[45] Kim C.W., Kim J.H., Yu C.S., Shin U.S., Park J.S., Jung K.Y., Kim T.W., Yoon S.N., Lim S.B. & Kim J.C. (2010) Complications after sphincter-saving resection in rectal cancer patients according to whether chemoradiotherapy is performed before or after surgery. *Int J Radiat Biol Phys;* 78: 156-63.

[46] Guillem J.G., Díaz-Gonzalez J.A., Minsky B.D., Valentini V., Jeong S.Y., Rodriguez-Bigas M.A., Coco C., Leon R., Hernandez-Lizoain J.L., Aristu J.J., Riedel E.R., Nitti D., Wong W.D. & Pucciarelli S. (2008) cT3N0 rectal cancer: potential overtreatment with preoperative chemoradiotherapy is warranted. *J Clin Oncol;* 26:368-373.

[47] Peeters K.C.M.J., Marijnen C.A.M., Nagtegaal I.D., Klein Kranenbarg E., Putter H., Wiggers T., Rutten H., Pahlman L., Glimelius B., Leer J.W. & van de Velde C., for the Dutch Colorectal Cancer Group. (2007) The TME Trial after a median follow-up

of 6 years. Increased local control but no survival benefit in irradiated patients with resectable rectal carcinoma. *Ann Surg;* 246:693-701.

[48] Nagtegaal I.D. & Quirke P. (2008) What is the role for the circumferential margin in the modern treatment of rectal cancer? *J Clin Oncol;* 26:303-12.

20

New Option for Metastatic Colorectal Cancer: Oxaliplatin and Novel Oral S-1 Combination Chemotherapy

Dae Young Zang
Division of Hematology-Oncology, Department of Internal Medicine
Hallym University Medical Center and Hallym University College of Medicine, Anyang
South Korea

1. Introduction

The combination of oxaliplatin or irinotecan with bolus and infusional fluorouracil (FU) and folinic acid (FA) is considered the standard regimen for the first-line treatment of metastatic colorectal cancer [1-4]. However, this regimen is inconvenient owing to its requirement for continuous infusion of FU via vascular access.

To overcome this drawback, oral fluoropyrimidines such as capecitabine have been used as a substitute for infused FU/FA [5], and recent data have shown that capecitabine plus oxaliplatin (XELOX) was not inferior to infused FU/FA plus oxaliplatin (known as FOLFOX-4 or FUOX) [6, 7]. S-1, a novel dihydropyrimidine dehydrogenase-inhibitory oral fluoropyrimidine, has been used widely in patients with gastric cancer. In phase II studies, S-1 as a single agent showed an overall response rate (ORR) of 19–40% with tolerable toxicities in the first-line treatment of metastatic colorectal cancer [8-10].

To explore the possibility of using S-1 to replace the continuous FU infusion of the FOLFOX regimen, Korean investigators carried out a phase II clinical trial [11] and Japanese investigators performed a phase I/II clinical trial [12] with a regimen of oxaliplatin plus S-1 (OS) for the first-line treatment of metastatic colorectal cancer, respectively.

2. Patients and methods

2.1 Eligibility

Eligible patients met all of the following criteria: presence of unresectable, metastatic, histologically confirmed colorectal cancer; age from 18 to 70 years [11] or from 20 to 74 years [12]; Eastern Cooperative Oncology Group (ECOG) performance status (PS) of 0–2 [11] or 0–1 [12]; estimated life expectancy of more than 3 months; and adequate hematological, renal, and hepatic functions. The presence of a unidimensionally measurable lesion was also required for the phase II studies. Patients with a previous history of chemotherapy (except adjuvant or neoadjuvant chemotherapy not including oxaliplatin or S-1), central nervous system metastasis, obvious bowel obstruction, serous gastrointestinal bleeding, or serious comorbid conditions were excluded from the study.

Each patient gave written informed consent before entering the study. The protocol was approved by the institutional review board of each center.

2.2 Pretreatment evaluations

Baseline evaluations included medical history, physical examination, ECOG PS, complete blood count with differential count, serum chemistry and electrolytes, urine analysis, and three-dimensional computed tomography.

2.3 Treatment scheme

In phase I part of the Japanese phase I/II study, oxaliplatin was administered at a dose of 100 mg/m^2 (level 1) or 130 mg/m^2 (level 2) on day 1, and S-1 (40–60 mg) was given twice daily for 2 weeks followed by a 1-week rest [12]. This schedule was repeated every 3 weeks. Level 2 was determined to be the recommended dose (RD) for the phase II part of the study. In two Japanese and Korean phase II studies, oxaliplatin 130 mg/m^2 mixed with 250 mL of dextrose solution was administered intravenously over 2 h on day 1, and S-1 40 mg/m^2 [body surface area (BSA) < 1.25 m^2, 40 mg; 1.25 ≤ BSA < 1.5, 50 mg; BSA ≥ 1.5, 60 mg] was administered orally, twice daily from day 1 to 14, followed by a 7-day rest period [11, 12]. The treatment was repeated every 3 weeks until progression of the disease, the development of unacceptable toxicity, or consent withdrawal by the patient.

2.4 Dose modifications

The dose of a specific agent was adjusted when the cause of toxicity could be distinguished [11]. When both agents were believed to have caused the toxicity, the doses of both were reduced. Treatment was interrupted in the case of grade 2 or higher toxicity and was not resumed until the toxicity resolved or had improved to grade 0 or 1. The dose of oxaliplatin was reduced by 25% of the initial dose for related grade 3 toxicities or for the second occurrence of same grade 2 toxicity. The dose of S-1 was reduced by 20 mg/day for related grade 3 toxicities or for second occurrence of the same grade 2 toxicity. The dose of oxaliplatin was reduced by 50% of the initial dose for related grade 4 toxicities or for the second occurrence of same grade 3 toxicity. The initial dose of S-1 was reduced by 40 mg/day for related grade 4 toxicities or for second occurrence of the same grade 3 toxicity. No dose increase was allowed. Treatment was discontinued if, despite the dose reduction, the same toxicity occurred for a fourth time at grade 2, a third time at grade 3, or a second time at grade 4. In addition, if the toxicity had not improved to grade 0 or 1 after 3 weeks to allow the continuation of treatment, the patient was removed from the study.

Dose-limiting toxicity (DLT) was defined as any of the following findings during cycle 1: (1) a neutrophil count of less than 500/mm^3 for more than 4 days, (2) a platelet count of less than 50,000/mm^3, (3) diarrhea of grade 3 or more that occurred despite adequate supportive therapy, (4) grade 3 or 4 non-hematologic toxicity, excluding nausea, vomiting, anorexia, and electrolyte imbalance, or (5) a treatment delay longer than 1 week due to drug-related toxicity in the phase I part [12]. If DLT occurred, the dose of oxaliplatin in the subsequent course was reduced to 75% of the initial dose and that of S-1 was reduced by one dose level: from 80 to 50, 100 to 80, and 120 to 100. S-1 intake was interrupted mid-cycle if there was a neutrophil count less than 1,000/mm^3, a platelet count less than 75,000/mm^3, diarrhea, stomatitis, or hand foot syndrome occurred at grade 1 or more, aspartate aminotransferase (AST) or alanine aminotransferase (ALT) more than 150 IU/L, total bilirubin more than 1.5 times the upper limit of normal, or creatinine more than the upper limit of normal. The treatment in the subsequent cycle could be resumed if these adverse events resolved within 3 weeks after the last S-1 treatment. If peripheral neuropathy persisted between courses, the next treatment cycle was started at 75% of the previous dose of oxaliplatin.

2.5 Response and toxicity evaluation

The Response Evaluation Criteria in Solid Tumors guidelines [13] were used to evaluate tumor responses, and the National Cancer Institute Common Toxicity Criteria (version 3.0) were used to assess toxicity. Complete response (CR) was defined as the disappearance of all target and nontarget lesions. Partial response (PR) was a 30% or greater decrease in the sum of the longest diameter of target lesions, referenced against the baseline sum of the longest diameter of target lesions together with stabilization or decrease in size of nontarget lesions. Progressive disease (PD) required a 20% or greater increase in the sum of the longest diameter of target lesions, an unequivocal increase in the nontarget lesions, or appearance of any new lesions. Stable disease (SD) was defined as insufficient shrinkage to qualify for partial response and insufficient increase to qualify for progressive disease. Tumor responses were evaluated every two cycles [11] or every month [12] by three-dimensional computed tomography and were determined by an independent response review committee. All partial and complete responses were confirmed not less than 4 weeks after the criteria for response were first met. After completion of the study treatment, patients were followed up every 2 or 3 months until disease progression or death.

2.6 Statistical analysis

The primary aim of these phase II studies was to assess the ORR, and the secondary endpoints were safety profile, time to progression (TTP) or progression free survival (PFS), overall survival time, and duration of response.

Simon's MinMax two-stage design [14] was used to calculate the sample size in the Korean study [11]. The first stage required at least seven of 19 patients to have a confirmed response, assuming $P_1 = 0.40$, $P_0 = 0.20$, $\alpha = 0.05$, and $\beta = 0.20$, before proceeding to the second stage. In the second stage, 20 additional patients were to be entered, to achieve a target sample size of 43 assessable patients. Assuming a dropout rate of 10%, 48 patients were initially enrolled for the study.

The sample size was calculated to be at least 28 patients on the assumption of the null hypothesis of overall response rate of $\leq$30% versus the alternative hypothesis of overall response rate of > 60%, power 80%, and a 2.5% (one-sided) in the Japanese study [12].

The duration of response, TTP, and survival time were estimated using the Kaplan-Meier method.

3. Results

3.1 Patient characteristics

Forty-eight patients were enrolled in the Korean study [11]. All patients were assessed for safety and survival. Response was evaluated in all patients, except one patient who died due to the rupture of an underlying aortic aneurysm after the second cycle but before the evaluation, and one patient who had only non-measurable lesions and peritoneal seeding with malignant ascites. Patient characteristics are listed in Table 1. There were 25 men, and the median age was 56 years (range, 24-70). Twenty-three (48%) had colon cancer, seven (15%) had rectosigmoid colon cancer, and 18 (38%) had rectal cancer. Thirty-one patients (65%) were diagnosed with metastatic disease. Seventeen patients (35%) had recurrent colorectal cancer that relapsed after surgery, with adjuvant chemotherapy or chemo-radiotherapy. The most common metastatic sites were distant lymph nodes (56%), liver (56%), and lung (31%). The median number of metastatic organs was two (range, 1-6).

Twenty-nine patients were treated at the RD in the Japanese study [12]. All 29 patients were evaluated for toxicity. Efficacy was evaluated in 28 patients. One patient was excluded from the analysis of efficacy due to symptoms of brain metastasis suspected to have existed before enrolment. There are 20 men, and the median age was 57 years (range 34–71). Eighteen (62%) had colon cancer and 11 (38%) had rectal cancer. Four patients had received adjuvant oral fluorouracil based therapy.

Characteristic	**No. of patients (%) [ref. 11]**	**No. of patients (%) [ref. 12]**
Total number of patients	48 (100)	29 (100)
Gender		
Male	25 (52)	20 (69)
Female	23 (48)	9 (31)
Age, years		
Median	56	57
Range	24–70	34–71
Eastern Cooperative Oncology Group performance status		
0	39 (81)	26 (90)
1	8 (17)	3 (10)
2	1 (2)	
Primary disease site		
Colon	23 (48)	18 (62)
Rectosigmoid colon	7 (15)	
Rectum	18 (38)	11 (38)
Surgery and adjuvant therapy		
None	12 (25)	
Resection only	19 (40)*	25 (86)
Resection + chemotherapy	8 (17)	4 (14)
Resection + chemotherapy + radiotherapy	9 (19)	
Metastatic sites		
Liver only	9 (19)	10 (35)
Lung	8 (17)	3 (10)
Liver and other lesions	18 (38)	10 (35)
Others	13 (27)	6 (21)
No. of metastatic sites		
1	19 (40)	15 (52)
≥2	29 (60)	14 (48)

*Palliative surgery only.

Table 1. Patient characteristics

3.2 Efficacy

In total, 413 treatment cycles were administered to 48 patients, with a median of six cycles (range, 2–24) per patient in the Korean study [11]. Tumor response data are listed in Table 2. There were three CRs, 23 PRs, 17 cases of SD, and three cases of progression. The confirmed ORR in the intention-to-treat (ITT) population was 54% (95% CI, 40–68%) and in the per protocol (pp) population was 57% (95% CI, 43–71%). The median time to response was 1.5 months (95% CI, 1.3–1.7), and the median duration of response was 9.3 months (95% CI, 6.5–12.1). The median duration of follow-up was 21.2 months (95% CI, 17.9–23.6). The median TTP in the ITT population was 8.5 months (95% CI, 6.2–10.9). The median survival time was 27.2 months (95% CI, 20.3–34.0), and the 2-year survival rate in the ITT group was 53%.

The median number of administered cycles was 6.5 (range: 2–14), and the total number of cycles for the 29 patients was 180 in the Japanese study [12]. The ORR was determined by the External Review Board. One of the 28 patients given the RD had CR and 13 patients had PRs, yielding a response rate of 50% (95% CI, 31–69%). In the 28 patients studied, the median PFS was 6.5 months (95% CI, 5.6–10.1). The median overall survival time was not reached when 1 year passed since the last patient enrolment, and the 1-year survival rate was 79% by the Kaplan–Meier method.

Response*	**No. of patients [ref. 11]**	**% (95% CI)**	**No. of patients [ref. 12]**	**% (95% CI)**
Total No. patients	48		29	
Overall response	26	57 (43–71)	14	50 (31–69)
Complete	3		1	
Partial	23		13	
Stable disease	17		9	
Disease control	43	93 (86–100)	23	82 (68–96)
Progression	3		5	
Not evaluable	2		1	
Median time to response (months)	1.5	(1.3–1.7)		
Median duration of response (months)	9.3	(6.5–12.1)		

* Response in evaluable patients.

Table 2. Analysis of response (independent response review committee assessed)

3.3 Safety

Safety was assessed in 48 patients based on a total of 413 cycles in the Korean study [11]. The adverse events are listed in Table 3. Thrombocytopenia, which developed in 13% of the patients, was the most common grade 3/4 adverse event. There was no case of symptomatic thrombocytopenia. Neutropenia, observed in 10% of the patients, was the second most common grade 3/4 toxicity, and febrile neutropenia developed in one patient. Anemia, observed in 6% of the patients, was the third most common grade 3/4 toxicity. Non-hematologic toxicities were usually mild (mostly grade 1/2) and manageable. The most common non-hematologic toxicities were anorexia, neuropathy, nausea, asthenia, and hyperbilirubinemia.

	No. of patients (n = 48) [ref. 11]				No. of patients (n = 29) [ref. 12]			
	NCI-CTC grade, version 3				NCI-CTC grade, version 3			
Event	**All**	**3**	**4**	**3/4 %**	**All**	**3**	**4**	**3/4 %**
Leukopenia	31	0	0	0	20	0	0	0
Neutropenia	34	5	0	10	18	4	0	14
Anemia	49	3	0	6	18	1	0	3
Thrombocytopenia	28	5	1	13	27	7	1	28
Anorexia	41	0	0	0	26	0	0	0
Nausea	35	0	0	0	21	0	0	0
Vomiting	16	0	0	0	7	0	0	0
Diarrhea	10	0	0	0	17	1	0	3
Neuropathy	36	0	0	0	29	0	0	0
Abnormal AST/ALT	29	0	0	0	n/a			
Hyperbilirubinemia	23	1	0	2	n/a			
Asthenia/ fatigue	27	0	0	0	26	0	0	0
Allergic reaction	0	0	0	0	1	1	0	3

NCI-CTC, National Cancer Institute—Common Toxicity Criteria; AST, aspartate aminotransferase; ALT, alanine aminotransferase.

Table 3. Observed adverse events according to number of patients

The median relative dose intensities (ratio of dose received to dose planned) of oxaliplatin and S-1 for all cycles administered were 0.82 (range, 0.46–1.00) and 0.82 (range, 0.52–1.00), respectively [11]. The mean relative dose intensities of oxaliplatin and S-1 for all cycles administered were 0.79 and 0.83, respectively. The mean relative dose intensities of both drugs in each cycle during one to nine treatment cycles are shown in Figure 1. The dose reductions and delays during one to nine treatment cycles (total, 311 cycles in 48 patients) were as follows. Oxaliplatin was reduced in 37 cycles (12%), primarily because of thrombocytopenia (18 cycles), neutropenia (10 cycles), and thrombocytopenia with neutropenia (9 cycles). S-1 was reduced in 28 cycles (9%), primarily because of thrombocytopenia (14 cycles), neutropenia (8 cycles), and thrombocytopenia with neutropenia (6 cycles). Eighty-six cycles (28%) were delayed owing to thrombocytopenia (39 cycles), neutropenia (34 cycles), thrombocytopenia with neutropenia (10 cycles), and other reasons (3 cycles).

After identification of tolerability at level 2 (130 mg/m^2) of oxaliplatin, 29 other patients received the RD at 130 mg/m^2, including the phase I part patients, to further evaluate the tolerability and toxicity of the study regimen [12]. Oxaliplatin could be administered at the RD without dose reduction in 57% of 28 patients. At the RD, grade 3 neutropenia was observed in four patients (14%), and grade 3 and 4 thrombocytopenia in seven patients (24%) and one patient (3%), respectively. The median relative dose intensity was 0.83 for oxaliplatin and 0.75 for S-1 at level 2. The causes of treatment discontinuation at the RD were PD in 13 patients (36%), delayed recovery from toxicity such as neutropenia, thrombocytopenia, and slight hyperbilirubinemia in 8 patients, discretion of the investigator in 2 patients, allergic reaction in 1 patient, and symptomatic deterioration in 1 patient. The treatment was discontinued due to prolonged thrombocytopenia in eight patients after a median of seven cycles (range, 3–8). No treatment-related death was observed.

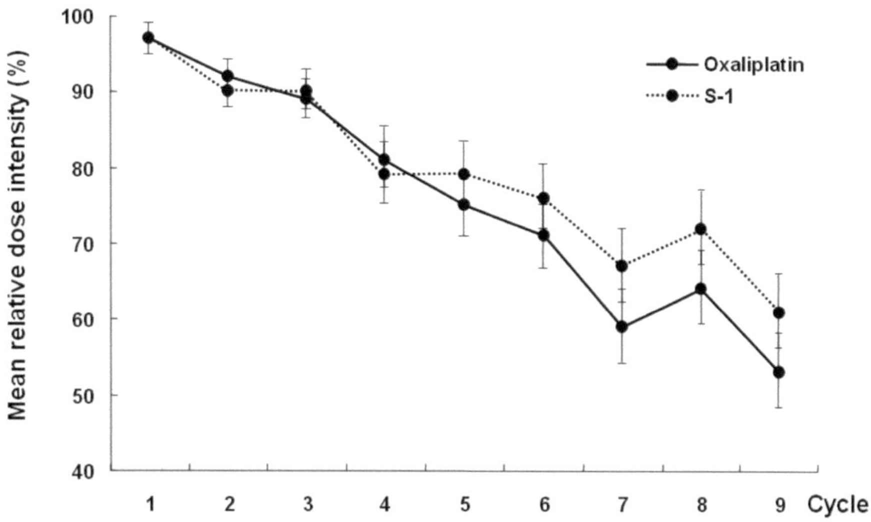

Fig. 1. Mean relative dose intensities of oxaliplatin and S-1 in each cycle between the 1st and 9th treatment cycles.

Sensory neuropathy occurred in all patients [12]. However, no functional impairment was observed in this study. The most common non-hematologic toxicities were anorexia, nausea, and diarrhea. One patient had grade 3 diarrhea at the RD. Another mild adverse event related to treatment was injection site reactions (45%). One patient had severe allergic reactions such as skin rash and fever, which are typical platinum-related reactions during the sixth cycle.

4. Discussion

The primary outcome of these two studies was the ORR, and the secondary outcomes were safety, TTP or PFS, and overall survival time [11, 12]. These studies demonstrated an ORR of 57% [11] and 50% [12], a median TTP of 8.5 months [11] and PFS of 6.5 months [12], and a median survival time of 27.2 months [11] in patients with metastatic colorectal cancer treated with the combination of oxaliplatin with S-1. Although these two studies were phase II studies, these efficacy results compare favorably to an ORR of 37–54%, a PFS or TTP of 8.0–9.5 months, and a median survival time of 16.2–20.8 months obtained with infused FU/FA and oxaliplatin (FOLFOX or FUFOX) as first-line chemotherapy for metastatic colorectal cancer in phase III studies [1, 2, 6, 7, 15-17]. Capecitabine plus oxaliplatin (XELOX or CAPOX) is another regimen commonly used in treating colorectal cancer. When oxaliplatin 130 mg/m^2 (day 1) or 70 mg/m^2 (days 1, 8) was administered intravenously, and capecitabine 1,000 mg/m^2 was administered orally, twice daily on days 1–14, every 3 weeks, the ORR, median PFS or TTP, and median overall survival with the XELOX or CAPOX regimen were 37–55%, 6.0-8.9, and 16.8–19.8 months, respectively [5–7, 16, 18–20]. Those efficacy data for oxaliplatin combined with infused 5-FU/FA or capecitabine are similar to the data for oxaliplatin combined with S-1 in the present studies [11, 12].

The median age of the subjects was 56 [11] and 57 years [12], which was relatively younger than in other studies, which typically had median ages between 60 and 66 years [6, 7, 15, 16, 18, 20]. The inclusion criterion for the age of the patients was 18–70 years old [11] and 20–74 years old [12], while the criterion used in many other studies was age ≥18 years old. This might explain the relatively young median age of 56 (range 24–70) years and 57 (range 34–71) years in Korean and Japanese studies, respectively [11, 12].

The treatment was generally well tolerated by most patients. The most common and second most common grade 3/4 adverse events were thrombocytopenia (13% [11] and 28% [12] of all patients) and neutropenia (10% [11] and 14% [12]), respectively. There was no symptomatic thrombocytopenia, and only one patient experienced febrile neutropenia [11]. Although peripheral neuropathy was commonly observed (75% [11] and 100% [12]), most cases were grade 1 or 2. Hand-foot syndrome was rarely observed in these studies. The toxicity profile observed in the present study is different from those of the FOLFOX/FUFOX and XELOX/CAPOX regimens. Diarrhea, neutropenia, and neuropathy are major toxicities of FOLFOX/FUFOX regimens, and diarrhea, hand-foot syndrome, and neuropathy occur most commonly with XELOX/CAPOX regimens [6, 7, 16]. There were few observed grade 3/4 non-hematologic toxicities, with just one grade 3 hyperbilirubinemia [11], and one grade 3 diarrhea and one grade 3 allergic reaction [12]. Possible explanations for the reduced occurrence of severe non-hematologic toxicities compared to other studies using the XELOX regimen include the younger patient population, greater dose reduction or delay, or real reduced toxicity of the OS regimen. In contrast, the median age was between 60 and 66 years (range, 24–88) in many other studies, while the median age in these studies was 56 and 57 years (range, 24–71) due to the lower upper limit for patient inclusion. Perhaps younger patients can better tolerate the treatment. In addition, strict dose modifications according to the toxicities in previous cycles might have reduced the chance of developing more severe toxicities in subsequent cycles. Large comparative studies are needed to confirm the more favorable toxicity profiles of the OS regimen.

As expected, the administration of the OS regimen was convenient for the patients. Unlike the inconvenient, 2-day, continuous infusion of 5-FU in the FOLFOX regimen, the OS regimen requires only a 2-h infusion of oxaliplatin and oral administration of S-1 every 3 weeks. Thus, the OS regimen was as convenient as the XELOX regimen and required fewer clinic visits than the FOLFOX regimen [21].

5. Conclusion

The OS regimen can be an effective, well tolerated, and convenient therapeutic strategy in patients with metastatic colorectal cancer. Two comparative clinical trials with the XELOX regimen in advanced colorectal cancer are ongoing in Korea.

6. References

[1] de Gramont A, Figer A, Seymour M et al. Leucovorin and fluorouracil with or without oxaliplatin as first-line treatment in advanced colorectal cancer. J Clin Oncol 2000; 18: 2938–2947.

[2] Giacchetti S, Perpoint B, Zidani R et al. Phase III multicenter randomized trial of oxaliplatin added to chronomodulated fluorouracil-leucovorin as first-line treatment of metastatic colorectal cancer. J Clin Oncol 2000; 18: 136–147.
[3] Douillard JY, Cunningham D, Roth AD et al. Irinotecan combined with fluorouracil compared with fluorouracil alone as first-line treatment for metastatic colorectal cancer: a multicentre randomised trial. Lancet 2000; 355: 1041–1047.
[4] Meyerhardt JA, Mayer RJ. Systemic therapy for colorectal cancer. N Engl J Med 2005; 352: 476–487.
[5] Cassidy J, Tabernero J, Twelves C et al. XELOX (capecitabine plus oxaliplatin): active first-line therapy for patients with metastatic colorectal cancer. J Clin Oncol 2004; 22: 2084–2091.
[6] Cassidy J, Clarke S, Díaz-Rubio E et al. Randomized phase III study of capecitabine plus oxaliplatin compared with fluorouracil/folinic acid plus oxaliplatin as first-line therapy for metastatic colorectal cancer. J Clin Oncol 2008; 26: 2006–2012.
[7] Díaz-Rubio E, Tabernero J, Gómez-España A et al. Phase III study of capecitabine plus oxaliplatin compared with continuous-infusion fluorouracil plus oxaliplatin as first-line therapy in metastatic colorectal cancer: final report of the Spanish Cooperative Group for the Treatment of Digestive Tumors Trial. J Clin Oncol 2007; 25: 4224–4230.
[8] Ohtsu A, Baba H, Sakata Y et al. Phase II study of S-1, a novel oral fluoropyrimidine derivative, in patients with metastatic colorectal carcinoma. S-1 Cooperative Colorectal Carcinoma Study Group. Br J Cancer 2000; 83: 141–145.
[9] Van den Brande J, Schöffski P, Schellens JH et al. EORTC Early Clinical Studies Group early phase II trial of S-1 in patients with advanced or metastatic colorectal cancer. Br J Cancer 2003; 88: 648–653.
[10] Shirao K, Ohtsu A, Takada H et al. Phase II study of oral S-1 for treatment of metastatic colorectal carcinoma. Cancer 2004; 100: 2355–2361.
[11] Zang DY, Lee BH, Park H et al. Phase II study with oxaliplatin and S-1 for patients with metastatic colorectal cancer. Ann Oncol 2009; 20: 892–896.
[12] Yamada Y, Tahara M, Miya T et al. Phase I/II study of oxaliplatin with oral S-1 as first-line therapy for patients with metastatic colorectal cancer. Br J Cancer 2008; 98: 1034–1038.
[13] Therasse P, Arbuck SG, Eisenhauer EA et al. New guidelines to evaluate the response to treatment in solid tumors. European Organization for Research and Treatment of Cancer, National Cancer Institute of the United States, National Cancer Institute of Canada. J Natl Cancer Inst 2000; 92: 205–216.
[14] Simon R. Optimal two-stage designs for phase II clinical trials. Control Clin Trials 1989; 10: 1–10.
[15] Goldberg RM, Sargent DJ, Morton RF et al. A randomized controlled trial of fluorouracil plus leucovorin, irinotecan, and oxaliplatin combinations in patients with previously untreated metastatic colorectal cancer. J Clin Oncol 2004; 22: 23–30.
[16] Porschen R, Arkenau HT, Kubicka S et al. Phase III study of capecitabine plus oxaliplatin compared with fluorouracil and leucovorin plus oxaliplatin in

metastatic colorectal cancer: a final report of the AIO Colorectal Study Group. J Clin Oncol 2007; 25: 4217–4223.

[17] Tournigand C, André T, Achille E et al. FOLFIRI followed by FOLFOX6 or the reverse sequence in advanced colorectal cancer: a randomized GERCOR study. J Clin Oncol 2004; 22: 229–237.

[18] Makatsoris T, Kalofonos HP, Aravantinos G et al. A phase II study of capecitabine plus oxaliplatin (XELOX): a new first-line option in metastatic colorectal cancer. Int J Gastrointest Cancer 2005; 35: 103–109.

[19] Scheithauer W, Kornek GV, Raderer M et al. Randomized multicenter phase II trial of two different schedules of capecitabine plus oxaliplatin as first-line treatment in advanced colorectal cancer. J Clin Oncol 2003; 21: 1307–1312.

[20] Shields AF, Zalupski MM, Marshall JL, Meropol NJ. Treatment of advanced colorectal carcinoma with oxaliplatin and capecitabine: a phase II trial. Cancer 2004; 100: 531–537.

[21] Mayer RJ. Should capecitabine replace infusional fluorouracil and leucovorin when combined with oxaliplatin in metastatic colorectal cancer? J Clin Oncol 2007; 25: 4165–4167.

21

Bone Metastasis of Rectal Carcinoma

Germán Borobio León, Asunción García Plaza, Roberto González Alconada, Ignacio García Cepeda, Jorge López Olmedo, Alberto Moreno Regidor and David Pescador Hernández
Complejo Asistencial de Salamanca
Spain

1. Introduction

Bone metastases are the most common cause of osteolytic lesions of bones in adults. Cancers most likely to metastasize to bone include breast, lung, kidney and prostate, while metastases are rare in colorectal cancer (although they cannot be dismissed). In this last case, metastases usually appear in advanced stages of the disease. Most of the metastatic lesions in women derive from breast cancer, and in the case of men, they derive from prostate cancer. Primary sarcomas of the bone do not usually metastasize to bone.

Metastatic lesions are usually multiple, and they tend to appear on the axial skeleton and the proximal segments of the limbs. Their location, in decreasing order, is the following: dorso-lumbar spine, sacrum, pelvis, ribs, sternum, proximal third of the femur, proximal third of the humerus and cranium.

Metastases affect the cancellous bone more, but they have a larger repercussion if they affect a cortical bone, because if load-bearing bones are involved, pathological fractures may appear. Colorectal carcinoma may generate metastasis on the cancellous and cortical bone.

According to the statistics, three out of every four patients who die of cancer present a bone metastasis, and an estimated 90% of cancer patients die of metastasis. Therefore, this is one of the final causes of the high mortality rates associated to cancer, and there is a limited amount of therapeutic and clinical resources to deal with it.

The most common locations for these metastases are: spinal column, pelvis, ribs and pectoral and pelvic girdles. Acral metastases are rare and for this reason they will be analyzed separately.

2. Physiopatology

Bone destruction secondary to metastasis is not caused by the tumor cells, but by the activation of the osteoclasts. The tumor cells secrete an osteoclast activating factor, and the osteoclasts induce the loss of cortical bone and trabecular bone. This process is divided in four stages (Mundy&Yoneda,1995):

1. The tumor cells adhere to the basement membrane (laminin, E-cadherin, integrins).
2. The tumor cells produce proteolytic enzymes that damage the basement membrane.
3. The tumor cells migrate via the basement membrane under the specific control of chemotactic factors.

4. The tumor cells can stimulate the activity of the osteoclasts.

Clohisy et al. have described four mechanisms that stimulate osteoclast-mediated bone destruction (Clohisy et al. ,2000):

1. Stimulation of the union between the osteoclasts and the bone.
2. Stimulation of the osteoclast-mediated bone resorption.
3. Extension of the survival time of osteoclasts.
4. Acceleration of the production of osteoclasts by precursor cells.

3. Clinical presentation

a. *Constitutional symptoms*: Some patients report anorexia, nausea, vomiting, asthenia, malaise, and weight loss.
b. *Symptoms derived from the primary location*: Colorectal carcinoma usually presents itself accompanied by an alteration of the intestinal rhythm and by the expulsion of blood originated in the rectum. In advanced stages of the disease, the patient presents constipation, and a transabdominal mass can be perceived by palpation. A rectal examination needs to be performed, because tumors of the lower part of the rectum can be easily found.
c. *Symptoms derived from the metastatic disease*: Regardless of the symptoms that metastases may produce on other regions, bone metastases can lead to:
    a. PAIN in the affected area, or referred pain, which may be of insidious, and either progressive or sudden onset, and it may be slight and intermittent or continuous and activity-related. Night pain is a typical symptom, and it does not always disappear with oral analgesics, unlike the pain that derives from degenerative processes, such as osteoarthritis, which increases with loads and articular mobility. When pain affects a long bone, it is easily located by the patient, but when it affects the pelvis or the spinal column, the pain makes it difficult to properly locate the lesion. When it affects the femur or the tibia (load-bearing bones), the patients report pain on walking, although the pain usually appears when the bone destruction levels are over 50% and they indicate an imminent fracture.
    b. SWELLING: It may be a sign of lesion aggressiveness when the tumor invades the cortical bone and affects soft tissue. This presentation is characteristic from colorectal carcinoma, renal carcinoma and melanoma.
    c. FUNCTIONAL DEFICIT: it appears as a consequence of pain. It may be a result of a medullary or radicular involvement in the case of spinal metastases.
    d. IMMINENT FRACTURE: It is a fracture that can appear as a result of a physiological load. Anamnesis and plain X-ray are necessary for the diagnosis, and the cortical involvement, the location and characteristics of the lesion (lytic, sclerotic or mixed) and the existence of fracture lines must be assessed. Permeative and lytic lesions of the proximal third of the femur are prone to fractures. Pain after radiation is also a sign of an imminent fracture. In cases in which an imminent fracture is expected on an active patient, a prophylactic fixation is recommended, especially in load-bearing bones.

4. Diagnostic assessment

In the context of colorectal carcinoma, bone metastases normally appear when the disease is already in an advanced stage (with metastases on other areas), and when the diagnosis has

already been established. For this reason, a histological diagnosis is not usually necessary, and the treatment can be planned. However, we must also take into account the fact that in 1-2% of the cases, the osteolytic lesion is unrelated to the primary tumor, which means that a biopsy is advisable. Myelomas can represent an exception, because they can be diagnosed with an electrophoresis test. Nevertheless, there are also cases in which the diagnosis of the primary tumor has not been yet established, and the orthopedic surgeon is asked to assess and treat an imminent or pathological fracture, or to perform the biopsy of a bone lesion for its final diagnosis, before the surgical stabilization.
In the case of an osteolytic lesion without diagnosis of the primary tumor, the differential diagnosis must be performed with benign conditions (Paget's disease, hyperparathyroidism, myeloma, lymphoma, chondrosarcoma, malignant fibrous histiocytoma, sarcomas) and an approach that includes:

4.1 Complete physical examination

including the thyroid gland, breasts, lungs and digestive system.

4.2 Laboratory analysis

1. COMPLETE BLOOD COUNT: Anemia, leukopenia or thrombocytopenia may be a sign of medullary involvement.
2. ESR: High levels may indicate a myeloma or an active process.
3. ELECTROPHORESIS OF SERUM PROTEINS: They can show a monoclonal gammopathy and they can confirm a possible myeloma diagnosis.
4. BIOCHEMICAL ANALYSIS: It can rule out hyperparathyroidism.
5. ALKALINE PHOSPHATASE: It shows high levels in cases of advanced metastatic disease. Very high levels show an unfavorable prognostic factor.
6. CARCINOEMBRYONIC ANTIGEN: Its levels are high in digestive or hepatocellular carcinomas.
7. PROSTATE-SPECIFIC ANTIGEN: It can detect a prostate carcinoma.
8. HEPATIC ENZYMES AND SERUM ELECTROLYTES: They can show bone and liver involvement.

4.3 Imaging tests

1. ANTEROPOSTERIOR AND LATERAL X-RAYS OF THE LESION: In order to assess an imminent fracture and to analyze the information they provide.
2. THORACIC X-RAY: In order to see the existence of carcinoma or lung metastases.
3. THORACIC AND ABDOMINAL CT SCAN: In order to assess the existence of possible visceral metastases.
4. Tc^{99m} BONE SCINTIGRAPHY: In order to assess bone lesions.

Data from the clinical record, an exhaustive physical examination, blood tests and imaging tests identify more than 85% of all the primary tumors that appear as a bone metastasis. The following tests could also be performed, albeit only when required:
-NMR: It is seldom recommended in cases of isolated bone lesions (fig. 1) , but it may be useful in cases of a single metastasis in which a resection can be performed, in order to rule out *skip metastases* or metastases inside the bone and on the vertebrae, due to its excellent properties for the exploration of the bone marrow.

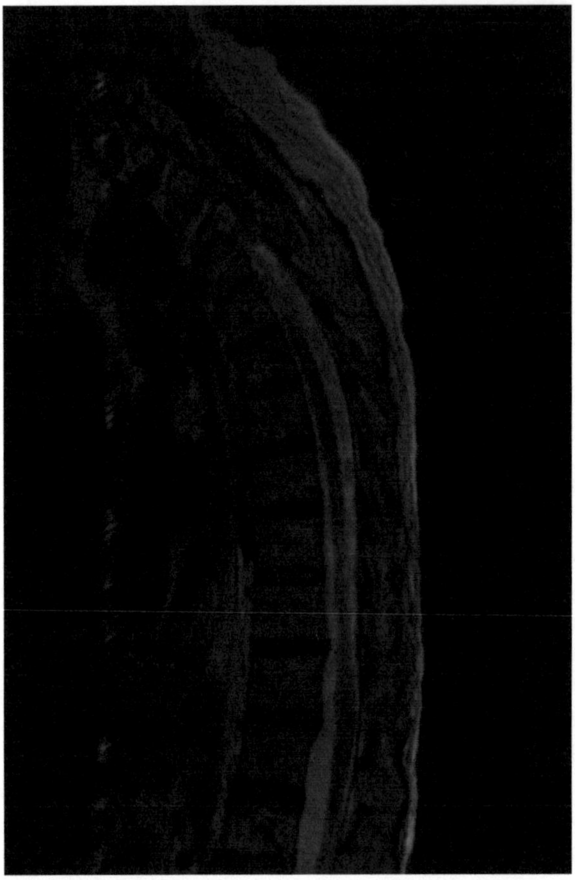

Fig. 1. Metastatic lesion on T12

-POSITRON EMISSION TOMOGRAPHY (PET): This imaging technique is becoming more and more important in the field of orthopedic oncology. It uses [18F]2-fluoro-2-deoxy-D-glucose (FDG) as a tracer. This is a glucose analog which is taken to the cells by a group of proteins. This marker is absorbed by malignant tissue with an increased metabolic activity. PET scans have a very high sensitivity, and it is an important technique for the identification of primary lesions and other metastases. It can establish the difference between a local recurrence and a scar, and it is also useful in the assessment of response to treatment.

4.4 Biopsy

Puncture biopsy is an excellent way to confirm a diagnosis of bone metastasis. CT-guided fine-needle aspiration and thick- or trephine-needle biopsies are very precise techniques, and they are easy to use. The orthopedic surgeon must choose the exact location, taking into account the location of the lesion, viable access routes and, whenever possible, the final incision line of the operation, in case of resection surgery, excising all the area of the biopsy, because it might be contaminated.

When finding certain locations (usually on the pelvis), a CT scan may be necessary in order to identify the best point and route of access that will reach the metastatic area and to avoid regions with reactive sclerotic bone, because these parts may not have tumor cells.

If there is more than one metastasis, the most accessible one will be chosen.
The anatomopathological analysis requires several tissue samples. For this reason, the pathologist should attend the biopsy in order to confirm that enough tissue has been extracted.
With regard to colorectal carcinoma, if it presents itself with a bone metastasis and the lesion is biopsied, the biopsy may not always provide a diagnosis for the primary tumor, because a tissue compatible with adenocarcinoma does not always tell the difference between primary tumors of the digestive system, prostate, breast and lung.

5. Imaging tests for the metastasic bone lesion

5.1 Plain radiography

Plain radiographies are useful in the characterization of known lesions or in lesions at risk of imminent fracture, but they are not helpful in the detection of a metastatic bone disease, because this condition is undetectable if the bone mineral loss is below 30-50% (fig. 2)

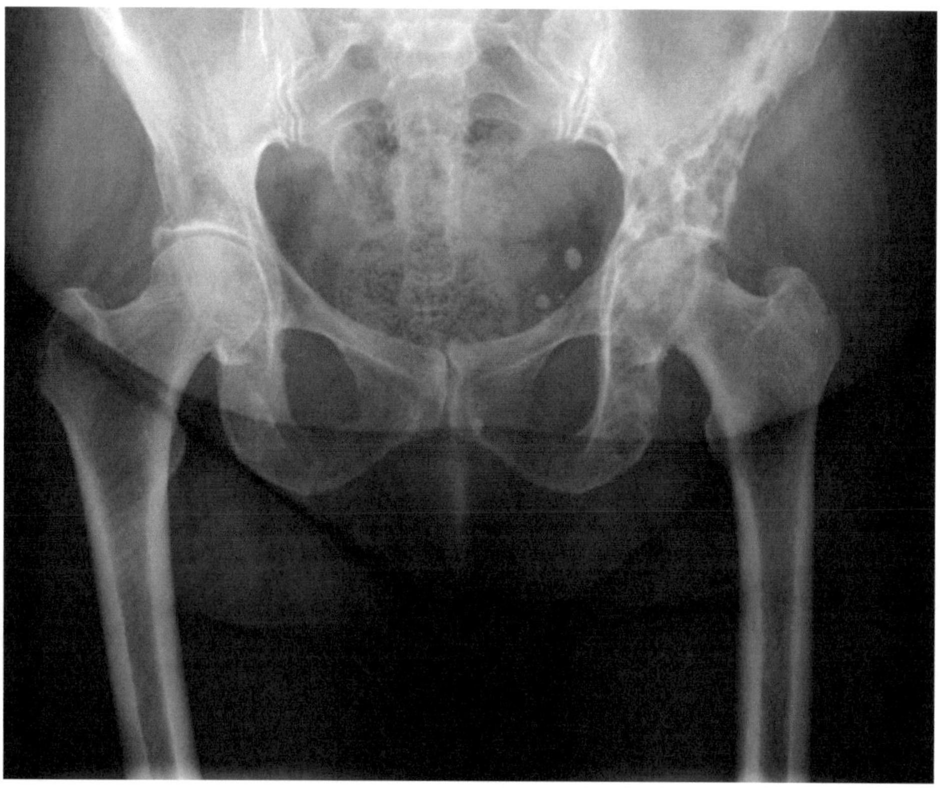

Fig. 2. Metastasic periacetabular lesion

A bone X-ray series, in the case of a metastasis, includes anteroposterior and lateral radiographies of the dorso-lumbar spine (fig. 3) and the pelvis, as well as lateral radiographies of the skull and the cervical spine and anteroposterior radiographies of the thorax, the humerus and the femur. However, in view of their low sensitivity, bone series have largely been replaced by scintigraphy.

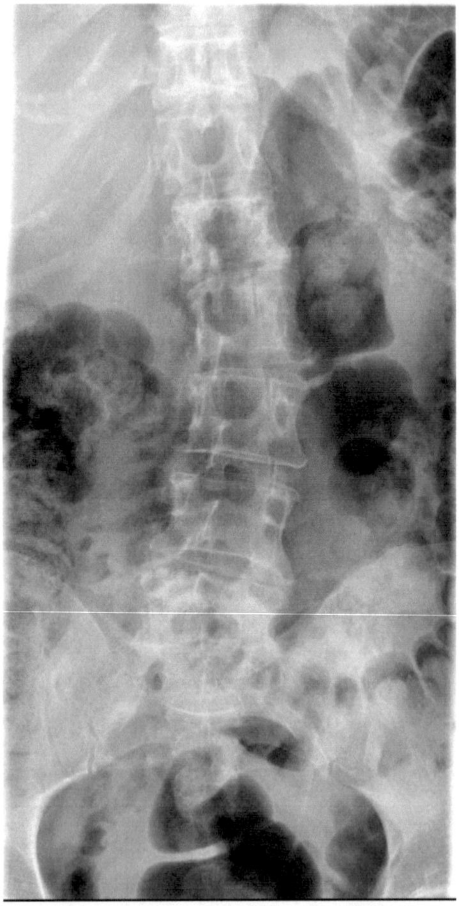

Fig. 3. Lytic vertebral lesions, mainly on L1

The radiological aspects of the bone lesion will depend on the bone response. In the case of malignant digestive tumors, metastases are usually either lytic or mixed. Reactive bones represent an attempt at reparation, which usually takes place. Osteolysis is mediated by osteoclastic resorption, and it may be geographical, moth-eaten or pervious, and the margins may be well- or ill-defined. They can occasionally present themselves with a periosteal reaction and a soft-tissue mass. Metastases that invade the cortical bone or that show a pervious or moth-eaten pattern are more aggressive than metastasis with a geographic pattern.

Another useful aspect of plain radiographies is the assessment of response to treatment. Osteolytic metastases create a sclerotic edge of reactive bone, followed by an increase in sclerosis, moving from the edges towards the center. In then becomes even and finally reduces its size. Comparisons with earlier radiographies make it possible to tell the difference between progression and a positive response to treatment.

The detection or prediction of fracture risk is another objective of this technique. It requires a detailed assessment of the size, reach and character of the bone destruction. Osteolytic lesions are associated to a higher risk than mixed and osteoblastic lesions, just as lesions that invade more than half of the diameter of the cortical bone, lesions located on the trochanteric region or lesions that affect a load-bearing bone. All these findings, together with clinical data, define the need for a prophylactic osteosynthesis.

5.2 Bone scintigraphy

Tc-99m bone scintigraphy offers certain advantages (Galasko, 1995)

- High sensitivity.
- It provides information for the staging of the lesion.
- It assesses the entire skeleton simultaneously.
- It assesses the response to treatment.

The isotope is absorbed by areas with increased blood flow and increased exchange of reactive bone. It shows enhanced areas in osteolytic and osteoblastic lesions, due to the bone renewal that takes place at the periphery of the lesion.

A group of randomly dispersed lesions with scintigraphic enhancement on the axial skeleton may be a sign of metastatic disease. However, isolated lesions may be difficult to interpret. There are certain considerations that we must take into account with regard to the interpretation of potential false positive and false negative results:

- Fractures and surgical operations can be enhanced up to 1-3 years after they have taken place (fig. 4)
- Enhancement of the ribs is difficult to interpret: If the enhancement follows the longitudinal axis of the rib, it can be a sign of metastasis.
- The scintigraphy should be assessed in combination with NMR and CT scans in order to reduce the rate of false positive and false negative results.
- Highly anaplastic carcinomas or diffuse metastatic disease may lead to false negatives, due to an increased enhancement in the entire skeleton.
- Other related processes that increase enhancement, such as radiation-induced osteonecrosis or steroid abuse, must be also taken into account.

Scintigraphy is also useful in the assessment of recovery: At first, an increase in enhancement can be observed as a consequence of an increased local blood flow, followed by a gradual decrease in enhancement.

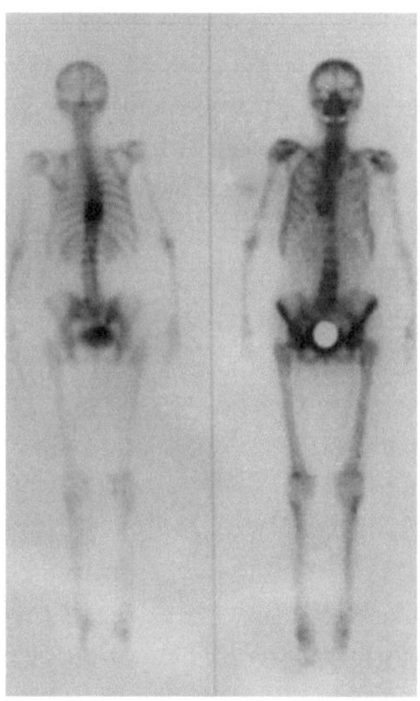

Fig. 4. Enhancement of vertebral column because of vertebral fracture

5.3 CT

It is a useful tool that complements radiographies and provides more information on the presence of hematomas, cortical involvement or the possibility of an imminent fracture. It is useful in the assessment of the vertebral column and the pelvis (fig. 5).

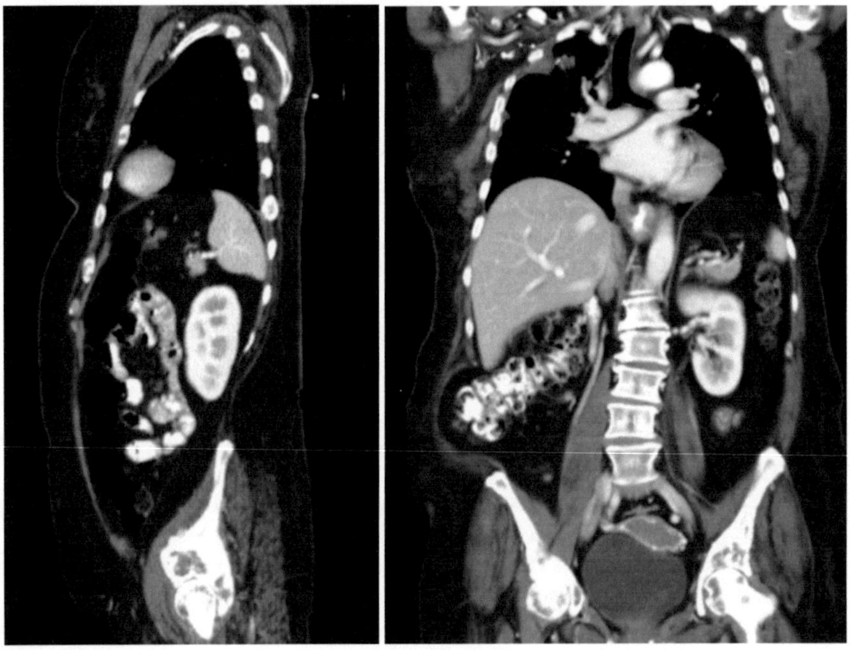

Fig. 5. Periacetabular metastatic lesions and femoral head metastatic lesions

This technique is also very useful for guided biopsies.

5.4 RMN

NMR presents high sensitivity for the detection of metastasis, and high specificity for the characterization of lesions. Metastatic lesions show low intensity in T1-weighted images, while they present high intensity in T2-weighted images. Fat suppression techniques are required in order to increase the visibility of T2-weighted images. The characteristics of the signal may vary according to the type of tissue, its cellularity, its water contents, and the presence of fibrosis, necrosis, hematoma or inflammation. This technique presents certain advantages:

- It assesses peritumoral soft tissue.
- If offers a more accurate assessment of neurovascular compression.
- It provides a better characterization of the bone marrow and the possibility of skip metastases.
- It assesses the risk of medullary compression (fig.6)

The differential diagnosis between a metastatic bone lesion and an osteoporotic spinal fracture is very interesting: old fractures present normal fat signal, but the intensity of acute fractures is similar. Multiple lesions, the presence of soft-tissue masses, the involvement of posterior elements, a convex shape and a sharp edge between normal marrow and affected marrow are signs of metastasis.

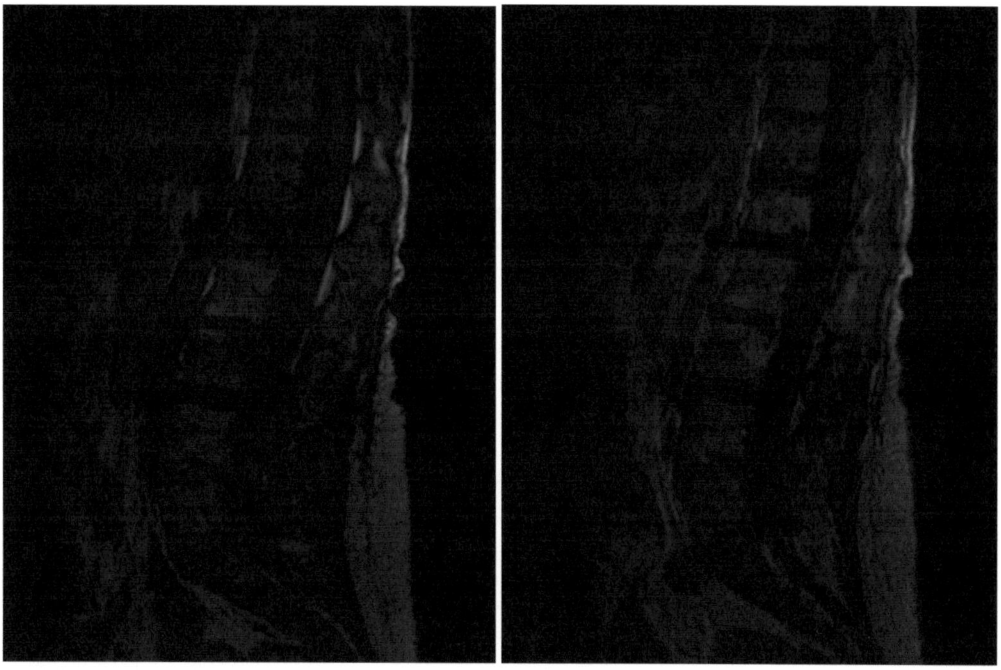

Fig. 6. Lumbar metastases

5.5 Angiography

It is a useful technique in the case of a preoperative embolization of highly vascularized lesions.

6. Treatment

The therapeutic approach for bone metastases, as in any neoplastic pathology, is a multidisciplinary one. A joint effort between oncologists, anatomopathologists, interventional radiologists, pain therapeutics and orthopedic surgeons is of paramount importance.

6.1 Supportive measures

6.1.1 Analgesic therapy

Around 70% of all patients with a bone metastasis report pain at some point along the course of the disease. The physiopathological pain may be due to medullary compression, distension of the periosteum or peripheral neurovascular involvement, as well as to pathological fractures, whenever they are present and mediated by substances such as histamine, substance P or other cytokines.

Other important factors are the characterization of the intensity of pain, its topography and nature and the factors that alleviate or worsen it, as well as a complete clinical record, an exhaustive clinical examination and adequate imaging tests.

Pain, fatigue and psychological angst have been proven to be the most common symptoms in cancer patients.

The therapeutic plan will begin with a simple posological scheme and with non-invasive or minimally invasive treatment. Patients with slight or moderate pain will be started on non-

opioid analgesics, such as paracetamol, acetylsalicylic acid or NSAIDs. If the pain does not disappear with maximum doses of these drugs, a mild opioid, such as codeine or hydrocodone. Patients who suffer moderate or intense pain in spite of the opioids should be treated with third-step analgesics, that is, narcotics and NSAIDs administered separately.
Although they are ideally administered orally, in cases of dysphagia, digestive disorders or lack of adherence to treatment, they can be applied via transdermal, rectal, endovenous, subcutaneous or intrathecal administration. If the patients do not respond to opioids, there are other strategies that include nerve block and neurostimulation and rehabilitation surgery.

6.1.2 Biphosphonates

Metastatic osteolysis is caused by the stimulation of osteoclast activity. For this reason, bisphosphonates can play an important role in this process, because they inhibit the osteoclast activity. They bind with the mineral bone matrix and they have a great physico-chemical impact on the hydroxylapatite crystals.
Some authors have suggested that they are not only useful in the treatment of pain and the prevention of osteolytic complications, but that they can also modify the natural course of evolution of cancer in some cases, due to the effect they have on some intermediate products, such as growth factors.
Ross et al. carried out a systematic review of all randomized essays on patients with bone metastasis. It is a meta-analysis based on 18 randomized studies in which different bisphosphonates have been compared with a placebo or between themselves. Most of these studies were performed on patients with breast carcinoma (Ross et al, 2004). The review showed a decrease in the incidence and an increase in the time until the appearance of bone complications, with a better evolution of pain and functional capacity, with regard to the control group who received a placebo. Treatment with oral bisphosphonates (clodronate, etidronate) caused a decrease in the number of spinal and non-spinal fractures, but it had no effect on the indications of radiotherapy or in hypercalcaemia.
The American Society of Clinical Oncology (ASCO) recommends treatment with bisphosphonates in patients with breast carcinoma and bone metastasis whenever there is radiological evidence of a lytic lesion, regardless of whether it causes pain or not.

6.1.3 Treatment of hypercalcaemia

Hypercalcaemia affects 10-40% of cancer patients at some point, and it causes anorexia, nausea, vomiting, polydipsia, polyuria, dehydration, constipation, confusion and coma.
It is the result of PTHrP production, which activates bone metabolism and induces an excess of osteoclast activity. Osteoclasts are then stimulated by local factors produced by tumor cells, such as interleukin 6. Moreover, calcium levels are also increased due to lower levels of renal calcium elimination, because PTHrP acts on the renal receptors of the parathyroid hormone and it increases calcium resorption on the renal tubule. Polyuria and reduction of intravascular volume appear as a consequence, and for this reason, the initial treatment with these patients is rehydration with intravenous saline serum in order to balance the intravascular volume and to improve glomerular filtration and renal secretion of calcium.
Calcitonin inhibits osteoclasts and it has a rapid effect, although for a brief period of time. For this reason, it is mainly used in emergency treatments.
Plicamycin normalizes calcium levels in up to 50% of the cases, but its serious adverse effects make it unadvisable to use it.

Bisphosphonates represent the cornerstone of hypercalcaemia treatment: The intravenous pamidronate balances serum calcium in 70-100% of the cases, and serum calcium, phosphate, magnesium, electrolytes and creatinine levels need to be measured.
In any case, the best possible treatment for hypercalcaemia is the remission of the cancer.

6.2 Non-surgical treatment

6.2.1 Treatment of metastatic bone disease secondary to colorectal carcinoma

The treatment of bone metastases derived from colorectal tumors is the same as the treatment for other metastases caused by other tumors. Surgical resection of the primary tumor, together with chemotherapy and radiotherapy for the rectal cancer is the treatment of choice, depending on the cases.

6.2.2 Radiotherapy

Radiotherapy is the most widely used palliative treatment for bone metastasis. It is the treatment of choice for painful lytic bone metastases without short-term risk of fracture, and it is combined with surgery when there is an imminent fracture or when the fracture has already taken place. It leads to the necrosis of tumor cells, which makes it possible for the bone tissue to regenerate afterwards. The result is pain relief and, later on, a re-calcification of the destroyed areas of the bone, which is important for the functional recovery of the patient and the prevention of pathological fractures.
Two different radiation methods are used: external radiation therapy and systemic or metabolic radiation therapy.

a) External radiation therapy

Radiation therapy causes pain relief in 80-90% of the patients, and in 55-60% of them, the effect lasts for at least a year. Tong et al. presented a study in which 50-70% of the patients who showed pain relief on the radiated area did not report pain on that same location for the rest of their life. Bone re-calcification can be observed in X-rays between one and three months after radiation in 60-80% of the patients. For this reason, a period for the protection and prevention of mechanical interventions that may endanger the integrity of the affected bone needs to be observed.
Radiotherapy is applied on the bone lesion with variable margins according to the location of the lesion and the type of tumor. The imaging techniques that were described before are needed in the treatment planning, in order to define the area of the bone lesion, as well as a possible soft-tissue involvement.
Several courses of action and treatment fractions have been applied. In the eighties, the results of a study that compared several fraction systems were published (15 fractioned doses of 275cGy, 15 fractioned doses of 300 cGy, 10 fractioned doses of 300 cGy, 5 fractioned doses of 400 cGy, and 5 fractioned doses of 500 cGy). No significant differences were found with regard to pain control, although the most fractioned schemes were the most effective in the long term: 15 fractioned doses of 275 cGy and 10 fractioned doses of 300 cGy.
Some European groups of scientists have carried out studies with radiation therapy administration in a single fraction, and they observed a symptomatic pain relief in 70% of the patients. When fractioned radiation therapy studies were compared with one-fraction radiation therapy, this last option required more re-treatments and a greater number of pathological fractures.

b) Sistemic radiation therapy

Systemic treatment with radiopharmaceuticals is the recommended approach for patients with symptomatic diffuse bone involvement, and as an adjuvant therapy for patients who receive localized radiation therapy and also present diffuse involvement.

Patients must present a positive scintigraphy, progressive pain on several locations or pain on an area that had been previously radiated. It cannot be applied on the acute stage of a pathological fracture or a medullary compression, but it can be administered when the emergency treatment has already been resolved.

The most common radiopharmaceuticals are strontium-89 and samarium-153. Both of them accumulate on the bone tissue with a 10:1 preference over soft tissues. This makes it possible to provide a very specific treatment for bone lesions.

Treatment with systemic radiation therapy shows pain relief in 70-75% of the patients, and it lasts for 2-4 months. In patients with a good clinical response, the treatment can be repeated. Clinical results have been tested on different studies over the last 10-15 years. A significant improvement in pain control after the administration of radiopharmaceuticals has been observed, when compared with a placebo.

6.2.3 Orthopedic therapy

With a few exceptions, curative surgery is not a realistic objective for these patients. Their general condition needs to be assessed, together with the type and location of the tumor. Generally speaking, the treatment of pathological fractures is similar to the treatment of conventional fractures.

In view of the fact that these patients are prone to prolonged pain, the usual treatment for pathological fractures is early osteosynthesis for a precocious mobilization. However, this is not always possible, and the fractures can be controlled with radiation, hormonal therapy and chemotherapy.

There are several types of immobilization, depending on the area involved, including figure-of-eight bandages, slings or Velpeau bandage, hanging casts, splints and orthotics.

In the case of spinal involvement, patients with a neurological deficit associated to instability require early decompression and stabilization. In the case of stable lesions, they can benefit from radiotherapy and orthotics, like braces or corsets.

If the pelvis is involved, in cases in which surgery is not possible or in which it represents a high risk, the loads supported by the bone need to be limited with a walking support or with crutches.

Lesions on the femur and the tibia are usually treated surgically, but in cases in which this is not possible, the usual immobilization systems will be used.

6.3 Surgical treatment

Surgery for bone metastases requires a previous complete general and local assessment. It presents its own indications, objectives, techniques and means, and it is associated to a program for postoperative radiotherapy that follows the lines that have been previously described.

Before the operation, we must know whether the general condition of the patient allows it, as well as the estimated survival rates according to the stage of the disease and the type of original tumor. There are some carcinomas, such as thyroid carcinoma, with high long-term survival rates, in spite of the appearance of bone metastases, whereas in lung cancer, the short-term prognosis is quite poor, with a life expectancy of a few months. The surgical approach may vary according to these data and other information regarding the metastasis, such as its location, its size and the areas it affects.

6.3.1 Spinal metastases

The objective in this case is to improve the patient's quality of life as much as possible. In view of its associated morbidity and its recovery rates, many practitioners think that patients with a minimum life expectancy of 6-12 weeks are candidates for surgery. We can divide the role of surgery into diagnostic procedures (biopsy) and therapeutic procedures.

-BIOPSY: The most accessible lesions should be biopsied, and all the areas of the spine can be easily reached. A percutaneous core-needle biopsy shows positive results in 65% of all osteolytic lesions, and in open biopsy this rate goes up to 85% of the cases.

-THERAPEUTIC PROCEDURES: Laminectomy provides an excellent improvement of pain in 75-100% of the patients, as well as neurological improvement in 50-75% of the cases. More than 95% of the patients who did not present a preoperative deficit maintained their function, more than 95% maintains mobility and 90% maintains the continence ability 3 months after surgery, while less than 40% of the patients recover these abilities once they have lost them. Risks derive from the basal situation of the patients, because of their poor nutrition and the fact that they are usually affected by thrombocytopenia and leukopenia and that they have been previously exposed to radiotherapy. For these reasons, the risk of infections or complications in the wound reaches 10-15%.

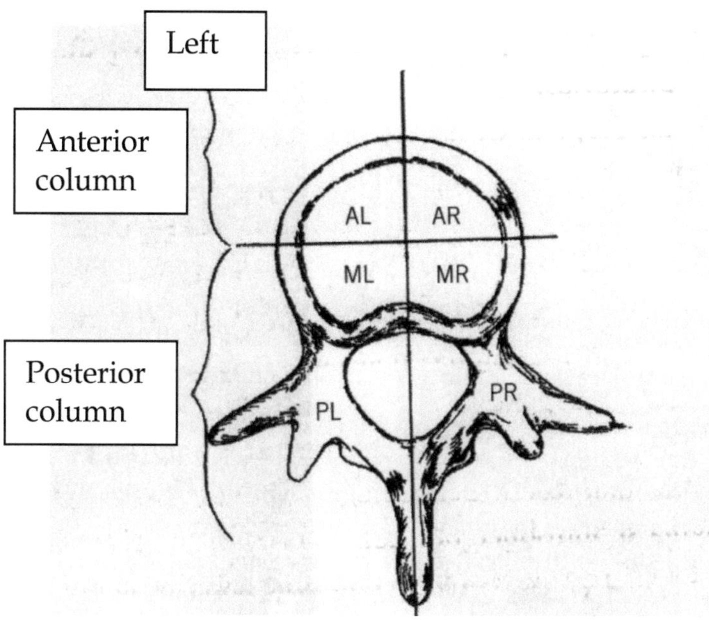

Fig. 7. Modification of Denis classification: Divison into 6 areas

With regard to indications, we can use a modification of Denis (fig. 7) classification as a reference, which subdivides each one of the three regions of the column into two parts: medial column and lateral column, thus creating 6 areas of the column. With this basis, the destruction of less than 3 areas shows a stable situation, the destruction of 3-4 areas is considered unstable (fig. 8) and requires surgical stabilization, and destruction of 5-6 areas reveals extreme instability and requires combined antero-posterior stabilization.

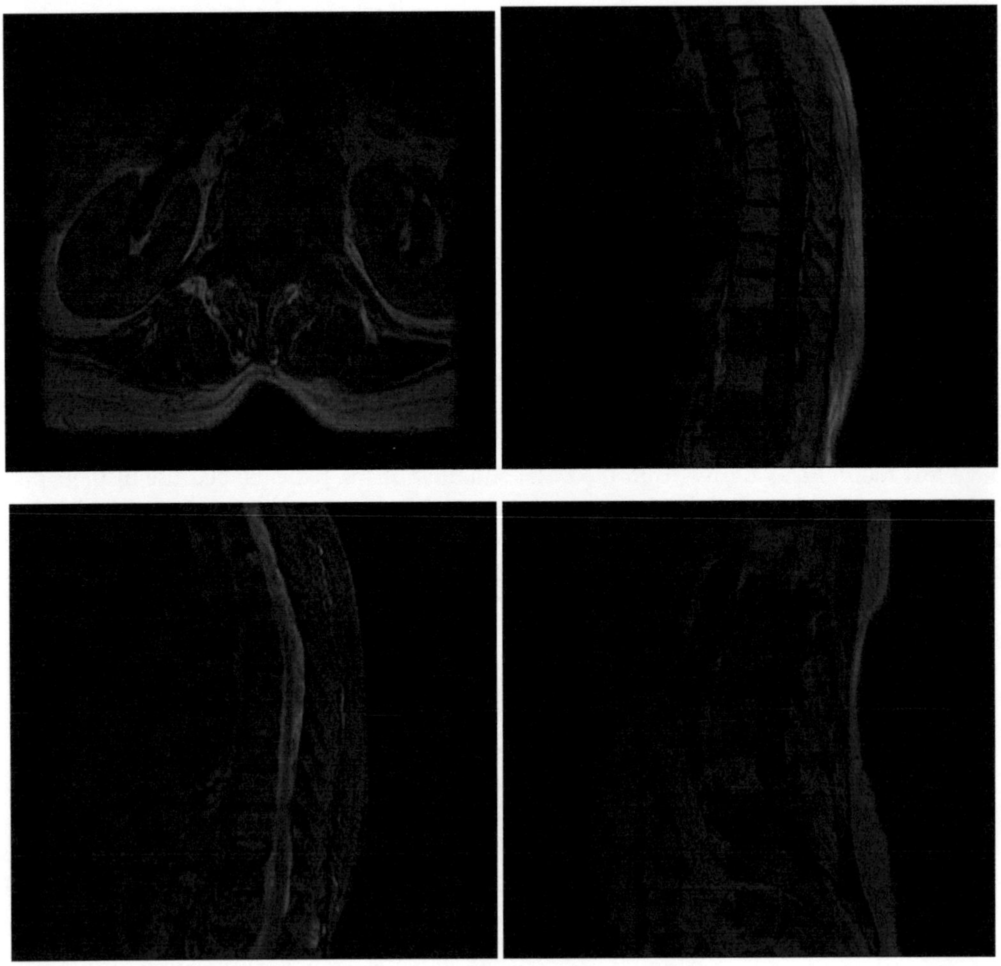

Fig. 8. Unstable vertebral lesion on L1, in a patient with multiple metastases

Primary surgical intervention is indicated when the chances of an adjuvant therapy providing a long-term response are low. Secondary surgery is indicated when symptoms are still present in spite of treatment of fractures or instability after treatment, as well as for the post-therapeutic progression of the tumor and medullary compression.

Corticoids are used due to their anti-edema effect on neurological lesions, and they are never used alone, except in cases in which the general condition of the patient does not allow a different choice.

Radiotherapy is indicated in patients with intense pain with no medullary involvement or with a neurological deficit that shows a slow and incomplete onset and progression, whenever osteoarticular spinal instability (which is the key element for the indication of surgery) has been ruled out. In cases in which short-term prognosis is poor or when surgery is contraindicated due to the general condition of the patient, radiotherapy is the only option.

6.3.2 Non-spinal metastases

The surgical treatment of pathological fractures has been proven to reduce the complications associated to metastatic bone disease, and to improve the patient's pain, independence and ability to walk, as well as longer survival rates.

-PELVIS AND ACETABULUM: The complex anatomy and approach of the pelvis make surgery a difficult task, and other palliative techniques, such as arterial embolization of the metastasis or radiotherapy may be indicated in the first place. These treatments are an ideal choice if the lesion affects isolated areas of the ischium, the pubis, the sacro-iliac region and the iliac wing. However, they are not effective on the periacetabular area, which is subject to lots of mechanic efforts, and which requires surgical reconstruction

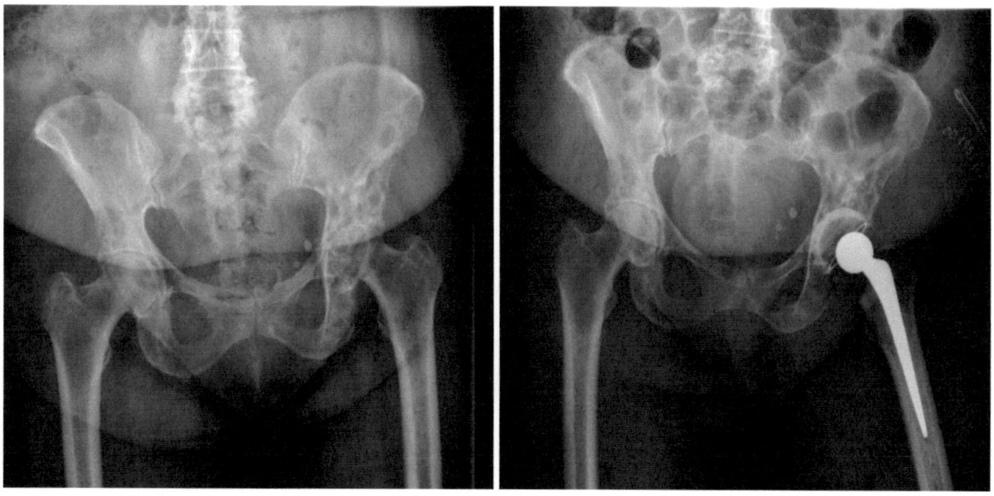

Fig. 9. Total hip arthroplasty

The reconstruction of periacetabular destructive lesions is extremely rare and complex. The results are not as fast or as spectacular as those achieved in other areas, and complications may be more frequent and serious. For these reasons, the choice of patients and techniques must be particularly careful.

The possibilities of surgery will depend on the extent of the periacetabular destruction. In cases of slight or moderate destruction, the initial treatment may be isolated radiotherapy, and if it fails, then curettage of the lesion is indicated. The new space should be filled with bone cement and a conventional total hip replacement should be inserted. There are several different metallic materials that can provide stability for the area, such as acetabular anti-protrusio rings and mails that prevent the pelvic invasion of bone cement. In cases of serious or severe destruction, the same methods can be applied, and there is also the possibility of performing wide resections associated with the implantation of massive bone allografts as a replacement, taking into account the fact that a total hip replacement will always be inserted in the end.

- PROXIMAL THIRD OF THE FEMUR: This is the most common location for metastases that affect long bones. The most common techniques used are hip arthroplasty (fig. 9) , pin osteosynthesis or open osteosynthesis
- DIAPHYSEAL LESIONS: The most commonly affected bones are the femur and the humerus, in order of frequency, and the proximal and medial portions are more

common than the distal area. In the femur, the functional impact is more relevant, because this bone is subject to more demanding mechanic efforts, particularly when walking.

In diaphyseal bone metastases, the treatment of choice is an osteosynthesis of the bone as wide and stable as possible, covering all weak areas, even anticipating the foreseeable progression of the disease.

Already during the 50s and 60s, some authors published studies that highlighted the advantages of internal fixation of pathological fractures, compared with other classic procedures, such as complete rest for a long period of time and orthotics or external immobilization techniques that were more or less complicated. These authors proposed the stabilization of pathological fractures with intramedullary nails as well as their prophylactic use in some cases of lithic lesions that were at risk of fracture, associated with postoperative radiotherapy. These are the same grounds observed in the current treatments, albeit with the materials and procedures of that time. The results in the improvement of pain and immediate function were already promising back then.

The subsequent introduction of endomedullary locking nails represented a qualitative step towards the rotational and global stability of the result. It prevented a collapse of the bone defect that was created by the metastasis with a short, safe and barely aggressive intervention that did not require a surgical approach of the metastatic. Also, early radiation therapy could be applied, because the scars were not near the radiated area.

Giannoudis used locking nails in 30 pathological and imminent fractures of the femoral diaphysis and he achieved enough stability for a painless or almost painless mobilization of the patients in all cases. Other authors present case series with similar results. The results of this technique are the same for humeral diaphysis.

The potential dissemination of tumor cells due to endomedullary procedures is a matter of some controversy. Although some authors report isolated cases of local spreading after the use of these techniques, other studies proved that the moment in which the pathological fracture takes place is the one in which the possibility of tumor dispersion via the blood significantly increases. For this reason, when the prophylactic nailing reduces the risks of a fracture, it also reduces the possibility of dissemination. There are few reported cases with these complications in the clinical practice.

The effectiveness of surgical stabilization of diaphyseal bone metastases of the long bones is out of question, as well as the value of associated radiation therapy after surgery. Townsend presents better functional and long-term results, a lower number of re-interventions due to malfunctioning of the internal fixation and a higher average survival rate in patients that arte treated with surgical stabilization and radiation therapy, compared with patients who only underwent surgery for pathological and imminent fractures of the femur.

In spite of the excellent results obtained with internal fixation followed by radiation therapy. These results are not always stable. The progression of the tumor leads to a failure of surgical stabilization in more than 10% of the cases. The most important risk factor is prolonged survival after surgery. There are other factors that tend to increase the risk of a re-intervention, such as kidney carcinoma as a primary tumor, femoral location, due to a higher mechanic effort, and osteosynthesis surgery, compared with prosthesis.

After an analysis of these data we can observe the need to identify patients with prolonged survival prospects, in order to adapt the therapeutic approach. In these cases, an intervention on the metastatic site and a resection of the affected bone fragment and subsequent reconstruction are indicated. The reconstruction with bone cement was common during the

80s and 90s, but massive intercalary bone allografts are more common nowadays. Postoperative radiation therapy is more effective, because it reduces the size of the tumor mass. There is a clear improvement in the mechanic capability and the stability of the internal fixation, with better and more durable results regarding the function of the bone.
This approach changes in epiphyseal and metaphyseal lesions. Osteosynthesis becomes less effective, and it is replaced by prosthesis. Whenever there is a mainly epiphyseal involvement, the solution is its resection and the implantation of a conventional articular cemented graft, both on the hip and the shoulder. The use of cement and long rods is useful in the prevention of the consequences of a later appearance of other metastatic sites. In cases in which the affected metaphyseal area is large and requires a wide bone resection, there are special resection grafts or composite bone allografts (prosthesis plus graft).
-HUMERUS: This is the second most commonly affected bone in the limbs after the femur. The initial symptom is usually a pathological fracture or pain associated to an imminent fracture. However, as this is not a load-bearing bone, sometimes the lesions reach a very large size. Standard procedures include arthroplasty and osteosynthesis.

7. Discussion

Colorectal cancer affects 6% of the population in western countries along their lives, and it is the third cause of cancer-related death in the world, both for men and women. More than one third of the patients develop a metastasis during the course of the disease, but only a small fraction of them would benefit from a potentially curative surgery. Approximately 50% of the patients with cancer die within 5 years after the diagnosis, due to cancer-related problems. These deaths are due to complications in distant metastases. (Schlüter, et al. 2006)
The most common locations for these metastases are the liver, the peritoneum and the lung. Bone metastases in colorectal cancer are rare. (Kose, et al 2009).
The skeleton is the most common organ for metastasis of other tumors, however, and it has a high prevalence in breast and prostate cancers. These two tumors represent 80% of all cases, and the high incidence of bone metastases leads to high morbidity rates. There are other types of cancer that also tend to present bone metastasis, although not as often, such as multiple myeloma and lung cancer. Bone metastases, however, are rare in colorectal cancer. In general terms, the incidence of these metastases, according to the literature, ranges between 5.6% and 10.1%. (Kose, et al 2009).
Malignant colorectal tumors do not evolve with a primary extension to the bone. Thus, bone metastases are less common than in other types of cancer. 70% of patients with a stage IV breast cancer present bone metastasis, compared with 10% of patients with colorectal cancer. Bone metastases of colorectal cancer do not appear if the tumor has not metastasized on the liver or the lung first.
The location of colorectal cancer established a recurrence pattern and a dissemination mechanism of the tumor. The colon has intra-peritoneal segments (covered with serous membrane) in the cecum, the transverse colon and the sigmoid colon, as well as extra-peritoneal segments (without a serous membrane) in the posterior area, the ascending colon, the descending colon and both flexures.
When the colon carcinoma is located on the intra-peritoneal areas, it has a high risk of peritoneal dissemination. Tumors located on the extra-peritoneal segments tend to a direct dissemination towards the retroperitoneal organs, such as the kidney, the ureter or the pancreas. (García Plaza, 2003)

Tumors of the rectum usually invade perirectal tissue, such as the base of the bladder, the prostate or the vagina. Tumors located on the lower third of the rectum drain the superior hemorrhoidal vein towards the portal venous system, via the inferior mesenteric vein. These tumors commonly lead to hepatic metastases.

The recurrence pattern for rectal cancer is not the same as for the colon cancer. The local recurrence of the rectal colon is usually isolated, and it is not accompanied by a disseminated disease, contrary to colon cancer, in which local recurrence is associated to a disseminated disease in most of the cases. This phenomenon is explained by the fact that the recurrence of colon is detected at the same time that dissemination, whereas in rectal cancer, the detection of the recurrence takes place before that stage, due to the limited pelvic space and the accessibility of the exploration. (García Plaza, 2003).

The recurrence pattern of colon cancer is characterized by a rate of local recurrence that ranges between 1 and 19%, a 5-16% rate of local recurrence associated to distant metastasis, and a 12-22% rate of systemic recurrence. The recurrence pattern of rectal cancer is: local recurrence rate of 7-33%, local and systemic recurrence rate of 7-30% and systemic recurrence rate of 6-19%. The increase in the incidence of local recurrence can be attributed to an increased difficulty in securing safe margins in the pelvis, and to the high number of lymphatic ducts located on the mesorectum. The location for the recurrence of rectal cancer depends on the location of the primary tumor. Local recurrence is predominant in lesions of the middle and lower third, and the systemic recurrence is more common in lesions of the upper third, similarly to the recurrence pattern of colon cancer (García Plaza, 2003).

Bone metastases are more common in patients with primary rectal cancer than in patients with primary colon cancer. (Bonnheim, et al.1986)

A higher incidence of patients with pulmonary and bone metastases (16.1%) has been observed, compared with the number of patients with bone metastases alone (6.4%). There has been a decrease in the number of patients with hepatic metastases. (Sundermeyer et al. 2004, 2005).

A study carried out by Roth et al. showed that there is no time pattern, in spite of the individual variables of the degree and sequence of involvement of organs affected by metastasis between colorectal cancer patients. Colorectal tumors do not spread mainly towards the bones. This is a particular characteristic in colorectal cancer; bone metastases are more common in other types of cancer.(Roth et al 2008).

A lower incidence of bone metastases in colorectal cancer with regard to other carcinomas suggests that the behavior of colon cancer is different to other types of tumors. (Roth et al 2008).

An experimental study carried out by Schlüter et al. shows for the first time that the organ-specific formation of colorectal metastases appears to be mainly mediated by specific interactions between circulating carcinoma cells and the vessel wall of potential target organs. (Schlüter et al 2006). On the other hand, a correlation was found between the metastatic potential of colon carcinoma cells and their ability for cell adhesion within potential target organs. For the first time, they directly observed circulating tumor cells within the pulmonary microcirculation in situ and they found specific cell adhesions without size restriction comparable to the liver sinusoids, whereas cells were unable to arrest within the renal and other capillaries in situ. Further studies are required to investigate the underlying molecular mechanisms of these specific adhesive interactions in metastatic target organs.

A review of literature shows that colorectal cancer metastasizes first on the liver or the lung, which contain dense capillary beds that can trap the tumor cells and insert them in these organs. The environment of a specific organ and its influence on the adherence of tumor cells can also have an influence on the effectiveness of the spreading of the tumor. This is what happens more frequently with colorectal cancer patients in the liver and the lungs.(Schlüter et al 2006).

Recent studies have revealed that the patients who receive adjuvant or neo-adjuvant therapy show an increased rate of bone metastases. A rare location is the brain: an estimated 6% of the patients present bone and brain metastases. The prognosis is closely related to the dissemination potential of the tumor through lymph and blood. This dissemination occurs in 10-15% of the cases, regardless of the existence of a complete resection of the primary tumor, and it is closely related to the histological degree of the lesion. It affects the liver via the portal system, and the liver is the organ in which metastases are mainly detected. However, higher survival rates in colon cancer have led to an increasingly frequent appearance of metastases in locations that were previously rare. Sundermeyer et al., in a review of 1,020 patients diagnosed with colon cancer, found up to 10% of bone metastases and a 3% of brain metastases, mainly in patients that had been subject to multiple systemic treatments and with pulmonary involvement. (Sundermeyer et al. 2004, 2005). The development of bone metastases is associated to more precocious stages at diagnosis or with metachronic metastases, compared with patients who were diagnosed with a stage IV disease. Time between diagnosis and the development of a metastatic disease was long in patients with bone and brain metastases, although survival rates for the development of metastatic disease was similar. There are two possible explanations: On the one hand, the microscopic metastatic disease may be present at diagnosis and it remains inactive for long periods of time due to the particular interaction between the tumor and its microenvironment. On the other hand, it may very well be that many patients with bone and brain metastases will never develop a clinical metastatic disease in these areas. (Sundermeyer et al. 2004, 2005).

8. Acrometastasis

Acrometastases are metastases to the hands or the feet. They are very rare, and they represent between 0.3% and 3% of all bone metastases, and their frequency is variable according to different authors, between 15% and 84%. Hand metastases of a colorectal cancer are even rarer (fig. 10), and there are almost no references to it in the medical literature (Ben Abdelghani et al., 2008; Flynn CJ et al., 2008)

Benign lesions are common on the hand, but malignant lesions are very rare. Acrometastases are usually the first manifestation of a hidden neoplasia that, in most cases, leads to a diagnostic error and a wrong treatment. (Desmanet et al, 1991)

Acrometastases are difficult to diagnose. They are frequently mistaken for a benign disease, osteomyelitis, rheumatoid arthritis, gout, fractures, synovitis or glomus tumor, among others. Most of the bone metastases located on the hands affects the phalanges and they come from a lung cancer in the first place, followed by breast cancer. Acrometastases of colon cancer and urinary tract cancer are usually found on the foot; hand acrometastases are exceptionally rare. (Méndez López et al, 1997)

Nozue et al. reviewed the treatment and prognosis of patients with colorectal cancer and bone metastases. Out of 928 patients in the study, only 1.3% of the patients (12 patients) presented these metastases, which were in an advanced stage in all cases. Most of the primary tumors were located in the spine and the pelvis. The survival rate for these patients was very poor, with an average of 5 months and a 1-year survival rate of 20%. (Nozue et al, 2002)

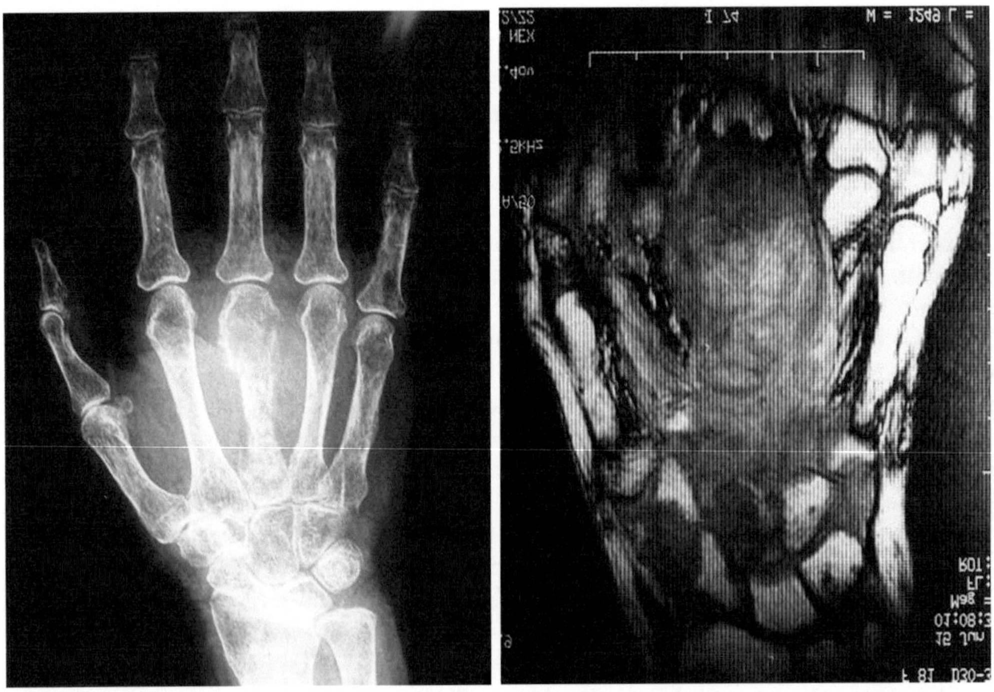

Fig. 10. a) Osteolytic lesion on the third metacarpal bone with permeative pattern and pathological fracture, b)The lesion shows large involvement of soft tissue

The mechanisms of dissemination are not well known. Some authors have stated that they spread via the lymphatic nodes, whereas others say that they spread via the blood. The embolization of the tumor requires certain conditions for the development of a metastasis. There are different factors that have been suggested for the accumulation of tumor cells on the limbs, such as traumatisms, temperature gradients, hormonal factors, local hemodynamic factors or immune factors, as well as the properties inherent to the metastasizing cell. These metastases usually leave the articulations intact. (Chang et al., 2001)

The most common location on the hands is the phalanges, and the right hand is more common than the left hand, although 10% of the patients showed bilateral metastases. (Healey et al, 1986) showed that most of the patients presented lesions on their dominant hand, because it receives more blood and it is more prone to traumatisms. It seems that the chemotactic factors that come after traumatisms may cause the cellular migration and the bone adherence. The third finger is the most common one in the medical literature, and the distal phalange is the most commonly affected. The metacarpus, the proximal phalange and the middle phalange are the next most common locations for acrometastasis.

Acrometastasis is more common in men, with a 2:1 ratio, probably due to a higher incidence of lung carcinoma.

The acrometastases usually appear in an advanced stage of the disease (Borobio, et al. 2010). For this reason, the prognosis is poor, and the objective is to alleviate pain. The therapeutic options include amputation, radiation therapy, curettage, cementation, chemotherapy and wide excision. (Spiteri et al., 2008)
The median age of acrometastasis patients was 58 years.

9. Conclusion

Bone metastasis from colorectal cancer are uncommon (10-23% in autopsy cases), usually present late in the natural history of metastasic disease, and is associated with liver or lung metastasis. Acrometastasis are reported to be 0,3-3% of all the bone metastasis.
Cancers to the rectum and cecum are accompanied by bone metasatasis more frecuently than cancers of other porcions of the colon. Signet-ring cell carcinoma show a high incidence of bone metastasis.
Pain is the most common symptom of bone metastasis. As a result of the loss of bone density, bones affected become prone to fracture and injury.
Testing for bone metastasis includes X-ray, bone scanning; open biopsy is necessary to establish the diagnosis, exclude osteomyelitis and allow treatment. Early diagnosis is important for improving quality of life in this patients.
Therapeutic management of this condition includes chemotherapy, radiotherapy and surgery, but because of survival after onset of bone metastasis is very poor, palliative treatment is the aim.

10. References

Ben Abdelghani, K; Chekili;, Hajri, R; Laater, A; Zakraoui, L.(2008). Adénocarcinome colique et acrométastase du talus: à propos d´un cas. *Gastroentérologie Clinique et Biologique 2008; 32: 835-838.*

Borobio León, G; García Plaza, A; García Cepeda, I; González Alconada, R.; Hernández Cosido, L. (2010). Metástasis en mano de adenocarcinoma de recto. Un caso excepcional. *Cirugía Española 2010;88:195-7.-vol. 88 núm. 03*

Bonnheim, D.C; Petrelli, N.J; Herrera, L.; Walsh, D; Mittelman, A.(1986). Osseous metastases from colorectal carcinoma. *Am J Surg*, vol. 151(4), (April 1986), 457-459.

Chang, H.C; Lew, K.H; Low, C.O .(2001). Metastasis of an adenocarcinoma of the stomach to the 4th metacarpal bone. *Hand Surgery 2001 December; 6(2): 239-242.*

Clohisy, DR; Perkins, SL; Ramnaraine ML. Review of cellular mechanisms of tumor osteolysis (2000). *Clin Orthop 2000;3743:104-114*

Desmanet, E; Amrani, M; Fievez, R; Six Ch. Les acrométastases. A propos de deux cas.(1991). *Revue de la littérature. Ann Chir Main 1991; 10, nº2: 154-157.*

Flynn, CJ; Danjoux, C; Wong, J; Christakis, M; Rubenstein, J; Yee, A; et al.(2008). Two cases of acrometastasis to the hands and review of the literature. *Curr Oncol 2008 October; 15 (5): 51-58.*

Galasko, CS. Diagnosis of skeletal metastases and assessment of response to treatment.(1995). *Clin Orthop 1995;312:64-75*

García Plaza, A. (2003). *Aspectos terapéuticos y pronósticos del carcinoma colorrectal.* Ediciones Universidad de Salamanca. (Marzo 2003). Colección Vitor 105.

Healey, J.H; Turnbull, A.D; Miedema, M; Lane, J.M.(1986). Acrometastases. A study of twenty-nine patients with osseous involvement of the hands and feet. .*J Bone Joint Surg Am. 1986; 68:743-746.*

Kose, F; Sakalli, H ; Sezer, A; Mertsoylu, H; Pourbagher, A; Reyhan, M; Ozyilkan, O. (2008). Colon adenocarcinoma and solitary tibia metastasis: Rare entity. *J Gastrointest Canc*, vol.39, (February 2008), 146-148.

Méndez López, JM; García Mas, R; Salvà Coll, G. (1997). Metastasis of an adenocarcinoma of the colon to the 1st metacarpal bone. *Ann Chir Main Memb Super 1997; 16(2): 134-7.*

Mundy, JR & Yoneda, T. Facilitation and supresion of bone metastasis (1995). *Clin Orthop 1995;312:34-44*

Nozue, M; Oshiro, Y; Kurata, M; Seino, K; Koike, N; Kawamoto, T et al (2002). Treatment and prognosis in colorectal cancer patients with bone metastasis. *Oncol Rep 2002 Jan-Feb; 9(1): 109-112.*

Ross, J.R; Saunders ,Y; Edmonds, P.M; Patel, S; Wonderling, D; Normand, C. (2004). A systematic review of the role of bisphosphonates in metastatic disease. *Health Technol Assess*. vol 8. (August 2004). 1-176.

Roth, E.S; Fetzer, D.T; Barron,B.J; Usha, A; Joseph, U. A; Isis, W; Gayed, I. W; Wan, D.Q. (2009). Does colon cancer ever metastasize to bone first? a temporal analysis of colorectal cancer progression. *BMC Cancer*. vol. 9, (August 2009), 274.

Schlüter, K; Gassmann, P; Enns, A.(2006) Organ-Specific Metastatic Tumor Cell Adhesion and Extravasation of Colon Carcinoma Cells with Different Metastatic Potential. *The American Journal of Pathology. vol.169,* (September 2006),1064–1073.

Schlüter, K; Gassmann, P; Enns, A; Korb, T; Hemping-Bovenkerk, A; Hölzen, J; Haier,J. (2006). Organ-Specific Metastatic Tumor Cell Adhesion and Extravasation of Colon Carcinoma Cells with Different Metastatic Potential. *American Journal of Pathology.* Vol 169, (September 2006), 1064-1073.

Spiteri, V; Bibra, A; Ashwood, N; Cobb, J. Managing acrometastases treatment strategy with a case illustration (2008). *Ann R Coll Surg Engl 2008 October; 90(7): 8-11.*

Sundermeyer, M. L; Meropol, N.J; Rogatko, A; Wang, H; Cohen, S.J. (2004). Changing patterns of colorectal cancer metastases: A 10-year retrospective review. *Journal of Clinical Oncology*, vol 22, nº 14S ,(July 15 Supplement 2004), 3548.

Sundermeyer, M. L; Meropol, N.J; Rogatko, A; Wang, H; Cohen, S.J. (2005).Changing Patterns of Bone and Brain Metastases in Patients with Colorectal Cancer. Clinical Colorrectal Cancer. vol 5, nº 2 (July 2005). 108-113.